The Companion to Specialist Surgical Practice eLibrary

Series edited by

O. James Garden and Simon Paterson-Brown

The content of all eight volumes of the Fifth Edition of the **Companion to Specialist Surgical Practice** is now available both in print and as part of an electronic library. Your purchase of this book allows you to download the fully searchable contents to your desktop, laptop, tablet or smartphone.

Your **Companion to Specialist Surgical Practice eLibrary** is portable: the titles in the series download to your device or you can access online so they are with you whenever you need them.

Your eBook is much more than just 'pictures of pages':

- customize your page views
- search in single books that you have purchased or across any volumes in the series in your collection
- highlight and take searchable notes, and even print and copy-and-paste with bibliographic support
- utilize reference lists linked where available to Medline citations (including authors, title, source, and often an abstract) to journal articles and an indication of free electronic full-text availability.

To purchase other eBooks in the **Companion to Specialist Surgical Practice eLibrary** please visit www.elsevierhealth.com/companionseries

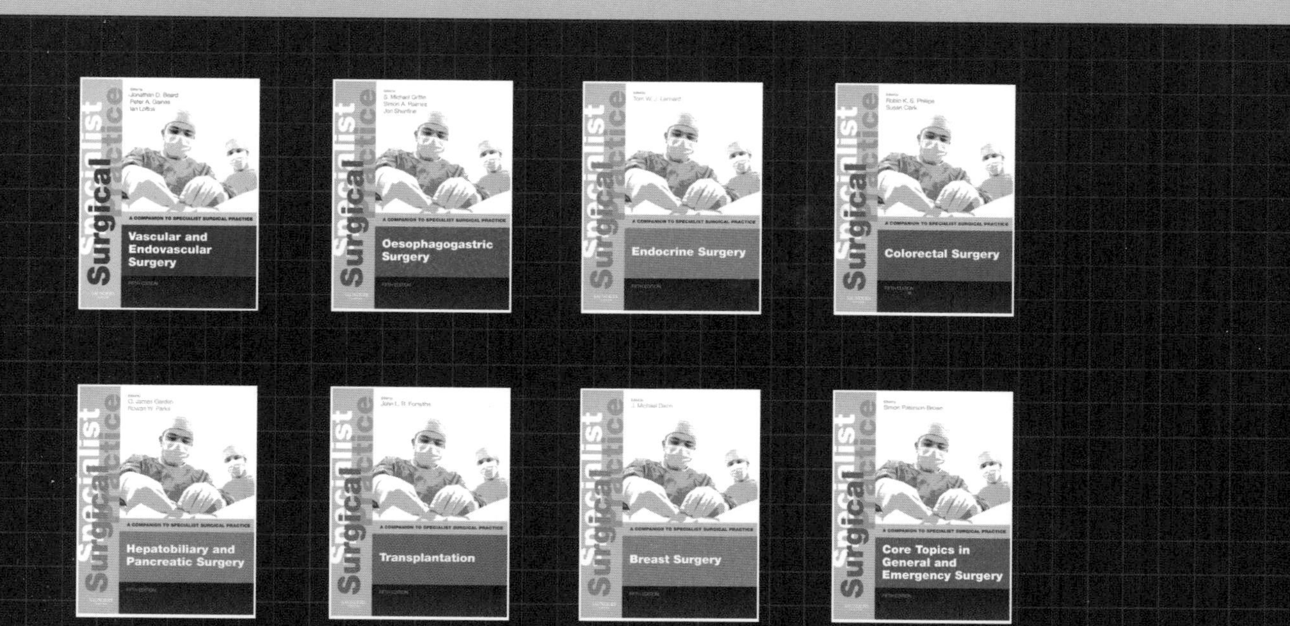

Oesophagogastric Surgery

A COMPANION TO SPECIALIST SURGICAL PRACTICE

Series Editors
O. James Garden
Simon Paterson-Brown

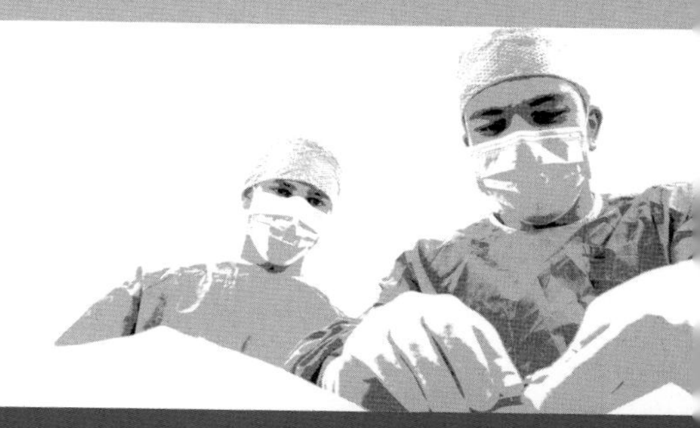

Oesophagogastric Surgery

FIFTH EDITION

Edited by
S. Michael Griffin
MD FRCS
Professor of Surgery, Northern Oesophago-gastric Unit,
Royal Victoria Infirmary, Newcastle upon Tyne, UK

Assistant Editors
Simon A. Raimes
MD FRCS
Consultant Upper Gastrointestinal Surgeon,
Northern Oesophago-gastric Unit, Cumberland Infirmary, Carlisle, UK

Jon Shenfine
PhD FRCS
Consultant Oesophago-Gastric Surgeon,
Northern Oesophago-gastric Unit, Royal Victoria Infirmary, Newcastle upon Tyne, UK

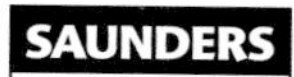

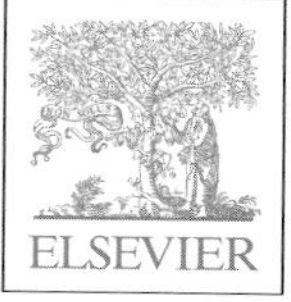

Edinburgh London New York Oxford Philadelphia St Louis Sydney Toronto 2014

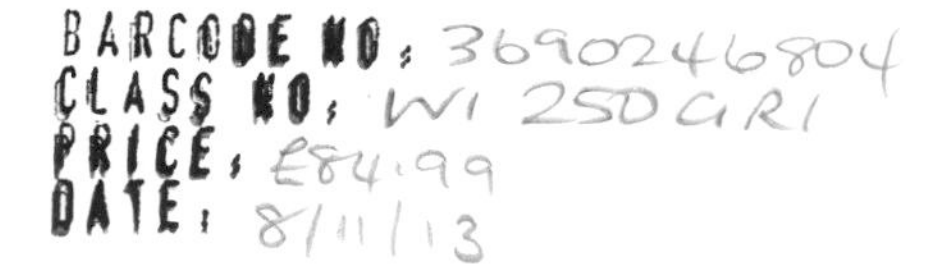

SAUNDERS
ELSEVIER

First edition 1997
Second edition 2001
Third edition 2005
Fourth edition 2009
Fifth edition 2014

ISBN 978-0-7020-4962-0
e-ISBN 978-0-7020-4970-5

British Library Cataloguing in Publication Data
A catalogue record for this book is available from the British Library

Library of Congress Cataloging in Publication Data
A catalog record for this book is available from the Library of Congress

Notice

Knowledge and best practice in this field are constantly changing. As new research and experience broaden our understanding, changes in research methods, professional practices, or medical treatment may become necessary.

Practitioners and researchers must always rely on their own experience and knowledge in evaluating and using any information, methods, compounds, or experiments described herein. In using such information or methods they should be mindful of their own safety and the safety of others, including parties for whom they have a professional responsibility.

With respect to any drug or pharmaceutical products identified, readers are advised to check the most current information provided (i) on procedures featured or (ii) by the manufacturer of each product to be administered, to verify the recommended dose or formula, the method and duration of administration, and contraindications. It is the responsibility of practitioners, relying on their own experience and knowledge of their patients, to make diagnoses, to determine dosages and the best treatment for each individual patient, and to take all appropriate safety precautions.

To the fullest extent of the law, neither the Publisher nor the authors, contributors, or editors, assume any liability for any injury and/or damage to persons or property as a matter of products liability, negligence or otherwise, or from any use or operation of any methods, products, instructions, or ideas contained in the material herein.

Printed in China

Commissioning Editor: Laurence Hunter
Development Editor: Lynn Watt
Project Manager: Vinod Kumar Iyyappan
Designer/Design Direction: Miles Hitchen
Illustration Manager: Jennifer Rose
Illustrator: Antbits Ltd

Contents

Contributors

Derek Alderson, MBBS, MD, FRCS
Barling Professor of Surgery, University of Birmingham, Birmingham, UK

William H. Allum, BSc, MD, FRCS
Consultant Surgeon, Royal Marsden NHS Foundation Trust, London, UK

Max Almond, MRCS, DM
Department of Oesophagogastric Surgery, Gloucestershire Royal Hospital, Gloucester, UK

Hugh Barr, MD, ChM, FRCS, FRCSE, FHEA
Professor and Consultant Upper Gastrointestinal Surgeon, Gloucestershire Royal Hospital, Gloucester, UK

Richard G. Berrisford, ChM, FRCS
Consultant Thoracic Surgeon, Peninsula Oesophagogastric Centre, Derriford Hospital, Plymouth, UK

Jane M. Blazeby, BSc, MD, FRCS(Gen Surg)
Professor of Surgery and Honorary Consultant Surgeon, Centre for Surgical Research, School of Social and Community Medicine, University of Bristol; Division of Surgery, Head and Neck, University Hospitals Bristol NHS Foundation Trust, Bristol Royal Infirmary, Bristol, UK

Natalie Blencowe, BMedSci, BMBS, MRCS
NIHR Doctoral Research Fellow, Centre for Surgical Research, School of Social and Community Medicine, University of Bristol; Division of Surgery, Head and Neck, University Hospitals Bristol NHS Foundation Trust, Bristol Royal Infirmary, Bristol, UK

Nathan W. Bronson, MD
Department of Surgery, Oregon Health and Science University, Portland, OR, USA

Graeme Couper, MD, MBChB, FRCS
Consultant Upper Gastrointestinal Surgeon, Royal Infirmary of Edinburgh, Edinburgh, UK

Adrian Crellin, MA, FRCR, FRCP
Consultant Clinical Oncologist, St James's Institute of Oncology, St James's University Hospital, Leeds, UK

Tom Crosby, MBBS, MRCP, FRCR
Consultant Oncologist, Velindre Cancer Centre, Cardiff, UK

John M. Findlay, BMedSci, BMBS(Hons), MRCS
Oxford OesophagoGastric Centre, Churchill Hospital, Oxford University Hospitals Trust, Oxford, UK

Heike I. Grabsch, MD, PhD, FRCPath
Senior Lecturer in Gastrointestinal Pathology and Honorary Consultant Histopathologist, Pathology and Tumour Biology, Leeds Institute of Molecular Medicine, University of Leeds, Leeds, UK

S. Michael Griffin, MD, FRCS
Professor of Surgery, Northern Oesophago-gastric Unit, Royal Victoria Infirmary, Newcastle upon Tyne, UK

Richard H. Hardwick, MBBS, MD, FRCS
Consultant Upper GI Surgeon, Cambridge Oesophago-Gastric Centre, Addenbrookes Hospital, Cambridge, UK

James Helman, FACA
Virginia Mason Medical Center, Seattle, WA, USA

John G. Hunter, MD
Professor and Chair of Surgery, Oregon Health and Science University, Portland, OR, USA

Janusz Jankowski, MSc(Oxford), MD(Dundee), PhD(London), FRCP(UK), FACG(USA), AGAF(USA)
Acting Associate Dean for Research, Sir James Black Professor of Medicine, Plymouth University Peninsula Schools of Medicine and Dentistry, Plymouth, UK

Arjun D. Koch, MD
Gastroenterology and Hepatology, Erasmus MC – University Medical Center, Rotterdam, The Netherlands

J. Jan B. van Lanschot, MD, PhD, FRCSEd(Hon)
Professor of Surgery, Erasmus MC – University Medical Center, Rotterdam, The Netherlands

Donald E. Low, MD, FACS, FRCS(C)
Head, Thoracic Oncology and Thoracic Surgery, Department of General and Thoracic Surgery, Virginia Mason Medical Center; Clinical Assistant Professor of Surgery, University of Washington School of Medicine, Seattle, WA, USA

Sheraz R. Markar, MRCS, MA
Thoraco-Esophageal Fellow, Virginia Mason Medical Center, Seattle, WA, USA

Robert Mason, BSc, ChM, MD, FRCSEd
Professor of GI Surgery, Guy's and St Thomas' NHS Foundation Trust, King's Health Partners AHSC, London, UK

Nicholas D. Maynard, BA (Hons Oxon), MBBS, MS, FRCS
Oxford OesophagoGastric Centre,
Churchill Hospital, Oxford University Hospitals Trust, Oxford, UK

Kyle A. Perry, MD
Assistant Professor of Surgery, Division of General and Gastrointestinal Surgery, The Ohio State University, Columbus, OH, USA

Joost Rothbarth, MD, PhD
Department of Surgery, Erasmus MC – University Medical Center, Rotterdam, The Netherlands

Takeshi Sano, MD, PhD, FRCSEd
Director, Department of Gastroenterological Surgery, Cancer Institute Hospital, Tokyo, Japan

Jon Shenfine, PhD, FRCS
Consultant Oesophago-Gastric Surgeon, Northern Oesophago-gastric Unit, Royal Victoria Infirmary, Newcastle upon Tyne, UK

B. Mark Smithers, MBBS, FRACS, FRCS(Eng), FRCSEd
Associate Professor, Surgery, Princess Alexandra Hospital; Director, Upper GI / Soft Tissue Unit, Princess Alexandra Hospital, Brisbane, Australia

Iain Thomson, MBBS, FRACS
Division of Surgery, University of Queensland, Princess Alexandra Hospital, Brisbane, Australia

David I. Watson, MBBS, MD, FRACS
Professor and Head of Surgery, Flinders University; Head of Oesophago-Gastric Surgery Unit, Flinders Medical Centre, Bedford Park, Australia

John Wayman, MD, FRCS
Consultant Surgeon, Cumberland Infirmary, Carlisle, UK

Richard Welbourn, MBBS, MD, FRCS
Consultant Surgeon, Department of Upper Gastrointestinal and Bariatric Surgery, Musgrove Park Hospital, Taunton; Honorary Visiting Researcher, Department Metabolic Medicine, Imperial College London, London, UK

Series Editors' preface

It is now some 17 years since the first edition of the *Companion to Specialist Surgical Practice* series was published. We set ourselves the task of meeting the educational needs of surgeons in the later years of specialist surgical training, as well as consultant surgeons in independent practice who wished for contemporary, evidence-based information on the subspecialist areas relevant to their general surgical practice. The series was never intended to replace the large reference surgical textbooks which, although valuable in their own way, struggle to keep pace with changing surgical practice. This Fifth Edition has also had to take due account of the increasing specialisation in 'general' surgery. The rise of minimal access surgery and therapy, and the desire of some subspecialties such as breast and vascular surgery to separate away from 'general surgery', may have proved challenging in some countries, but has also served to emphasise the importance of all surgeons being aware of current developments in their surgical field. As in previous editions, there has been increasing emphasis on evidence-based practice and contributors have endeavoured to provide key recommendations within each chapter. The eBook versions of the textbook have also allowed the technophile improved access to key data and content within each chapter.

We remain indebted to the volume editors and all the contributors of this Fifth Edition. We have endeavoured where possible to bring in new blood to freshen content. We are impressed by the enthusiasm, commitment and hard work that our contributors and editorial team have shown and this has ensured a short turnover between editions while maintaining as accurate and up-to-date content as is possible. We remain grateful for the support and encouragement of Laurence Hunter and Lynn Watt at Elsevier Ltd. We trust that our original vision of delivering an up-to-date affordable text has been met and that readers, whether in training or independent practice, will find this Fifth Edition an invaluable resource.

O. James Garden, BSc, MBChB, MD, FRCS(Glas), FRCS(Ed), FRCP(Ed), FRACS(Hon), FRCSC(Hon), FRSE
Regius Professor of Clinical Surgery, Clinical Surgery School of Clinical Sciences, The University of Edinburgh and Honorary Consultant Surgeon, Royal Infirmary of Edinburgh

Simon Paterson-Brown, MBBS, MPhil, MS, FRCS(Ed), FRCS(Engl), FCS(HK)
Honorary Senior Lecturer, Clinical Surgery School of Clinical Sciences, The University of Edinburgh and Consultant General and Upper Gastrointestinal Surgeon, Royal Infirmary of Edinburgh

Editor's preface

The Fifth Edition of *Oesophagogastric Surgery* includes the latest opinions of world experts on complicated and rapidly changing disciplines in surgery. Whilst we have not changed the number of chapters from the Fourth Edition, we have over half of the chapters written by new authors. The advances in endoscopic and laparoscopic investigation, management and treatment of oesophagogastric disease have required us to re-design many of the submissions. The contribution to the oesophagogastric volume is now truly international from all around the world. In particular, I am delighted to welcome Professor Takeshi Sano from Tokyo, Professor Don Low from Seattle and Professor Mark Smithers from Brisbane to our team. Each edition of this volume has been put together within a relatively short timeframe in order to keep right up to date with current practice. The authors who provided the input into the Fourth Edition have been specifically asked to update the detail and specifically to focus on areas where practice has changed. All authors have incorporated the most up-to-date references for their subjects to highlight key points and expert opinion. We have continued using the strong recommendations summary to aid in the learning process.

I wish to thank all of our contributors for providing their expertise and experience in contemporary practice and for remaining true to the criteria set for the series in general. I trust that this book truly reflects current oesophagogastric surgical practice and not only supplies the demand for trainees studying for the exit exam but also for established oesophagogastric specialists around the world.

Acknowledgements

The Fifth Edition has greatly benefited from the significant change in authorship and I am particularly indebted to those from overseas who have provided insight into cutting-edge practice. I acknowledge the unstinting support of my secretary, Alison Hood, and my colleagues, Simon Raimes and Jon Shenfine. I dedicate this work to my mother, Joan Griffin, who died recently, without whom none of this would have been possible.

S. Michael Griffin
Newcastle upon Tyne

Evidence-based practice in surgery

Critical appraisal for developing evidence-based practice can be obtained from a number of sources, the most reliable being randomised controlled clinical trials, systematic literature reviews, meta-analyses and observational studies. For practical purposes three grades of evidence can be used, analogous to the levels of 'proof' required in a court of law:

1. **Beyond all reasonable doubt.** Such evidence is likely to have arisen from high-quality randomised controlled trials, systematic reviews or high-quality synthesised evidence such as decision analysis, cost-effectiveness analysis or large observational datasets. The studies need to be directly applicable to the population of concern and have clear results. The grade is analogous to burden of proof within a criminal court and may be thought of as corresponding to the usual standard of 'proof' within the medical literature (i.e. $P<0.05$).
2. **On the balance of probabilities.** In many cases a high-quality review of literature may fail to reach firm conclusions due to conflicting or inconclusive results, trials of poor methodological quality or the lack of evidence in the population to which the guidelines apply. In such cases it may still be possible to make a statement as to the best treatment on the 'balance of probabilities'. This is analogous to the decision in a civil court where all the available evidence will be weighed up and the verdict will depend upon the balance of probabilities.
3. **Not proven.** Insufficient evidence upon which to base a decision, or contradictory evidence.

Depending on the information available, three grades of recommendation can be used:

a. Strong recommendation, which should be followed unless there are compelling reasons to act otherwise.
b. A recommendation based on evidence of effectiveness, but where there may be other factors to take into account in decision-making, for example the user of the guidelines may be expected to take into account patient preferences, local facilities, local audit results or available resources.
c. A recommendation made where there is no adequate evidence as to the most effective practice, although there may be reasons for making a recommendation in order to minimise cost or reduce the chance of error through a locally agreed protocol.

✔✔ Evidence where a conclusion can be reached '**beyond all reasonable doubt**' and therefore where a **strong recommendation** can be given.
This will normally be based on evidence levels:
- Ia. Meta-analysis of randomised controlled trials
- Ib. Evidence from at least one randomised controlled trial
- IIa. Evidence from at least one controlled study without randomisation
- IIb. Evidence from at least one other type of quasi-experimental study.

✔ Evidence where a conclusion might be reached '**on the balance of probabilities**' and where there may be other factors involved which influence the recommendation given. This will normally be based on less conclusive evidence than that represented by the double tick icons:
- III. Evidence from non-experimental descriptive studies, such as comparative studies and case–control studies
- IV. Evidence from expert committee reports or opinions or clinical experience of respected authorities, or both.

Evidence which is associated with either a **strong recommendation** or **expert opinion** is highlighted in the text in panels such as those shown above, and is distinguished by either a double or single tick icon, respectively. The references associated with double-tick evidence are highlighted in the reference lists at the end of each chapter along with a short summary of the paper's conclusions where applicable.

The reader is referred to Chapter 1, 'Evidence-based practice in surgery' in the volume, *Core Topics in General and Emergency Surgery* of this series, for a more detailed description of this topic.

1

Pathology of oesophageal and gastric tumours

Heike I. Grabsch

Oesophagus

Introduction

Patients with neoplastic processes of the oesophagus most commonly present clinically at an advanced disease stage with strictures, plaque-like or polypoid masses protruding into the lumen, diffuse thickening of the mucosa and wall or deeply penetrating ulcers. Oesophageal neoplasms can be broadly divided into epithelial and mesenchymal subtypes according to the cell of origin. Whilst epithelial neoplasms are more common and can be recognised endoscopically due to mucosal irregularities, mesenchymal neoplasms are usually located subepithelially with an intact overlying mucosa. Precursor lesions have been recognised for malignant epithelial tumours and will be discussed in this chapter together with the histopathological features and molecular pathology of oesophageal tumours.

Epithelial tumours of the oesophagus and the gastro-oesophageal junction

Benign tumours and tumour-like lesions

Squamous cell papillomas are the most frequent benign epithelial tumours of the oesophagus, with a distinctive endoscopic appearance. They are most commonly located in the middle or lower third of the oesophagus, are exophytic, sessile or partly pedunculated, well demarcated and measure usually less than 5 mm in diameter. Only patients with very large lesions become clinically symptomatic. True **adenomas** of the oesophagus are benign tumours that develop from the submucosal oesophageal glands and are exceedingly rare.

Developmental cysts and congenital oesophageal duplications are benign lesions that may clinically mimic a tumour because of their mass effect, causing compression of the neighbouring respiratory tract. Similarly, patients with **giant fibrovascular polyps**, an entirely benign neoplasm, may present with severe dysphagia and respiratory symptoms and a large pedunculated mass obliterating the oesophageal lumen.

Malignant tumours

Squamous cell carcinoma

Squamous cell carcinoma is the most common malignant tumour of the oesophagus worldwide and affects men two to ten times more often than females, with an average age between 50 and 60 years at time of diagnosis. There is a marked geographic and ethnic variation in incidence. Incidence rates are highest in Iran, China, South America and Eastern Africa and are higher in African-Americans than Caucasian-Americans regardless of gender.

✔ The aetiology and predisposing factors for oesophageal squamous cell carcinoma vary significantly in different regions of the world.[1] Tobacco smoking and alcohol consumption are major risk factors for oesophageal squamous cell carcinoma.[2,3]

The intake of hot beverages has been shown to increase the risk of squamous cell carcinoma. Furthermore, dietary factors such as a lack of fresh fruit and vegetables and high intake of barbecued meat or pickled vegetables most likely play a role in the aetiology of squamous cell carcinoma. Human papilloma virus infection has been implicated in the pathogenesis of oesophageal squamous cell carcinoma, but its precise role is still controversial at present. Patients with achalasia have an increased risk of developing cancer compared to the normal population.[4] The risk of developing oesophageal carcinoma is also increased in patients with coeliac disease,[5] Plummer–Vinson syndrome (also called Paterson–Kelly syndrome),[6] tylosis (also called focal non-epidermolytic palmoplantar keratoderma),[7,8] previous ingestion of corrosive substances,[9] Zenker's diverticulum[10] or after ionising radiation.[11] In the Asian population, polymorphisms in *ALDH1B1* and *ALDH2*, both genes encoding aldehyde dehydrogenases, are associated with squamous cell carcinoma.[12]

Oesophageal squamous cell carcinomas are found in the upper, middle and lower third of the oesophagus in a ratio of approximately 1:5:2. The macroscopic appearance depends on the depth of tumour invasion and is classified into four different types according to the Japanese classification for oesophageal cancer,[13] which is similar to the macroscopic classification of gastric cancer (see Fig. 1.8 below). Approximately 60% of squamous cell carcinomas show an exophytic or fungating growth pattern, 25% are ulcerative and 15% are infiltrative (**Fig. 1.1**). However, the macroscopic appearance of all cancers can significantly change as a result of neoadjuvant chemotherapy or chemoradiation, with tumour shrinkage, extensive necrosis and fibrosis.

Squamous cell carcinomas invade both horizontally and vertically. In the West, 60% of patients have carcinomas that have invaded beyond the muscularis propria and have regional lymph node metastases at the time of diagnosis, whereas in Japan up to 40% of all resected carcinomas are superficial or early carcinomas involving mucosa and submucosa only.[14] The frequency of lymph node metastases is related to the depth of tumour invasion and has been reported as less than 5% for intramucosal carcinomas and up to 45% for submucosal carcinomas. Although tumours located in the upper third of the oesophagus are more likely to spread to cervical and upper mediastinal nodes, a significant proportion will also spread to perigastric nodes.

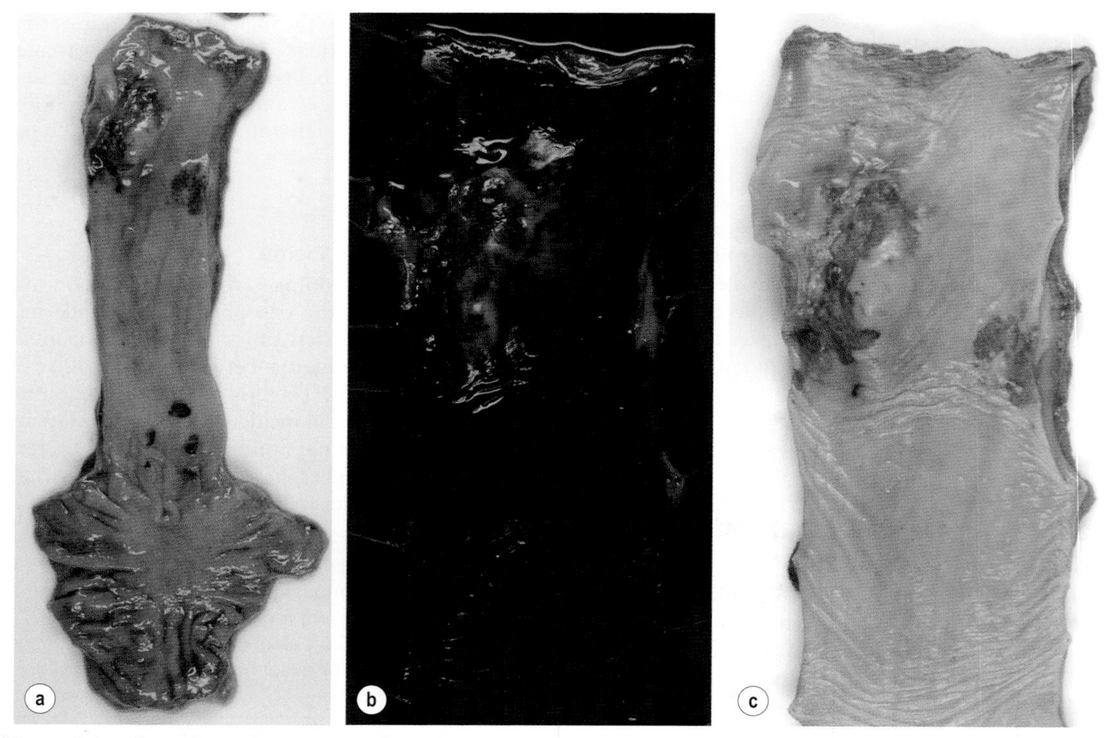

Figure 1.1 • Oesophageal squamous cell carcinoma located in the middle oesophagus. **(a)** Fresh oesophagectomy specimen with a polypoid exophytic tumour growth and a smaller flat (red coloured) mucosal abnormality. **(b)** Lack of (dark) iodine staining in the abnormal areas. **(c)** Same specimen after fixation. Courtesy of Dr Tomio Arai, Tokyo.

✔ Tumours located in the middle and lower oesophagus can spread to upper mediastinal and perigastric nodes, and patients with lymph node metastases on both sides of the diaphragm have been shown to have a poorer prognosis.[15–17]

Distant metastases due to haematogenous spread are most commonly found in liver, lung, adrenal gland and kidney.[18]

Histologically, squamous cell carcinomas are characterised by keratinocyte-like cells that may or may not have intercellular bridges and show a variable degree of keratinisation (**Fig. 1.2**). Depending on the extent of mitotic activity, nuclear atypia and degree of squamous differentiation including degree of keratinisation, squamous cell carcinomas are graded as well, moderately or poorly differentiated.[12] The histology of squamous cell carcinoma can change dramatically after neoadjuvant chemo(radio)therapy and then typically shows extensive necrosis, inflammation, fibrosis and foreign body-type granulomas around keratin pearls. There is currently no consensus on how to grade tumour regression. The regression grading according to Mandard et al.[19] considers the relative proportion of residual viable tumour cells and fibrosis in the primary cancer and is probably currently the one most commonly used in the UK. Very recently, a grading system to assess tumour regression in lymph nodes has been proposed and showed prognostic significance in a small series of patients.[20]

Three main variants of squamous cell carcinoma have been described:[12]

1. **Verrucous carcinoma** of the oesophagus is a rare, locally aggressive tumour that is more common in males. Macroscopically, the tumour has an exophytic papillary appearance and tumours are usually very large before they become clinically apparent. Microscopically, the tumour is very well differentiated with minimal atypia. Superficial biopsies are often insufficient to distinguish between a squamous papilloma, pseudoepitheliomatous hyperplasia and verrucous carcinoma.[21]
2. **Spindle cell carcinoma** (also known as carcinosarcoma, sarcomatoid carcinoma and polypoid carcinoma) is a polypoid tumour located in the middle or lower third of the oesophagus. Histologically, the tumour is a mixture of a well-differentiated squamous cell carcinoma and a high-grade spindle cell component that can show osseous, cartilaginous or skeletal muscle differentiation.[22] Spindle cell carcinomas are highly aggressive carcinomas, with 5-year survival rates of 10–15%.[23]
3. **Basaloid squamous cell carcinoma** is an unusual variant of squamous cell carcinoma that needs to be distinguished from 'pure' squamous cell carcinoma, adenoid cystic carcinoma and neuroendocrine tumours. It is a highly aggressive carcinoma with a very poor prognosis. Histologically, this tumour shows the characteristic basaloid cells together with a mucoid hyaline-like substance, as well as multiple other components.

Precursor lesions of squamous cell carcinoma

Oesophageal squamous cell carcinoma development is believed to be a multistep process from normal squamous epithelium via intraepithelial

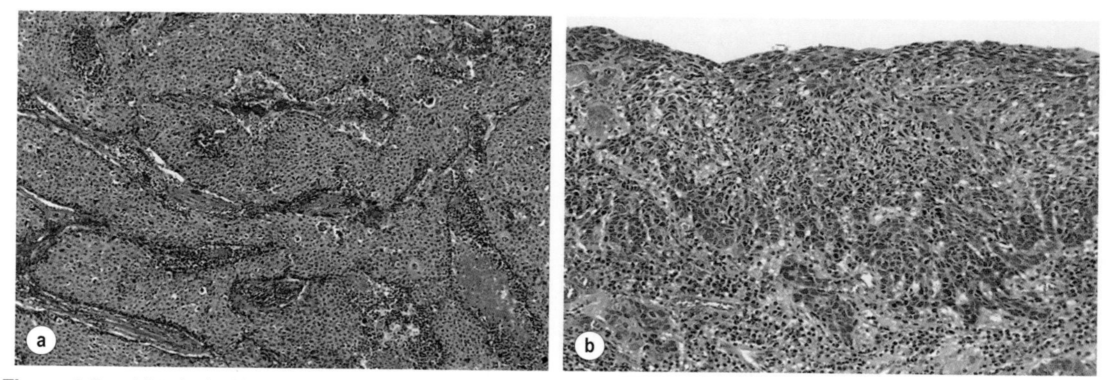

Figure 1.2 • Histological images from specimen in Fig. 1.1. **(a)** Histology of the nodule shows poorly differentiated squamous cell carcinoma with no evidence of keratin formation and necrosis (pink material) between strands of neoplastic cells. **(b)** Histology of the flat lesion shows early infiltrative squamous cell carcinoma. Courtesy of Dr Tomio Arai, Tokyo.

neoplasia (synonym: dysplasia) to invasive carcinoma based on findings in high-risk populations where dysplasia predates the development of carcinoma by approximately 5 years.[24,25] In general, dysplasia is defined as the presence of unequivocal neoplastic cells within the epithelium. Squamous cell dysplasia is classified as 'low grade' when architectural and cytological abnormalities are seen in the basal half of the squamous epithelium with preserved maturation of the upper half, and as 'high grade' when more than the bottom half shows architectural and cytological abnormalities. Full-thickness dysplasia of the squamous epithelium is referred to as 'carcinoma in situ' by some authors.

Molecular pathology of squamous cell carcinoma

Up to 80% of squamous cell carcinomas show mutation with consecutive loss or inactivation of the tumour suppressor gene *p53* (the 'guardian' of the genome located on the short arm of chromosome 17), of the retinoblastoma gene *RB* and of *p16*.[26] Amplification (e.g. an increase in gene copy number) and subsequent protein overexpression of *cyclin D1*, a cell cycle regulating gene, occurs in 20–40% of squamous cell carcinomas. Inactivation of *FHIT* (fragile histidine triad gene, a presumed tumour suppressor gene on chromosome 3p14), *DLEC1* (deleted in lung and oesophageal cancer-1) and *DEC1* (deleted in oesophageal cancer-1) by genetic or epigenetic mechanisms promoting cancer cell growth has recently been shown. Amplifications of several proto-oncogenes and growth factors such as *FGF4* and *FGF6* (fibroblast growth factors 4 and 6), *EGFR* (epidermal growth factor receptor) and *MYC* have also been found in oesophageal squamous cell carcinoma. Some of these changes, such as *p53* mutations, appear to be an early event as they have also been demonstrated in squamous cell dysplasia. The presence of such genetic changes may be used to select patients for targeted therapy with antibodies or small-molecule inhibitors in the near future.

Adenocarcinoma

Population-based studies in the USA and Europe indicate that the incidence of oesophageal adenocarcinoma, adenocarcinoma of the gastro-oesophageal junction and proximal stomach has doubled between the 1970s and late 1980s, and continues to increase by 5% every year.[2,27] Countries with the highest incidence of oesophageal adenocarcinoma are the UK, Australia, the Netherlands and the USA. Oesophageal adenocarcinoma is much more common in males (male:female ratio 4:1 to 7:1) and 80% of oesophageal adenocarcinomas occur in the white population.

✔ Ninety-five per cent of oesophageal adenocarcinomas are associated with Barrett's oesophagus, which has been identified as the single most important risk factor.

The relative risk of developing adenocarcinoma in patients with Barrett's oesophagus is of the order of 30–60,[27] but only 5% of patients with oesophageal adenocarcinoma have had a previous diagnosis of Barrett's oesophagus.[28] Other risk factors of oesophageal adenocarcinoma are tobacco smoking, obesity (which may promote gastro-oesophageal reflux), and use of medications that relax the gastro-oesophageal sphincter. No clear association has been found between alcohol consumption or diet and adenocarcinoma. Case–control studies seem to indicate that infection with *Helicobacter pylori* is protective against oesophageal adenocarcinoma.

There is an ongoing debate whether adenocarcinoma in the proximity of the oesophagogastric junction should be classified as oesophageal or gastric carcinoma. This is mainly related to the fact that there is no consensus on the definition of the 'gastro-oesophageal junction' and ten different definitions are listed in the fourth edition of the WHO classification of digestive cancer 2010.[12] Siewert and Stein[29] defined adenocarcinoma of the gastro-oesophageal junction as 'tumours that have their centre within 5 cm proximal and distal of the anatomical cardia' and suggested three tumour types based on the anatomical location of the tumour centre determined by a combination of radiography, endoscopy, computed tomography and intraoperative appearance:

- **Type I.** Adenocarcinoma of the distal oesophagus, which usually arises from an area with specialised intestinal metaplasia (i.e. Barrett's oesophagus) and which may infiltrate the gastro-oesophageal junction from above. This entity is also referred to as 'Barrett carcinoma'. These adenocarcinomas have their centre within 1–5 cm above the cardia.
- **Type II.** True carcinoma of the cardia arising from the gastric cardia epithelium or from short segments with intestinal metaplasia at the gastro-oesophageal junction. This entity is also referred to as 'junctional carcinoma'. These adenocarcinomas have their centre within 1 cm above and 2 cm below the cardia.
- **Type III.** Subcardial gastric carcinoma that infiltrates the oesophagogastric junction and distal oesophagus from below. This entity is

also referred to as 'proximal gastric carcinoma'. These adenocarcinomas have their centre within 2–5 cm below the cardia.

Adenocarcinoma associated with Barrett's oesophagus

Columnar epithelium in the oesophagus in combination with ulceration and oesophagitis was first described by Norman Barrett in 1950, who was convinced that this was due to a congenitally short oesophagus.[30] Moersch et al.[31] and Hayward[32] were the first to suggest that the columnar lining of the oesophagus might be an acquired condition due to gastro-oesophageal reflux. Experiments conducted by Bremner et al.[33] in 1970 in a dog model of gastro-oesophageal reflux strongly supported this concept.

✔ **Barrett's oesophagus is defined as the replacement of the squamous epithelium by specialised columnar epithelium, which is characterised by intestinal metaplasia.[34]**

The risk of developing adenocarcinoma appears to be related to the length of the metaplastic mucosa, with 3 cm being used as the cut-off between a 'short' and a 'long' segment Barrett's oesophagus. Further details of Barrett's oesophagus including the proposed metaplasia–dysplasia–adenocarcinoma sequence can be found in Chapter 15.

Barrett's associated adenocarcinomas are located almost exclusively in the distal third of the oesophagus and often infiltrate into the proximal stomach (**Fig. 1.3**). Up to 50% of adenocarcinomas show a macroscopic infiltrative growth pattern and only 5–10% are polypoid. Histologically, oesophageal adenocarcinomas are typically papillary and/or tubular (intestinal type according to the Laurén classification[35]) and are graded as well, moderately or poorly differentiated according to the proportion of tumour that is composed of glands.[12] Approximately 10% of all oesophageal adenocarcinomas are of mucinous or signet-ring cell type. Most patients present with locally advanced disease, where the adenocarcinoma has infiltrated beyond the deep muscle layer into the perioesophageal tissue and involves regional lymph nodes in up to 75% of cases. Should the patient present with early disease, it is important to remember that there is a double muscularis mucosae in almost all cases with Barrett's oesophagus. Carcinomas infiltrating between the two layers of the muscularis mucosae are still to be classified as 'intramucosal' pT1a cancers. However, carcinomas that have infiltrated into this double muscularis mucosae layer may be associated with a higher frequency of lymphoangioinvasion and lymph node metastases.[36] This has implications for endoscopic treatments.

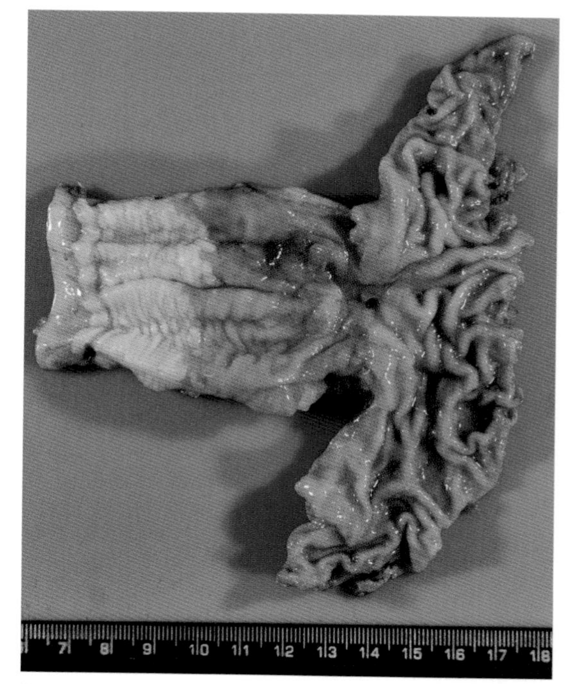

Figure 1.3 • Barrett's oesophagus with adenocarcinoma is seen on the left. An irregular, partly ulcerated tumour is located at the gastro-oesophageal junction. Between the proximal edge of the tumour and the squamous lined oesophagus is metaplastic columnar epithelium. The squamocolumnar junction (border between the pale appearing squamous epithelium and brownish-appearing metaplastic epithelium) is located at least 2.5 cm proximal to the gastro-oesophageal junction. Courtesy of Dr B. Disep, Newcastle.

Variants of oesophageal adenocarcinoma

1. Truly **non-Barrett's oesophagus-associated adenocarcinoma** of the oesophagus is rare and arises either from heterotopic gastric mucosa (so called 'gastric inlet'), which can be anywhere in the oesophagus or from the epithelium of submucosal oesophageal glands.
2. **Adenoid cystic carcinoma** is also very rare. These carcinomas are histologically identical to salivary gland-type adenoid cystic carcinoma and occur more frequently in females.[37] These carcinomas arise from submucosal oesophageal glands. They usually form well-circumscribed solid nodules in the submucosa and the overlying squamous epithelium shows no abnormalities. Most tumours show some differentiation towards squamous, glandular or even small cell elements which could indicate an origin from a multipotential stem cell.

Precursor lesions of oesophageal adenocarcinoma and molecular pathology of oesophageal adenocarcinoma are discussed in more detail in Chapter 15.

Neuroendocrine tumours of the oesophagus

Oesophageal neuroendocrine tumours are very rare, representing less than 8% of all oesophageal carcinomas. The majority of them are poorly differentiated neuroendocrine carcinomas (also known as small cell carcinomas) that are highly aggressive and median survival is usually 6–12 months or less. Macroscopically, they appear as exophytic or ulcerative growths measuring on average 6 cm at presentation. Histologically, these may appear as homogeneous tumours (**Fig. 1.4**) or as a mixture of squamous and mucoepidermoid elements. The histological features including immunohistochemical markers are similar to small cell carcinoma of the lung and the possibility of metastatic or direct spread from the lung should always be considered in the differential diagnosis.

Mesenchymal tumours of the oesophagus

Leiomyoma

Leiomyoma is the most common benign mesenchymal tumour of the oesophagus, which is twice as frequent in males as females. Leiomyomas are typically located in the distal or middle oesophagus. Most are less than 3 cm in size and form a hard white-greyish mass. In contrast to gastrointestinal stromal tumours, leiomyomas are immunoreactive for desmin and smooth muscle actin and negative for KIT (CD117) and DOG1.

Granular cell tumour

Granular cell tumours are found in the skin, mouth and throughout the gastrointestinal tract, but most frequently in the oesophagus. Nearly two-thirds of these tumours have been found in the lower third of the oesophagus and arise in the submucosa. The covering squamous epithelium is often thickened and may show pseudoepitheliomatous hyperplasia. The characteristic tumour cells are uniform plump cells with granular cytoplasm that stain with periodic acid–Schiff and S-100 protein.

Lymphoma of the oesophagus, melanoma, choriocarcinoma and secondary tumours (metastases) are not discussed here.

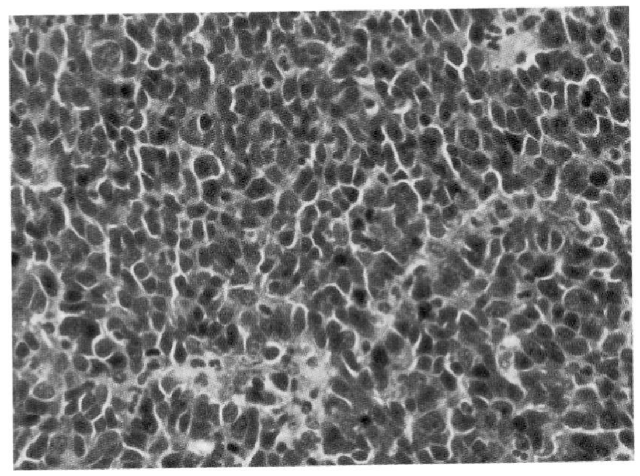

Figure 1.4 • Microscopic image of a neuroendocrine carcinoma.

Stomach

Gastric polyps

Gastric polyps are usually found incidentally during endoscopy. According to the cell of origin polyps can be epithelial (fundic gland polyp, hyperplastic polyp, adenomatous polyp), neuroendocrine, lymphohistiocytic (xanthelasma, lymphoid hyperplasia), mesenchymal (gastrointestinal stromal tumour, neural or vascular tumours) or mixed. They can be sporadic or occur as part of a disease syndrome.

Fundic gland polyps

Fundic gland polyps are the most common type of gastric polyps and were originally described in patients with familial adenomatous polyposis (FAP) syndrome.[38] Sporadic fundic gland polyps are found in up to 11% of patients, are more common in middle-aged women and are typically single or few, measuring less than 0.5 cm. The incidence of fundic gland polyps is low in patients with *H. pylori* infection and high in patients taking proton-pump inhibitors.[39] While low-grade dysplasia is frequent in FAP patients with fundic gland polyps, dysplasia is rare in sporadic cases.[40]

✔ Seventy-five per cent of FAP-associated fundic gland polyps show an *APC* mutation, whereas sporadic fundic gland polyps are devoid of *APC* mutations and harbour *CTNNB1* (β-catenin) mutations in up to 90%.[41]

Fundic gland polyps have been considered as being hamartomatous lesions in the past, a view that has been challenged recently.

Hyperplastic polyps are composed of epithelial and stromal components, and are most frequently found in the antrum of patients with inflamed or atrophic gastric mucosa. A recent review of more than 8000 gastric polyps showed that only 14% were hyperplastic polyps.[39] Hyperplastic gastric polyps are thought to arise as a hyperproliferative response of the gastric foveolae to tissue injury.

Removal of the underlying injury such as *H. pylori* infection resulted in regression of the hyperplastic polyps in 70% of patients.[42] 1–20% of hyperplastic polyps show foci of dysplasia, *p53* mutations, chromosomal aberrations and microsatellite instability, which seem to be related to larger size (>2 cm).[43] Hyperplastic polyps should be regarded as surrogate markers of cancer risk and synchronous or metachronous gastric carcinomas have been reported in up to 6% of cases.

Adenomatous polyps are subdivided into classic intestinal-type adenomas and non-intestinal-type adenomas. The latter are less common and are characterised by gastric-type differentiation. Non-intestinal-type gastric adenomas such as pyloric gland adenoma, foveolar adenoma and chief cell adenoma are relatively rare and are not further discussed here.

Sporadic intestinal-type adenomas are most common in patients over 50 years of age, three times more frequent in men and most commonly found on the lesser curve of the antrum. They are usually solitary, less than 2 cm in diameter, well circumscribed, pedunculated or sessile, and their prevalence varies widely from 4% in Western countries to 27% in Japan. Adenomatous polyps are precursors of gastric adenocarcinomas and the risk of adenocarcinoma seems to increase with increasing size. Fifty per cent of adenomatous polyps >2 cm harbour an adenocarcinoma.[44]

Other lesions that can endoscopically appear as polyps in the stomach are: inflammatory fibroid polyps, which consist of benign submucosal proliferations of spindle cells, small vessels and inflammatory cells; xanthomas, which consist of aggregates of lipid-laden macrophages embedded in the lamina propria; and lipomas, which are circumscribed masses of adipose tissue without atypia usually located in the submucosa and pancreatic heterotopias.

Polyposis syndromes

Hamartomatous polyps in the stomach have been found in patients with Peutz–Jeghers syndrome, juvenile polyposis, Cronkite–Canada syndrome and Cowden disease. With the exception of Peutz–Jeghers polyps, the histological features of these polyps overlap with those of sporadic hyperplastic polyp and the pathological diagnosis of a 'syndromic polyp' will require knowledge of the suggestive clinical context. All patients with the above mentioned polyposis syndromes have an increased risk of developing gastric carcinoma that appears to be highest in patients with Peutz–Jeghers syndrome at 30%.[45] Up to 80% of patients with Peutz–Jeghers syndrome have a germ-line mutation of the *STK11/LKB1* gene that encodes an enzyme responsible for cell division, differentiation and signal transduction. The most common genetic alterations in patients with juvenile polyposis are germline mutation of *SMAD4* or *BMPR1A*, both genes implicated in the transforming growth factor (TGF)-β signalling pathway. Cowden disease is caused by germline mutations of *PTEN* resulting in multiple hamartomas involving multiple different organs. Cronkite–Canada syndrome is a non-inherited polyposis syndrome of unknown pathogenesis.

Gastric carcinoma

Epidemiology of gastric carcinoma

Despite a steady decline of gastric carcinoma incidence at a rate of approximately 5% per year since the 1950s,[46] gastric carcinoma is still the fourth most common carcinoma in the world, with one million people newly diagnosed per year, representing 8% of all new cancers diagnosed per year in the world. Age-standardised incidence rates of gastric carcinoma are twice as high in males as in females and show prominent geographical variation, ranging from 3.9 in Northern Africa to 42.4 in Eastern Asia per 100 000 males.[47] Seventy-five per cent of all new gastric carcinoma cases are diagnosed in Asia. Gastric carcinoma is the second leading cause of cancer death in both sexes worldwide, being responsible for 10% of all cancer deaths. A male:female ratio of 2:1 has been reported for non-cardia gastric carcinoma in contrast to a male:female ratio of 5:1 for gastric cardia carcinoma.[48]

Aetiology and risk factors of gastric carcinoma

Ten per cent of gastric carcinomas show familial clustering, but only 1–3% of gastric carcinomas are related to identified inherited gastric carcinoma predisposition syndromes such as hereditary diffuse gastric carcinoma, hereditary non-polyposis colon cancer (Lynch syndrome), familial adenomatous polyposis, Peutz–Jeghers syndrome, Li–Fraumeni syndrome, and familial breast and ovarian cancer.[49,50]

One of the defining characteristics of the **hereditary diffuse gastric carcinoma syndrome** (HDGC) is the presence of a germline *CDH1* (E-cadherin) mutation.[51] *CDH1* mutations have been found in hereditary as well as sporadic diffuse-type gastric carcinomas, but not in intestinal-type gastric carcinomas. *CDH1* mutations in sporadic diffuse-type gastric carcinoma cluster in exons 7–9, whereas *CDH1* germline mutations are spread over the whole length of the gene in HDGC patients, making genetic testing very time consuming as the whole *CDH1* gene might need to be sequenced.[52] Patients diagnosed with HDGC have an increased risk of lobular breast cancer and signet-ring colon cancer, and should undergo appropriate surveillance for these diseases.[53] The penetrance of the gene varies between 70% and 80%, and the lifetime risk of developing gastric carcinoma in mutation carriers is 67% in men and 83% in women. In order to identify patients that should be offered *CDH1* mutation testing, including appropriate genetic counselling, the updated recommendations of the International Gastric Cancer Linkage Consortium (IGCLC) should be followed[51] (Box 1.1).

Box 1.1 • Criteria to identify patients who require testing for *CDH1* mutation[51]

1. Two or more documented cases of gastric cancer in first degree relatives with at least one documented case of diffuse-type gastric cancer diagnosed before the age of 50 years OR
2. Three or more cases of documented diffuse gastric cancer in first or second degree relatives independent of age of onset OR
3. Diffuse gastric cancer before the age of 40 without family history OR
4. Families with diagnoses of both, diffuse-type gastric cancer and lobular breast cancer with one case before the age or 50 years OR
5. In cases where expert pathologists detect carcinoma *in situ* adjacent to diffuse-type gastric cancer, genetic testing should be considered as this is rarely, if ever, seen in sporadic diffuse-type gastric cancer cases.

✔ Total gastrectomy with or without perioperative chemotherapy as appropriate is recommended for patients diagnosed with hereditary diffuse-type gastric carcinoma irrespective of tumour location or disease stage.

The resection specimen should be worked up and reported according to the recommendations of the IGCLC.[51]

Helicobacter pylori **infection** increases the risk of gastric carcinoma up to sixfold and hence represents one of the most important environmental risk factors for the development of gastric carcinoma. Humans are the only known host for *H. pylori* that can colonise the body and the antrum (**Fig. 1.5**). The development of gastric carcinoma after *H. pylori* infection has been considered as a multistep process progressing from chronic active pan- or corpus predominant gastritis to increasing loss of gastric glands (atrophy), replacement of the normal mucosa by intestinal metaplasia and malignant transformation.[54–56] Most *H. pylori*-infected individuals will remain asymptomatic and only 1–5% of the infected population will develop gastric carcinoma, a phenomenon that has been attributed to different bacterial strains, host-inflammatory genetic susceptibility and in particular the *H. pylori* virulence factors vacuolating cytotoxin antigen (VacA) and cytotoxin-associated gene A antigen (CagA).[54,57,58]

It has been estimated that 10% of gastric carcinomas are associated with **Epstein–Barr virus (EBV) infection.**[59] Considering the worldwide incidence of gastric carcinoma, EBV-associated gastric carcinoma is the largest group of carcinomas within

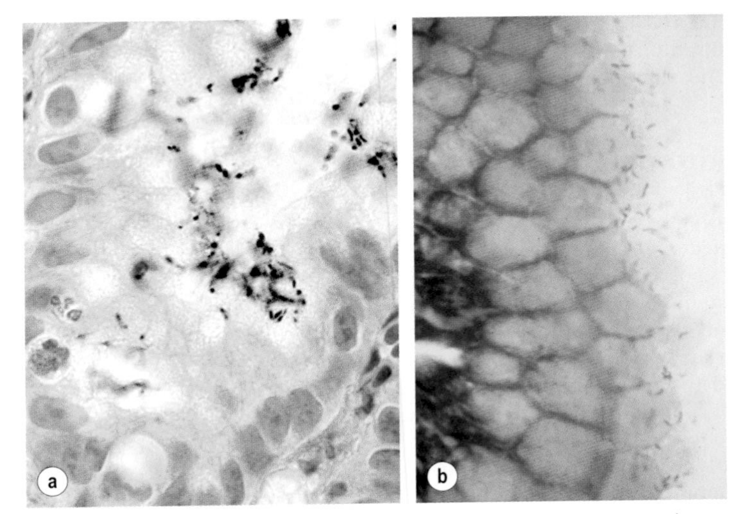

Figure 1.5 • *Helicobacter pylori.* The Gram-negative, spiral-shaped, 2.5 to 5 μm long bacterium can be found on the gastric surface epithelium within the mucous layer. **(a)** Immunohistochemical staining demonstrates the organisms as brown rods. **(b)** In the modified Giemsa staining, the organisms appear light blue.

all EBV-associated malignancies. In contrast to *H. pylori*, which has a role in the early stage of gastric carcinoma development as it binds to the surface of the normal gastric epithelial cell but cannot bind to the surface of gastric carcinoma cells, EBV is absent in normal or dysplastic gastric epithelial cells but present in all gastric carcinoma cells.[60] For unknown reasons, EBV prevalence is higher in gastric stump cancer.[61]

The prominent geographical variation in gastric carcinoma incidence suggests that other environmental factors such as diet might play an important aetiological role. However, evidence for all areas like fruit and vegetable consumption, dietary supplementation with antioxidants such as vitamin C, dietary salt and nitroso compounds is still conflicting.[62–64]

A dose dependent relationship between smoking and gastric carcinoma risk has been shown in prospective studies and it has been estimated that 18% of gastric carcinomas in the European population were attributable to smoking.[65] There is currently no conclusive evidence for an association between alcohol consumption and gastric carcinoma.[66] An increased risk of gastric carcinoma after previous gastric surgery for benign peptic ulcer disease has been reported.[67] Another potential source of gastric stump carcinoma is the Roux-en-Y gastrojejunostomy used to treat morbid obesity and gastric carcinoma after bariatric surgery has already been reported.

Lesions predisposing to gastric carcinoma

The natural history of sporadic gastric carcinoma is thought to be a multistep process. Correa postulated a sequence from chronic atrophic gastritis, intestinal metaplasia, dysplasia and gastric carcinoma based on histopathological findings[68] (for more details, see Chapter 2). Ten years later, this model was expanded by Yasui et al.[69] to include stepwise molecular alterations.

Chronic atrophic gastritis and intestinal metaplasia

Inflammation of the gastric mucosa is the result of bacterial infection (most commonly due to *H. pylori* infection), chemical agents (non-steroidal anti-inflammatory drugs (NSAIDs), alcohol, bile reflux) or the consequence of an autoimmune process (i.e. autoimmune gastritis due to parietal cell antibodies). Depending on the underlying aetiology, chronic inflammation can result in (a) the shrinkage or complete disappearance of the typical gastric glands followed by replacement fibrosis of the lamina propria or (b) replacement of the native glands by metaplastic glands (i.e. intestinal and/or pseudopyloric metaplasia). In both conditions there is 'atrophy' (loss of appropriate glands), but only (b) is considered a condition with an increased risk of developing carcinoma (**Fig. 1.6**).

Two main types of intestinal metaplasia have been identified depending on whether the epithelium is similar to small bowel epithelium or large bowel epithelium and on the histochemical characteristics of the mucin. Type I is complete, small bowel type, positive for neutral mucin and sialomucin, and negative for sulfomucin; type II/III is incomplete, large bowel type, positive or negative for neutral mucin, and positive for sialomucin and sulfomucin (**Fig. 1.7**).

✔ Some but not all studies indicate that there is a positive correlation between cancer risk and degree and extent of incomplete intestinal metaplasia.[12]

Chronic gastric ulcer

Chronic gastric ulcers are typically located near the border of atrophic mucosa. If a chronic gastric ulcer is detected on endoscopy, it should be suspected of being neoplastic until histology has proven otherwise.

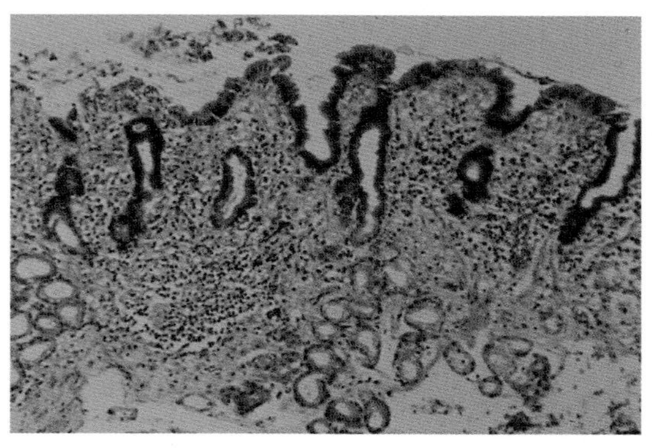

Figure 1.6 • Microscopic image showing gastric atrophy.

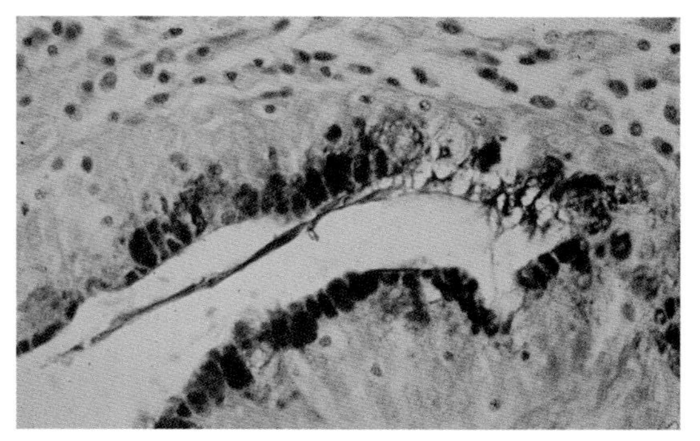

Figure 1.7 • Intestinal metaplasia (type III). The pits show both large solitary and multiple smaller secretory vacuoles with the apical positions of the cells. Stained with Alcian Blue and High Iron Diamine.

Patients with gastric ulcer have an increased risk for gastric carcinoma as gastric ulcer and gastric carcinoma have the same risk factors. Five per cent of endoscopically benign ulcers eventually prove to be malignant. However, overall, less than 1% of all gastric carcinomas develop in pre-existing peptic ulcers.[70]

Gastric dysplasia

Gastric dysplasia (synonym: intraepithelial neoplasia) can have a flat, slightly depressed or polypoid growth pattern. In Europe and North America polypoid dysplasia is termed 'adenoma', whereas in Japan dysplasia with any growth pattern is called 'adenoma'.

The prevalence of gastric dysplasia varies, depending on the underlying aetiology, between 20% in high risk areas and 4% in Western countries, where gastric carcinoma is less common.[71] Dysplasia is more frequent in males, patients over 70 years of age, and most commonly affects the lesser curve and the antrum. Histologically, dysplasia is characterised by architectural as well as cytological atypia and is stratified into two grades, low and high. Low grade dysplasia progresses to adenocarcinoma in up 23% of cases within 10 months to 4 years, whereas malignant transformation of high grade dysplasia has been reported to occur in 60–80% of cases.

✔ The diagnosis of dysplasia shows significant interobserver variability due to the low specificity of the abnormalities used to establish the diagnosis and in particular the difficulties in distinguishing regenerative atypia from dysplasia and high grade dysplasia from intramucosal carcinoma. In an attempt to standardise the terminology used to describe the morphological spectrum of lesions, several proposals including the Padova and Vienna classifications have been made.[72–74]

Whilst chromosomal and microsatellite instability, *APC* and *p53* mutations, as well as CpG-island methylation, have all been found in gastric dysplasia, none of these molecular findings is specific enough to establish and support the diagnosis of dysplasia in routine clinical practice.

Early and advanced gastric carcinoma

Early gastric carcinoma is defined as adenocarcinoma limited to either the mucosa or submucosa irrespective of the presence of lymph node metastases.[75] The term 'early' does not refer to the size or age of the lesion. Conversely, gastric carcinomas infiltrating into the muscularis propria and beyond are defined as 'advanced'. These two categories of gastric carcinoma differ not only in prognosis, but also with respect to morphology and clinical aspects. Gastric carcinoma limited to the mucosa and submucosa has an excellent prognosis, with a 5-year survival rate exceeding 90% in Japan.[76,77] Five-year survival rate of advanced gastric carcinomas, the most frequent presentation in the West, is around 23% when treated by surgery alone and around 36% when treatment includes perioperative chemotherapy.[78] Retrospective and prospective long-term follow up studies showed that the tumour growth rate differs significantly between early and advanced carcinomas, and estimated a doubling time of early carcinomas of several years but less than a year for advanced carcinomas.[79,80]

✔ The macroscopic growth pattern of advanced carcinomas is classified according to Borrmann into four major types.[81] Type 5 is used for unclassifiable cancers. Early gastric carcinomas are macroscopically Borrmann type '0' and classified according to Murakami as protruding, superficial elevated/flat/depressed and excavated (**Figs 1.8** and **1.9**).

The classification of the macroscopic growth pattern is applicable to radiological and endoscopic images as well as the macroscopic appearance of the resected specimen, and consistent use of this macroscopic classification can greatly improve the communication among surgeons, endoscopists, radiologists and pathologists, as demonstrated in Japan. Interestingly, approximately 10% of gastric carcinomas retain their endoscopic and radiological 'early cancer' appearance as they progress to advanced stage.[82] This can lead to a potential underestimation of the 'true' clinical disease stage.

In Japan, approximately 2% of early gastric carcinomas recur after curative resection. Submucosal invasion, lymph node metastases and differentiated-type histology have been associated with increased risk of recurrence.[83] Differentiated histology is a risk factor for recurrence as cancers with differentiated histology show a higher incidence of haematogenous spread compared to undifferentiated cancer that is more prone to recur in lymph nodes or serosa lined cavities. The incidence of lymph node metastases is 2–3% for intramucosal carcinomas[84,85] and 20–30% for submucosal carcinomas.[86]

✔ Risk factors of lymph node metastasis in early gastric carcinoma include age at time of diagnosis size greater than 20 mm, depressed macroscopic type, undifferentiated histology, presence of an ulcer or scar, lymphatic invasion and submucosal invasion by more than 500 µm.[84,86]

For advanced gastric carcinoma, depth of infiltration into the wall (T category of the TNM classification) and number of lymph nodes with metastatic tumour (N category of the TNM classification) remain the strongest prognostic indicators.

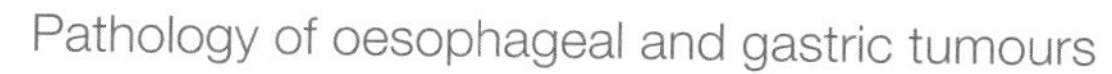

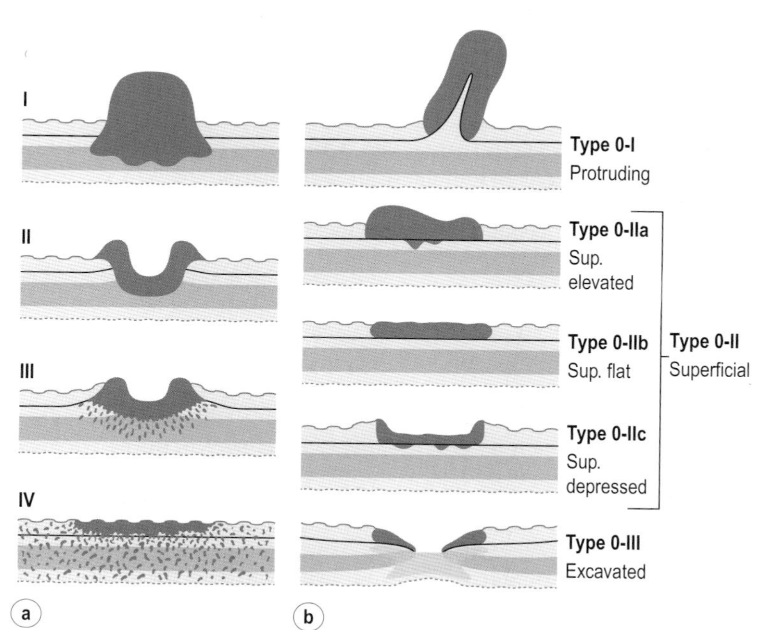

Figure 1.8 • **(a)** Borrmann classification for advanced cancers. Type I: polypoid with a broad base, may be superficially ulcerated. Type II: excavated ulcerated lesion with elevated borders, sharp margin with no definitive infiltration into adjacent mucosa. Type III: ulcerative, diffusely infiltrating base. Type IV: diffusely infiltrative thickening of the wall (linitis plastica). **(b)** Murakami classification for early cancers. Modified from Japanese Gastric Cancer Association. Japanese classification of gastric carcinoma, 3rd English edn. Gastric Cancer 2011; 14(2):101–12.

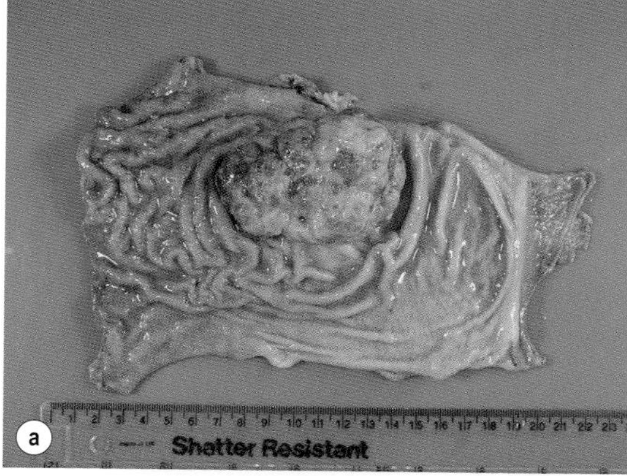

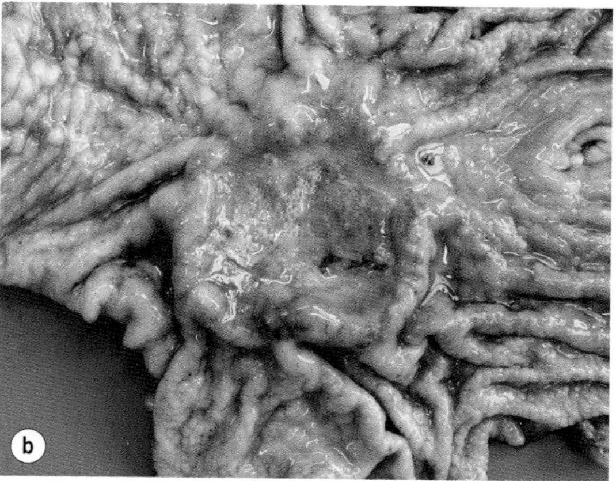

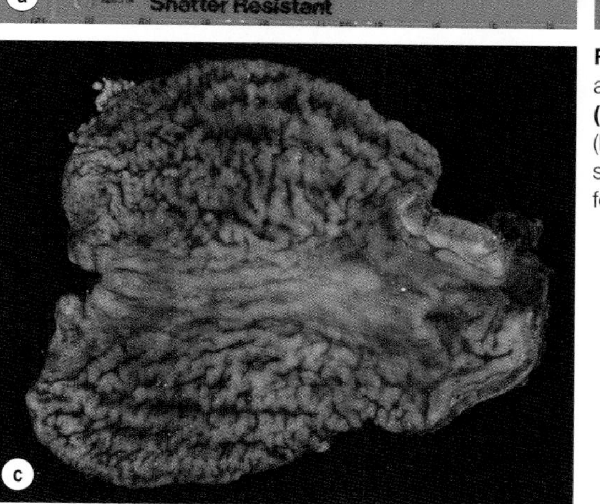

Figure 1.9 • The macroscopic appearances of advanced gastric cancer. **(a)** Polypoid (Borrmann type I). **(b)** Ulcerating (Borrmann type III). **(c)** Linitis plastica (Borrman type IV) with diffuse infiltration of the wall of the stomach by tumour and apparent thickening of the rugal folds.

Morphological subtypes of gastric carcinoma

The histology of gastric carcinoma is characterised by marked heterogeneity. The variability of the histological appearance increases with increasing depth of infiltration into the wall and increasing age at time of diagnosis. As a result of this marked morphological diversity, a number of different classification systems have been advocated by different authors such as Laurén,[35] Ming,[87] Nakamura et al.,[88] Mulligan,[89] Goseki et al.,[90] Carneiro[91] and the World Health Organisation (WHO).[12]

> ✔ The histological classification according to Laurén (intestinal-type versus diffuse-type versus mixed-type gastric carcinoma), Ming (expanding type versus infiltrative type) and WHO (tubular versus papillary versus mucinous versus poorly cohesive including signet ring) are the classifications most commonly used outside of Japan.

In Japan, the recommended histological typing is similar but not 100% identical to the WHO classification.[92] In the West, 60–70% of gastric carcinomas are classified as intestinal-type according to Laurén (**Fig. 1.10a**), which is characterised by a predominance of glandular epithelium with cells similar to intestinal columnar cells. There is good cellular cohesion, the carcinoma is usually sharply demarcated and has a pushing margin according to Ming's classification. Laurén's diffuse-type is composed of scattered, poorly cohesive cells or small clusters of cells and is diffusely infiltrative (**Fig. 1.10b**). Cells may contain mucus and can have a signet ring cell appearance (**Fig. 1.10c**). Gastric carcinomas that consist of approximately 50% diffuse and 50% intestinal-type, solid type carcinomas and others that cannot be classified as diffuse or intestinal are called either indeterminate, unclassifiable or mixed. Intestinal-type carcinomas are more common in men over 60 years of age and in highrisk countries, are located in the antrum, are

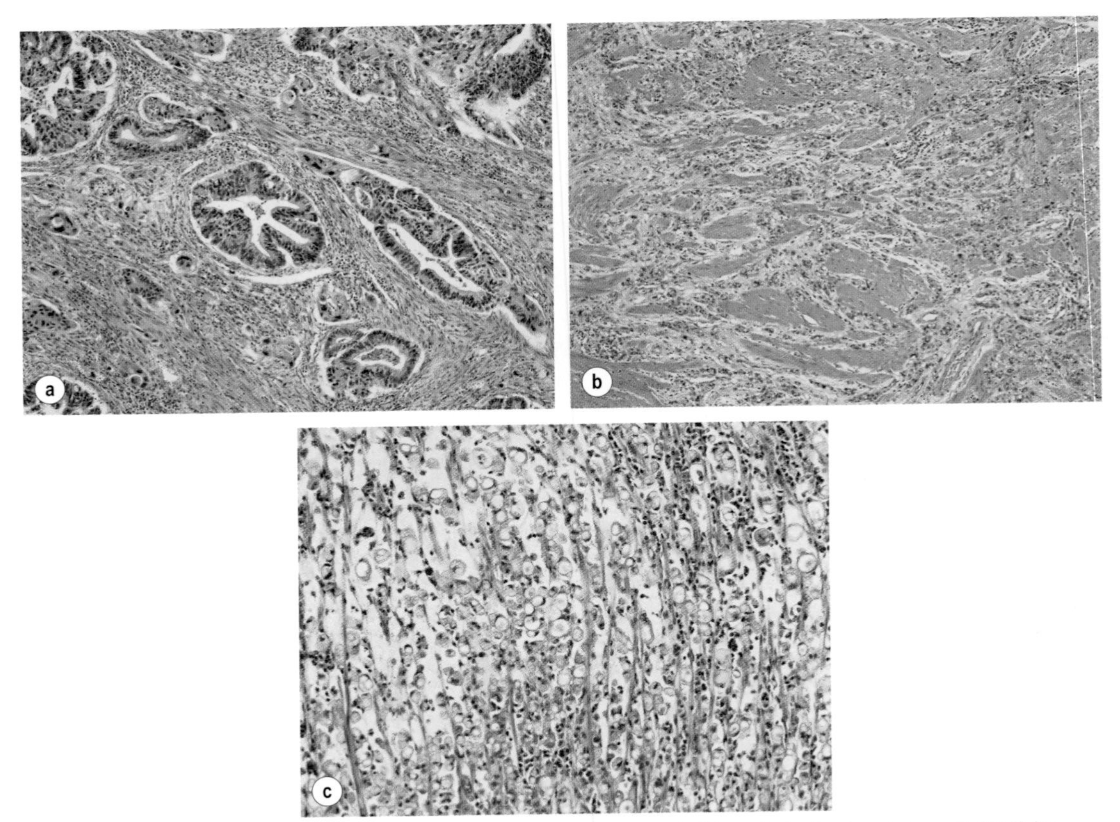

Figure 1.10 • (a) Intestinal-type carcinoma tubular subtype composed of irregularly sized and shaped glandular structures with mildly pleomorphic nuclei. However, this tumour is admixed with poorly differentiated tubular structures with large cells and bizarre shaped nuclei. **(b)** Diffuse-type carcinoma. Poorly cohesive single cells are diffusely infiltrating the smooth muscle wall. **(c)** Signet ring cell carcinoma. The neoplastic cells are characterised by large amounts of intracytoplasmic mucin (almost 'clear' cytoplasm) with eccentrically located and mostly flattened nuclei.

Borrmann type II and show metastases in the liver. In contrast, diffuse-type carcinomas are more common in younger females, have a similar incidence in most countries, are located predominantly in the proximal body of the stomach and show a linitis plastica type growth pattern with transperitoneal metastases.

Gastric carcinomas are graded as well differentiated (more than 90% of the carcinoma consists of well-formed glands resembling intestinal epithelium), moderately differentiated (intermediate between well and poor) and poorly differentiated (highly irregular glands that may be difficult to be recognised as glands). According to the WHO classification,[12] this grading system should only be applied for tubular- and papillary-type carcinomas, not for other morphological subtypes and not after neoadjuvant therapy. However, grading of tumour differentiation is prone to considerable interobserver variation and the value of the histological subtyping and/or tumour grading in predicting patient prognosis is still controversial.

Molecular pathology of gastric carcinoma

The first gene found to be amplified in gastric carcinoma was *c-MYC* in 1984,[93] while the first oncogene discovered in gastric carcinoma was *FGF4* in 1986.[94] Ten years later, Yasui et al.[69] proposed a multistep model of molecular alterations, refining the multistep model of histological changes proposed by Correa[56] (**Fig. 1.11**). This refined model by Yasui et al. suggests that the two main morphological gastric carcinoma subtypes, intestinal and diffuse, are characterised by different underlying molecular mechanisms. However, some alterations such as genetic instability, hypermethylation and telomere reduction have been identified in both histological subtypes and therefore appear to occur during the early stages of cancer development. Others are supposedly unique or at least predominant in a particular histological subtype, such as *CDH1* mutations in diffuse-type and *KRAS* mutations in intestinal-type gastric carcinoma.

c-*MET* is a transmembrane tyrosine kinase receptor and was found to be amplified at higher frequency in diffuse-type gastric carcinoma compared to intestinal-type gastric carcinoma (39% *vs.* 19% gastric carcinoma).[95] Overexpression of c-*MET* has been related to tumour stage.[96] With the advent of c-*MET* inhibitors, the interest in this molecule has been revived and a very recent large study conducted in Korea demonstrated that c-*MET* was amplified in 21% of gastric carcinomas, identifying c-*MET* as a potential new drug target.[97] Fibroblast growth factor receptor 2 (FGFR2) is another potential drug target and *FGFR2* amplification has been detected in gastric carcinoma.

✔ The only targeted therapy that is currently approved for use in patients with metastatic gastric carcinoma is trastuzumab, which targets the human epidermal growth factor receptor 2 (HER2), also known as c-erbB2 or HER2/neu. HER2 is preferentially amplified and overexpressed in intestinal-type carcinoma.

p53 is frequently inactivated in gastric carcinoma by loss of heterozygosity (LOH) or mutations. *p53* mutations have been identified in 60% of gastric carcinomas, with approximately equal frequency in different histological subtypes, and thus make it the most frequently mutated gene in gastric carcinoma.[98] *APC* mutations have been observed in 30–40% of well and moderately differentiated intestinal-type gastric carcinomas and in less than 2% diffuse-type gastric carcinomas.[99]

Alterations (mutations or gene silencing by methylation) of any of the five human DNA mismatch repair genes, *MSH2*, *MLH1*, *MSH6*, *PMS1* and *PMS2*, result in defective mismatch repair. Tumours with DNA mismatch repair deficiency show variations in the number of short tandem repeat units contained within microsatellites, a phenomenon called microsatellite instability. Cells with defective mismatch repair also display substantially elevated numbers of mutations thought to accelerate carcinogenesis. The reported frequency of microsatellite instability varies between 15% and 38% of gastric carcinomas, is higher in intestinal-type gastric carcinoma and is more common in cancers from older age females and cancers in the antrum.[100]

Neuroendocrine tumours of the stomach

The gastric mucosa contains several types of neuroendocrine cells, which produce neurotransmitter, neuromodulator or neuropeptide hormones and release them into the bloodstream. These cells are usually immunoreactive for chromogranin A and synaptophysin.[101] Neuroendocrine tumours (previously known as 'carcinoids') arise most commonly from enterochromaffin-like (ECL) cells. Hypergastrinaemia due to unregulated hormone release by a gastrinoma or due to hyperplasia of gastrin producing cells in the antrum secondary to achlorhydria is consistently associated with hyperplasia of the ECL cells.[102] A multistep progression from simple hyperplasia through nodule formation to dysplasia and tumour formation is thought to occur.

The incidence of gastric neuroendocrine tumours has been increasing over the last decades and accounts for 6% of all gastrointestinal neuroendocrine tumours.[103] Neuroendocrine tumours of the stomach are almost exclusively located in the body of the stomach.

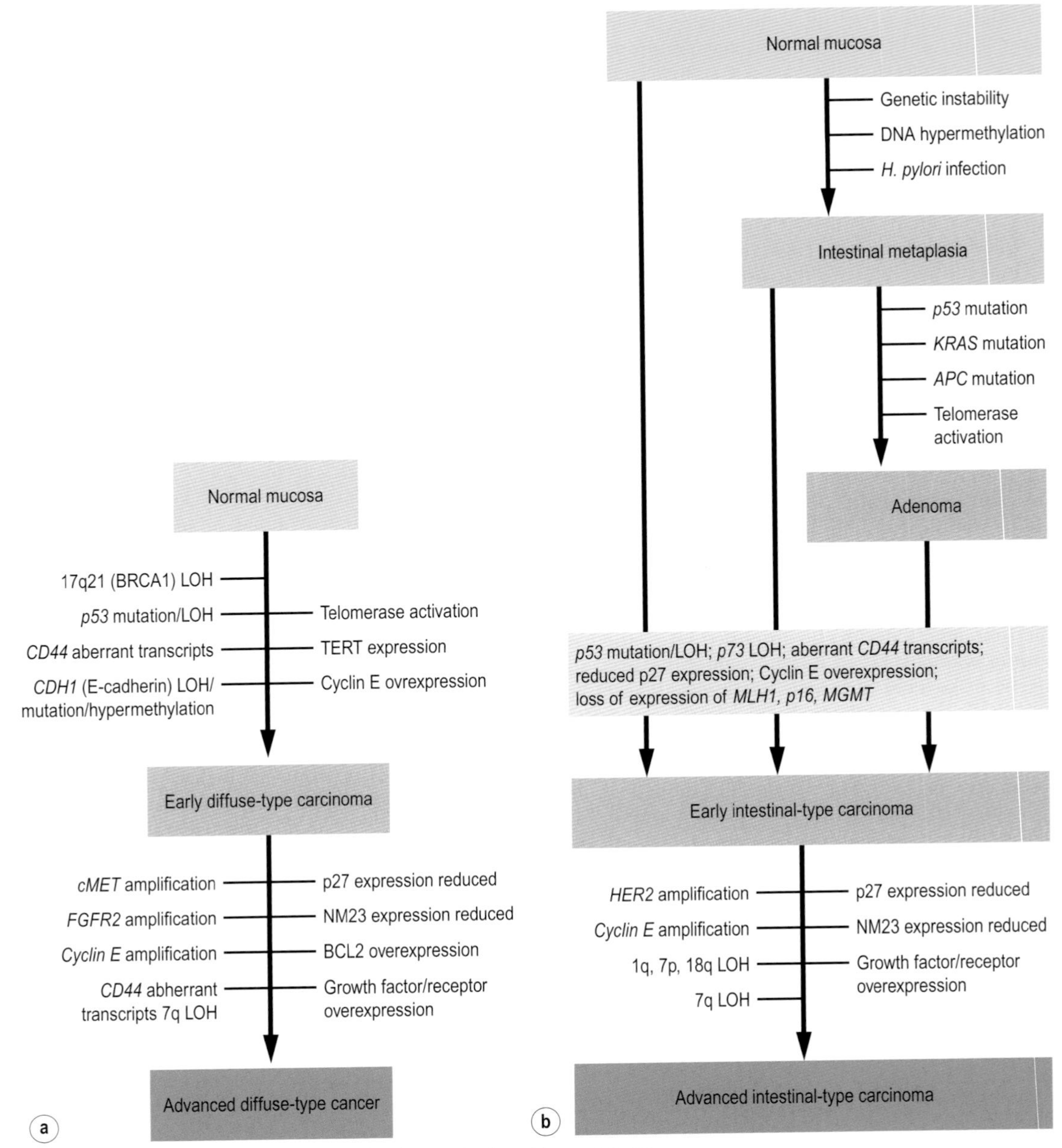

Figure 1.11 • Genetic pathway of the development of gastric carcinoma.

Three distinct types of neuroendocrine tumours can be distinguished based on their pathogenesis (Table 1.1):[12]

- **Type 1.** Multiple well-differentiated neuroendocrine tumours affecting predominantly middle-aged females are associated with autoimmune chronic atrophic gastritis and pernicious anaemia due to auto-antibodies against parietal cells. This type is the most common type of gastric neuroendocrine tumour. Tumours tend to be limited to the submucosa. Metastases can be found in 7–12% of cases and are usually confined to the local lymph nodes. A reduction in the number of ECL cells can be achieved by treatment with octreotide.[104]
- **Type 2.** Neuroendocrine tumours associated with the Zollinger–Ellison syndrome (gastrinoma-related syndrome) in patients with

Table 1.1 • Characteristics of gastric neuroendocrine tumours

	Type 1	Type 2	Type 3
Percentage (%)	70–85	5–10	15–25
Tumour characteristics	Often small, multiple, polypoid, multicentric	Often small, multiple, polypoid, multicentric	Single, >1–2 cm, polypoid and often ulcerated
Mean age at diagnosis (years)	63	50	55
Gender	Females >males	Females = males	Males > females
Associated conditions	Chronic atrophic gastritis type A	ZES/MEN-1	Sporadic
Serum gastrin levels	Increased	Increased	Normal
pH of gastric juice	Increased	Low	Normal
Ki67 (%)	Usually <2	Usually <2	Usually >2
Metastases (%)	2–5	<10	>50

MEN, multiple endocrine neoplasia; ZES, Zollinger–Ellison syndrome.
Reproduced from Massironi S, Sciola V, Spampatti MP et al. Gastric carcinoids: between underestimation and overtreatment. World J Gastroenterol 2009; 15:2177–83.

multiple endocrine neoplasia (MEN) type 1 have no sex predilection. The tumours tend to be multicentric with minimal gastritis in the background, but both ECL hyperplasia and dysplasia are present. These tumours often extend deep into the muscle wall, have lymph node metastases and have occasionally caused death. The loss of the tumour suppressor gene *MEN1* on chromosome 11q13 is seen in the majority of these tumours, a defect also found in those tumours of the gut, pancreas and parathyroid associated with MEN-1.[105]

- **Type 3.** Sporadic neuroendocrine tumours are neither associated with atrophic gastritis nor with MEN-1 syndrome. These tumours are usually solitary lesions that occur in middle-aged men. They tend to be larger (>2 cm) and have a more aggressive behaviour. The background mucosa shows no evidence of atrophic gastritis and no evidence of neuroendocrine hyperplasia or dysplasia. Serosal infiltration with lymphatic and vascular invasion and liver metastasis with an accompanying carcinoid syndrome are common. Metastases are present in 52% of cases and approximately one third of patients will have died within 51 months.

✔ Grading of neuroendocrine tumours using a combination of the morphological features and the proliferation fraction (mitotic index or Ki67 index) has been shown to be of prognostic value.[12]

Grade 1 neuroendocrine tumours have typically a Ki67 index below 2%, whereas grade 3 tumours are poorly differentiated, have a Ki67 index above 20%, show necrosis and are therefore classified as neuroendocrine carcinomas. Guidelines for the management of gastric neuroendocrine tumours have been updated very recently.[106]

Mesenchymal tumours of the stomach

Non- epithelial tumours such as glomus tumour, inflammatory myofibroblastic tumours, leiomyoma, leiomyosarcoma, schwannoma, synovial sarcoma and Kaposi sarcoma are all relatively rare in the stomach and will not be discussed here.

This chapter will focus on **gastrointestinal stromal tumours** (GISTs), which are the most common primary mesenchymal tumours of the gastrointestinal tract, and 60–70% of GISTs occur in the stomach. Most GISTs are sporadic, but they can also be part of syndromes, namely Carney's triad, Carney Stratakis syndrome, neurofibromatosis type 1 or can be familial due to germline mutations of the *KIT* and *PDFGFR* genes.

GISTs can occur in any part of the stomach and vary from small nodules in the wall that are covered by intact mucosa to large masses leading to gastric outlet obstruction. Histologically, most GISTs show a spindle cell morphology with little atypia. Twenty per cent of GISTs show epithelioid histology. GISTs are immunoreactive for KIT (CD117), DOG1 and often also for CD34. Even if all common immunohistochemical markers are unexpectedly negative, it is still legitimate to make the diagnosis of a GIST based on morphology alone. However, those cases should be investigated for relevant mutations. GISTs contain *KIT*- or *PDGFRA*-activating mutations. *KIT*-activating mutations are most frequently found in exon 11 and most GISTs with

Table 1.2 • Prediction of malignant potential of gastrointestinal stromal tumours

Tumour parameters		Risk of progressive disease (metastasis or tumour-related death)			
Mitotic index	**Size**	**Gastric**	**Duodenum**	**Jejunum/ileum**	**Rectum**
≤5(in 5 mm²)	≤2 cm	None (0%)	None (0%)	None (0%)	None (0%)
	≤2 to ≤5 cm	Very low (1.9%)	Low (8.3%)	Low (4.3%)	Low (8.5%)
	>5 to ≤10 cm	Low (3.6%)	(Insufficient data)	Moderate (24%)	(Insufficient data)
	>10 cm	Moderate (10%)	High (34%)	High (52%)	High (57%)
>5 (in 5 mm²)	≤2 cm	(Insufficient data)	(Insufficient data)	High (limited data)	High (54%)
	≤ 2 to ≤5 cm	Moderate (16%)	High (50%)	High (73%)	High (52%)
	>5 to ≤10	High (55%)	(Insufficient data)	High (85%)	(Insufficient data)
	>10 cm	High (86%)	High (86%)	High (90%)	High (71%)

Reproduced from Royal College of Pathologists Dataset for gastrointestinal stromal tumours, published February 2012, with permission from the Royal College of Pathologists.

KIT mutations are imatinib sensitive, whereas GISTs with *PDGFRA*-activating mutations are usually imatinib resistant.

With the exception of very small tumours, all GISTs have the potential to become malignant.

✓ A combination of site of origin, size and mitotic index has been shown to predict the risk of progressive disease in patients with GISTs (Table 1.2).[107]

Lymphoma of the stomach

Any type of lymphoma can also occur in the gastrointestinal tract, which is the commonest extranodal site.[12] Within the gastrointestinal tract, 50–75% of lymphomas are located in the stomach; 5–10% of all gastric malignancies are primary lymphomas. The two most common subtypes of primary gastric lymphomas are extranodal marginal zone lymphoma of the mucosa associated lymphoid tissue (so-called MALT lymphoma) and diffuse large B-cell lymphoma. The incidence of primary gastric lymphoma is similar in men and women.

MALT lymphoma

The majority of MALT lymphomas occur in patients over the age of 50 years, with equal sex distribution, who present clinically with symptoms suggesting a diagnosis of gastritis or peptic ulcer disease. The tumours appear macroscopically as an ill defined thickening of the mucosa with erosions, sometimes ulcerated (**Fig. 1.12**) and frequently multifocal. Gastric MALT lymphoma can spread to the regional nodes. MALT lymphoma is composed of neoplastic B cells that resemble follicle centre cells and are termed centrocyte-like, whereas other cells

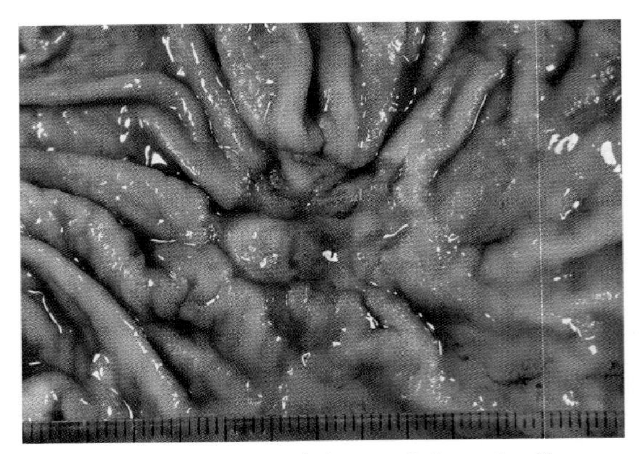

Figure 1.12 • Macroscopic image of stomach with lymphoma.

show plasma cell differentiation and occasionally there are blast cells. The characteristic lympho-epithelial lesion (**Fig. 1.13**) is composed of small to medium-sized tumour cells with irregular nuclei that infiltrate the pit epithelium. This lesion is not pathognomonic of a lymphoma as it can also be demonstrated in an *H. pylori*-associated gastritis, Sjögren's syndrome and Hashimoto's thyroiditis.

It is thought that the development of MALT lymphoma is a multistage process initiated by chronic active inflammation due to *H. pylori* infection. Eradication of *H. pylori* with antibiotics has been shown to be associated with MALT lymphoma remission in up to 77% of patients within 12 months. Less than 10% relapse and this could be due to reinfection with *H. pylori*; in the absence of reinfection the relapse appears to be self-limiting.

Cytogenetic studies show that three major translocations are seen in MALT lymphomas: t(11,18)(q21;q21)/*API2-MALT1* (30–40% of cases), t(14:18)(q32:q21)/*IGH-MALT1* and t(1:14)(p22:q32)/*IGH-BCL10*.

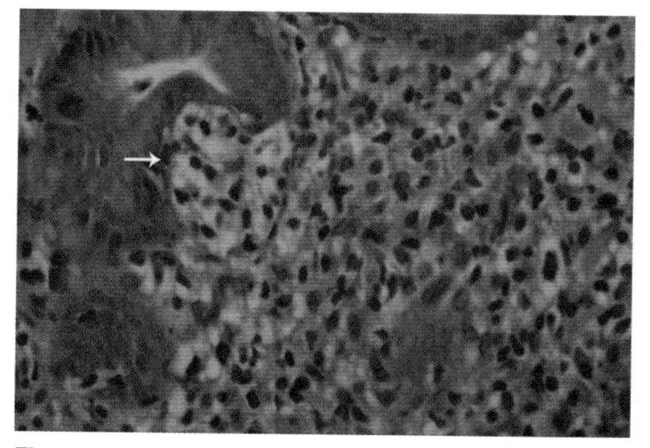

Figure 1.13 • Microscopic image of lymphoepithelial lesion.

Some of the translocations have been related to unresponsiveness to *H. pylori* eradication. Other translocations are associated with the juxtaposition of *BCL10* to the immunoglobulin heavy chain gene, resulting in deregulation of the immunoglobulin. In addition, there is loss or mutation of *p53*, c-*MYC* mutation, inactivation of *p15/p16* by hypermethylation and *FAS* gene mutation.

Most low grade MALT lymphomas are associated with disease confined to the gastric mucosa with slow dissemination. The favourable clinical behaviour may reflect the partial dependence on the *H. pylori* antigenic drive. The progression to the more common high grade MALT lymphoma is thought to require the acquisition of further genetic abnormalities.[108] Gastric MALT lymphoma with the t(11;18)(q21;q21) translocation should be treated with chemotherapy or radiation, as *H. pylori* eradication alone is ineffective. The other lymphomas that are resistant to *H. pylori* eradication are those with abnormalities of the *BCL10* locus or those associated with an autoimmune gastritis. These can be identified by strong nuclear staining with anti-*BCL10* in the former and in the latter by staining with the product of the *FAS* oncogene. These non-responsive lymphomas can be treated surgically or in combination with chemoradiotherapy. The 5-year survival for localised cases is 90–100%. Continued follow up of these patients is recommended as it is now recognised that synchronous and metachronous adenocarcinomas can occur.[109]

Diffuse large B cell lymphoma

Primary gastric diffuse large B cell lymphoma is composed of B cells with a nuclear size equivalent to a macrophage nucleus of at least twice the size of a normal lymphocyte. Similar to MALT lymphoma, the neoplastic cells destroy the gastric glandular architecture. Up to 50% of diffuse large B cell lymphomas have foci of MALT lymphomas and regression of diffuse large B cell lymphoma after eradication of *H. pylori* has been reported. Macroscopically, this lymphoma appears as a large ulcerated mass mimicking advanced gastric carcinoma. Chromosomal translocations involving the immunoglobulin heavy chain gene locus are frequent in diffuse large cell lymphomas, resulting in deregulation of *BCL6*, *BCL2* and *MYC*.[110] In the presence of EBV, diffuse large B cell lymphomas are more likely to be resistant to chemoradiotherapy.[111]

Key points

- The multistep progression from normal mucosa to cancer shows that the *p53* gene has been found to be abnormal in up to half the cases of oesophageal squamous cell carcinoma. Different mutations of *p53* are found in adenocarcinoma of the oesophagus. The mutations allow abnormal cell growth and are associated with further damage to the genome, especially to the important tumour suppressor genes.
- Squamous cell dysplasia is regarded as a precancerous condition of the oesophagus. In screened high risk populations, the finding of dysplasia predates the development of carcinoma by approximately 5 years.
- It is difficult to distinguish between distal oesophageal adenocarcinoma and proximal gastric cancer in advanced cancers based on the location of the tumour with respect to the gastro-oesophageal junction. Intestinal metaplasia can indicate the presence of Barrett's oesophagus, but can also occur in the stomach.
- Although it is possible to reverse the inflammation and some of the intestinal metaplastic changes associated with *H. pylori* infection, atrophy and the colonic type intestinal metaplasia (type III – incomplete metaplasia) are regarded as irreversible. There is continuing controversy as to the value of identifying the colonic type mucin and its predictive value in identifying patients at risk of developing cancer.

- There are several problems associated with histological interpretation of grades of glandular oesophageal and gastric dysplasia; these include high interobserver variation, distinguishing regenerative atypia from true dysplasia, the ability to differentiate high grade dysplasia from intramucosal carcinoma, and a lack of experience due to the relative rarity of dysplasia, especially in low incidence areas.
- There are several classifications for gastric adenocarcinoma, the most widely used being Laurén's classification. The tumours are divided into two main types: those that form glandular structures are known as intestinal-type, while those without glandular structures are referred to as diffuse-type carcinomas. Those with a mixed, solid or unusual appearance are regarded as unclassifiable/ indeterminate.
- The molecular features characterising intestinal-type and diffuse-type gastric cancer (Fig. 1.13) suggest that the different histological phenotype is related to a different underlying genetic phenotype and most likely different aetiology.
- Abnormalities of the *CDH1* (E-cadherin) gene and aberrant expression of this protein have been found in up to 90% of sporadic gastric carcinomas, especially the diffuse-type. Germline *CDH1* mutations are the defining molecular defect in hereditary diffuse gastric cancer.
- The stomach is the commonest site for gastrointestinal lymphomas, which are mostly B cell non-Hodgkin's lymphomas. The most common lymphoma is low grade MALT lymphoma, which is thought to be initiated by *H. pylori* infection. Several different chromosomal translocations have been identified, some of them conferring therapy resistance.
- Three subgroups of patients with neuroendocrine tumours (formerly called 'carcinoids') can be identified. Most are benign and associated with overgrowth of the ECL cells. Solitary lesions frequently metastasise and can be highly malignant.

References

1. Munoz N, Crespi M, Grassi A, et al. Precursor lesions of oesophageal cancer in high-risk populations in Iran and China. Lancet 1982;1:876–9.
2. Blot W, McLaughlin J, Fraumeni J. Esophageal cancer. In: Schottenfeld D, Fraumeni J, editors. Cancer epidemiology and prevention. New York: Oxford University Press; 2006. p. 697–706.
3. Boffetta P, Hashibe M. Alcohol and cancer. Lancet Oncol 2006;7:149–56.
4. Leeuwenburgh I, Haringsma J, Van Dekken H, et al. Long-term risk of oesophagitis, Barrett's oesophagus and oesophageal cancer in achalasia patients. Scand J Gastroenterol 2006;43(Suppl. 2):7–10.
5. Swinson CM, Slavin G, Coles EC, et al. Coeliac disease and malignancy. Lancet 1983;1:111–5.
6. Chisholm M. The association between webs, iron and post-cricoid carcinoma. Postgrad Med J 1974;50:215–9.
7. Risk JM, Evans KE, Jones J, et al. Characterization of a 500kb region on 17q25 and the exclusion of candidate genes as the familial Tylosis Oesophageal Cancer (TOC) locus. Oncogene 2002;21:6395–402.
8. O'Mahony MY, Ellis JP, Hellier M, et al. Familial tylosis and carcinoma of the oesophagus. J R Soc Med 1984;77:514–7.
9. Appelqvist P, Salmo M. Lye corrosion carcinoma of the esophagus: a review of 63 cases. Cancer 1980;45:2655–8.
10. Huang BS, Unni KK, Payne WS. Long-term survival following diverticulectomy for cancer in pharyngoesophageal (Zenker's) diverticulum. Ann Thorac Surg 1984;38:207–10.
11. Micke O, Schafer U, Glashorster M, et al. Radiation-induced esophageal carcinoma 30 years after mediastinal irradiation: case report and review of the literature. Jpn J Clin Oncol 1999;29:164–70.
12. World Health Organisation. WHO classification of tumours of the digestive system. 4th ed. Lyon: IARC; 2010.
13. Japan Esophageal Society. Japanese classification of esophageal cancer, tenth edition: part I. Esophagus 2009;6:1–25.
14. Takubo K, Aida J, Sawabe M, et al. Early squamous cell carcinoma of the oesophagus: the Japanese viewpoint. Histopathology 2007;51:733–42.
15. Peters CJ, Hardwick RH, Vowler SL, et al. Generation and validation of a revised classification for oesophageal and junctional adenocarcinoma. Br J Surg 2009;96:724–33.
16. Ando N, Ozawa S, Kitagawa Y, et al. Improvement in the results of surgical treatment of advanced squamous esophageal carcinoma during 15 consecutive years. Ann Surg 2000;232:225–32.

17. Akiyama H, Tsurumaru M, Udagawa H, et al. Radical lymph node dissection for cancer of the thoracic esophagus. Ann Surg 1994;220:364–73.

18. Sarbia M, Porschen R, Borchard F, et al. Incidence and prognostic significance of vascular and neural invasion in squamous cell carcinomas of the esophagus. Int J Cancer 1995;61:333–6.

19. Mandard AM, Dalibard F, Mandard JC, et al. Pathologic assessment of tumor regression after preoperative chemoradiotherapy of esophageal carcinoma. Clinicopathologic correlations. Cancer 1994;73:2680–6.

20. Bollschweiler E, Holscher AH, Metzger R, et al. Prognostic significance of a new grading system of lymph node morphology after neoadjuvant radiochemotherapy for esophageal cancer. Ann Thorac Surg 2011;92:2020–7.

21. Chu Q, Jaganmohan S, Kelly B, et al. Verrucous carcinoma of the esophagus: a rare variant of squamous cell carcinoma for which a preoperative diagnosis can be a difficult one to make. J La State Med Soc 2011;163:251–3.

22. Handra-Luca A, Terris B, Couvelard A, et al. Spindle cell squamous carcinoma of the oesophagus: an analysis of 17 cases, with new immunohistochemical evidence for a clonal origin. Histopathology 2001;39:125–32.

23. Lauwers GY, Grant LD, Scott GV, et al. Spindle cell squamous carcinoma of the esophagus: analysis of ploidy and tumor proliferative activity in a series of 13 cases. Hum Pathol 1998;29:863–8.

24. Wang GQ, Abnet CC, Shen Q, et al. Histological precursors of oesophageal squamous cell carcinoma: results from a 13 year prospective follow up study in a high risk population. Gut 2005;54:187–92.

25. Crespi M, Munoz N, Grassi A, et al. Precursor lesions of oesophageal cancer in a low-risk population in China: comparison with high-risk populations. Int J Cancer 1984;34:599–602.

26. Lin J, Beerm DG. Molecular biology of upper gastrointestinal malignancies. Semin Oncol 2004;31:476–86.

27. Lagergren J. Adenocarcinoma of oesophagus: what exactly is the size of the problem and who is at risk? Gut 2005;54:i1–5.

28. Dulai GS, Guha S, Kahn KL, et al. Preoperative prevalence of Barrett's esophagus in esophageal adenocarcinoma: a systematic review. Gastroenterology 2002;122:26–33.

29. Siewert JR, Stein HJ. Classification of adenocarcinoma of the oesophagogastric junction. Br J Surg 1998;85:1457–9.

30. Barrett NR. Chronic peptic ulcer of the oesophagus and 'oesophagitis'. Br J Surg 1950;38:175–82.

31. Moersch RN, Ellis Jr. FH, McDonald JR. Pathologic changes occurring in severe reflux esophagitis. Surg Gynecol Obstet 1959;108:476–84.

32. Hayward J. The treatment of fibrous stricture of the oesophagus associated with hiatal hernia. Thorax 1961;16:45–55.

33. Bremner CG, Lynch VP, Ellis Jr. FH. Barrett's esophagus: congenital or acquired? An experimental study of esophageal mucosal regeneration in the dog. Surgery 1970;68:209–16.

34. Haggitt RC. Barrett's esophagus, dysplasia, and adenocarcinoma. Hum Pathol 1994;25:982–93.

35. Lauren P. The two histological main types of gastric carcinoma: diffuse and so-called intestinal-type carcinoma. An attempt at a histo-clinical classification. Acta Pathol Microbiol Scand 1965; 64:31–49.

36. Abraham SC, Krasinskas AM, Correa AM, et al. Duplication of the muscularis mucosae in Barrett esophagus: an underrecognized feature and its implication for staging of adenocarcinoma. Am J Surg Pathol 2007;31:1719–25.

37. Na YJ, Shim KN, Kang MJ, et al. Primary esophageal adenoid cystic carcinoma. Gut Liver 2007;1:178–81.

38. Bianchi LK, Burke CA, Bennett AE, et al. Fundic gland polyp dysplasia is common in familial adenomatous polyposis. Clin Gastroenterol Hepatol 2008;6:180–5.

39. Carmack SW, Genta RM, Schuler CM, et al. The current spectrum of gastric polyps: a 1-year national study of over 120,000 patients. Am J Gastroenterol 2009;104:1524–32.

40. Stolte M, Vieth M, Ebert MP. High-grade dysplasia in sporadic fundic gland polyps: clinically relevant or not? Eur J Gastroenterol Hepatol 2003;15:1153–6.

41. Abraham SC, Nobukawa B, Giardiello FM, et al. Sporadic fundic gland polyps: common gastric polyps arising through activating mutations in the beta-catenin gene. Am J Pathol 2001;158:1005–10.

42. Ohkusa T, Takashimizu I, Fujiki K, et al. Disappearance of hyperplastic polyps in the stomach after eradication of *Helicobacter pylori*. A randomized, clinical trial. Ann Intern Med 1998;129:712–5.

43. Zea-Iriarte WL, Sekine I, Itsuno M, et al. Carcinoma in gastric hyperplastic polyps. A phenotypic study. Dig Dis Sci 1996;41:377–86.

44. Kolodziejczyk P, Yao T, Oya M, et al. Long-term follow-up study of patients with gastric adenomas with malignant transformation. An immunohistochemical and histochemical analysis. Cancer 1994;74:2896–907.

45. Giardiello FM, Brensinger JD, Tersmette AC, et al. Very high risk of cancer in familial Peutz–Jeghers syndrome. Gastroenterology 2000;119:1447–53.

46. Howson CP, Hiyama T, Wynder EL. The decline in gastric cancer: epidemiology of an unplanned triumph. Epidemiol Rev 1986;8:1–27.

47. Ferlay J, Shin HR, Bray F, et al. Estimates of worldwide burden of cancer in 2008: GLOBOCAN 2008. Int J Cancer 2010;127:2893–917.

48. El-Serag HB, Mason AC, Petersen N, et al. Epidemiological differences between adenocarcinoma of the oesophagus and adenocarcinoma of the gastric cardia in the USA. Gut 2002;50:368–72.

49. Zanghieri G, Di Gregorio C, Sacchetti C, et al. Familial occurrence of gastric cancer in the 2-year experience of a population-based registry. Cancer 1990;66:2047–51.

50. Palli D, Galli M, Caporaso NE, et al. Family history and risk of stomach cancer in Italy. Cancer Epidemiol Biomarkers Prev 1994;3:15–8.

51. Fitzgerald RC, Hardwick R, Huntsman D, et al. Hereditary diffuse gastric cancer: updated consensus guidelines for clinical management and directions for future research. J Med Genet 2010;47:436–44.

52. Oliveira C, Suriano G, Ferreira P, et al. Genetic screening for familial gastric cancer. Hered Cancer Clin Pract 2004;2:51–64.

53. Pharoah PD, Guilford P, Caldas C. Incidence of gastric cancer and breast cancer in CDH1 (E-cadherin) mutation carriers from hereditary diffuse gastric cancer families. Gastroenterology 2001;121:1348–53.

54. Suzuki H, Iwasaki E, Hibi T. *Helicobacter pylori* and gastric cancer. Gastric Cancer 2009;12:79–87.

55. Correa P, Haenszel W, Cuello C, et al. A model for gastric cancer epidemiology. Lancet 1975;2:58–60.

56. Correa P. *Helicobacter pylori* and gastric carcinogenesis. Am J Surg Pathol 1995;19(Suppl. 1):S37–43.

57. Peek Jr. RM, Blaser MJ. *Helicobacter pylori* and gastrointestinal tract adenocarcinomas. Nat Rev Cancer 2002;2:28–37.

58. Atherton JC, Peek Jr. RM, Tham KT, et al. Clinical and pathological importance of heterogeneity in vacA, the vacuolating cytotoxin gene of *Helicobacter pylori*. Gastroenterology 1997;112:92–9.

59. Fukayama M, Ushiku T. Epstein–Barr virus-associated gastric carcinoma. Pathol Res Pract 2011;207:529–37.

60. Tokunaga M, Land CE, Uemura Y, et al. Epstein–Barr virus in gastric carcinoma. Am J Pathol 1993;143:1250–4.

61. Zur Hausen A, van Rees BP, van Beek J, et al. Epstein–Barr virus in gastric carcinomas and gastric stump carcinomas: a late event in gastric carcinogenesis. J Clin Pathol 2004;57:487–91.

62. Tsugane S. Salt, salted food intake, and risk of gastric cancer: epidemiologic evidence. Cancer Sci 2005;96:1–6.

63. Gonzalez CA, Pera G, Agudo A, et al. Fruit and vegetable intake and the risk of stomach and oesophagus adenocarcinoma in the European Prospective Investigation into Cancer and Nutrition (EPIC-EURGAST). Int J Cancer 2006;118:2559–66.

64. Bjelakovic G, Nikolova D, Simonetti RG, et al. Antioxidant supplements for preventing gastrointestinal cancers. Cochrane Database Syst Rev 2008;CD004183.

65. Gonzalez CA, Pera G, Agudo A, et al. Smoking and the risk of gastric cancer in the European Prospective Investigation into Cancer and Nutrition (EPIC). Int J Cancer 2003;107:629–34.

66. Franceschi S, La Vecchia C. Alcohol and the risk of cancers of the stomach and colon–rectum. Dig Dis 1994;12:276–89.

67. Stalnikowicz R, Benbassat J. Risk of gastric cancer after gastric surgery for benign disorders. Arch Intern Med 1990;150:2022–6.

68. Correa P. A human model of gastric carcinogenesis. Cancer Res 1988;48:3554–60.

69. Yasui W, Yokozaki H, Shimamoto F, et al. Molecular-pathological diagnosis of gastrointestinal tissues and its contribution to cancer histopathology. Pathol Int 1999;49:763–74.

70. Lee S, Iida M, Yao T, et al. Long-term follow-up of 2529 patients reveals gastric ulcers rarely become malignant. Dig Dis Sci 1990;35:763–8.

71. Farinati F, Rugge M, Di Mario F, et al. Early and advanced gastric cancer in the follow-up of moderate and severe gastric dysplasia patients. A prospective study. I.G.G.E.D. – Interdisciplinary Group on Gastric Epithelial Dysplasia. Endoscopy 1993;25:261–4.

72. Schlemper RJ, Riddell RH, Kato Y, et al. The Vienna classification of gastrointestinal epithelial neoplasia. Gut 2000;47:251–5.

73. Rugge M, Correa P, Dixon MF, et al. Gastric dysplasia: the Padova international classification. Am J Surg Pathol 2000;24:167–76.

74. Dixon MF. Gastrointestinal epithelial neoplasia: Vienna revisited. Gut 2002;51:130–1.

75. UICC. TNM classification of malignant tumors. 7th ed Wiley-Blackwell: Oxford; 2009.

76. Everett SM, Axon AT. Early gastric cancer in Europe. Gut 1997;41:142–50.

77. Hirota T, Ming SC, Itabashi M. Pathology of early gastric cancer. In: Nishi M, Ichikawa H, Nakajima Y, editors. Gastric cancer. Tokyo: Springer-Verlag; 1993. p. 66–85.

78. Cunningham D, Allum WH, Stenning SP, et al. Perioperative chemotherapy versus surgery alone for resectable gastroesophageal cancer. N Engl J Med 2006;355:11–20.

79. Kohli Y, Kawai K, Fujita S. Analytical studies on growth of human gastric cancer. J Clin Gastroenterol 1981;3:129–33.

80. Tsukuma H, Oshima A, Narahara H, et al. Natural history of early gastric cancer: a non-concurrent, long term, follow up study. Gut 2000;47:618–21.

81. Borrmann R. Handbuch der speziellen pathologischen Anatomie und Histologie. In: von Henke F, Lubarch O, editors. IV/erster Teil. Berlin: Julius Springer Verlag; 1926. p. 864–71.

82. Mori M, Adachi Y, Nakamura K, et al. Advanced gastric carcinoma simulating early gastric carcinoma. Cancer 1990;65:1033–40.

83. Saka M, Katai H, Fukagawa T, et al. Recurrence in early gastric cancer with lymph node metastasis. Gastric Cancer 2008;11:214–8.

84. Yamao T, Shirao K, Ono H, et al. Risk factors for lymph node metastasis from intramucosal gastric carcinoma. Cancer 1996;77:602–6.

85. Hirasawa T, Gotoda T, Miyata S, et al. Incidence of lymph node metastasis and the feasibility of endoscopic resection for undifferentiated-type early gastric cancer. Gastric Cancer 2009;12:148–52.

86. Tajima Y, Murakami M, Yamazaki K, et al. Risk factors for lymph node metastasis from gastric cancers with submucosal invasion. Ann Surg Oncol 2010;17:1597–604.

87. Ming SC. Gastric carcinoma. A pathobiological classification. Cancer 1977;39:2475–85.

88. Nakamura K, Sugano H, Takagi K. Carcinoma of the stomach in incipient phase: its histogenesis and histological appearances. Gann 1968;59:251–8.

89. Mulligan RM. Histogenesis and biologic behavior of gastric carcinoma. Pathol Annu 1972;7:349–415.

90. Goseki N, Takizawa T, Koike M. Differences in the mode of the extension of gastric cancer classified by histological type: new histological classification of gastric carcinoma. Gut 1992;33:606–12.

91. Carneiro F. Classification of gastric carcinoms. Curr Diagn Pathol 1997;4:51–9.

92. Japanese Gastric Cancer Association. Japanese classification of gastric carcinoma, 3rd English edn. Gastric Cancer 2011;14:101–12.

93. Nakasato F, Sakamoto H, Mori M, et al. Amplification of the c-myc oncogene in human stomach cancers. Gann 1984;75:737–42.

94. Sakamoto H, Mori M, Taira M, et al. Transforming gene from human stomach cancers and a noncancerous portion of stomach mucosa. Proc Natl Acad Sci U S A 1986;83:3997–4001.

95. Kuniyasu H, Yasui W, Kitadai Y, et al. Frequent amplification of the c-met gene in scirrhous type stomach cancer. Biochem Biophys Res Commun 1992;189:227–32.

96. Kuniyasu H, Yasui W, Yokozaki H, et al. Aberrant expression of c-met mRNA in human gastric carcinomas. Int J Cancer 1993;55:72–5.

97. Lee J, Seo JW, Jun HJ, et al. Impact of MET amplification on gastric cancer: possible roles as a novel prognostic marker and a potential therapeutic target. Oncol Rep 2011;25:1517–24.

98. Yokozaki H, Kuniyasu H, Kitadai Y, et al. p53 point mutations in primary human gastric carcinomas. J Cancer Res Clin Oncol 1992;119:67–70.

99. Nakatsuru S, Yanagisawa A, Ichii S, et al. Somatic mutation of the APC gene in gastric cancer: frequent mutations in very well differentiated adenocarcinoma and signet-ring cell carcinoma. Hum Mol Gen 1992;1:559–63.

100. Wirtz HC, Mueller W, Noguchi T, et al. Prognostic value and clinicopathological profile of microsatellite instability in gastric cancer. Clin Cancer Res 1998;4:1749–54.

101. Fahrenkamp AG, Wibbeke C, Winde G, et al. Immunohistochemical distribution of chromogranins A and B and secretogranin II in neuroendocrine tumours of the gastrointestinal tract. Virchows Arch 1995;426:361–7.

102. Bordi C, D'Adda T, Azzoni C, et al. Hypergastrinemia and gastric enterochromaffin-like cells. Am J Surg Pathol 19(Suppl. 1):S8–19.

103. Modlin IM, Lye KD, Kidd M. A 5-decade analysis of 13,715 carcinoid tumors. Cancer 2003;97:934–59.

104. Ferraro G, Annibale B, Marignani M, et al. Effectiveness of octreotide in controlling fasting hypergastrinemia and related enterochromaffin-like cell growth. J Clin Endocrinol Metab 1996;81:677–83.

105. Debelenko LV, Emmert-Buck MR, Zhuang Z, et al. The multiple endocrine neoplasia type I gene locus is involved in the pathogenesis of type II gastric carcinoids. Gastroenterology 1997;113:773–81.

106. Ramage JK, Ahmed A, Ardill J, et al. Guidelines for the management of gastroenteropancreatic neuroendocrine (including carcinoid) tumours (NETs). Gut 2012;61:6–32.

107. Miettinen M, Lasota J. Histopathology of gastrointestinal stromal tumor. J Surg Oncol 2011;104:865–73.

108. Zucca E, Bertoni F, Roggero E, et al. Molecular analysis of the progression from *Helicobacter pylori*-associated chronic gastritis to mucosa-associated lymphoid-tissue lymphoma of the stomach. N Engl J Med 1998;338:804–10.

109. Bacon CM, Du MQ, Dogan A. Mucosa-associated lymphoid tissue (MALT) lymphoma: a practical guide for pathologists. J Clin Pathol 2007;60:361–72.

110. Nakamura S, Ye H, Bacon CM, et al. Translocations involving the immunoglobulin heavy chain gene locus predict better survival in gastric diffuse large B-cell lymphoma. Clin Cancer Res 2008;14:3002–10.

111. Yoshino T, Nakamura S, Matsuno Y, et al. Epstein–Barr virus involvement is a predictive factor for the resistance to chemoradiotherapy of gastric diffuse large B-cell lymphoma. Cancer Sci 2006;97:163–6.

2

Epidemiology, genetics and screening for oesophageal and gastric cancer

William H. Allum

Introduction

There are three main types of oesophageal and gastric cancer: squamous cell carcinoma of the oesophagus (SCC), adenocarcinoma of the oesophagogastric junction including the cardia (ACA) and non-cardia adenocarcinoma of the stomach of either diffuse or intestinal type. Each presents a major health problem in different parts of the world, and much effort has been directed to improving our understanding of aetiology and natural history and methods of detecting disease at an early and treatable stage. Preventative strategies have been studied with varying degrees of success. More recently, as understanding of cancer genetics has evolved, there has been considerable interest in evaluating genetic mutations within gastric cancer families and patients who develop gastric cancer at an early age.

The poor overall results of treatment have reflected the advanced stage of most cases at presentation. Those parts of the world with a high incidence have developed and pursued active mass screening programmes. These have certainly identified precursor lesions and premalignant conditions. Indeed, application of these programmes has produced a significant improvement in survival rates for gastric cancer, particularly in Japan. Knowledge of these changes and underlying conditions has enabled areas of lower incidence to pursue examination of those assessed to be at high risk and as a result to increase the number of cancers diagnosed at an early stage.

Definitions

The concentration of disease around the oesophagogastric junction has created differences in opinion with regard to classification. This partly reflects differences in the pathological behaviour of tumours arising at the different sites. In addition, the recent change in the TNM classification[1] has described cancers as either oesophageal, including all within 5 cm of the oesophagogastric junction, or gastric. In epidemiology it is important to ensure a clear classification in order to understand differences in incidence and to appreciate aetiological evidence for the observed changes in these cancers.

For the purposes of the following discussion, carcinoma of the oesophagus will include cancers of the thoracic and abdominal oesophagus but will exclude the cervical oesophagus. Oesophagogastric junctional cancers will be considered according to the Siewert and Stein classification:[2]

- **Type I** is adenocarcinoma of the distal oesophagus, which usually arises from an area of Barrett's metaplasia and which may infiltrate the oesophagogastric junction from above.
- **Type II** is true carcinoma of the cardia arising from the cardiac epithelium or short segments with intestinal metaplasia at the oesophagogastric junction, often referred to as 'junctional carcinoma'.
- **Type III** is subcardial gastric carcinoma that infiltrates the oesophagogastric junction and distal oesophagus from below.

Non-cardia gastric cancer will include all cancers of the fundus, body and pyloric antrum.

Epidemiology

Incidence

Cancer epidemiology studies are often limited by the nature of data collection, frequently being retrospective and by necessity incomplete and not standardised. An apparent increase in disease incidence may be influenced by improvements in registration efficiency, an effect of the increasing age of the population or by an overall increase in the incidence of the disease itself. As such, changes in incidence and the actual burden of new cases over time are the result of changes in the size and composition of population and in the actual risk for a specific cancer. Cancer registration may be based upon clinical details alone without histological confirmation or on histology of 'cancer' rather than specific reference to squamous cell or adenocarcinoma. These approaches will cause bias to incidence data, although latterly more thorough standardised approaches have reduced these influences.

Oesophageal cancer

Carcinoma of the oesophagus (ICD code 150) was the eighth commonest cancer in 2008.[3] Worldwide there were 481 000 new cases representing 7% of the total cases of cancer. Mortality was high, with 406 000 deaths or 84% of all registered cases. Incidence varies across the world, with the highest risk in the so-called Asian 'oesophageal cancer belt', which extends from Northern Iran through Central Asia to North Central China. SCC predominates in these less developed countries, reflecting low socioeconomic status and poor diet. Overall, the male to female ratio is 2.1:1, although there are variations. In more developed countries the incidence of SCC has declined, with age-specific rates in white males in the USA at 2.2 per 100 000.[4] However, there have been increasing trends in some regions; for example, in Scotland rates are increasing in women and decreasing in men, possibly reflecting the changing patterns of tobacco and alcohol consumption.

Oesophageal and oesophagogastric junctional adenocarcinoma

Adenocarcinoma of the oesophagus and junction accounts for variable proportions of oesophageal cancer across the world, ranging from 0% in parts of China to 10% in Northern Europe to 48% in the UK.[4] Adenocarcinoma of the oesophagogastric junction includes cancer located in the distal third of the oesophagus and the cardia of the stomach. Although there is a male predominance there are differences according to organ of origin. For oesophageal tumours the male to female ratio is 2.6:1 and for gastric origin tumours 4:1. Recent data from England show an increase in incidence of lower third oesophageal cancer from 8.1 per 100000 in 1998 to 10.1 per 100 000 in 2007, although the rate of increase has stabilised since 2002.[5] Over the same period there has been a slight decrease in cardia cancer incidence. The peak age group affected is between 50 and 60 years of age.

Gastric cancer

Gastric cancer (ICD code 151) is the fourth most frequent cancer worldwide.[3] In 2008 there were 988 000 new cases with 737 000 deaths. This represents 14% of all new cases of malignancy and 10.3% of all cancer deaths. Crude numbers are still increasing in relation to demographic changes of the ageing population throughout the world. The majority of cases occur in less developed countries, where the male to female ratio is 1.8:1. This contrasts with a ratio of 1.6:1 in more developed countries. Highest incidence rates are found in Japan (male 69.2 per 100 000 and female 28.6 per 100 000). Other countries with high incidence include East Asia, Korea, Eastern Europe, and Central and South America. Although distal cancers still predominate in countries with highest incidence, there has been a fall in mid and distal gastric cancer, with a progressive increase in cardia cancer.

Inter-country variations are well known between the Far East and the West. There are, however, significant intra-country variations. These largely reflect a north to south gradient, which is particularly apparent in the northern hemisphere. In both Japan and China mortality rates in the northern provinces are almost double those in the south. Similar differences are observed in the UK, with higher standardised mortality rates in north and northwestern regions. In the southern hemisphere, however, the gradient is reversed. Indeed, the higher geographical latitudes in both hemispheres are more temperate or colder and have a higher risk of gastric cancer, thus implicating environmental and particularly dietary factors in aetiology.

Aetiology

Squamous cell carcinoma of the oesophagus

Smoking and alcohol

Smoking and alcohol are established risk factors for SCC, particularly in the West. Smokers have a fivefold higher risk than non-smokers, which doubles again in heavy smokers. There is a positive dose–response effect for both duration and intensity of smoking, although long-term use of tobacco appears to be the stronger influence. The risk reduces after stopping. In the USA tobacco consumption decreased between the 1960s and 1990s, and this is reflected in the decrease in disease incidence. However, the reduction in smoking was less apparent in the black population, in which SCC rates have remained high.

The effect of alcohol is similar to smoking, although the amount consumed appears to be the greater risk factor. Several studies have demonstrated relative risks ranging from 2.9 to 7.4 for heavy drinkers. As with smoking, abstention from alcohol does appear to decrease the risk. Alcohol and smoking seem to have both synergistic and independent effects. The mechanism of action for the damaging effect of alcohol is unclear: it may directly damage the oesophageal mucosa or increase its susceptibility to other carcinogens, or may have its effect via the secondarily associated dietary deficiencies. There also seem to be individual influences reflecting variations on genes coding for enzymes involved in alcohol metabolism (see below).

Socio-economic and dietary influences

Areas of highest incidence are those countries of low socio-economic status where poverty and malnutrition predominate. The development of SCC appears to be related to a type of chronic oesophagitis that is different from that found in the West and is often complicated by atrophy and dysplasia (see Chapter 1). It is not usually associated with gastro-oesophageal reflux and is often asymptomatic.

SCC has been associated with ingestion of very hot beverages, a family history of oesophageal cancer, prevalence of oesophagitis among siblings, and a low intake of fresh fruits and wheat flour products.[6] Furthermore, riboflavin deficiency and vitamin A and C deficiency[7] have been identified as risk factors that are particularly important at a young age. By contrast, vitamin C intake confers a protective benefit; Hu et al.,[8] in a case–control study, found that 100 mg of vitamin C per day decreased risk by 39%.

Associated conditions

SCC is associated with a variety of uncommon conditions that relate to some form of inflammatory injury. Oesophageal strictures developing after ingestion of corrosive agents, particularly in childhood, are associated with a 1000-fold increase in the risk of carcinoma. There is a time delay of 20–40 years after ingestion of the corrosive, and as a result tumours are seen at a younger age than normal.

Achalasia is associated with SCC, but the magnitude of the risk is unclear. Brucher et al.[9] report from their single institution series that the risk of developing a carcinoma in long-standing achalasia is increased 140-fold when compared with the general population. The risk appears to relate to retention oesophagitis secondary to stasis and exposure to possible carcinogens in fermenting food residue. There is a lead time of approximately 15–20 years and these cases probably warrant long-term surveillance. Treatment of the achalasia does not seem to reduce the risk.

Tylosis palmarum is a rare inherited autosomal dominant condition in which there is a very high incidence of SCC. Perhaps of greater significance is the finding of the increased risk in low-risk areas for offspring of parents with oesophageal cancer.[10] There are numerical and structural chromosomal aberrations in patients with a family history not seen in those without a family history (see below).

Adenocarcinoma of the oesophagus and junctional cancers

Gastro-oesophageal reflux disease (GORD)

Gastro-oesophageal reflux is now the most common symptomatic presentation of all conditions affecting the upper gastrointestinal tract. Estimates suggest that 4–9% of all adults experience daily heartburn and up to 20% experience symptoms on a weekly basis.[11] Of these, 60% have no endoscopic abnormality, 30% have oesophagitis and 10% have Barrett's columnar lined oesophagus. Many are self-treated and do not attend for further investigation, yet 80% with Barrett's are asymptomatic. The relationship of GORD and oesophageal ACA has been evaluated in case–control studies.[12] The individual cancer risk is small because of the high frequency of GORD. Lagergen et al.[13] have estimated the risk of developing ACA of the oesophagus by scoring symptoms of heartburn and regurgitation (alone or in combination), timing of symptoms (particularly at night) and frequency of symptoms. Among those with recurrent symptoms of reflux, the odds ratio of developing cancer was 7.7 in comparison with those without symptoms. More frequent, more severe and longer-lasting symptoms of reflux were associated with a much greater risk (odds ratio 44). The risk associated with GORD is related to the development of Barrett's metaplasia, which is greatest among Caucasian males with a history of alcohol consumption and continuous smoking. Further detailed discussion of the role of Barrett's in the aetiology of ACA is presented in Chapter 15.

Obesity and dietary factors

In the last 20 years the incidence of junctional cancer has increased in parallel with the epidemic of obesity. There is a three- to sixfold excess risk among overweight individuals.[14] Obesity predisposes to hiatus hernia and reflux, and hence contributes mechanically to increase risk. However, data from a number of studies demonstrate an effect independent of reflux. Lindblad et al.[15] have reported a 67% increase in the risk of oesophageal ACA in patients with a body mass index (BMI) greater than 25, and this increases with increasing BMI. This effect was noted irrespective of the presence of reflux symptoms.

There appears to be a sex difference in that the effect was only found in women with a BMI greater than 30, whereas in men it was observed in both overweight and obese individuals. Recently this effect in women has been confirmed, with 50% of cases of oesophageal adenocarcinoma in postmenopausal women in the Million Women study being attributed to obesity.[16]

Evidence is accumulating to support different types of obesity. The distribution of abdominal fat tends to be central and retroperitoneal. This acts as a potent source of growth factors, hormones and regulators of the cell cycle. Such individuals develop the metabolic syndrome, which is linked to raised serum cholesterol and triglycerides, hypertension and hyperglycaemia. In the general population the metabolic syndrome occurs in 10–20%. Power et al.[17] have demonstrated that 46% of those with Barrett's oesophagus and 36% of those with GORD have features of the metabolic syndrome.

The factors released by centrally deposited fat may have an effect on the process of metaplasia transforming to dysplasia. Vaughan et al.[18] have examined the potential relationship between a series of biological markers of progression from metaplasia to cancer in obese and overweight patients. There was little evidence of change in the biomarkers in association with increasing obesity. However, abnormalities in the biomarkers were observed in individuals with high anthropometric measures of abdominal fat. The study concluded that increased BMI contributed to reflux and development of metaplasia but it was the 'male pattern' of abdominal obesity that was actually associated with malignant transformation.

Helicobacter pylori

The role of *Helicobacter pylori* infection in the aetiology of junctional cancer is unclear but appears to be evolving. Gastric infection with *H. pylori* is characterised by gastric atrophy and hypochlorhydria. It has been suggested that this reduction in acid production could, in association with ammonia production from urea by the bacteria, protect the lower oesophagus by changing the content of the refluxing gastric juice. In countries with an increase in junctional cancer, there has been a corresponding decrease in incidence of *H. pylori* infection. Furthermore, community-based approaches to eradicate *H. pylori* infection in the treatment of ulcer and non-ulcer dyspepsia may be inadvertently contributing to the increase in these cancers.

There is accumulating evidence that there may be two distinct types of junctional cancer reflecting the two potential sites of origin. McColl and Going[19] have suggested that one is similar to oesophageal cancer and the other gastric cancer. In a series of studies of patients with junctional cancer, they evaluated *H. pylori* infection from serology, gastric atrophy from pepsinogen I and II ratios, symptoms of reflux and histological subtype of diffuse or intestinal type. They also included biopsies of the distal stomach to document atrophy associated with *Helicobacter*. Tumours of oesophageal origin are intestinal type with no evidence of gastric atrophy or *Helicobacter* infection and occur in the context of reflux. By contrast, tumours of gastric origin are diffuse type or intestinal but with evidence of atrophy and *Helicobacter* infection and without a history of reflux (Table 2.1). Such different characteristics would imply a different carcinogenic process at the two sites and should be considered in prognosis and patient management.

Socio-economic factors

Lifestyle has an effect on the risk for junctional cancers. There is an association with lower socio-economic class but this is not as strong as for SCC. Powell and McConkey[20] demonstrated that the increase of ACA of the lower third of the oesophagus and the cardia was mainly in social classes I and II – that is, in professional and managerial occupations. In addition, in a large surgical series, Siewert and Ott[21] reported that patients with ACA were more

Table 2.1 • Oesophageal and gastric origin of junctional adenocarcinoma

	Reflux history	Tumour histology	Gastric atrophy	*Helicobacter pylori* infection
Oesophageal	Yes	Intestinal	No	No
Gastric	No	Diffuse Intestinal	Yes	Yes

frequently from an educated background, a characteristic not present in the population with SCC. However, the effect of socio-economic class may not be independent as, when adjusted for GORD, BMI and smoking, Jansson et al.[22] found the effect to be less apparent.

Gastric cancer

The Correa hypothesis[23] (**Fig. 2.1**) describes the steps in the process of malignant transformation for gastric cancer. It highlights where environmental factors stimulate changes, particularly in the development of intestinal-type gastric cancer (see Chapter 1). These include socio-economic and dietary influences, as well as exposure to carcinogens.

Socio-economic influences

Gastric cancer is a disease of lower socio-economic groups. The incidence of tobacco smoking tends to be higher in these groups and there is a 1.6-fold risk of developing stomach cancer for smokers in comparison to non-smokers.

An excess risk has been linked to certain occupations such as coalmining. Evidence for such a relationship is circumstantial, and as certain occupations reflect social background the risk may equally reflect lifestyle, particularly dietary habits, rather than actual occupational risk.

Exposure to potentially carcinogenic agents at an early age is clearly crucial to the risk of developing both precursor lesions and subsequent gastric cancer. Evidence for this risk is available from migrant studies. Japanese migrants to the USA had a far lower rate of intestinal-type cancers than the equivalent population who remained in Japan, indicating environmental or dietary aetiology, whereas the rates of diffuse-type cancer remained the same, suggesting a hereditary component.[24]

Diet

The prevalence of gastric cancer in poor communities reflects both malnutrition and intake of a poor-quality diet. Foodstuffs that are cheap prevail, as well as low-cost methods of food preservation and preparation. High carbohydrate intake has been

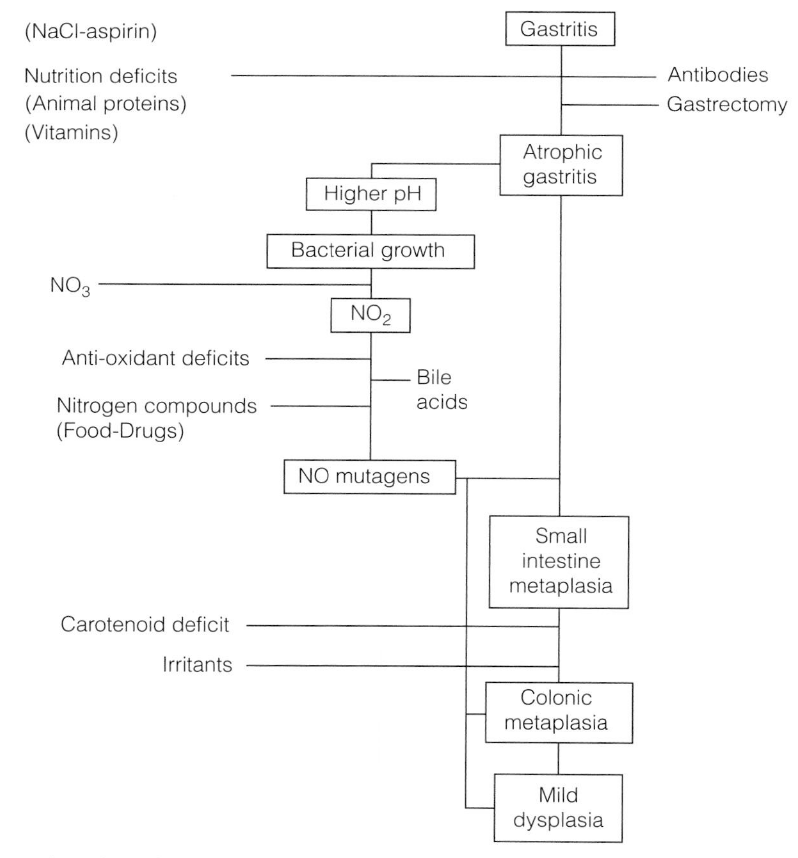

Figure 2.1 • Correa hypothesis for gastric carcinogenesis.

implicated. Areas with a high dietary carbohydrate content have a low protein intake. Protein deficiency will impair gastric mucosal repair and indeed high carbohydrate/low protein may impair defence mechanisms against injurious agents.

Salt preservation of food was common during the early years of the 20th century throughout the world; in some landlocked parts of the world this still occurs. In such areas and in those still using salt preservation there have been high rates of gastric cancer. The consumption of salted and pickled fish is high in Japanese and Colombians and correlates with their disease incidence. On the basis that salt induces injury to the gastric mucosa it may act like high carbohydrate intake, as an initiator to allow access for more potent carcinogens. By contrast, the rapid and widespread adoption of refrigerators in the 1950s and 1960s has significantly affected the preservation of fresh foods. The reduction in mortality observed in Japan shows an inverse relationship with the increase in ownership of domestic refrigerators.[25]

Fresh vegetables and fruit theoretically act to protect against gastric carcinogenesis. Vitamin C inhibits intragastric formation of nitrosamines from nitrite and amino precursors. Both vitamins A and E act as antioxidants within cells, as well as regulating cell differentiation and protecting the gastric mucosal barrier. However, dietary studies have failed to confirm these proposed effects. An inter-country variation in fruit and vegetable intake has not paralleled differences in gastric cancer incidence. It is possible, however, that prolonged exposure is more relevant, again supporting the philosophy of a balanced diet rather than one supplemented with a potentially beneficial foodstuff.

Helicobacter pylori

In 1994 the International Agency for Research on Cancer designated *H. pylori* to be a type I carcinogen[26] for gastric cancer. The initial effect of *H. pylori* is acute inflammation. Since the infection does not resolve spontaneously, an effect is likely to persist and may proceed to chronic gastritis and associated mucosal atrophy and intestinal metaplasia, dysplasia and eventually cancer. The evidence for its role is from a number of sources. Areas of high cancer incidence have a high rate of *H. pylori* infection. In a prospective population-based study in Japan, 2.9% of those infected developed gastric cancer compared with none from the uninfected population; 4.7% of those infected who had non-ulcer dyspepsia progressed to cancer.[27] In high incidence areas *H. pylori* infection tends to occur early in life. These early rates of infection are linked to low income, poor education, poor sanitation and overcrowding. There has, however, been a progressive fall in rates of *H. pylori* serology positivity in longitudinal studies, which have paralled the decline in gastric cancer incidence.

Although the evidence for *H. pylori* inducing gastric cancer is convincing, not all those infected develop the disease. The risk of malignant transformation appears to be enhanced by bacterial virulence and host factors (see below). *Helicobacter pylori* with cytotoxin-associated gene A (*cagA*) appears to be associated with the greatest risk.[28] In the West, 60% of *H. pylori* infections are *cagA* positive compared with 100% in Japan.[29,30] It is likely that *H. pylori* induces an environment that is susceptible to malignant transformation. It induces tissue monocytes to produce reactive oxygen intermediates, which are potent carcinogens. Infection is associated with a significant reduction in gastric juice ascorbic acid,[31] which acts to scavenge and suppress *N*-nitroso compounds and oxygen free radicals. It also facilitates the proliferation of nitrosating bacteria, which promote the development of *N*-nitroso compounds.

Precancerous conditions

Pernicious anaemia imposes a three- to fourfold increased risk of gastric cancer compared with the normal population. Patients who have undergone gastric resection for benign disease are considered to have a greater risk, possibly because of increased alkaline reflux.

Prevention of oesophageal and gastric cancer

Prevention strategies are either primary or secondary. Primary approaches aim to prevent cancer developing, whereas secondary prevention is intended to identify precancerous processes and conditions and to intervene to prevent progression to cancer.

In oesophageal and gastric cancer primary prevention approaches are currently limited to population education to alter social habits (such as decreasing or stopping tobacco or alcohol consumption) and dietary habits (such as maintaining a diet containing fresh fruit and vegetables with a low or minimal salt intake). In addition, the need to prevent obesity is now well established. The role of *H. pylori* eradication is important but programmes of eradication should only be considered according to the level of risk for oesophageal or gastric cancer in the population. In populations with a high risk of gastric cancer, eradication is indicated; however, in populations in which oesophageal ACA is common, eradication may have an adverse effect. The overall benefit of these approaches would be greatly enhanced if specific markers of risk could be identified to focus prevention strategies (see Chapter 15).

Secondary prevention depends upon understanding the natural history and detection of premalignant conditions. In SCC there is limited evidence that secondary measures could be effective because of lack of understanding of the histological changes leading to cancer. In oesophageal ACA, surveillance of Barrett's metaplasia to identify progression to dysplasia is theoretically a positive approach (see Chapter 15). Identification of *p53* expression and aneuploidy in biopsies of Barrett's has been shown to predict the risk of progression.[32] In both gastric and oesophageal cancer there is a potential role for chemoprevention. Increasing levels of cyclo-oxygenase-2 (COX-2) are present in the progression of atrophic gastritis to intestinal metaplasia and gastric cancer.[33] Smoking, acid and *H. pylori* are all associated with COX-2 expression. Aspirin and other non-steroidal agents inhibit COX-2 and their use may act as a chemopreventive for gastric cancer. Aspirin also seems to have an effect in Barrett's metaplasia and in combination with acid suppression may minimise progression to dysplasia. The ASPECT trial in the UK is assessing whether such a strategy can have a secondary preventive effect.[34]

Genetics of oesophageal and gastric cancer

The majority of the available evidence for the aetiology of oesophageal and gastric cancer implicates environmental factors. In oesophageal adenocarcinoma this is consistent with the sequence of Barrett's metaplasia to dysplasia and on to cancer, and in gastric cancer with the Correa hypothesis of atrophic gastritis, intestinal metaplasia, dysplasia and cancer. There is, however, an increasing body of evidence supporting a genetic predisposition. In oesophageal cancer there is some evidence of genetic effects from study of rare coexistent conditions such as tylosis palmaris. Epidemiology studies have shown a familial clustering in approximately 10% of gastric cancers, with 1–3% related to a hereditary gastric cancer precancer syndrome (hereditary diffuse gastric cancer). Gastric cancer is also one of the cancers in hereditary tumour syndromes. In addition, certain genes have been implicated with a greater risk for oesophageal and gastric carcinogenesis from environmental factors, suggesting a link between host genetic make-up and established aetiological agents.

Oesophageal cancer

Evidence for an inherited type of oesophageal cancer is limited. However, the rare skin condition of tylosis palmaris and familial clustering for Barrett's cancer raise the possibility of an hereditary risk. The relationship of tylosis palmaris with SCC had been recognised from epidemiological studies. Investigation of a group of families in Liverpool including several generations has identified a specific tylosis oesophageal cancer gene.[35] Subsequent studies have detected this gene in 69% of cases of sporadic SCC. Recently, more specific proteins coded for by this gene have been reported to be related to poorly differentiated SCC and potentially predict for those with a poorer prognosis.[36]

There have been a number of reports of families with Barrett's metaplasia who have developed adenocarcinoma. In these families the frequency of Barrett's was more than 20% and the frequency of GORD was approximately 40%. In a case–control study, 24% of those with Barrett's, oesophageal or junctional ACA had a family history compared to 5% in the control group.[37] Multivariate analysis confirmed that family history was an independent risk factor with equal weighting to age, male gender, obesity and alcohol consumption. Further analysis of similar families is required to evaluate possible genetic linkages.

Studies into sporadic SCC have identified gene polymorphisms in relation to genes involved in alcohol metabolism, detoxification of environmental carcinogens and folate metabolism. Some are protective and others promote malignant transformation. Most studies in SCC have been undertaken in Japanese and Chinese populations with a high incidence of alcohol consumption.

There are very few studies examining polymorphisms in sporadic adenocarcinoma and those that have been done show weak associations with risk of cancer development. In Barrett's it is likely that there are host polymorphisms, which interact with the environmental factors to promote progression to malignant transformation. The largest body of evidence supports a role for *p53* and aneuploidy as markers of risk (see Chapter 15).

Gastric cancer

Hereditary diffuse gastric carcinoma (HDGC)

The first description of a germ-line mutation was in 1998 in three New Zealand Maori families. Mutations in the *CDH1* tumour suppressor gene (the E-cadherin gene) have since been described in several families of different ethnic backgrounds. The *CDH1* mutation occurs along the gene in these families as opposed to clustering in one site as observed in sporadic cases. In order to develop a common approach for HDGC, the International Gastric Cancer Linkage Consortium defined HDGC as including families with more than two pathologically proven diffuse gastric cancers in individuals under 50 and families with more than three close relatives with pathologically proven diffuse gastric cancer at any age.[38]

HDGC is an autosomal dominantly inherited syndrome. Carriers of the *CDH1* mutation have in excess of 70% lifetime risk of developing diffuse gastric cancer. Female carriers have an additional risk of lobular breast cancer in about 40% of patients. Screening for *CDH1* mutations in the research setting has shown its presence in 40% of families with multiple gastric cancers and at least one diffuse gastric cancer in a member under 50. The criteria for potential screening have been extended to include a number of other combinations of presentation (Box 2.1).

The proportion of HDGC families that have the *CDH1* germ-line mutation, however, is only approximately 30%. In the remaining two-thirds either the detection methods to identify the mutation have been insensitive or there are other, as yet unidentified, HDGC susceptibility genes. A number of genes have been proposed, including those coding for other cell adhesion molecules such as β-catenin and γ-catenin and those involved in other hereditary cancer syndromes. Although some data support a role, this remains investigational.

The clinical issue for these families is their optimal management. In view of the 70% or more chance of developing diffuse gastric cancer with its attendant poor long-term survival, the options are either prophylactic total gastrectomy or endoscopic surveillance. There have been a number of reports of the pathology of resected stomachs after prophylactic gastrectomy. In clinically, endoscopically 'normal' stomachs, supported by biopsy, diffuse multifocal intramucosal disease was identified in all specimens.[39,40] Some studies have shown concentration of disease in the distal third, whereas others have more widespread involvement.[41] The question arises, however, as to the appropriateness of total gastrectomy in essentially a young population for whom the nutritional sequelae will be lifelong. Furthermore, the morbidity and mortality of such a procedure must be minimal. Therefore the role for endoscopy must be explored. Standard surveillance is limited but the distribution of disease from the pathology studies indicates where biopsies should be concentrated. Advances in endoscopy, which include endoscopic autofluorescence spectroscopy and chromoendoscopy, have the potential to enhance accuracy. A further point is that 20–30% of *CDH1* germ-line mutations do not progress to clinically diffuse gastric cancer. There are some data to suggest intramucosal disease may not progress and be of biological rather than clinical importance, analogous to prostatic cancer in elderly men. Thus, counselling of individuals from HDGC families produces very difficult questions, particularly as knowledge is incomplete as to risk, most appropriate management and the role of genetic intervention, as well as the sequelae of life following total gastrectomy.

Box 2.1 • Criteria for screening for *CDH1* in HDGC

- Three or more cases of gastric cancer at any age with at least one case of diffuse gastric cancer
- Isolated individual with diagnosis of diffuse gastric cancer <40
- Isolated individual with both diffuse gastric cancer and lobular breast cancer
- One family member with diffuse gastric cancer and another with lobular breast cancer
- One family member with diffuse gastric cancer and another with signet-ring colon cancer

Hereditary cancer syndromes

The development of molecular genetics has allowed confirmation of primary genetic aetiology for a spectrum of cancers which epidemiology studies had suggested were inherited (Table 2.2). Gastric cancer has been found to be coexistent in these syndromes, further supporting a genetic basis for its development.[42] There are differences across the world, consistent with evidence that the gene pool varies within different populations. In patients with familial adenomatous polyposis (FAP) there is an excess of gastric cancer in Japanese families that is not observed in US non-oriental families. Similarly, in the Lynch syndrome, gastric cancer is more common in China and Korea yet rare in Caucasians. Thus, screening surveillance in such populations should be directed accordingly. Unless there is gastric cancer in the family then upper gastrointestinal endoscopy is not routinely required in those with the Lynch syndrome.

Moderate cancer risk

Worldwide studies have shown that approximately 5–10% of patients with gastric cancer have a family history but without other features to suggest an inherited aetiology. However, it is possible that in this population there is some hereditary predisposition to increased susceptibility to environmental factors such that their risk is increased. Studies have shown increased rates of *H. pylori* infection with atrophic gastritis and hypochlorhydria in first-degree relatives of gastric cancer patients compared with normal controls. This could of course be purely due to environmental factors. Alternatively, normal

Table 2.2 • Hereditary cancer syndromes

Syndrome	Main tumours	Associated tumours
Lynch syndrome (hereditary non-polyposis colorectal cancer)	Colon carcinoma	Endometrial, gastric, small bowel and urothelial cancer
Li–Fraumeni syndrome	Breast cancer, osteosarcoma, brain tumours, soft tissue sarcoma	Gastric and colon cancer, adrenocortical carcinoma, haematological and gynaecological
Familial adenomatous polyposis coli	Colon cancer	Gastric cancer, papillary thyroid cancer, desmoid tumours, medulloblastoma and hepatoblastoma
Peutz–Jeghers syndrome	Hamartomatous polyps of the small bowel, colon and stomach	Gastrointestinal carcinomas, breast, testicular and ovarian cancers
Juvenile polyposis	Hamartomatous polyps of the colon and occasionally stomach and small bowel	Gastrointestinal cancer

variations in the genetic coding sequence of multiple genes (polymorphisms), which are inheritable, may lead to differential inflammatory responses to agents such as *H. pylori* or tobacco. Thus, the combined effect of inflammation promoting host genetic polymorphisms and different microbiological genotypes such as CagA *H. pylori* may increase the risk in a particular population. Specific studies including *p53* have shown certain polymorphisms to be associated with the production of variant proteins.[43] These have been identified more frequently in patients with diffuse gastric cancer than in matched controls. DNA polymorphism in the interleukin-1 gene cluster has been associated with a response to *H. pylori* infection. It is postulated that the polymorphism increases the production of interleukin-1β, a proinflammatory cytokine, which inhibits gastric acid secretion and hence achlorhydria and gastric atrophy.

Molecular genetics of oesophageal and gastric cancer

The development and progression of oesophageal and gastric cancer has been clearly demonstrated in numerous studies to have a genetic basis. Alterations in tumour suppressor genes and oncogenes have been identified in both cancers. Specifically genes, which have roles in diverse functions such as cell adhesion, signal transduction, differentiation, development, gene transcription or DNA repair, have been demonstrated in both oesophageal and gastric cancer. **Figure 2.2** shows some of the changes described in oesophageal cancer arising in Barrett's metaplasia, and **Fig. 2.3** shows the changes in gastric cancer and highlights different mechanisms for the intestinal and diffuse types. Studies of cDNA microarrays for gastric cancer have reported characteristic patterns of gene expression in chronic

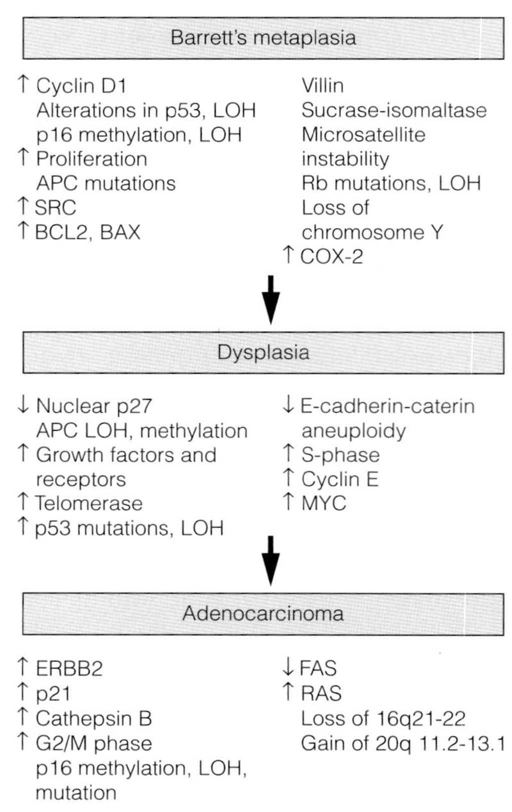

Figure 2.2 • Genetic changes described in the progression from Barrett's metaplasia to oesophageal adenocarcinoma. Reproduced from Lin J, Beer DG. Molecular biology of upper gastrointestinal malignancies. Semin Oncol 2004; 31:476–86. With permission from Elsevier.

gastritis, intestinal metaplasia, and intestinal and diffuse gastric cancer. These raise opportunities for identification of molecular markers and gene profiling in cancer progression and for the prediction of

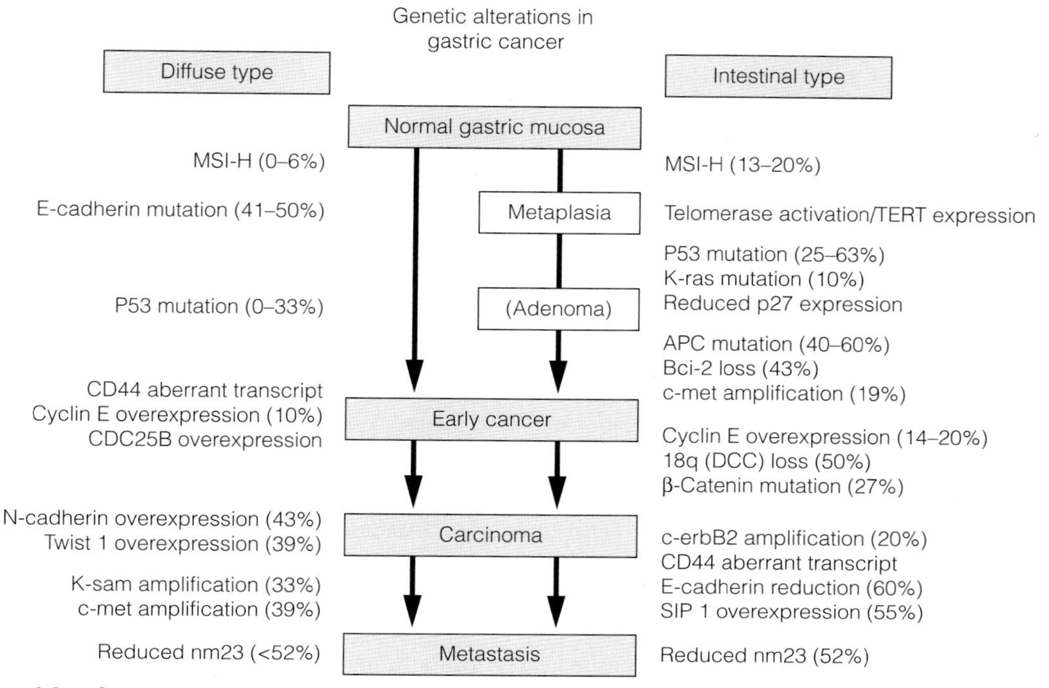

Figure 2.3 • Genetic alterations described in gastric cancer. Abbreviations: *APC*, adenomatous polyposis coli; Bcl-2, B-cell CLL/lymphoma 2; CD44, CD44 antigen; CDC25B, cell division cycle 25B; c-*erbB2*, v-*erb-B2* erythroblastic leukaemia viral oncogene homologue 2; c-*met*, met proto-oncogene (hepatocyte growth factor receptor); *DCC*, deleted in colon cancer; K-*ras*, v-Ki-*ras* 2 Kirsten rat sarcoma viral oncogene homologue; K-*sam*, encodes fibroblast growth factor receptor 2; MSI-H, microsatellite instability – high; nm23, non-metastatic cells 1 (protein, NM23, expressed in); p53, tumour protein p53 (Li–Fraumeni syndrome); SIP-1, SMAD-interacting protein 1; TERT, telomerase reverse transcriptase; TWIST 1, twist homologue 1. Reproduced from Keller G, Hofler H, Becker K-F. Molecular medicine of gastric adenocarcinomas. Expert Rev Mol Med 2005; 7:1–13. With permission from Cambridge University Press.

prognosis and treatment sensitivity.[42,44] Studies of host genetic factors are likely to provide vital information to explain the diverse risks in differing populations. This may require whole genome sequencing studies but these may be limited by the capability of bioinformatics to cope with the associated vast amounts of data.

Screening for oesophageal and gastric cancer

Screening programmes for any disease are dependent on a number of criteria. Firstly, the disease must be common in the target population. Secondly, a reliable and accurate test that is as sensitive and specific as possible is required, and the test should be acceptable to the screened population. There should be an effective treatment for the screened abnormality with minimum morbidity and mortality. Finally, not only does the treatment need to show an improvement in results, but implementation of the screening programme should also result in an overall benefit for the screened population.

The worldwide differences in incidence of oesophageal and gastric cancer allow the implementation of screening programmes for asymptomatic populations only in those areas where the incidence is high. However, lessons from these programmes have increased knowledge of natural history and have allowed high-risk groups to be targeted in low-risk areas in order to detect disease at an earlier stage.

Asymptomatic screening

Oesophageal cancer

Evaluation of asymptomatic screening for carcinomas of the oesophagus has centred on those parts of China with the highest incidence. The screening test involves swallowing a small deflated balloon, which is then inflated at the lower end of the oesophagus. The balloon surface is covered with a fine mesh; on withdrawal from the oesophagus, this scrapes the mucosa to collect cells. A cytological smear is then made from the scrapings for microscopic examination. Those individuals found to have abnormalities are then subjected to endoscopy and appropriate biopsy. In 132 subjects with early oesophageal cancer detected in this way, 26% had normal radiological appearances.[45]

The efficiency of this technique has had varying reports. Reviewing data based on 500 000 examinations, Shu[46] suggested an accuracy for the differentiation of benign from malignant of 90%. Mass surveys have shown that 73.8% of detected cancers were either in situ or minimally invasive. In a provincial review, Huang[47] reported on 17000 examinations screened during a 1-year period. Abnormalities were found in 68% of the population, with low-grade dysplasia in 37%, high-grade in 26% and in situ cancer in 2%. A group with high-grade dysplasia were followed for up to 8 years. Regression to normal or low-grade change was observed in 40%, 20% remained as high grade, 20% fluctuated between high and low grade, and 20% developed cancer. In the absence of dysplasia, 0.12% developed cancer. Progression from dysplasia to in situ cancer occurred over 3–12 years and from in situ to invasive cancer over 3–7 years. Tumour risk was consistent, with a known distribution of middle-third chronic oesophagitis in 76%. It would seem that the duration of severe dysplasia is the greatest risk for malignant transformation. Follow-up by endoscopy is therefore important and in order to ensure biopsy of the same site vital stains have been used. Huang[48] reported that staining with toluidine blue was effective for identifying neoplastic epithelium; 84% of cancers were identified in positively staining areas.

The problem associated with this approach is the management of dysplasia. Oesophageal dysplasia is a dynamic process with both spontaneous regression and progression. Furthermore, even if in situ cancer develops, progress to advanced disease is often prolonged and may be associated with prolonged survival. In one series of 23 untreated patients, 11 developed late-stage disease at a mean of 55 months. In the remainder there was no change for over 6 years and the 5-year survival of the group was 78%.[49] Five-year survival needs to be considered with caution as detection of asymptomatic slowly progressive disease introduces lead-time bias and this can falsely give the impression that treatment results for screen-detected cases are better.

As a result an International Union Against Cancer (UICC) recommendation has been to limit oesophageal cancer screening to areas of high risk.[50] The aim is to identify the natural history of dysplasia more completely. Common standards are required for the classification of dysplasia to identify those changes with greatest risk. Once the assessment is more reliable, control studies should be developed to determine whether screening intervention could reduce mortality for oesophageal squamous cell cancer.

Gastric cancer

The prominence of gastric cancer as a public health problem in Japan led to the development during the 1960s of a mass screening programme for all men over the age of 40 years. The programme has been based on double-contrast radiology with endoscopic assessment of any abnormalities.[51] Members of the public are invited to undergo radiology in mobile units at which seven films are taken after the ingestion of an effervescent contrast agent. Screening is undertaken annually or biannually depending on the area of Japan and the associated risk of disease. Government recommendations set a target of 30% for the annual examination rate. Despite the recognition of gastric cancer as a public health problem, attendance for screening is low. In 1985 over 5 million were examined, representing 13% of the at-risk population. Therein lies one of the problems with any screening programme, namely the cooperation of the public.

Approximately half the cases diagnosed are limited to the mucosa or submucosa (early gastric cancer). Half of those detected are symptomatic and an alternative approach could be envisaged. In keeping with the criteria for a screening programme there has been a highly significant decrease in mortality. However, as already discussed, there may be other reasons for the decline in mortality.

Oshima et al.[52] compared screened and unscreened populations to determine whether screening was important over and above the other influences on the decrease in mortality. In a case-controlled study they found that the risk of dying from gastric cancer among screened cases was at least 50% less than that for non-screened cases. Other Japanese groups have reported similar results. However, the actual effect on mortality remains to be proven as none of the studies have been randomised or controlled. As a result the UICC recommended that studies should be continued in Japan to resolve the problem, but screening in this way should not be adopted as public health programmes in other parts of the world.[50]

Symptomatic screening and early detection

The rate of dyspepsia and reflux in the general population and the non-specific nature of the symptoms do not justify endoscopic assessment for newly presenting patients of all ages. In the UK, in order to improve rates of early diagnosis a programme under the National Awareness and Early Diagnosis Initiative (NAEDI) is currently under way. This includes increasing patient awareness of symptoms and reporting them rather than self treating, improving primary care and pharmacist awareness by careful review of repeat prescriptions for acid-suppressing medication and ensuring adequate resources for evaluation of symptomatic patients.

Studies have evaluated methods of selecting those potentially at higher risk of having a significant diagnosis. Dyspepsia has been classified as uncomplicated or complicated by alarm symptoms including weight loss, anorexia, vomiting, dysphagia and signs of anaemia or an abdominal mass. Further classification according to age has also been studied as early gastric cancer tends to present approximately 10 years younger than advanced disease.[53] Although such studies have increased rates of detection of early gastric cancer to approximately 15–20%, many patients with uncomplicated dyspepsia have undergone normal examinations. In a series of 25 patients under 55 years with gastric cancer, 24 had complicated dyspepsia.[54] Furthermore, in a population database of 3293 oesophageal and gastric cancers, 290 were under 50 and 21 (7%) had uncomplicated dyspepsia.[55] The simple conclusion of this evidence is to restrict endoscopy for those under 55 years to complicated dyspepsia. However, the alarm symptoms used to define complicated dyspepsia are those of established locally advanced disease with the expected poor prognosis. This has been confirmed in a large case series of open access endoscopy from Newcastle upon Tyne.[56] It could be argued that the low index of suspicion for the significance of simple dyspepsia in younger patients had led to a delay in investigation until they developed more significant or alarm symptoms. The failure to diagnose earlier cancers in younger patients may be a result of a failure to initiate investigations until the cancer is advanced and raising the age threshold to 55 for uncomplicated dyspeptics would decrease the rate of diagnosis of upper gastrointestinal cancer. Indeed, the effect of early intervention in unselected dyspepsia not only increases the rate of earlier diagnoses of cancer, but this is also translated into a survival advantage (**Fig. 2.4**).[57]

A pragmatic approach has been adopted in the UK.[58] Urgent specialist referral or endoscopic investigation (within 2 weeks) is indicated for people with dyspepsia of any age when presenting with chronic gastrointestinal bleeding, progressive unintentional weight loss, iron-deficiency anaemia, progressive dysphagia, persistent vomiting, epigastric mass or suspicious barium meal. In addition to these alarm symptoms, similar referral is required for a dyspeptic patient over 55 years with onset of symptoms within the last year and/or continuous symptoms since onset. The advantage of referral within 2 weeks is largely procedural and has only limited support from the literature. For example, gastric cancers limited to the mucosa and submucosa have a doubling time of 1.5–10 years, whereas advanced disease has a doubling time of between 2 months and 1 year.[59,60] Reducing symptomatic delay is unlikely to alter outcome for early disease significantly, but may render more advanced disease amenable to resection. In a comparative audit of 2-week referrals (TWRs) with conventional presentations, Radbourne et al.[61] have found that although the TWR produced more cancers, the stage of disease was equivalent at diagnosis and survival was comparable between the two groups.

High-risk groups

GORD and Barrett's oesophagus

A variety of approaches have been assessed for early diagnosis in patients with GORD and at risk of Barrett's oesophagus. Small-calibre nasal

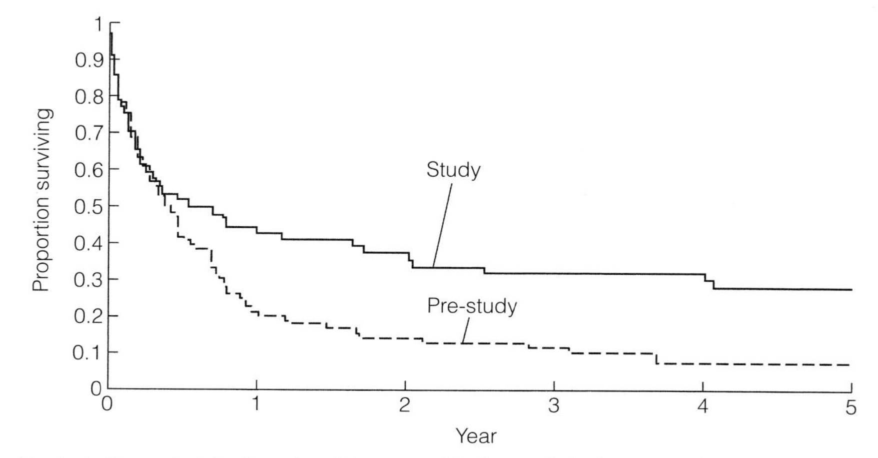

Figure 2.4 • Survival after early detection of gastric cancer (study population) compared with historical control population (pre-study population).

endoscopy in unsedated patients has been evaluated for accuracy of detecting Barrett's in patients with GORD. It was found to be well tolerated, technically feasible and accurate, despite producing smaller biopsy samples.[62]

A modification of the Chinese wire mesh covered balloon used to screen for SCC has recently been reported as a non-endoscopic screening test for Barrett's oesophagus in a population with a history of GORD.[63] The device, Cytosponge, has a similar design in which the patient swallows a gelatin capsule attached to a length of string. The capsule contains a compressed mesh, which expands to 3 cm in diameter once the outer gelatin coating dissolves in the proximal stomach. The string is withdrawn and the mesh takes samples of cells from the oesophageal mucosa. The mesh is processed to produce a cytological preparation, which is stained with a marker for Barrett's oesophagus. Further evaluation is required of this novel technique to determine if this has a role in selecting those with GORD for surveillance.

Helicobacter pylori

The role of *H. pylori* as a marker for endoscopy has received considerable attention. Both serological estimation and breath tests depending on exhalation of urea have been investigated. Serology has been assessed for concordance with the underlying histological presence of *H. pylori*. Farinati et al.[64] found 82% agreement between a measurable antibody response and histological evidence of *H. pylori* infection. Urea breath tests are in routine use in *Helicobacter* eradication programmes for duodenal ulceration. Again, the problem is one of specificity and sensitivity.

Helicobacter pylori seropositivity does not necessarily imply active infection. Equally, seropositivity is a common finding and may not be specific for the at-risk population. It increases with age and to a certain extent parallels gastric atrophy, which is equally an age-related phenomenon and in the majority does not progress to cancer. There is also evidence that seroreversion may occur, with seropositivity frequently seen in early gastric cancer and seronegativity in more advanced disease.[65] Whiting et al.[66] reported a retrospective analysis of *H. pylori* seropositivity in cancer patients compared with a group of undiagnosed dyspeptics. Although the cancer patients were significantly more likely to be seropositive, this was very much site related; cardia cancers were not usually seropositive. Thus, any screening programme based on *H. pylori* serology could miss proximal tumours, which are currently the more common cancers. Further investigation is required and longitudinal studies may resolve the issue of whether patients with *H. pylori* seropositivity warrant close endoscopic follow-up.

Gastric atrophy and intestinal metaplasia

Those found at endoscopic biopsy to have gastric atrophy and columnar-type gastric intestinal metaplasia may also form a risk group. Whiting et al.[67] have followed a group of patients by annual endoscopy who were found to have chronic atrophic gastritis and intestinal metaplasia at diagnostic endoscopy for dyspepsia. This group was reported to have an 11% risk of developing gastric cancer and the authors suggest that such patients should be considered a high-risk group.

Summary and future

Worldwide oesophageal and gastric cancer remain very common. There are differences in the pattern of these diseases reflecting environmental and genetic influences within populations. In the UK adenocarcinomas at the oesophagogastric junction now predominate. Although the incidence of junctional cancers has latterly risen faster than any other cancer, the rate of rise seems to be stabilising. Population demographics indicate this will remain a significant health burden in view of the ageing population. Junctional disease is aetiologically related to GORD and obesity. Greater understanding of those at risk of developing Barrett's oesophagus and subsequent cancer is essential to identify those who need careful surveillance. This will require careful evaluation of genetic and molecular markers. For the present, public awareness and professional education are required to attempt to increase rates of early diagnosis.

Key points

- Oesophageal and gastric cancer are the eighth and fourth most common cancers worldwide. The patterns of disease are variable in different population groups.
- The incidence of oesophageal squamous cell cancer has decreased slightly in recent years in Western countries. The incidence of adenocarcinoma of the oesophagogastric junction has risen rapidly, while that of non-cardia gastric cancer has decreased in most Western countries.

- The aetiology of squamous cancer of the oesophagus is linked to chronic oesophagitis and strongly influenced by diet, smoking and the ingestion of nitrosamines.
- The link between gastro-oesophageal reflux disease (GORD), Barrett's oesophagus and adenocarcinoma of the oesophagus is now proven. Obesity is closely linked to GORD but is also considered to have a primary role in the aetiology of junctional cancer.
- Adenocarcinoma of cardia of the stomach may have two aetiologies, one similar to non-cardia gastric cancer and the other similar to oesophageal ACA.
- The intestinal type of gastric cancer is strongly linked to environmental factors, in particular to diet (especially nitrate ingestion) and *Helicobacter pylori*-induced gastric atrophy.
- The International Agency for Cancer Research has classified *H. pylori* as a group I carcinogen for gastric cancer.
- Genetic studies confirm that oesophageal and gastric cancer can be inherited either as the sole cancer or as part of hereditary cancer syndromes.
- Sporadic oesophageal and gastric cancer may be caused by interactions between genetic polymorphisms and exogenous toxins.
- Asymptomatic screening for oesophageal squamous cell cancer is only justified in high-risk populations and in those with conditions known to predispose to this cancer, such as achalasia.
- Asymptomatic screening for gastric cancer is only justified in high-risk populations.
- Screening of dyspeptic patients remains controversial, as the number of malignancies detected is small. However, novel strategies for high-risk groups may increase rates of detection of premalignant conditions.

References

1. UICC, International Union Against Cancer. TNM classification of malignant tumours. 7th ed New York: Wiley-Blackwell Press; 2009.
2. Siewert JR, Stein HJ. Classification of adenocarcinoma of the oesophago-gastric junction. Br J Surg 1998;85:1457–9.
3. Globocan 2008. Online. Available at http://globocan.iarc.fr; [accessed 16.11.12].
4. Lambert R, Hainaut P. Epidemiology of oesophagogastric cancer. Best Pract Res Clin Gastroenterol 2007;21:921–45.
5. Coupland VH, Allum W, Blazeby J, et al. Incidence and survival of oesophageal and gastric cancer in England between 1998 and 2007, a population-based study. BMC Cancer 2012;12:11.
6. Chang-Claude JC, Wahrendorf J, Liang QS, et al. An epidemiological study of precursor lesions of oesophageal cancer among young persons in a high risk population in Huixian. China. Cancer Res 1990;50:2268–74.
7. Iran – IARC Study Group. Oesophageal cancer studies in the Caspian Littoral of Iran: results of population studies. A prodrome. J Natl Cancer Inst 1979;59:1127–38.
8. Hu J, Nyren O, Wolk A, et al. Risk factors for oesophageal cancer in northeast China. Int J Cancer 1994;57:38–46.
9. Brucher BL, Stein HJ, Bartels H, et al. Achalasia and oesophageal cancer: incidence, prevalence and prognosis. World J Surg 2001;25:745–9.
10. Li JY, Ershaw AG, Chen ZJ, et al. A case–control study of cancer of the oesophagus and gastric cardia in Linxian. Int J Cancer 1989;43:755–61.
11. Cameron AJ. Epidemiology of columnar-lined oesophagus and adenocarcinoma. Gastroenterol Clin North Am 1997;26:487–94.
12. Chow WH, Finkle WD, McLaughlin JK, et al. The relation of gastro-oesophageal reflux disease and its treatment to adenocarcinomas of the oesophagus and gastric cardia. JAMA 1995;274:474–7.
13. Lagergen J, Bergstrom R, Londgren A, et al. Symptomatic gastro-oesophageal reflux as a risk factor for oesophageal adenocarcinoma. N Engl J Med 1999;340:825–31.
14. Cheng KK, Sharp L, McKinney PA, et al. A case–control study of oesophageal adenocarcinoma in women: a preventable disease. Br J Cancer 2000;83:127–32.
15. Lindblad M, Rodriguez LA, Lagergen J. Body mass, tobacco and alcohol and risk of oesophageal, gastric cardia and gastric non-cardia adenocarcinoma among men and women in a nested case control study. Cancer Causes Control 2005;16:285–94.
16. Reeves GK, Pirie K, Beral V, et al. Cancer incidence and mortality in relation to body mass index in the Million Women Study; cohort study. Br Med J 2007;335:1134–9.

17. Power DG, Ryan AM, Healy LA, et al. Barrett's oesophagus: prevalence of central adiposity, metabolic syndrome and a pro-inflammatory state. In: Proceedings of Gastrointestinal Cancer Symposium.; American Society for Clinical Oncology; 2008. p. 70.

18. Vaughan TL, Kristal AR, Blount PL, et al. Non steroidal anti-inflammatory drug use, body mass index and anthropometry in relation to genetic and flow cytometric abnormalities in Barrett's oesophagus. Cancer Epidemiol Biomark Prev 2002;11:745–52.

19. McColl KEL, Going JJ. Aetiology and classification of adenocarcinoma of the gastro-oesophageal junction/cardia. Gut 2010;59:282–4.

20. Powell J, McConkey CC. The rising trend in oesophageal adenocarcinoma and gastric cardia. Eur J Cancer Prev 1992;1:265–9.

21. Siewert JR, Ott K. Are squamous and adenocarcinoma of the oesophagus the same disease? Semin Radiat Oncol 2006;17:38–44.

22. Jansson C, Johansson AL, Nyren O, et al. Socioeconomic factors and risk of oesophageal adenocarcinoma within the European Prospective Investigation into Cancer and Nutrition (EPIC). J Natl Cancer Inst 2006;98:345–54.

23. Correa P. A human model of gastric carcinogenesis. Cancer Res 1988;48:3554–60.

24. Correa P, Sasano N, Stemmerman N, et al. Pathology of gastric carcinoma in Japanese populations: comparisons between Miyagi prefecture, Japan, and Hawaii. J Natl Cancer Inst 1973;51:1449–59.

25. Hirayama T. Actions suggested by gastric cancer epidemiological studies in Japan. In: Reed PI, Hill MJ, editors. Gastric carcinogenesis. Amsterdam: Excerpta Medica; 1988. p. 209–28.

26. International Agency for Research on Cancer Working Group on the Evaluation of Carcinogenic Risks to Humans. Schistosomes, liver flukes and Helicobacter pylori. Luon: International Agency for Research on Cancer; 1994.

27. Uemara N, Okamoto S, Yamamoto S, et al. *Helicobacter pylori* infection and the development of gastric cancer. N Engl J Med 2001;345:784–9.

28. Tomb JF, White O, Kerlavage AR, et al. The complete genome sequence of the gastric pathogen *Helicobacter pylori*. Nature 1997;388:539–47.

29. Vicari JJ, Peek RM, Falk GW, et al. The seroprevalence of cagA-positive *Helicobaster pylori*: strains in the spectrum of gastro-oesophageal reflux disease. Gastroenterology 1998;115:50–7.

30. Ito Y, Azuma T, Ito S, et al. Analysis and typing of the vacA gene from cagA-positive strains of *Helicobacter pylori* isolated in Japan. J Clin Microbiol 1997;35:1710–4.

31. Sobala GM, Schorah CJ, Shires S. Gastric ascorbic acid concentration and acute *Helicobacter pylori* infection. Rev Esp Enf Digest 1990;78(Suppl. 1):63.

32. Fitzgerald RC. Molecular basis of Barrett's oesophagus and oesophageal adenocarcinoma. Gut 2006;55:1810–8.

33. Ristimaki A, Houkanen N, Jankala H, et al. Expression of cyclo-oxygenase-2 in human gastric carcinoma. Cancer Res 1997;57:1276–80.

34. Jankowski J, Barr H. Improving surveillance for Barrett's oesophagus: AspECT and BOSS trials provide an evidence base. Br Med J 2006;332:1512.

35. von Brevern M, Hollstein MC, Risk JM, et al. Loss of heterozygosity in sporadic oesophageal tumours in the tylosis oesophageal cancer gene region of chromosome 17q. Oncogene 1998;17:2101–5.

36. Moodley R, Reddi A, Chetty R, et al. Abnormalities of chromosome 17 in oesophageal cancer. J Clin Pathol 2007;60:990–4.

37. Chak A, Lee T, Kinnard MF, et al. Familial aggregation of Barrett's oesophagus, oesophageal adenocarcinoma, and oesophago-gastric junctional adenocarcinoma in Caucasian adults. Gut 2002;51:323–8.

38. Fitzgerald RC, Hardwick R, Huntsman D, et al. Hereditary diffuse gastric cancer: updated consensus guidelines for clinical management and directions for future research. (International Gastric Cancer Linkage Consortium) J Med Genet 2010;47:436–44.

39. Huntsman DG, Carneiro F, Lewis FR, et al. Early gastric cancer in young asymptomatic carriers of germline E cadherin mutation. N Engl J Med 2001;344:1904–9.

40. Chun YS, Linder NM, Smyrk TC, et al. Germline E-cadherin germ mutations. Is prophylactic total gastrectomy indicated? Cancer 2001;92:181–7.

41. Charlton A, Blair V, Shaw D, et al. Hereditary diffuse gastric cancer: predominance of multiple foci of signet ring cell carcinoma in distal stomach and transitional zone. Gut 2004;53:814–20.

42. Keller G, Hofler H, Becker KF. Molecular mechanisms of gastric adenocarcinoma. Expert Rev Mol Med 2005;7:1–13.

43. Hiyama T, Tanaka S, Kitadai Y, et al. p53 codon 72 polymorphism in gastric cancer susceptibility in patients with *Helicobacter pylori* associated chronic gastritis. Int J Cancer 2002;100:304–8.

44. Lin J, Beer DG. Molecular biology of upper gastrointestinal malignancies. Semin Oncol 2004;31:476–86.

45. Wang G-Q. Endoscopic diagnosis of early oesophageal carcinoma. J R Soc Med 1981;74:502–3.

46. Shu Y-J. Cytopathology of the oesophagus. Acta Cytol 1983;27:7–16.

47. Huang G-J. Recognition and treatment of the early lesion. In: Delarae NC, Wilkins EW, Wong J, editors. Oesophageal cancer. International trends: general thoracic surgery. 4th ed St Louis: Mosby; 1988. p. 149–52.

48. Huang GJ. Early detection and surgical treatment of oesophageal carcinoma. Jpn J Surg 1981;11:399–405.

49. Yanjun M, Li G, Xianzhil G, et al. Detection and natural progression of early oesophageal carcinoma – preliminary communication. J R Soc Med 1981;74:884–6.

50. Chamberlain J, Day NE, Hakama M, et al. UICC workshop of the project on evaluation of screening programmes for gastrointestinal cancer. Int J Cancer 1986;37:329–34.

51. Hisamichi S. Screening for gastric cancer. World J Surg 1989;13:31–7.

52. Oshima A, Hirata N, Ubakata T, et al. Evaluation of a mass screening programme for stomach cancer with a case–control study design. Int J Cancer 1986;38:829–34.

53. Fielding JWL, Ellis DJ, Jones BG, et al. Natural history of 'early' gastric cancer: results of a 10-year regional survey. Br Med J 1980;281:965–7.

54. Christie J, Shepherd NA, Codling BW, et al. Gastric cancer below the age of 55: implications for screening patients with uncomplicated dyspepsia. Gut 1997;41:513–7.

55. Salmon CA, Park KGM, Rapson T, et al. Age threshold for endoscopy and risk of missing upper GI malignancy: data from the Scottish Audit of Gastric and Oesophageal Cancer. Gut 2003;52:A26.

56. Bowrey DJ, Griffin SM, Wayman J, et al. Using alarm symptoms to select dyspeptics for endoscopy which result in patients with curable oesophagogastric cancer being overlooked. Surg Endosc 2006;20:1725–8.

57. Hallissey MT, Jewkes AJ, Allum WH, et al. The impact of the dyspepsia study on deaths from gastric cancer. vol. 1 In: Nishi M, Sugano H, Takahashi T, editors. International gastric cancer congress. Bologna: Monduzzi Editore-International Proceedings Division; 1995. p. 264.

58. NHS Executive. Referral guidelines for suspected cancer. London: HMSO; 2000.

59. Martin IG, Young S, Sue-Ling H, et al. Delays in the diagnosis of oesophago-gastric cancer: a consecutive case series. Br Med J 1997;314:467–71.

60. Kohli Y, Kawai K, Fujita S. Analytical studies on growth of human gastric cancer. J Clin Gastroenterol 1981;3:129–33.

61. Radbourne D, Walker G, Joshi D, et al. The 2 week standard for suspected upper GI cancers: its impact on staging. Gut 2008;52:A116.

62. Jobe BA, Hunter JG, Chang EY, et al. Office-based unsedated small-caliber endoscopy is equivalent to conventional sedated endoscopy in screening and surveillance for Barrett's esophagus: a randomized and blinded comparison. Am J Gastroenterol 2006;101:2693–703.

63. Kadri SR, Lao-Sirieix P, O'Donovan M, et al. Acceptability and accuracy of a non-endoscopic screening test for Barett's oesophagus in primary care: cohort study. Br Med J 2010;341:c4372–80.

64. Farinati F, Valiante F, Germania B, et al. Prevalence of *Helicobacter pylori* infection in patients with precancerous changes and gastric cancer. Eur J Cancer Prev 1993;2:321–6.

65. Kikuchi S. Epidemiology of *Helicobacter pylori* and gastric cancer. Gastric Cancer 2002;5:6–15.

66. Whiting JL, Hallissey MT, Fielding JWL, et al. Screening for gastric cancer by *Helicobacter pylori* serology: a retrospective study. Br J Surg 1998;85:408–11.

67. Whiting JL, Sigurdsson A, Rowlands DC, et al. The long term results of endoscopic surveillance of premalignant gastric lesions. Gut 2002;50:378–81.

3

Staging of oesophageal and gastric cancer

Graeme Couper

Introduction

A review of this chapter from previous editions highlights the huge changes that have, and continue, to occur in the staging process of oesophageal and gastric cancer. The two diseases now have quite distinct staging protocols with an overlap in the often complex area of junctional tumours. The final aim for each patient must be to reach the best treatment option available with the recognition that for the majority of patients this will be a non-curative decision. The extent of change occurring in the last 20 years is clearly demonstrated if we compare the staging investigations employed in the two large MRC trials of neoadjuvant chemotherapy for oesophageal cancer patients undertaken in the UK.[1,2] Assessments before treatment in the OEO2 trial (recruitment from 1992 to 1998) included chest radiography, bronchoscopy for upper third and middle third tumours, and ultrasonography or computed tomography (CT) of the liver. In comparison, for entry into the OEO5 trial (recruitment from 2005 to 2011), staging investigations were spiral/multislice CT of chest and abdomen (neck and pelvis when indicated) with oral contrast or water, endoscopic ultrasonography (EUS), laparoscopy where clinically indicated with further options of bone scan, positron emission tomography (PET), laparoscopic ultrasonography and intraperitoneal cytology. Although patients rarely require all of these staging modalities, they do all require to be discussed in this chapter with the indications, benefits and limitations outlined for each.

The need for accurate staging is essential not only to achieve the highest standards of care for patients, but in addition to allow for comparison of outcomes on a stage-for-stage basis between units and between countries.

Staging classifications

The TNM ('tumour–node–metastasis') staging system was devised by Pierre Denoix between 1943 and 1952, where T represents the extent of the primary tumour, N the absence or presence and extent of regional lymph node involvement, and M the absence or presence of distant metastases.[3] A single TNM staging classification was agreed between the American Joint Committee on Cancer (AJCC), the Japanese Joint Committee (JJC) and the International Union Against Cancer (UICC) in 1987.[4] This classification system has been revised on several occasions with the latest version, TNM7, coming into effect in January 2010.[5] It is now routinely used by the majority of centres in Europe and North America and its use is strongly recommended.

The TNM staging can be based on either clinical or pathological information. All cases should be confirmed microscopically. A classification based on clinical grounds is designated with a 'c' prefix (cTNM) and represents the pre-treatment stage of disease. This is achieved by physical examination, imaging and other relevant investigations. The pathological classification (pTNM) incorporates all the information from the clinical classification and the additional evidence provided from histopathological analysis. Patients receiving neoadjuvant or preoperative treatment are prefixed by the letter 'y' to indicate that the final pathological stage may have been affected by the treatment given.

In general, the cTNM determines the choice of treatment and the pTNM the basis for prognostic assessment. The pTNM may also determine adjuvant treatment. Comparison between cTNM and pTNM can help in evaluating the accuracy of the clinical and imaging methods used to determine the cTNM.

After assigning T, N and M and/or pT, pN and pM categories, these may be grouped into stages. The TNM classification and stage grouping, once established, must remain unchanged in the medical records. The clinical stage is essential to select and evaluate therapy, while the pathological stage provides the most precise data to estimate prognosis and calculate end results. If there is doubt concerning the correct T, N or M category to which a particular case should be allotted, then the lower (i.e. less advanced) category should be chosen. This will also be reflected in the stage grouping. In the case of multiple simultaneous tumours in one organ, the tumour with the highest T category should be classified and the multiplicity or the number of tumours should be indicated in parentheses, e.g. T2 (m) or T2 (5).

✔✔ This system[5] was approved by the UICC and AJCC in 1985, and in Japan in 1986. Table 3.1 illustrates the 2009 update of the unified TNM staging system for gastric cancer. Use of this system is strongly recommended.

Gastric cancer staging

The development of a staging system for gastric cancer with a worldwide application is difficult as the location of the tumour within the stomach influences survival.[6] Distal gastric cancers carry a more favourable prognosis and are more common in Asian populations, with more proximal lesions seen more frequently in western countries. Two thirds of gastric cancers occur in developing countries and the inclusion of molecular or immunohistochemical features of the tumour as part of the staging system would prevent the majority of gastric cancers worldwide being available for

Table 3.1 • TNM7 categories for gastric cancer

T category: primary tumour	
TX	Primary tumour cannot be assessed
T0	No evidence of primary tumour
Tis	Carcinoma in situ: intraepithelial tumour without invasion of the lamina propria
T1	Tumour invades lamina propria, muscularis mucosae or submucosa
T1a	Tumour invades lamina propria or muscularis mucosae
T1b	Tumour invades submucosa
T2	Tumour invades muscularis propria
T3	Tumour penetrates subserosal connective tissue without invasion of visceral peritoneum or adjacent structures
T4	Tumour invades serosa (visceral peritoneum) or adjacent structures
T4a	Tumour invades serosa (visceral peritoneum)
T4b	Tumour invades adjacent structures
N category: regional lymph nodes	
NX	Regional lymph nodes cannot be assessed
N0	No regional lymph node involved
N1	1–2 regional lymph nodes involved
N2	3–6 regional lymph nodes involved
N3a	7–15 regional lymph nodes involved
N3b	16 or more regional lymph nodes involved
M category: distant metastasis	
MX	Distant metastasis cannot be assessed
M0	No distant metastasis
M1	Distant metastasis (positive peritoneal cytology is classified as metastatic disease)

comparison.[7,8] It is for this reason they do not form part of the current TNM7 classification.

TNM7 included major changes in the classification of gastric carcinomas in comparison to TNM6.[4,9] One of the most significant is the use of the oesophageal cancer staging system for junctional tumours or any tumour arising within the proximal 5 cm of the stomach and crossing the oesophagogastric junction. Previously, in TNM6, junctional tumours could be staged according to either the gastric or oesophageal system depending on the judgment of the clinician.[9]

Within the luminal gastrointestinal (GI) tract the T categories have been amalgamated for tumours occurring anywhere from oesophagus to rectum. The T stage classification for gastric cancer has changed significantly, with subdivision of the T1 category into T1a (tumour invades lamina propria or muscularis mucosae) and T1b (tumour invades submucosa) (Table 3.1). The distinction between these two stages has become increasingly important with the development of endoscopic resectional techniques for early-stage gastric tumours. T3 is now invasion of the subserosa without invasion of the visceral peritoneum (T2b in TNM6). T4a is tumour invasion of the serosa (visceral peritoneum), which was T3 disease in TNM6. T4 disease in TNM6 (invasion into adjacent structures) is T4b in the current classification.

The extent of lymph node involvement is the most important independent prognostic factor in gastric cancer.[10] In the history of the development of the TNM classification there has been a move from the location of lymph node metastases (less than or greater than 3 cm from the primary tumour in TNM4) to the total number of involved lymph nodes.[9,11–14] The latest edition categorises the number of involved lymph nodes into narrower groups with the aim of improving prognostic accuracy. The seventh edition of TNM will result in upstaging of patients in comparison to TNM6, with fewer nodes required for entry into the N2 and N3 groups.

The regional lymph nodes of the stomach are defined as the perigastric nodes situated along the greater and lesser curvatures (stations 1–6), left gastric artery (station 7), common hepatic artery (station 8), coeliac trunk (station 9), splenic hilum and splenic artery (stations 10 and 11), and hepatoduodenal nodes (station 12). Involvement of other intra-abdominal lymph nodes in stations 13–16 (retropancreatic, mesenteric and para-aortic) is classified as distant metastases. Distant metastases also include peritoneal seedlings, positive peritoneal cytology and omental tumour not part of continuous extension. Involvement of distal organs is also classified as M1 disease.

There is the potential for the N classification to be underestimated if the number of examined nodes is too small. To determine the minimum number required for a correct classification, 926 patients undergoing curative resection for gastric carcinoma were analysed in a study by Ichikura et al.[15] The number of metastatic lymph nodes correlated significantly with the number of examined lymph nodes. In patients with pN0 disease those with five to nine examined nodes had a significantly lower survival rate compared to those with 10–14 examined nodes. Interestingly, patients with 10–14 nodes examined had as good a prognosis as those with 15 or more. On the basis of this finding the authors concluded that the minimum number of lymph nodes examined for a correct pN0 classification can be reduced from 15 to 10. However, this is assuming that the cTNM stage of N0 disease is accurate and, although there are reports of improvement in the accuracy rates of preoperative diagnosis in cases of early-stage gastric cancer, it would always be the author's recommendation that a D2 gastrectomy is performed whenever possible.[16] In the pN1 and pN2 categories, patients with 29 or fewer examined nodes tended towards lower survival rates than patients with 30 or more examined nodes. The authors concluded that for pN1–3 classifications, 20 or more nodes should be examined, and examining 30 or more lymph nodes may be desirable.

However, many reports do not reach these numbers and only 31% of gastric resections in a UK-based study included 15 or more lymph nodes for histological analysis.[17]

The prognostic value of metastatic lymph node ratio (the ratio of the number of metastatic lymph nodes to the number of lymph nodes removed) after curative resection has been reported.[18,19] Both studies reported the metastatic lymph node ratio as an independent prognostic factor for survival. Among patients with pN2 by the UICC/TNM6 classification, survival in patients with a metastatic lymph node ratio less than 0.1 was significantly better than in those with a higher metastatic lymph node ratio.[19] Maximising the total number of lymph nodes removed at the time of resection could decrease the metastatic lymph node ratio below 0.1, adding further evidence for the need for extended lymphadenectomy. The TNM7 stage groupings for gastric cancer are outlined in Table 3.2.

Oesophageal cancer staging

It is important to again highlight the major change that has occurred in the classification of junctional adenocarcinomas with the introduction of TNM7. These are now included in the oesophageal staging system and this will undoubtedly increase the number of tumours that are classified

Table 3.2 • TNM7 stage groupings for gastric cancer

Stage 0	Tis	N0	M0
Stage IA	T1	N0	M0
Stage IB	T2	N0	M0
Stage IIA	T1	N1	M0
	T3	N0	M0
Stage IIB	T2	N1	M0
	T1	N2	M0
Stage IIIA	T4a	N0	M0
	T3	N1	M0
Stage IIIB	T2	N2	M0
	T1	N3	M0
Stage IIIC	T4a	N1	M0
Stage IV	T3	N2	M0
	T2	N3	M0
	T4b	N0, N1	M0
	T4a	N2	M0
	T3	N3	M0
	T4a	N3	M0
	T4b	N2, N3	M0
	Any T	Any N	M1

as oesophageal lesions. In comparison to stomach cancer, histological subtype and topographical location are used to divide cases.

The anatomical subsites are:

1. **Cervical oesophagus.** From the lower border of the cricoid cartilage to the thoracic inlet (suprasternal notch), approximately 18 cm from the upper incisor teeth.
2. **Intrathoracic oesophagus.**
   i. **Upper thoracic portion.** From the thoracic inlet to the level of the tracheal bifurcation, approximately 24 cm from the upper incisor teeth.
   ii. **Mid-thoracic portion.** The proximal half of the oesophagus between the tracheal bifurcation and the oesophagogastric junction. The lower level is approximately 32 cm from the upper incisor teeth.
   iii. **Lower thoracic portion.** The distal half of the oesophagus between the tracheal bifurcation and the oesophagogastric junction. The lower level is approximately 40 cm from the upper incisor teeth. This portion is approximately 8 cm in length and includes the abdominal oesophagus.
3. **Oesophagogastric junction.**

Regional lymph nodes (N stage) are those in the oesophageal drainage area including coeliac axis nodes and paraoesophageal nodes in the neck, but not supraclavicular nodes. It is recommended that at least six lymph nodes are examined from the lymphadenectomy specimen. If fewer than six lymph nodes are present and all are negative the classification remains N0. The TNM7 categories for oesophageal cancer are shown in Table 3.3.

The introduction of a stratified classification of nodal involvement has been welcomed by most surgeons. Prior to the publication of the latest TNM7 classification, evidence existed that survival may be predicted by the number of involved lymph nodes.[20–22] A review of 336 patients undergoing resection of previously untreated adenocarcinoma and squamous cell carcinoma of the oesophagus and gastro-oesophageal junction reported that patients

Table 3.3 • TNM7 categories for oesophageal cancer

T category: primary tumour	
TX	Primary tumour cannot be assessed
T0	No evidence of primary tumour
Tis	Carcinoma in situ/high-grade dysplasia
T1	Tumour invades lamina propria, muscularis mucosae or submucosa
T1a	Tumour invades lamina propria or muscularis mucosae
T1b	Tumour invades submucosa
T2	Tumour invades muscularis propria
T3	Tumour invades adventitia
T4	Tumour invades adjacent structures
T4a	Tumour invades pleura, pericardium or diaphragm
T4b	Tumour invades other adjacent structures such as aorta, vertebral body or trachea
N category: regional lymph nodes	
NX	Regional lymph nodes cannot be assessed
N0	No regional lymph node metastasis
N1	Metastasis in 1–2 regional lymph nodes
N2	Metastasis in 3–6 regional lymph nodes
N3	Metastasis in 7 or more regional lymph nodes
M: distant metastasis	
M0	No distant metastasis
M1	Distant metastasis

with more than four involved lymph nodes had survival similar to that of patients with M1 disease.[20] Patients with no involved lymph nodes had the best prognosis. The authors identified 18 lymph nodes as the minimal number required for accurate staging. In a multinational, retrospective review of 1053 patients with oesophageal cancer treated with resection alone, recurrent disease had occurred in 40% at 5 years.[21] The frequency of systemic disease after oesophagectomy was 16% for those without nodal involvement and progressively increased to 93% in patients with eight or more involved lymph nodes.

A recent UK study of oesophageal and junctional adenocarcinomas used a revised node (N) classification based on number of involved lymph nodes (N0, none; N1, one to five; N2, six or more) and location in relation to the diaphragm.[22] This demonstrated that a poorer prognosis was associated with increasing nodal involvement and involvement above and below the diaphragm. The TNM7 stage groupings for oesophageal cancer are outlined in Table 3.4.

Multidisciplinary team

Over time staging investigations have become more numerous and complex, and treatment options more varied. In order to keep abreast of current evidence and to ensure the highest level of expertise is afforded to all patients it is essential that all cancer patients are discussed at a multidisciplinary team (MDT) meeting. This meeting should include surgeons, gastroenterologists, radiologists, radiation and medical oncologists, pathologists, cancer nurse specialists and palliative care physicians. The improved accuracy of CT staging with the involvement of specialist radiologists within the MDT setting has been reported.[23] It has also been shown that involvement of the MDT improves overall clinical staging accuracy and is associated with improved outcomes after surgery for gastro-oesophageal cancer.[24–26] In a recent review on the introduction of an MDT for patients with oesophageal cancer, there was a significant increase in the percentage of patients receiving complete staging, a multidisciplinary evaluation and adherence to nationally accepted care guidelines.[27] The time from diagnosis to treatment significantly decreased, reducing from a mean of 27 to 16 days ($P < 0.0001$). Dutch guidelines similarly recommend discussion of patients with upper GI malignancies by an MDT. A recent study found that in over one-third of cases the diagnostic work-up or treatment plan proposed by the referring physician was altered after evaluation by the MDT.[28]

Table 3.4 • TNM7 stage groupings for oesophageal cancer

Stage 0	Tis	N0	M0
Stage IA	T1	N0	M0
Stage IB	T2	N0	M0
Stage IIA	T3	N0	M0
Stage IIB	T1, T2	N1	M0
Stage IIIA	T4a	N0	M0
	T3	N1	M0
Stage IIIB	T1, T2	N2	M0
Stage IIIC	T3	N2	M0
Stage IV	T4a	N1, N2	M0
	T4b	Any N	M0
	Any T	N3	M0
	Any T	Any N	M1

Staging investigations

Clinical assessment

Oesophageal and gastric cancer affects an increasingly wide age group of patients, often with a broad spectrum of comorbidities. It is therefore essential that a full clinical assessment is made as early as possible in the staging process to prevent unnecessary investigations if it is evident that the patient is either too unfit to be considered for curative treatment or has clinical evidence of metastatic disease. It also allows an assessment of nutritional status and the opportunity to intervene in those patients with significant weight loss. An assessment of fitness is also made at this time.

Contrast radiography

Contrast radiography must be mentioned but cannot be regarded as either a first-line or routine investigation in patients with suspected upper GI malignancy. While there is evidence that double-contrast radiology can diagnose oesophageal and junctional tumours with a sensitivity of 96%, it cannot provide the essential histological confirmation that is obtained at endoscopy and is required for staging purposes.[29] It must, however, be stated that in patients with dysphagia with a normal contrast study there is minimal chance that endoscopy will detect any missed oesophageal carcinomas.[30,31] If for whatever reason an endoscopy is impossible or not tolerated, a contrast examination may be useful (**Fig. 3.1**).

Endoscopy

Flexible upper GI endoscopy is the most important investigation in the diagnosis of oesophageal and gastric carcinoma. In experienced hands it is a

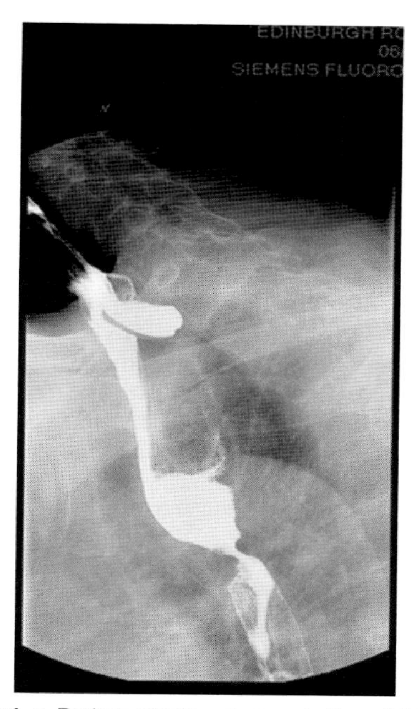

Figure 3.1 • Barium swallow demonstrating distal oesophageal adenocarcinoma with incidental finding of pharyngeal pouch.

safe procedure, with a large UK-based audit of 14 149 procedures reporting a perforation rate of 0.05% and an overall mortality rate of 0.008% during diagnostic endoscopy.[32] After cardiopulmonary complications, perforation is the second most important complication. Although historically the majority of endoscopies were performed under sedation, there is an ever increasing number being performed without sedation or under topical oropharyngeal anaesthesia with 100 mg lignocaine spray.[33–35] Endoscopy provides accurate information on the location and extent of the lesion and its relationship to anatomical landmarks. Crucially, it also provides the opportunity to obtain a tissue diagnosis with the acquisition of biopsies. It has been shown in patients with carcinoma of the oesophagus that two endoscopic biopsies will provide a positive diagnosis in 95.8% of cases, four biopsies in 97.9% and six biopsies in 100% of cases.[36] It is recommended that at least six to eight biopsies are taken at the time of endoscopy to improve the chances of reaching a definitive tissue diagnosis. Not all tumours are negotiable at the time of endoscopy and although dilatation can be performed, the risk of perforation is significantly increased with the risk of rendering a potentially operable tumour inoperable or greatly impairing the prognosis.[37] It is therefore advisable when a tumour is stenotic to first obtain an urgent tissue diagnosis before any consideration is given to dilatation.

✓✓ Endoscopy should be performed whenever possible in all patients suspected of having an oesophagogastric malignancy. It provides invaluable information on tumour characteristics, allows histological confirmation and is safe in experienced hands.

Computed tomography (CT)

Once a cancer diagnosis has been made, CT is recommended as the initial imaging investigation for both oesophageal and gastric lesions. This allows detection of nodal involvement and metastatic disease and is the most cost-effective investigation.[38] Recent progress in multi-detector row CT (MDCT) allows a thinner section thickness in a single breath hold to be obtained, with subsequent improvement in image quality.

Gastric cancer

Patients with gastric cancer require CT of chest, abdomen and pelvis. Scans are performed with intravenous contrast and oral ingestion of either effervescent granules or 1 litre of water to create gastric distention.[39,40] The CT appearances of gastric carcinoma are variable and can present with either focal or diffuse wall thickening (**Fig. 3.2**). Lesions may project into the lumen of the stomach or ulcerate into the wall. With MDCT the overall accuracy in determining the T stage is now in the region of 77–89%.[40–46] The ability of CT to detect organ invasion by the primary tumour remains disappointing even with modern scanners. A study from Japan that assessed high-resolution CT and adjacent organ invasion showed that the finding of an absence of fat plane or an irregularity of the border between the tumour and the adjacent organ was not significantly

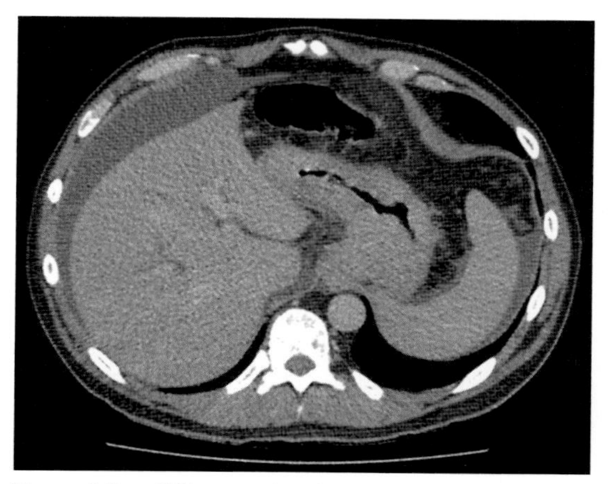

Figure 3.2 • CT image of patient with linitis plastica of stomach and ascites.

related to invasion.[47] However, when the mean densities at the region of interest were measured they were found to be significantly greater at invasion sites than at non-invasion sites. Although this allowed invasion of the pancreas, liver and colon to be assessed with an accuracy of 75%, 61% and 78%, respectively, these authors still found that CT had limited value in differentiating inflammatory adhesions with fibrosis or oedema from true invasion.

A recent study reported a marked improvement in T-stage accuracy using a new CT vessel probe reconstruction protocol using a 16-row MDCT.[48] When compared with standard axial images the overall accuracy rates for T stage improved from 68% to 94% when compared with final histology.

Virtual upper GI endoscopy is a minimally invasive test that utilises three-dimensional (3-D) CT to simulate conventional upper endoscopy images. Images are obtained using both oral and intravenous contrast. The detection rate of gastric lesions using virtual GI endoscopy has been reported to be between 78.7% and 96.7% in early gastric cancer and between 90% and 100% in advanced gastric cancer.[49,50] The overall accuracy, sensitivity and specificity for 3-D multi-detector row CT in the preoperative determination of depth of invasion of gastric cancer (T stage) have been reported to be 83.3%, 69.1% and 94.4%, respectively.[50] Conventional upper GI endoscopy provides direct visualisation of the mucosa, permits evaluation of colour changes that may be indicative of pathology, and suspicious lesions can be biopsied and the tissue sample evaluated histologically. While virtual upper GI endoscopy using CT is a promising method for the detection and evaluation of upper GI lesions, randomised controlled studies comparing it to conventional upper GI endoscopy are needed to determine its clinical value.

Accuracies ranging between 63% and 80% have been reported for N staging by CT when compared with histological staging of the resected specimen (sensitivity 74%, specificity 65%).[42–45,51,52] Limitations to CT nodal staging relate to the detection of involved perigastric nodes close to the primary tumour (**Fig. 3.3**). These lymph nodes often appear confluent with the primary tumour and therefore CT will continue to lack accuracy in nodal staging of some gastric cancers.

One study that retrospectively reviewed the histology of more than 23 000 lymph nodes from gastric cancer resections demonstrated that the mean diameter of a metastatic node was 7.8 mm, and if 5 mm was used as a cut-off, 38% of metastatic nodes would still be missed.[53] Improved image quality associated with modern scanners allows the identification of even smaller regional lymph nodes, but the pathological significance of these smaller lymph nodes remains unknown.

A recent study reported an accuracy rate of 93% in the identification of para-aortic lymph node metastases from gastric cancer using MDCT.[54] Thirteen of 92 (14%) patients undergoing potentially curative resection had para-aortic lymph node involvement on histological examination. Eleven of these were correctly staged preoperatively using MDCT, a sensitivity of 85%.

The accuracy, sensitivity and specificity of 3-D multi-detector row CT for lymph node staging were reported to be 75%, 57.4% and 89.3%, respectively.[51]

CT is useful in the detection of distant metastases and accuracy figures are similar to those seen for oesophageal malignancy (**Fig. 3.4**). CT, however, is limited in its ability to detect transcoelomic spread and the presence of peritoneal seedlings. In a study

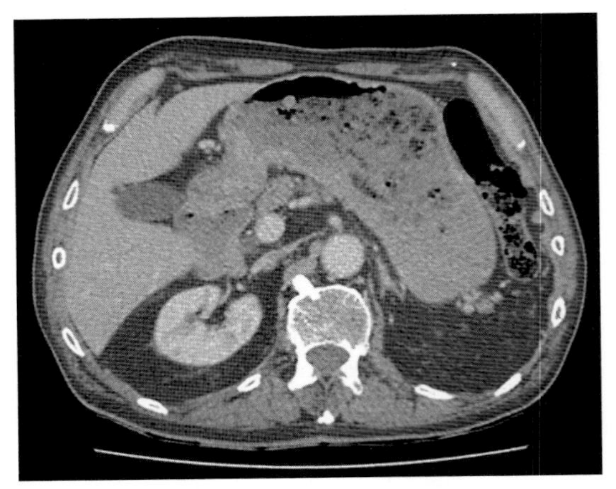

Figure 3.3 • CT image of patient with distal gastric cancer, gastric outlet obstruction and food residue within stomach.

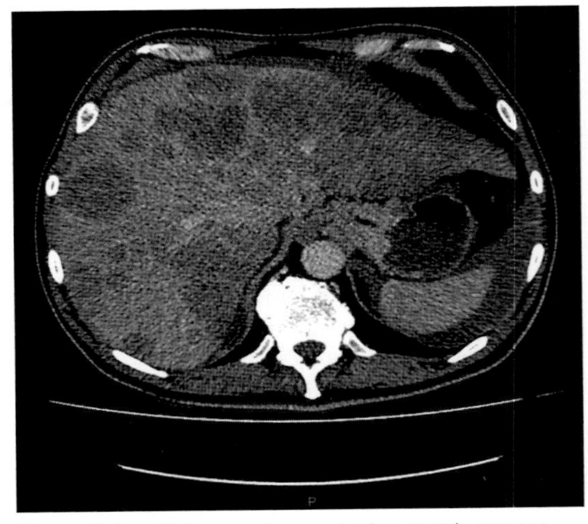

Figure 3.4 • CT image demonstrating gastric cancer with extensive liver metastases.

of 78 patients listed for curative gastrectomy for gastric cancer based on CT findings, 23 (29.5%) had undetected peritoneal spread at the time of laparoscopy.[55] It is recommended that all patients being considered for curative gastrectomy undergo a staging laparoscopy with peritoneal washings. The presence of CT-defined minimal ascites (<50 mL) has been reported not to affect survival on a stage-for-stage basis in patients with gastric cancer without peritoneal metastases.[56] Of those with CT-defined minimal ascites, 28.1% had peritoneal metastases confirmed at surgery.

Further improvements in the accuracy of CT staging may be achieved through establishment of radiologists with a special interest. One report demonstrated improved levels of sensitivity and specificity among radiologists who regularly stage patients with gastric cancer, with an associated reduction in the open-and-close laparotomy rate.[57] Such findings provide additional support for the formation of specialist multidisciplinary teams for the management of gastro-oesophageal cancer.

Oesophageal cancer

Conventional CT has historically diagnosed T4 lesions with high accuracy rates. This is because the criteria for staging T4 lesions are based on obliteration of the fat layer or the angle between the tumour and the adjacent organs (**Fig. 3.5**).[58–60] Oesophageal wall thickness has been used for earlier T stages because tumour cannot be sufficiently differentiated from normal oesophageal wall.[61,62] Accuracy rates for T-stage detection using spiral CT when compared with histopathological stage of resected specimens have been reported as between 43% and 92%.[63–65] Wu et al. reported the accuracies of T staging using the following criteria: T1 and T2, oesophageal wall thickness <5 mm; T3, oesophageal wall thickness >5 mm; and T4, invasion into adjacent organs.[66] In their study, the accuracy values of the respective T staging were 75% for T1/T2, 79% for T3 and 64% for T4. According to these criteria T1 lesions cannot be differentiated from either T2 lesions or from normal oesophageal wall. A recent study from Japan reported improved accuracy rates for T staging of early oesophageal carcinomas (T1a and T1b).[67] A dual-phase (arterial and venous phase) contrast-enhanced CT protocol with MDCT was used. All lesions classified as T1 lesions were T1b with no T1a lesions visualised. This differentiation is important as T1a lesions can be considered for endoscopic mucosal resection, with T1b requiring more radical treatment. In addition, the nodal involvement rate increases from 1.3% in T1a lesions to 22% in T1b lesions.[68]

Accuracy for N-stage disease ranges between 27% and 86% (sensitivity 48–68% with a specificity of 90–95%) (**Fig. 3.6**).[63–65,69,70] The difficulty in the accurate identification of involved lymph nodes is the reliance on size to differentiate between malignant and benign pathology.

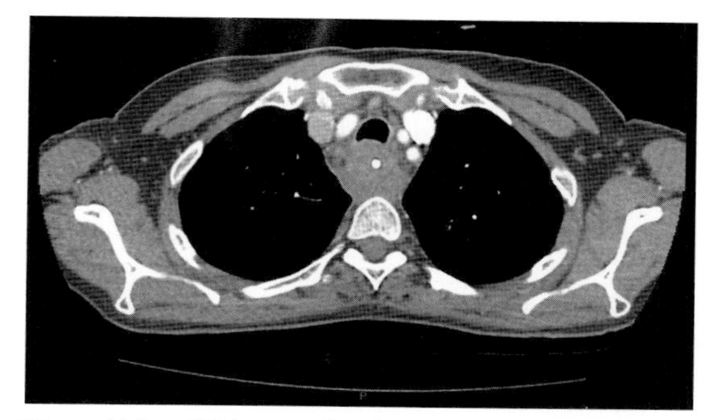

Figure 3.5 • CT image of patient with squamous cell carcinoma (SCC) of oesophagus from 20 to 27 cm with T4 invasion into trachea. A fine-bore feeding tube is in situ.

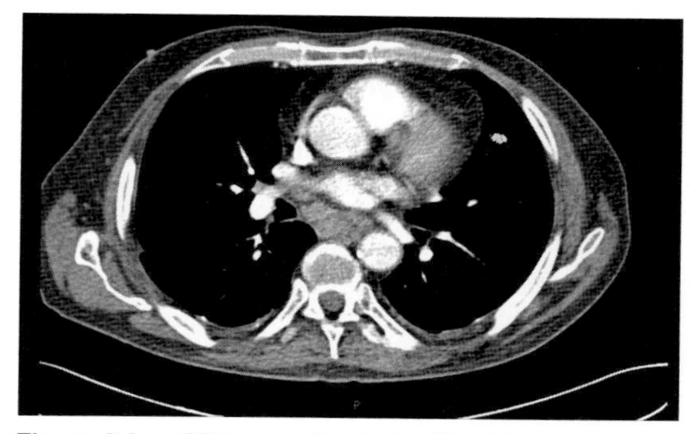

Figure 3.6 • CT image of patient with mid-oesophageal SCC staged as T3N3M0.

The size of the lymph node that different authors regard as a criterion for malignant involvement varies from 5 to 15 mm.[71] Lymph nodes of more than 1 cm in diameter can, however, be seen within the mediastinum in healthy people, particularly those with coexisting chest problems, and nodes of normal size may contain metastatic deposits.[72]

CT and EUS are complementary techniques in staging oesophageal cancer patients.[73,74] A comparison of EUS and CT identification of involved lymph node stations in 121 patients with squamous cell carcinoma of the oesophagus reported an overall accuracy of 64% for EUS (sensitivity 68%, specificity 58%, positive predictive value (PPV) 68%), 51% for CT (sensitivity 33%, specificity 75%, PPV 64%), and 64% for CT and EUS in combination (sensitivity 74%, specificity 50%, PPV 66%).[74] However, some metastatic lymph nodes in the neck and abdomen are only detectable by CT, and it was recommended that both EUS and CT should be undertaken for routine examination prior to treatment of oesophageal cancer.

The T and N stages of Siewert Type II junctional adenocarcinomas were more accurately predicted by EUS than CT. The T and N stages of Siewert Type III tumours were more difficult to assess, arguably because of anatomical constraints at the oesophagogastric junction. These results highlight the importance of multidisciplinary discussion in planning treatment.

✔✔ MDCT is the first-line imaging investigation in all patients with oesophageal and gastric cancer. Current scanners provide high levels of accuracy in TNM staging.

Positron emission tomography (PET)

Gastric cancer

The role of fluorodeoxyglucose (FDG)-PET in gastric cancer is not as well established as in oesophageal cancer. Reported detection rates of primary tumours vary between 60% and 90% and depend on the histopathological characteristics of the primary tumour.[75,76] Stahl et al. reported on a series of 40 gastric cancer patients and found that tumours with a non-intestinal growth type according to the Lauren classification showed significantly lower FDG uptake than tumours of the intestinal growth type.[77] Non-mucinous carcinomas accumulated significantly more FDG than mucinous ones. This finding has also been reported by Yamada et al., who found a higher standardised uptake value (SUV) in the tubular adenocarcinoma group than in the mucinous and signet-ring cell adenocarcinoma group.[78] These findings have been confirmed in a more recent study that also showed that the expression of the glucose transporter (GLUT-1) significantly correlated with the maximum calculated SUV: 76% of signet-ring cell carcinomas did not show GLUT-1 expression.[79]

Oesophageal cancer

Conflict still exists on the role of PET in the management of patients with oesophageal cancer, but it has been widely adopted in most large centres. The Scottish Intercollegiate Guidelines Network (SIGN) previously concluded that PET is not routinely indicated in staging gastro-oesophageal tumours.[80] To date, no randomised trial has been undertaken to determine the role of FDG-PET or PET/CT in staging upper GI cancer. Such a trial is unlikely to occur as it is now an established staging tool in upper GI cancer despite the lack of published evidence. In 2009 the Scottish National PET Advisory Group recommended the routine use of PET/CT in staging patients with potentially operable oesophageal cancer. Changes in management with the addition of FDG-PET to the staging protocol in patients with oesophageal cancer are reported to occur in anything from 3% to 41% of patients.[81–86] This huge variation may be related to the point in the staging pathway at which PET has been introduced. In a study of 199 patients, FDG-PET was performed only after a full preoperative staging protocol with MDCT, EUS and external ultrasonography of the neck, both combined with selective fine-needle aspiration cytology.[86] Only patients considered eligible for curative surgery after these investigations underwent FDG-PET. FDG-PET revealed suspicious hot spots in 15.1% of patients but metastases were confirmed in only 4.0%. All upstaged patients had clinical stage III–IV disease before FDG-PET. In 3.5% the hot spots appeared to be synchronous neoplasms, mainly colonic polyps. The remaining 7.5% were false positive, leading to unnecessary additional investigations. The authors concluded that the diagnostic benefit of the addition of PET is limited after state-of-the-art staging, and so broad implementation in daily clinical practice is questionable. However, it does not appear sensible on a cost basis to introduce PET at the end of the staging pathway. At the time of writing the costs of MDCT in the UK are approximately £500, PET/CT £1000 and EUS £1800. It would therefore seem reasonable to perform the investigations in this order, reserving the most expensive and invasive tests until the end of the pathway.

PET scans have a limited role in evaluating the T stage of a tumour due to their limited spatial resolution of approximately 6 mm (**Fig. 3.7**). In a comparison of CT, PET and EUS in the initial staging of patients with oesophageal cancer, Lowe et al. reported correct T staging by CT and PET in only 42% of patients compared with 71% with EUS.[87] Superficial and in-situ malignancies of the oesophagus can be difficult to detect with PET, with one study reporting 100% of tumours confined to the mucosa (Tis and T1a) being FDG negative.[88] Kato et al. reported that just 18% of T1a tumours and 61% of T1b tumours were FDG-PET positive.[89] Low FDG uptake has also been reported in tumours with undifferentiated or mucinous features.[90,91] Possible explanations for this include differences in the glucose transporter mechanism, reduced intracellular hexokinase activity resulting in a low rate of FDG phosphorylation, a low volume of metabolically active tumour cells or differences in tumour vascularity.

Early studies of FDG-PET in staging oesophageal cancer highlighted the difficulty in differentiating nodal disease adjacent to the primary tumour from the primary tumour itself.[92–94]

In a review of 12 published studies, pooled sensitivity and specificity for the detection of locoregional metastases were 0.51 (95% confidence interval (CI) 0.34–0.69) and 0.84 (95% CI 0.76–0.91), respectively.[95] For distant metastases, pooled sensitivity and specificity were 0.67

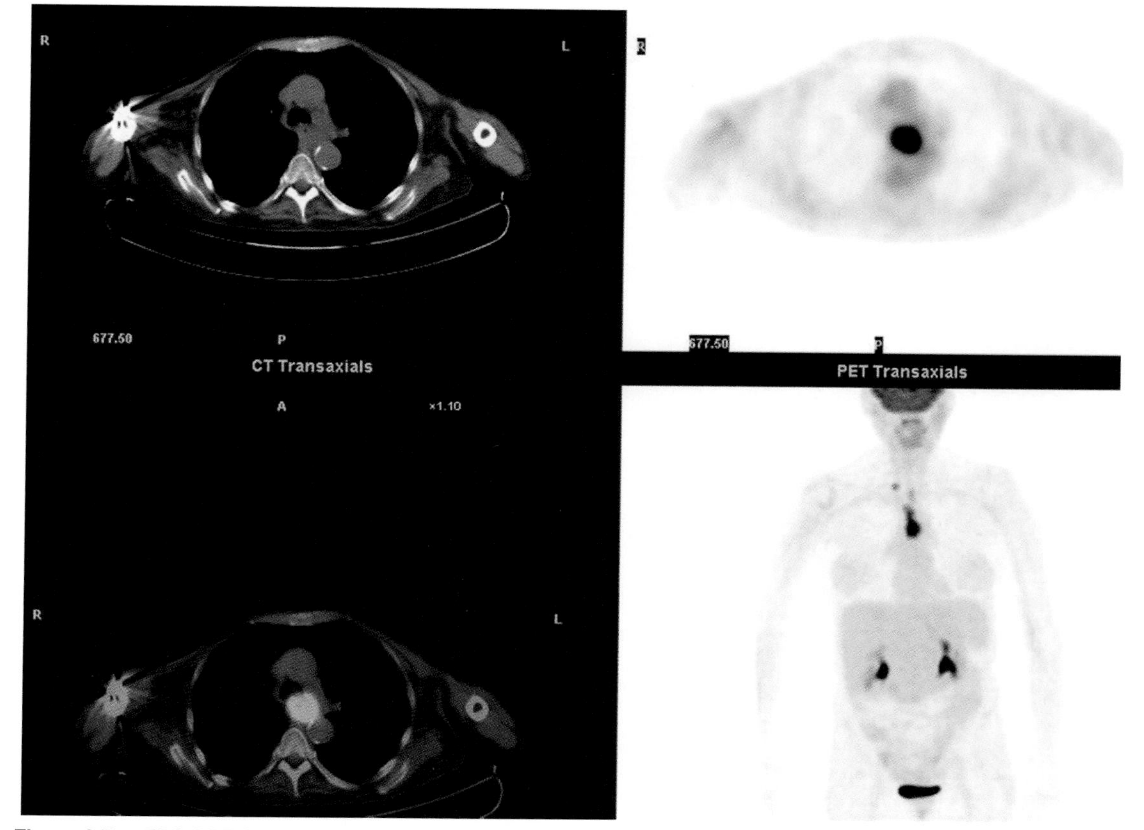

Figure 3.7 • FDG-PET/CT image demonstrating increased uptake in a mid-oesophageal SCC. Increased uptake is evident in a right supraclavicular lymph node.

(95% CI 0.58–0.76) and 0.97 (95% CI 0.90–1.0), respectively. A more recent meta-analysis reported similar results, where pooled sensitivity and specificity of FDG-PET for regional lymph node metastases were 0.57 (95% CI 0.43–0.70) and 0.85 (95% CI 0.76–0.95), respectively.[96]

The introduction of integrated CT and PET has improved the accuracy of staging for patients with oesophageal cancer.[97,98] In a study of 45 patients with thoracic oesophageal squamous cell cancer, PET/CT was superior to PET alone in the detection of locoregional nodal involvement.[98] Sensitivity, specificity and accuracy of PET/CT were 94%, 92% and 92%, respectively, whereas PET alone was 82% sensitive, 87% specific and 86% accurate.

The main role of PET/CT is the identification of distant metastases not evident on CT (**Figs 3.8** and **3.9**). This prevents unnecessary surgery in patients with incurable disease and allows for appropriate palliative treatments to be offered. In two similar sized meta-analyses, each of over 400 patients, the reported sensitivities and specificities for PET in the detection of distant metastases were similar.[95,96] Twelve studies were analysed in the study by van

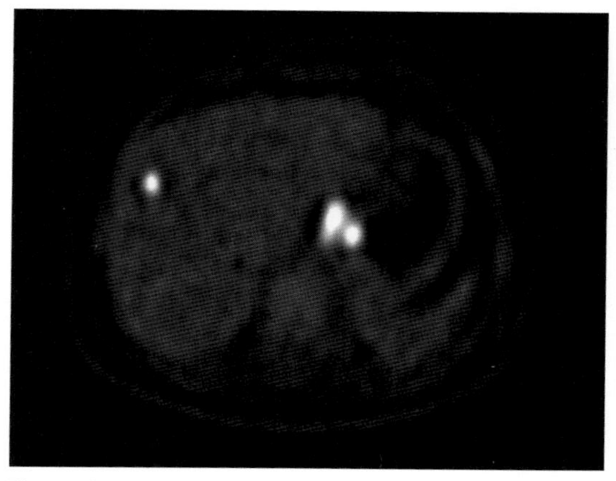

Figure 3.8 • FDG-PET/CT image demonstrating increased uptake in abdominal lymph nodes and a solitary metastasis in the right lobe of the liver. The primary lesion was a distal oesophageal adenocarcinoma.

Westreenen et al., with a pooled sensitivity of 67% (95% CI 58–76%) and a specificity of 97% (95% CI 90–100).[95] In the report by Van Vliet et al., nine

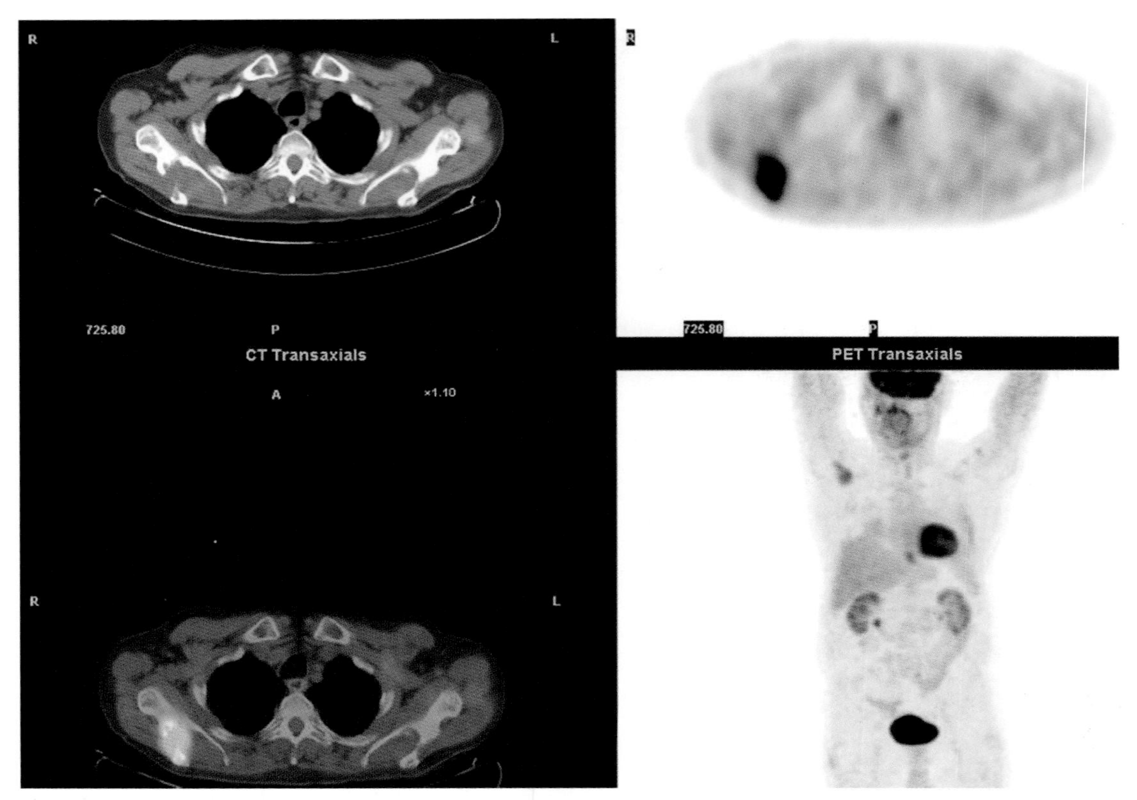

Figure 3.9 • FDG-PET/CT image demonstrating a bone metastasis in right scapula from a distal oesophageal adenocarcinoma. The bone lesion was not detected on original review of the CT images.

studies were analysed, with a pooled sensitivity of 71% (95% CI 62–79%) and a specificity of 93% (95% CI 89–97).[96] Interestingly, only three studies appeared in both meta-analyses.

Accepting that the main role of PET is the detection of metastatic disease, it is debatable whether the routine use of PET is justified in patients with early lesions that are often not visualised on PET and have a low risk of nodal involvement let alone metastatic disease.[68,88,89] It is possible that patients with no obvious lymph node involvement on CT gain little from PET but require EUS for confirmation of N0 status and if confirmed should be offered immediate surgery. Those patients with locoregional lymphadenopathy on CT are more likely to have undetected metastases and should be offered PET/CT.

✓ PET/CT should be the second-line imaging investigation following CT in patients with oesophageal cancer being considered for curative treatment. This is justified on the basis of cost and its ability to detect previously unrecognised metastatic disease.

Endoscopic ultrasonography (EUS)

Gastric cancer

The accuracy of EUS in staging gastric cancer has been varied, with reports that EUS under-stages the depth of invasion and over-stages the nodal invasion because of inflammation around the tumour or in the lymph nodes.[99] In a meta-analysis by Puli et al., 22 studies involving 1896 patients were analysed in relation to the accuracy of EUS for staging gastric cancer.[100] In relation to T stage, sensitivity and specificity for T1 lesions were 88.1% (95% CI 84.5–91.1) and 100.0% (95% CI 99.7–100.0), respectively. For T2 the sensitivity was 82.3% (95% CI 78.2–86.0) and specificity was 95.6% (95% CI 94.4–96.6). T3 sensitivity was 89.7% (95% CI 87.1–92.0) and specificity was 94.7% (95% CI 93.3–95.9), and T4 had a sensitivity of 99.2% (95% CI 97.1–99.9) and specificity of 96.7% (95% CI 95.7–97.6). The pooled sensitivity and specificity for N1 were 58.2% (95% CI 53.5–62.8) and 87.2% (95% CI 84.4–89.7), respectively. N2 had a pooled sensitivity of 64.9% (95% CI 60.8–68.8) and specificity of

92.4% (95% CI 89.9–94.4). The pooled sensitivity from four studies to diagnose distal metastasis was 73.2% (95% CI 63.2–81.7) and specificity was 88.6% (84.8–91.7).

The presence of low-volume ascites (LVA) on EUS has been shown to be indicative of inoperability in patients with gastric and junctional tumours.[101] In patients without evidence of metastatic disease on CT, 6.5% had LVA on EUS. Of these, 76% had either metastatic disease confirmed at laparoscopy or underwent a non-curative resection.

A recent comparison was made of the accuracy of staging using EUS and MDCT in comparison to postoperative pathology patients with gastric cancer undergoing gastrectomy or endoscopic resection.[102] In 277 patients the overall accuracy for T staging of EUS was 74.7% and for MDCT was 76.9%. The overall accuracy for N staging was 66% for EUS and 62.8% for MDCT. The performance of EUS and MDCT for large lesions and lesions at the cardia and angle of His had significantly lower accuracy than that of other groups. EUS had significantly lower accuracy rates for early gastric cancer lesions with ulcerative changes compared to those without.

Oesophageal cancer

While EUS has been in use for nearly 30 years, it has not been universally accepted as an essential, routine staging investigation in patients with oesophageal cancer.[103] Excellent results have been reported from units that rarely use EUS or have a targeted approach to its application.[104] In keeping with ultrasonographic examinations elsewhere its accuracy is operator dependent. Accepting that EUS and EUS-guided fine-needle aspiration (EUS-FNA) are the most accurate techniques for locoregional staging of oesophageal cancer, little evidence exists that they impact on clinical care.[105] Pooled sensitivities for the detection of regional lymph node metastases in oesophageal cancer were 0.80 for EUS (95% CI 0.75–0.84), 0.50 for CT (0.41–0.60) and 0.57 for FDG-PET (0.43–0.70) in a meta-analysis by Van Vleit et al.[96] Specificities were 0.70 (0.65–0.75), 0.83 (0.77–0.89) and 0.85 (0.76–0.95), respectively.

An excellent meta-analysis of the accuracy of EUS in the staging of oesophageal cancer was reported by Puli et al.[106] Forty-nine studies comprising 2558 patients were analysed. Pooled sensitivity and specificity of EUS to diagnose T1 were 81.6% (95% CI 77.8–84.9) and 99.4% (95% CI 99.0–99.7), respectively (**Fig. 3.10**). To diagnose T4, EUS had a pooled sensitivity of 92.4% (95% CI 89.2–95.0) and specificity of 97.4% (95% CI 96.6–98.0) (**Fig. 3.11**). The addition of fine-needle aspiration (FNA) improved the sensitivity to diagnose N stage from 84.7% with EUS alone (95% CI 82.9–86.4) to 96.7% with EUS-FNA (95% CI 92.4–98.9). They concluded that EUS should be strongly considered for staging oesophageal cancer.

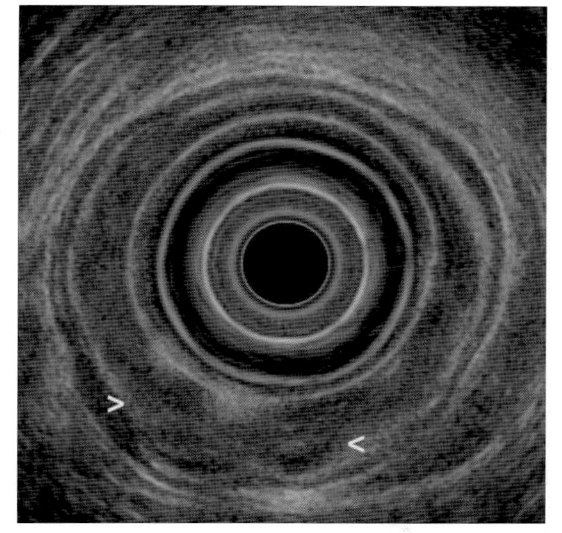

Figure 3.10 • EUS image of T1 oesophageal adenocarcinoma. With thanks to Dr Ian Penman, Royal Infirmary of Edinburgh.

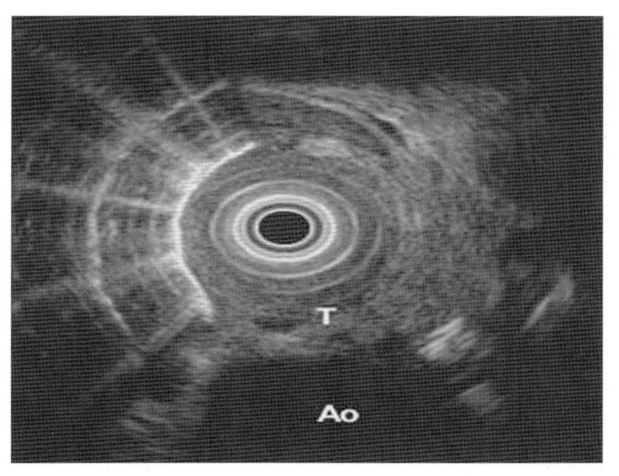

Figure 3.11 • EUS image of oesophagus showing a T4 tumour with extension into the aorta. With thanks to Dr Ian Penman, Royal Infirmary of Edinburgh.

An earlier review of 27 studies reported that EUS is highly effective for discrimination of stages T1 and T2 from stages T3 and T4 for primary gastro-oesophageal carcinomas.[103] This review included 13 papers for staging oesophageal cancer, 13 for gastric cancer and four for cancers at the gastro-oesophageal junction. The accuracy of EUS was lower for tumours at the gastro-oesophageal junction, thought to be possibly due to the anatomy at this site leading to a tendency to scan obliquely through the bowel wall, giving rise to artefactual misrepresentation of the true depth of penetration.

Failure to intubate and cross oesophageal tumours by EUS is reported to occur in up to 45% of cases and is thought to be associated with an especially poor prognosis.[107] It has been reported that over 80% of non-traversable oesophageal tumours are either T3 or T4.[108] However, a recent report of 411 consecutive patients undergoing EUS examination by a specialist radiologist reported a failure to cross the tumour in only 12 patients (2.9%).[109] Forty (10%) patients required a dilation.

The addition of EUS to history, physical examination, upper endoscopy and CT in patients with oesophageal cancer was reported to change management in 24% of cases (95% CI 12–36%), usually to a more resource-intensive approach.[105] EUS-FNA plus cytology results altered management in an additional 8% (95% CI 6–15%) of cases.

The differentiation between inflammatory and neoplastic lymphadenopathy within the mediastinum is essential to ensure patients receive the appropriate treatment. A meta-analysis and systematic review of the accuracy of EUS in evaluating mediastinal lymphadenopathy reported on 76 studies and included 9310 patients.[110] Of these, 44 studies used EUS alone and 32 studies used EUS-FNA. FNA improved the sensitivity of EUS from 84.7% (95% CI 82.9–86.4%) to 88.0% (95% CI 85.8–90.0%). With FNA, the specificity of EUS improved from 84.6% (95% CI 83.2–85.9%) to 96.4% (95% CI 95.3–97.4%). As part of the review the EUS studies with FNA were grouped into three time periods and analysed to standardise the criteria and the technology of EUS over two decades. During this time the sensitivity and specificity of EUS with FNA had substantially improved. EUS with FNA should be the diagnostic test of choice for evaluating mediastinal lymphadenopathy (**Fig. 3.12**).

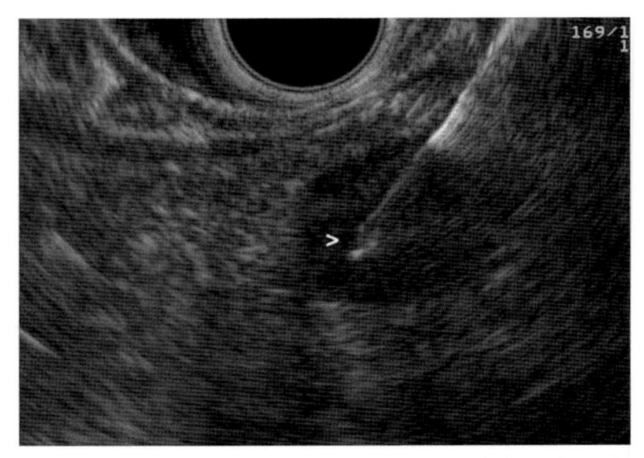

Figure 3.12 • EUS-FNA image of perigastric lymph node in a patient with gastric cancer. The 22G needle is visible within the node. With thanks to Dr Ian Penman, Royal Infirmary of Edinburgh.

All these results suggest that EUS, CT and FDG-PET each play a distinctive role in the staging of patients with oesophageal and gastric cancer.

✔ Performing FNA cytological analysis in conjunction with EUS is safe and is associated with improvements in local staging accuracy and may improve accuracy in detecting response to preoperative therapies and detecting disease recurrence.

Ultrasonography (US)

US is not widely adopted as a routine investigation in the staging of oesophagogastric cancer, although it has specific indications. It has an important role in clarifying liver lesions identified on CT or PET and in obtaining guided biopsies for tissue diagnosis where metastatic disease is suspected. External US of the neck has been recommended as part of the routine diagnostic work-up in patients with oesophageal cancer even after normal CT and PET scanning.[111] It has been estimated that 10–28% of patients with upper or mid oesophageal tumours have metastatic involvement of neck lymph nodes.[112–114] In 176 of 233 patients with oesophageal cancer, CT did not identify any lymphatic metastasis to the neck.[110] External US disagreed in 36 patients and FNA confirmed metastasis in nine cases, resulting in an additional value of external US after normal CT scanning of 5% (9/176). In 74 patients with normal CT and PET imaging of the neck, 3 of 74 (4%) had FNA-confirmed metastasis.

In a larger study of 567 patients with oesophageal or gastric cardia cancer US-FNA was the preferred diagnostic modality for the detection of supraclavicular lymph node metastases.[115] Sensitivities for US alone were 75%, US-FNA 72%, US plus CT 80%, and US-FNA plus CT 79%, in comparison to a sensitivity of CT alone of 25% ($P < 0.001$). Specificities were high for US-FNA (100%), CT (99%) and US-FNA plus CT (99%), whereas those of US alone (91%) and US plus CT (91%) were lower ($P < 0.001$). In 4 of 65 (6%) patients with true-positive malignant lymph nodes, CT was positive with US and/or US-FNA being negative. However, in 36 of 65 (55%) patients, US and/or US-FNA were positive with CT being negative.

Conversely, another group failed to demonstrate any additional staging benefit to performing routine neck US in 180 patients with oesophageal cancer.[116] All patients with cervical metastases had stage T3 or T4 disease on EUS. All cervical nodal metastases were detected by the combination of PET and MDCT. The main role of external US is to obtain cytological proof of suspected cervical lesions.

Laparoscopy

Staging laparoscopy should be considered in all patients with gastric cancer being considered for curative resection and in those with oesophageal or junctional cancers with evidence of a significant infradiaphragmatic component. The investigation is performed under general anaesthesia and involves the creation of a CO_2 pneumoperitoneum and the insertion of typically three laparoscopic ports. This allows thorough visualisation of the peritoneal cavity, and the opportunity to biopsy any suspicious lesions and obtain peritoneal washings for cytology. The detection of low-volume peritoneal disease remains difficult, with sensitivities for the detection of peritoneal disease by CT alone in the region of 58% for oesophageal cancer and 33% for gastric cancer.[117] De Graaf et al. reported on a large series of 416 patients with oesophagogastric cancer staged as having resectable tumours after preoperative staging with CT and/or US.[118] Staging laparoscopy changed treatment decision in 84 cases (20.2%), with locally advanced disease present in 17 patients, extensive lymph node disease in four and distant metastases (liver and peritoneum) in 63 cases. Of those patients deemed resectable by staging laparoscopy, 8.1% were found to be unresectable at laparotomy, 16 with locally advanced disease and 11 with metastases. They concluded that staging laparoscopy was most useful in adenocarcinoma, distal oesophageal, gastro-oesophageal junction and gastric cancers, and probably not necessary in lesions of the upper two-thirds of the oesophagus.

Further studies have shown that as a result of preoperative assessment by laparoscopy 10–29.5% of patients avoid unnecessary surgery.[119–122] A systematic review has previously recommended the use of laparoscopy for the staging of patients with oesophagogastric cancer.[123]

Peritoneal cytology

Positive peritoneal cytology is a predictor of poor survival in patients with gastric cancer (**Fig. 3.13**).[124–128] In a series of 118 patients with completely resected gastric carcinoma, 23 patients (20%) had free peritoneal tumour cells (FPTCs).[124] The median survival time for patients with positive cytology compared with negative cytology was significantly shorter (11 compared with >72 months), with estimated 5-year survival rates of 8% vs. 60%. None of the patients with FPTCs had an early gastric cancer. Recurrent disease occurred in 91% of positive and in 38% of negative patients.

A review of outcomes of 26 consecutive patients with gastric cancer with positive peritoneal washings without peritoneal dissemination reported 1-, 2- and 3-year survival rates of 69%, 35% and 0%, respectively.[125] Sixty-nine per cent of patients had peritoneal recurrences and the authors concluded that aggressive surgical resection does not provide any survival benefit for gastric cancer patients with positive peritoneal washings even in the absence of peritoneal dissemination.

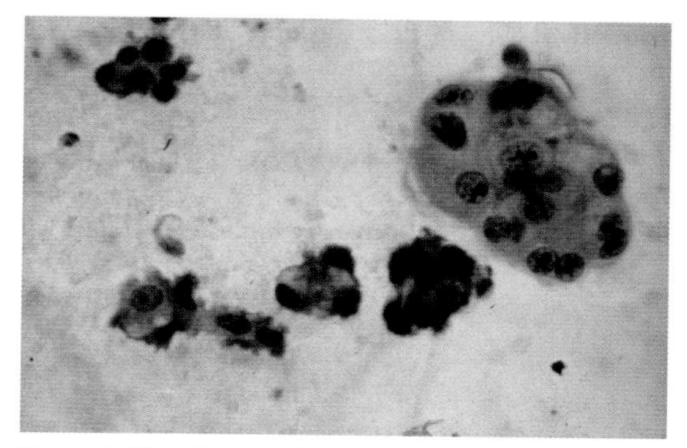

Figure 3.13 • Peritoneal washings demonstrating the presence of malignant cells in a patient with gastric adenocarcinoma.

In a larger study, 996 consecutive patients with advanced gastric cancer who underwent gastrectomy were studied.[126] The 2- and 5-year survival rates of the patients who underwent gastrectomy without any other non-curative factors besides positive peritoneal cytology were 25.3 and 7.8%, respectively. It was concluded that the prognosis of gastric cancer patients with positive peritoneal cytology is so poor that multimodality therapy, including perioperative chemotherapy, is essential.

In a recent report of 1241 patients with gastric cancer undergoing laparoscopy with peritoneal washings, 291 (23%) had positive cytology.[127] Of these, 198 patients (68%) had visible metastases but 93 patients (32%) were without gross evidence of advanced disease. The median disease-specific survival for patients with visible metastases was 0.8 years and for those with positive cytology only was 1.3 years. Forty-eight patients had repeat staging laparoscopy after chemotherapy. Compared with patients who had persistently positive cytology (n = 21), those who converted to negative cytology (n = 27) showed a significant improvement in disease-specific survival (2.5 years vs. 1.4 years, P = 0.0003).

It remains unclear whether neoadjuvant chemotherapy can eliminate free peritoneal tumour cells in the peritoneal lavage. In a study of 61 patients with resectable gastric cancer, peritoneal cytology was performed at staging laparoscopy and at the time of tumour resection following neoadjuvant chemotherapy.[128] FPTCs were detected immunohistochemically with Ber-EP4 antibody.

Forty-two patients (69%) were negative and 19 positive (31%) before chemotherapy. During chemotherapy, 10 (24%) of 42 patients developed FPTCs and 7 (37%) of 19 patients reverted from positive to negative. Patients who became FPTC negative (n = 7) showed an improved median survival (36.1 months) and a longer 2-year survival (71.4%) compared to FPTC-positive patients before and after NAC (n = 12), with a median survival of 9.2 months and a 2-year survival rate of 25%. In contrast, patients who reverted from FPTC negative to positive during NAC (n = 10) had a median survival of 18.5 months and a 2-year survival of only 20%. This study does raise the issue of potential progression during neoadjuvant chemotherapy and demonstrates that the stage of disease prior to starting treatment may be different to that at the time of resection. It is essential that peritoneal washings are obtained at the time of resection.

✓✓ Laparoscopy must be performed and peritoneal cytology obtained in all patients with gastric cancer being considered for resection. Accurate TNM7 classification includes positive peritoneal cytology as metastatic disease.

Laparoscopic ultrasonography (lapUS)

This technique is performed at the time of staging laparoscopy. Commonly used linear array probes have a frequency of 5–10 MHz with a depth of penetration of 4–10 cm. Early reports suggested that lapUS was more accurate at staging gastric and oesophageal cancer than CT or laparoscopy alone, with accuracies quoted between 80% and 90%.[129,130] It can provide additional information on tumour depth, regional lymphadenopathy, small metastases deep within the liver parenchyma and assessment of invasion of adjacent organs. In patients with gastric cancer the addition of lapUS to laparoscopy alone provided additional information in 1 of 28 patients.[131] The Society of American Gastrointestinal and Endoscopic Surgeons (SAGES) recently recommended staging laparoscopy with lapUS if routine preoperative staging investigations in patients with gastric cancer demonstrate no evidence of metastatic disease.[131] The evidence for its use in oesophageal cancer is limited.[131] Recent improvements in the quality of alternative imaging techniques have resulted in the increased detection of smaller liver lesions and enlarged lymph nodes. As such the additional benefit of performing lapUS over and above conventional laparoscopy is now less clear.

Magnetic resonance imaging (MRI)

MRI is mainly reserved as a complementary staging modality and is often used when additional information is required on particular abnormalities identified by CT, in particular liver and bone lesions or adrenal gland abnormalities (**Fig. 3.14**). A systematic review comparing local staging accuracy of MRI, EUS and spiral CT for stomach cancer found overall T-stage accuracies for EUS of 65–92%, for CT of 77–89% and for MRI of 71–83%.[132] A recent study reported similar accuracies for 64-slice multi-detector computed tomography (MDCT) and MRI in the T staging of gastric carcinoma in comparison with histopathology.[133] Forty patients were imaged. The accuracy of MRI was slightly higher than that of MDCT in identifying T1 lesions (50% vs. 37.5%), whereas the accuracy of MDCT was higher in differentiating T2 lesions (81.2% vs. 68.7%). The accuracy of MRI and MDCT did not differ significantly in the evaluation of T3–T4 lesions (P>0.05). Understaging was observed in 20% of cases with MR imaging and in 17.5% with MDCT.

MRI was significantly worse at assessing accuracy of T stage of oesophageal cancer (60%) when compared with EUS (84%).[134] A study comparing CT, MRI and endobronchial ultrasonography (EBUS) for the assessment of invasion of thyroid or oesophageal cancer in cases with suspected tracheobronchial invasion reported sensitivity and specificity of CT for invasion of 59% and 56%, for MRI 75% and 73%, and for EBUS 92% and 83%, respectively.[135]

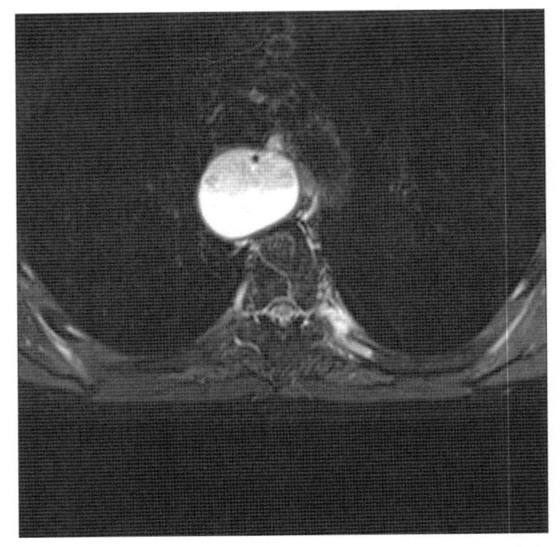

Figure 3.14 • MRI image of a bone metastasis in the left proximal sixth rib. This had arisen from an oesophageal adenocarcinoma and was not evident on CT but had appeared on PET/CT.

Currently MRI has a more limited availability and a higher cost than CT, which remains the preferred investigation for staging of both oesophageal and gastric tumours. MRI is limited in its ability to examine more than one organ system or one area of the body during a single examination. It is not as good as CT for evaluation of pulmonary metastases, and a high-quality study of the entire mediastinum and the upper abdomen in one sitting is difficult to obtain due to movement artefacts.

Endobronchial ultrasonography (EBUS)

EBUS is a technique that enables ultrasound examination of the endobronchial tree using a modified bronchoscope, similar in principle to EUS examination of the upper GI tract. Several studies have reported improved accuracy rates compared with CT assessment in cases where endobronchial invasion by the tumour is suspected. Accuracy rates in the region of 90–95% have been reported for EBUS (sensitivity values around 90%, specificity 80–100%), whereas the reported accuracy of CT in distinguishing endobronchial invasion from compression by the tumour is much lower, at around 50–60%.[135–137] EBUS may also be used to examine carinal and mediastinal lymph nodes and EBUS-directed FNA can also be performed on any suspicious nodes noted at the time of examination.

Restaging following neoadjuvant or radical therapy

With the increasing number of patients being offered neoadjuvant or radical non-surgical treatment, the requirement for repeat staging investigations is also increasing. A clinical improvement in swallowing ability in those patients with dysphagia may or may not be a useful indicator of tumour response.[138,139] A scoring system has been devised as follows: 0, no dysphagia; 1, mild, i.e. with solids, requiring modification of diet to soft foods; 2, moderate, i.e. difficulty with soft foods, predominantly liquid diet; 3, severe, i.e. obstructed, needing medical intervention for dilatation or bolus obstruction.[140] Clearly this will have limited application in patients without dysphagia.

A study assessing the impact of baseline nutritional status on treatment response and survival in 105 patients with locally advanced oesophageal cancer treated with definitive chemoradiotherapy reported that serum albumin level >35 g/L was the only independent predictive factor of complete response.[141]

Endoscopic assessment of response to neoadjuvant therapy has been reported in 100 consecutive patients with oesophageal cancer.[142] Thirty patients were considered to have had a complete response but this was confirmed pathologically in only 15 patients. Survival was improved in those with a pathologically confirmed complete response (3-year survival rate 62.4%, SE 12.9%) compared with non-responders (16.3%, SE 6.6%). Those with microscopic residual disease also had an improved 3-year survival rate (46.3%, SE 12.2%).

EUS assessment of response is limited by disintegration of the involved anatomical structures.[143] In a study of 40 patients who completed chemoradiotherapy and underwent oesophagectomy, EUS measurements of maximal tumour thickness were made pre- and post-chemoradiotherapy. A tumour thickness after chemoradiotherapy of less than or equal to 6 mm or a reduction in thickness greater than or equal to 50% correlated significantly with histopathological tumour regression grade and overall survival. However, the study was limited as 10 of 56 patients could not have repeat EUS due to the development of severe oesophageal stenosis.

The most commonly used assessment of response is follow-up CT, but historically the value of CT in predicting response to chemotherapy has been disappointing.[144] One study of patients with oesophageal cancer who underwent CT before and after preoperative chemotherapy found that 93% of patients had a reduction in tumour volume following chemotherapy, but this showed no correlation to histological evidence of tumour response or to survival.[145] One limitation with conventional imaging is the reliance on a large change in tumour volume, often requiring a greater than 50% reduction in tumour volume to reliably predict response.

In recent years there has been an increasing interest in the use of FDG-PET to identify evidence of response. Malignant tumours generally exhibit an increased rate of glycolysis that is most evident in rapidly growing, poorly differentiated neoplasms.[146] Malignant cells accumulate more glucose than normal cells due to a predominantly glycolytic catabolism instead of a citric acid cycle catabolism.[147] The original study of FDG-PET assessment of response to chemotherapy in patients with upper GI cancer reported that a wide range of changes in uptake were evident between pre-treatment scans and those performed on completion.[148] There are now several subsequent studies. In the first of these, Brucher et al. took a reduction of 52% in tumour FDG uptake as evidence of response on PET.[149] Histologically there were 11 non-responders and 13 responders. Using this cut-off, 5 of 11 patients determined as non-responders histologically would, on PET imaging, be classified as responders. In the histological partial response group the change in SUV ranged from +1% to −68%. This remains a major issue, with considerable overlap between PET identified and histologically identified responders and non-responders.

The level of reduction in FDG uptake chosen to identify response has varied from 30% to 80% in published studies.[148–153] There has been much recent debate on the MUNICON trial, which tailored patient management according to the change in FDG uptake following one cycle of platinum and fluorouracil-based induction chemotherapy.[154] Those patients with decreases of 35% or more were defined as metabolic responders and continued to receive neoadjuvant chemotherapy for 12 weeks and then surgery. Non-responders, according to PET, discontinued chemotherapy after the first cycle and proceeded to surgery. After a median follow-up of 2.3 years (interquartile range 1.7–3.0), median overall survival was not reached in metabolic responders, whereas median overall survival was 25.8 months (19.4–32.2) in non-responders (hazard ratio 2.13 (1.14–3.99), $P = 0.015$). No histological response was reported in metabolic non-responders, but this is perhaps not surprising as they did not receive a full course of chemotherapy. In addition, the PET non-responders essentially had surgery alone and, when compared to those receiving neoadjuvant chemotherapy and surgery, had a poorer overall survival, as would be expected from the results of the phase III trials of neoadjuvant chemotherapy.[1,155]

The overlap between metabolic and pathological responders has been widely reported and remains a major issue. In a study by Kim et al., a complete metabolic response to preoperative chemoradiotherapy on FDG-PET showed the highest correlation with pathological complete response when compared with endoscopic biopsies or CT.[156] However, the concordance was 71% and basing management decisions on FDG-PET response could result in incorrect and suboptimal management in some cases. Accuracy in predicting complete histological response has been reported as 89% for FDG-PET/CT, 67% for EUS-FNA and 71% for CT.[157] Other studies report no correlation between FDG-PET response and histopathological response.[158,159] More research is needed before FDG-PET can accurately determine which patients with oesophageal carcinoma should continue with neoadjuvant treatment or be offered early surgery.

A similar situation has been reported for assessment of response to neoadjuvant chemotherapy in patients with gastric cancer.[160] In a study by Vallbohmer et al., 40 patients underwent gastrectomy following neoadjuvant chemotherapy.[160] FDG-PET was performed before and 2 weeks after the end of neoadjuvant chemotherapy. There was no significant correlation between the pre-treatment SUV, post-treatment SUV or change in SUV and response or prognosis.

Sentinel lymph nodes

A sentinel lymph node (SLN) is the node in direct communication with the primary tumour and the first node to be involved in lymphatic metastasis. The role of SLN biopsy is well established in cancers of the breast and melanoma, but its role in oesophageal and gastric cancer is still evolving and is controversial.[161–163] The main aim of the SLN concept is to reduce the extent of dissection necessary to detect lymph node metastases. Ideally, the SLN is confined to a single lymph node or lymph node station but published studies show that this is not the case in oesophageal cancer, with a mean number of SLNs of 4.7 reported by Takeuchi et al. and a median of 4 by Grotenhuis et al.[164,165] In addition, the lymphatic drainage of the oesophagus is comprised of abundant lymph–capillary networks, especially in the submucosa. The resultant longitudinal lymphatic drainage can result in skipping metastases leading to positive distant nodes in the presence of negative local nodes.[165,166] The finding of multiple, dispersed SLNs in patients with oesophageal cancer would indicate that a radical lymphadenectomy is indicated in most patients.

This finding also applies to gastric cancer. In a review of 88 patients with gastric cancer with a solitary lymph node metastasis, 65 occurred in the perigastric nodes while 23 showed skipping metastases.[167] In relation to the location of the tumour, the authors identified several different lymph node stations that could be involved with identically placed tumours. The same finding was reported in a similar sized study by Kunisaki et al.[168] Of 102 patients with single lymph node metastases, over 60% occurred in specific lymph nodes for each tumour but the remainder were scattered in an unpredictable manner, including the para-aortic lymph nodes. With such an unpredictable pattern of spread a radical lymphadenectomy is essential to ensure that no residual disease is left in patients with potentially curable disease.

Future developments

The next version of this chapter will undoubtedly again require major revision as technology improves and available evidence on the role of each staging method is strengthened. One important study result awaited is the COGNATE trial, in which patients with oesophageal and gastric cancer without evidence of metastatic disease are randomised to receive EUS or not.[169] The two groups will be compared with regards to the treatment received and the rate of complete resection. Length and quality of survival will be compared between the two groups.

Hopefully, the worldwide introduction and acceptance of the TNM7 classification of oesophageal and gastric cancer will allow more meaningful comparison of results between units and may help in guiding clinicians towards a uniformly high standard of care. Ideally, the staging pathway should include a histopathological or biochemical marker of tumour behaviour, but this remains elusive.

Acknowledgements

The previous editions of this chapter have been written and contributed to by John Anderson, Jonathan Ferguson, Simon Paterson-Brown and Chris Deans. Some of the original background data from their text remains and I wish to acknowledge their contributions.

Key points

- All patients with oesophageal and gastric cancer should have the diagnosis confirmed histologically whenever possible and this should be by upper GI endoscopy.
- Multi-slice CT should be the first-line imaging investigation based on accessibility and cost-effectiveness.
- The TNM7 classification should be adopted worldwide to allow comparison of outcomes on a stage-for-stage basis between units and between countries.
- All patients should be discussed by an MDT with input from all involved specialities.
- Positive peritoneal cytology is classified as M1 disease in TNM7 and should be performed in all patients with gastric cancer being considered for curative treatment either at the time of staging laparoscopy or at the time of resection.
- FDG-PET/CT should now be the second-line imaging investigation in patients with oesophageal cancer based on its ability to detect metastatic disease, its non-invasiveness and cost.
- Although EUS has very high reported accuracy rates in detecting mediastinal lymph node involvement in patients with oesophageal cancer, it may no longer be routinely indicated. A more targeted approach using FNA analysis of lymph nodes to clarify CT and PET/CT findings is now an acceptable option.
- With a multitude of staging investigations available to clinicians we can no longer subject all patients to every investigation and there is a clear need to adopt 'bespoke staging' with a tailored approach to each patient's disease with subsequent investigations dependent on the results of the previous tests. This will avoid unnecessary discomfort to patients, unnecessary cost and delay in reaching a final clinical stage, thus allowing earlier commencement of treatment.

References

1. Medical Research Council Oesophageal Cancer Working Party. Surgical resection with or without preoperative chemotherapy in oesophageal cancer: a randomised controlled trial. Lancet 2002;359:1727–33.
2. Medical Research Centre Clinical Trials Unit. Available from www.ctu.mrc.ac.uk; 2012 accessed 12.09.12.
3. Denoix PF. Enquete permanente dans les centres anticancereaux. Bull Inst Nat Hyg 1946;1:70–5.
4. Hermanek P, Sobin LH. UICC TNM classification of malignant tumors. Berlin: Springer; 1987.
5. Sobin LH, Gospodarowicz MK, Wittekind CH, editors. TNM classification of malignant tumors. 7th ed. Oxford: Wiley-Blackwell; 2009.
   The current TNM classification that all units should adopt.
6. Hundahl SA, Phillips JL, Menck HR. The National Cancer Data Base Report on poor survival of U.S. gastric carcinoma patients treated with gastrectomy: Fifth Edition American Joint Committee on Cancer staging, proximal disease, and the "different disease" hypothesis. Cancer 2000;88(4):921–32.
7. Parkin DM, Bray F, Ferlay J, et al. Global cancer statistics, 2002. CA Cancer J Clin 2005;55(2):74–108.
8. Washington K. 7th edition of the AJCC cancer staging manual: stomach. Ann Surg Oncol 2010;17(12):3077–9.
9. Greene F, Page D, Morrow M. AJCC cancer staging manual. 6th ed. New York: Springer; 2002.
10. Siewert JR, Bottcher K, Stein HJ, et al. Relevant prognostic factors in gastric cancer: ten-year results of the German Gastric Cancer Study. Ann Surg 1998;228(4):449–61.
11. Oliver HB, Donald EH, Robert VP, et al. Manual for staging of cancer, American Joint Committee on Cancer. 4th ed. Philadelphia: JB Lippincott; 1992.

12. Fleming I, Cooper JS, Henson DE, et al. Manual for staging of cancer, American Joint Committee on Cancer. 5th ed. Philadelphia: JB Lippincott; 1997.
13. Sobin L, Wittekind C. UICC TNM classification of malignant tumors. 5th ed. New York: Wiley-Liss; 1997.
14. Sobin L, Wittekind C. International Union Against Cancer (UICC): TNM classification of malignant tumors. 6th ed. New York: Wiley; 2002.
15. Ichikura T, Ogawa T, Chochi K, et al. Minimum number of lymph nodes that should be examined for the International Union Against Cancer/American Joint Committee on Cancer TNM classification of gastric carcinoma. World J Surg 2003;27(3):330–3.
16. Tsujimoto H, Sugasawa H, Ono S, et al. Has the accuracy of preoperative diagnosis improved in cases of early-stage gastric cancer? World J Surg 2010;34(8):1840–6.
17. Mullaney PJ, Wadley MS, Hyde C, et al. Appraisal of compliance with the UICC/AJCC staging system in the staging of gastric cancer. Union Internacional Contra la Cancrum/American Joint Committee on Cancer. Br J Surg 2002;89:1405–8.
18. Saito H, Fukumoto Y, Osaki T, et al. Prognostic significance of level and number of lymph node metastases in patients with gastric cancer. Ann Surg Oncol 2007;14(5):1688–93.
19. Kunisaki C, Shimada H, Nomura M, et al. Clinical impact of metastatic lymph node ratio in advanced gastric cancer. Anticancer Res 2005;25(2B):1369–75.
20. Rizk N, Venkatramen E, Park B, et al. The prognostic importance of the number of involved lymph nodes in esophageal cancer: implications for revisions of the American Joint Committee on Cancer staging system. J Thorac Cardiovasc Surg 2006;132(6):1374–81.
21. Peyre CG, Hagen JA, DeMeester SR, et al. Predicting systemic disease in patients with esophageal cancer after esophagectomy: a multinational study on the significance of the number of involved lymph nodes. Ann Surg 2008;248(6):979–85.
A multinational trial of 1053 patients with oesophageal cancer treated by resection alone. Systemic disease occurred in 16% of node-negative patients and with increasing rates with increasing nodal involvement, occurring in 93% of patients with >8 nodes positive.
22. Peters CJ, Hardwick RH, Vowler SL, et al. Generation and validation of a revised classification for oesophageal and junctional adenocarcinoma. Oesophageal Cancer Clinical and Molecular Stratification Study Group. Br J Surg 2009;96(7):724–33.
23. Barry JD, Edwards P, Lewis WG, et al. Special interest radiology improves the perceived preoperative stage of gastric cancer. Clin Radiol 2002;57:984–8.
24. Davies AR, Deans DAC, Penman I, et al. The multidisciplinary team meeting improves staging accuracy and treatment selection for gastro-esophageal cancer. Dis Esophagus 2006;19(6):496–503.
25. Stephens MR, Lewis WG, Brewster AE, et al. Multidisciplinary team management is associated with improved outcomes after surgery for oesophageal cancer. Dis Esophagus 2006;19:164–71.
26. Adams R, Morgan M, Mukherjee S, et al. A prospective comparison of multidisciplinary treatment of oesophageal cancer with curative intent in a UK cancer network. Eur J Surg Oncol 2007;33(3):307–13.
27. Freeman RK, Van Woerkom JM, Vyverberg A, et al. The effect of a multidisciplinary thoracic malignancy conference on the treatment of patients with esophageal cancer. Ann Thorac Surg 2011;92(4):1239–42.
28. van Hagen P, Spaander MC, van der Gaast A, et al. Impact of a multidisciplinary tumour board meeting for upper-GI malignancies on clinical decision making: a prospective cohort study. Int J Clin Oncol 2011;Dec 23. Epub ahead of print.
29. Levine MS, Chu P, Furth EE, et al. Carcinoma of the esophagus and esophagogastric junction: sensitivity of radiographic diagnosis. AJR Am J Roentgenol 1997;168(6):1423–6.
30. DiPalma JA, Pretchter GC, Brady 3rd CE. X-ray-negative dysphagia: is endoscopy necessary. J Clin Gastroenterol 1984;6(5):409–11.
31. Halpert RD, Feczko PJ, Spickler EM, et al. Radiological assessment of dysphagia with endoscopic correlation. Radiology 1985;157(3):599–602.
32. Quine MA, Bell GD, McCloy RF, et al. Prospective audit of perforation rates following upper gastrointestinal endoscopy in two regions of England. Br J Surg 1995;82(4):530–3.
33. Quine MA, Bell GD, McCloy RF, et al. Prospective audit of upper gastrointestinal endoscopy in two regions of England: safety, staffing, and sedation methods. Gut 1995;36(3):462–7.
34. Fisher NC, Bailey S, Gibson JA. A prospective, randomized controlled trial of sedation vs. no sedation in outpatient diagnostic upper gastrointestinal endoscopy. Endoscopy 1998;30:21–4.
35. Al-Atrakchi HA. Upper gastrointestinal endoscopy without sedation: a prospective study of 2000 examinations. Gastrointest Endosc 1989;35:79–81.
36. Lal N, Bhasin DK, Malik AK, et al. Optimal number of biopsy specimens in the diagnosis of carcinoma of the oesophagus. Gut 1992;33:724–6.
37. Di-Franco F, Lamb PJ, Karat D, et al. Iatrogenic perforation of localised oesophageal cancer. Br J Surg 2008;95:837–40.
38. Hadzijahic N, Wallace MB, Hawes RH, et al. CT or EUS for the initial staging of esophageal cancer? A cost minimization analysis. Gastrointest Endosc 2000;52:715–20.
CT scan is the most cost-effective initial staging investigation.
39. Mani NB, Suri S, Gupta S, et al. Two-phase dynamic contrast-enhanced computed tomography with water-filling method for staging of gastric carcinoma. Clin Imaging 2001;25:38–43.

40. Park HS, Lee JM, Kim SH, et al. Three-dimensional MDCT for preoperative local staging of gastric cancer using gas and water distention methods: a retrospective cohort study. AJR Am J Roentgenol 2010;195(6):1316–23.
41. Kim HJ, Kim AY, Oh ST, et al. Gastric cancer staging at multi-detector row CT gastrography: comparison of transverse and volumetric CT scanning. Radiology 2005;236(3):879–85.
42. Kim AY, Kim HJ, Ha HK. Gastric cancer by multidetector row CT: preoperative staging. Abdom Imaging 2005;30(4):465–72.
43. Yang DM, Kim HC, Jin W, et al. 64 multidetector row computed tomography for preoperative evaluation of gastric cancer: histological correlation. J Comput Assist Tomogr 2007;31(1):98–103.
44. Chen CY, Hsu JS, Wu DC, et al. Gastric cancer: preoperative local staging with 3D multidetector row CT – correlation with surgical and histopathologic results. Radiology 2007;242(2):472–82.
45. Hur J, Park MS, Lee JH, et al. Diagnostic accuracy of multidetector row computed tomography in T and N staging of gastric cancer with histopathologic correlation. J Comput Assist Tomogr 2006;30(3):372–7.
46. Hwang SW, Lee DH, Lee SH, et al. Preoperative staging of gastric cancer by endoscopic ultrasonography and multidetector-row computed tomography. J Gastroenterol Hepatol 2010;25(3):512–8.
47. Tsubnraya A, Naguchi Y, Matsumoto A, et al. A preoperative assessment of adjacent organ invasion by stomach carcinoma with high resolution computed tomography. Jpn J Surg 1994;24:299–304.
48. Moschetta M. Stabile Ianora AA, Anglani A, et al. Preoperative T staging of gastric carcinoma obtained by MDCT vessel probe reconstructions and correlations with histological findings. Eur Radiol 2010;20(1):138–45.
49. Kim JH, Eun HW, Choi JH, et al. Diagnostic performance of virtual gastroscopy using MDCT in early gastric cancer compared with 2D axial CT: focusing on interobserver variation. AJR Am J Roentgenol 2007;189(2):299–305.
50. Bhandari S, Shim CS, Kim JH, et al. Usefulness of three-dimensional, multidetector row CT (virtual gastroscopy and multiplanar reconstruction) in the evaluation of gastric cancer: a comparison with conventional endoscopy, EUS, and histopathology. Gastrointest Endosc 2004;59(6):619–26.
51. Cho JS, Kim JK, Rho SM, et al. Pre-operative assessment of gastric carcinoma: value of two-phase dynamic CT with mechanical i.v. injection of contrast material. AJR Am J Roentgenol 1994;163:69–75.
52. Inamoto K, Kouzai K, Ueeda T, et al. CT virtual endoscopy of the stomach: comparison study with gastric fiberscopy. Abdom Imaging 2005;30(4):473–9.
53. Noda N, Sasako M, Yamaguchi N, et al. Ignoring small lymph nodes can be a major cause of staging error in gastric cancer. Br J Surg 1998;85:831–4.
54. Marrelli D, Mazzei MA, Pedrazzani C, et al. High accuracy of multislices computed tomography (MSCT) for para-aortic lymph node metastases from gastric cancer: a prospective single-center study. Ann Surg Oncol 2011;18(8):2265–72.
55. Kapiev A, Rabin I, Lavy R, et al. The role of diagnostic laparoscopy in the management of patients with gastric cancer. Isr Med Assoc J 2010;12(12):726–8.
56. Lee H, Hwang HS, Chang DK, et al. Clinical significance of minimal ascites of indeterminate nature in gastric adenocarcinoma without peritoneal carcinomatosis: long-term follow-up stud. Hepatogastroenterology 2011;58(105):137–42.
57. Barry JD, Edwards P, Lewis WG, et al. Special interest radiology improves the perceived preoperative stage of gastric cancer. Clin Radiol 2002;57:984–8.
58. Vilgrain V, Mompoint D, Palazzo L, et al. Staging of esophageal carcinoma: comparison of results with endoscopic sonography and CT. AJR Am J Roentgenol 1990;155:277–81.
59. Picus D, Balfe DM, Koehler RE, et al. Computed tomography in the staging of esophageal carcinoma. Radiology 1983;146:433–8.
60. Kumbasar B. Carcinoma of esophagus: radiologic diagnosis and staging. Eur J Radiol 2002;42:170–80.
61. Botet JF, Lightdale CJ, Zauber AG, et al. Preoperative staging of esophageal cancer: comparison of endoscopic US and dynamic CT. Radiology 1991;181:419–25.
62. Iyer RB, Silverman PM, Tamm EP, et al. Diagnosis, staging, and follow-up of esophageal cancer. AJR Am J Roentgenol 2003;181:785–93.
63. Kim SH, Lee JM, Han JK, et al. Three-dimensional MDCT imaging and CT esophagography for evaluation of esophageal tumors: preliminary study. Eur Radiol 2006;16(11):2418–26.
64. Panebianco V, Grazhdani H, Iafrate F, et al. 3D CT protocol in the assessment of the esophageal neoplastic lesions: can it improve TNM staging? Eur Radiol 2006;16(2):414–21.
65. Onbas O, Eroglu A, Kantarci M, et al. Preoperative staging of esophageal carcinoma with multidetector CT and virtual endoscopy. Eur J Radiol 2006;57(1):90–5.
66. Wu LF, Wang BZ, Feng JL, et al. Preoperative TN staging of esophageal cancer: comparison of miniprobe ultrasonography, spiral CT and MRI. World J Gastroenterol 2003;9:219–24.
67. Umeoka S, Koyama T, Watanabe G, et al. Preoperative local staging of esophageal carcinoma using dual-phase contrast-enhanced imaging with multidetector row computed tomography: value of the arterial phase images. J Comput Assist Tomogr 2010;34(3):406–12.
68. Leers JM, DeMeester SR, Oezcelik A, et al. The prevalence of lymph node metastases in patients with T1 esophageal adenocarcinoma: a retrospective review of esophagectomy specimens. Ann Surg 2011;253(2):271–8.

69. Moorjani N, Junemann-Ramirez M, Judd O, et al. Endoscopic ultrasound in oesophageal carcinoma: comparison with multislice computed tomography and importance in the clinical decision making process. Minerva Chir 2007;62(4):217–23.

70. Pfau PR, Perlman SB, Stanko P, et al. The role and clinical value of EUS in a multimodality esophageal carcinoma staging program with CT and positron emission tomography. Gastrointest Endosc 2007;65(3):377–84.

71. Fekete F, Gayet B, Frija J. CT scanning in the diagnosis of oesophageal disease. In: Jamieson GG, editor. Surgery of the oesophagus. Edinburgh: Churchill Livingstone; 1988. p. 85–9.

72. Schnyder PA, Gamsu G. CT of the pretracheal retrocaval space. AJR Am J Roentgenol 1981;136:303–8.

73. Blackshaw G, Lewis WG, Hopper AN, et al. Prospective comparison of endosonography, computed tomography, and histopathological stage of junctional oesophagogastric cancer. Clin Radiol 2008;63(10):1092–8.

74. Takizawa K, Matsuda T, Kozu T, et al. Lymph node staging in esophageal squamous cell carcinoma: a comparative study of endoscopic ultrasonography versus computed tomography. J Gastroenterol Hepatol 2009;24(10):1687–91.

75. Chen J, Cheong JH, Yun MJ, et al. Improvement in preoperative staging of gastric adenocarcinoma with positron emission tomography. Cancer 2005;103:2383–90.

76. Mochiki E, Kuwano H, Katoh H, et al. Evaluation of ^{18}F-2-deoxy-2-fluoro-D-glucose positron emission tomography for gastric cancer. World J Surg 2004;28:247–53.

77. Stahl A, Ott K, Weber WA, et al. FDG PET imaging of locally advanced gastric carcinomas: correlation with endoscopic and histopathological findings. Eur J Nucl Med Mol Imaging 2003;30:288–95.

78. Yamada A, Oguchi K, Fukushima M, et al. Evaluation of 2-deoxy-2-[^{18}F]fluoro-D-glucose positron emission tomography in gastric carcinoma: relation to histological subtypes, depth of tumor invasion, and glucose transporter-1 expression. Ann Nucl Med 2006;20:597–604.

79. Alakus H, Batur M, Schmidt M, et al. Variable ^{18}F-fluorodeoxyglucose uptake in gastric cancer is associated with different levels of GLUT-1 expression. Nucl Med Commun 2010;31(6):532–8.

80. http:www.sign.ac.uk, website of SIGN, [accessed 10.10.12].

81. Blackstock AW, Farmer MR, Lovato J, et al. A prospective evaluation of the impact of 18-F-fluoro-deoxy-D-glucose positron emission tomography staging on survival for patients with locally advanced esophageal cancer. Int J Radiat Oncol Biol Phys 2006;64:455–60.

82. Heeren PA, Jager PL, Bongaerts F, et al. Detection of distant metastases in esophageal cancer with ^{18}F-FDG PET. J Nucl Med 2004;45:980–7.

83. Katsoulis IE, Wong WL, Mattheou AK, et al. Fluorine-18 fluorodeoxyglucose positron emission tomography in the preoperative staging of thoracic oesophageal and gastro-oesophageal junction cancer: a prospective study. Int J Surg 2007;5(6):399–403.

84. Lerut T, Flamen P. Role of FDG-PET scan in staging of cancer of the esophagus and gastroesophageal junction. Minerva Chir 2002;57(6):837–45.

85. Meltzer CC, Luketich JD, Friedman D, et al. Whole-body FDG positron emission tomographic imaging for staging esophageal cancer: comparison with computed tomography. Clin Nucl Med 2000;25:882–7.

86. van Westreenen HL, Westerterp M, Sloof GW, et al. Limited additional value of positron emission tomography in staging oesophageal cancer. Br J Surg 2007;94(12):1515–20.

87. Lowe VJ, Booya F, Fletcher JG, et al. Comparison of positron emission tomography, computed tomography, and endoscopic ultrasound in the initial staging of patients with esophageal cancer. Mol Imaging Biol 2005;7:422–30.

88. Himeno S, Yasuda S, Shimada H, et al. Evaluation of esophageal cancer by positron emission tomography. Jpn J Clin Oncol 2002;32:340–6.

89. Kato H, Miyazaki T, Nakajima M, et al. The incremental effect of positron emission tomography on diagnostic accuracy in the initial staging of esophageal carcinoma. Cancer 2005;103:148–56.

90. Sihvo EI, Rasanen JV, Knuuti MJ, et al. Adenocarcinoma of the esophagus and the esophagogastric junction: positron emission tomography improves staging and prediction of survival in distant but not in locoregional disease. J Gastrointest Surg 2004;8:988–96.

91. Flamen P, Lerut T, Haustermans K, et al. Position of positron emission tomography and other imaging diagnostic modalities in esophageal cancer. Q J Nucl Med Mol Imaging 2004;48:96–108.

92. Strauss LG. Fluorine-18 deoxyglucose and false-positive results: a major problem in the diagnostics of oncological patients. Eur J Nucl Med Mol Imaging 1996;23:1409–15.

93. Flanagan FL, Dehdashti F, Siegel BA. Staging of esophageal cancer with 18-F-fluorodexoglucose positron emission tomography. AJR Am J Roentgenol 1997;64:770–7.

94. McAteer D, Wallis F, Couper GW, et al. Evaluation of ^{18}F-FDG positron emission tomography in gastric and oesophageal cancer. Br J Radiol 1999;72:525–9.

95. van Westreenen HL, Westerterp M, Bossuyt PM, et al. Systematic review of the staging performance of ^{18}F-fluorodeoxyglucose positron emission tomography in esophageal cancer. J Clin Oncol 2004;22(18):3805–12.

96. Van Vliet EP, Heijenbrok-Kal MH, Hunink MG, et al. Staging investigations for oesophageal cancer: a meta-analysis. Br J Cancer 2008;3:547–57.

97. Bar-Shalom R, Guralnik L, Tsalic M, et al. The additional value of PET/CT over PET in FDG imaging of oesophageal cancer. Eur J Nucl Med Mol Imaging 2005;32(8):918–24.

98. Yuan S, Yu Y, Chao KS, et al. Additional value of PET/CT over PET in assessment of locoregional lymph nodes in thoracic esophageal squamous cell cancer. J Nucl Med 2006;47:1255–9.

99. Pollack BJ, Chak A, Sivak Jr. MV. Endoscopic ultrasonography. Semin Oncol 1996;23:336–46.

100. **Puli SR, Reddy JB, Bechtold ML, et al. How good is endoscopic ultrasound for TNM staging of gastric cancers? A meta-analysis and systematic review. World J Gastroenterol 2008;14(25):4011–9.**
Twenty-two studies involving 1896 patients with gastric cancer.

101. Sultan J, Robinson S, Hayes N, et al. Endoscopic ultrasonography-detected low-volume ascites as a predictor of inoperability for oesophagogastric cancer. Br J Surg 2008;95(9):1127–30.

102. Hwang SW, Lee DH, Lee SH, et al. Preoperative staging of gastric cancer by endoscopic ultrasonography and multidetector-row computed tomography. J Gastroenterol Hepatol 2010;25(3):512–8.

103. Kelly S, Harris K, Berry E, et al. A systematic review of the staging performance of endoscopic ultrasound in gastro-esophageal carcinoma. Gut 2001;49:534–9.

104. Smithers BM, Gotley DC, Martin I, et al. Comparison of the outcomes between open and minimally invasive esophagectomy. Ann Surg 2007;245(2):232–40.

105. Gines A, Cassivi SD, Martenson Jr. JA, et al. Impact of endoscopic ultrasonography and physician specialty on the management of patients with esophagus cancer. Dis Esophagus 2008;21(3): 241–50.

106. Puli SR, Reddy JB, Bechtold ML, et al. Staging accuracy of esophageal cancer by endoscopic ultrasound: a meta-analysis and systematic review. World J Gastroenterol 2008;14(10):1479–90.
This study analysed 49 studies comprising 2558 patients. It reported high accuracy rates for EUS for both T and N staging in patients with oesophageal cancer.

107. Heintz A, Höhne U, Schweden F, et al. Preoperative detection of intrathoracic tumour spread of esophageal cancer: endosonography versus computed tomography. Surg Endosc 1991; 5:75–8.

108. Hordijk ML, Zander H, van Blankenstein M, et al. Influence of tumour stenosis on the accuracy of endosonography in preoperative T staging of esophageal cancer. Endoscopy 1993;25:171–5.

109. Morgan MA, Twine CP, Lewis WG, et al. Prognostic significance of failure to cross esophageal tumors by endoluminal ultrasound. Dis Esophagus 2008;21(6):508–13.

110. Puli SR, Reddy JB, Bechtold ML, et al. Endoscopic ultrasound: its accuracy in evaluating mediastinal lymphadenopathy? A meta-analysis and systematic review. World J Gastroenterol 2008;14(19):3028–37.
A meta-analysis of 9310 patients with mediastinal lymphadenopathy demonstrating improved accuracy rates with the addition of EUS-FNA.

111. Omloo JM, van Heijl M, Smits NJ, et al. Additional value of external ultrasonography of the neck after CT and PET scanning in the preoperative assessment of patients with esophageal cancer. Dig Surg 2009;26(1):43–9.

112. Bressani Doldi S, Lattuada E, Zappa MA, et al. Ultrasonographic evaluation of the cervical lymph nodes in preoperative staging of eosphageal neoplasms. Abdom Imaging 1998;23:275–7.

113. Van Overhagen H, Lameris JS, Zonderland HM, et al. Ultrasound and ultrasound-guided fine needle aspiration biopsy of supraclavicular lymph nodes in patients with esophageal carcinoma. Cancer 1991;67:585–7.

114. Bonvalot S, Bouvard N, Lothaire P, et al. Contribution of cervical ultrasound and ultrasound fine-needle aspiration biopsy to the staging of thoracic oesophageal carcinoma. Eur J Cancer 1996;32A:893–5.

115. Van Vliet EP, van der Lugt A, Kuipers EJ, et al. Ultrasound, computed tomography, or the combination for the detection of supraclavicular lymph nodes in patients with esophageal or gastric cardia cancer: a comparative study. J Surg Oncol 2007;96(3):200–6.

116. Schreurs LM, Verhoef CC, van der Jagt EJ, et al. Current relevance of cervical ultrasonography in staging cancer of the esophagus and gastroesophageal junction. Eur J Radiol 2008;67(1):105–11.

117. Lightdale CJ. Endoscopic ultrasonography in the diagnosis, staging and follow-up of esophageal and gastric cancer. Endoscopy 1992;24:297–303.

118. De Graaf GW, Ayantunde AA, Parsons SL, et al. The role of staging laparoscopy in oesophagogastric cancers. Eur J Surg Oncol 2007;33(8):988–92.

119. Yau KK, Siu WT, Cheung HY, et al. Immediate preoperative laparoscopic staging for squamous cell carcinoma of the esophagus. Surg Endosc 2006;20(2):307–10.

120. Smith A, Finch MD, John TG, et al. Role of laparoscopic ultrasonography in the management of patients with oesophagogastric cancer. Br J Surg 1999;86:1083–7.

121. Molloy RG, McCourtney JS, Anderson JR. Laparoscopy in the management of patients with cancer of the gastric cardia and oesophagus. Br J Surg 1995;82:352–4.

122. Kapiev A, Rabin I, Lavy R, et al. The role of diagnostic laparoscopy in the management of patients with gastric cancer. Isr Med Assoc J 2010;12(12):726–8.

123. Rao B, Hunerbein M. Diagnostic laparoscopy: indications and benefits. Langenbecks Arch Surg 2005;390(3):187–96.

124. Nekarda H, Gess C, Stark M, et al. Peritoneal cytology. Immunocytochemically detected free peritoneal tumour cells (FPTC) are a strong prognostic factor in gastric carcinoma. Br J Cancer 1999;79(3–4):611–9.

125. Nakagohri T, Yoneyama Y, Kinoshita T, et al. Prognostic significance of peritoneal washing cytology in patients with potentially resectable gastric cancer. Hepatogastroenterology 2008;55(86–87):1913–5.

126. Fukagawa T, Katai H, Saka M, et al. Significance of lavage cytology in advanced gastric cancer patients. World J Surg 2010;34(3):563–8.

127. Mezhir JJ, Shah MA, Jacks LM, et al. Positive peritoneal cytology in patients with gastric cancer: natural history and outcome of 291 patients. Ann Surg Oncol 2010;17(12):3173–80.

128. Lorenzen S, Panzram B, Rosenberg R, et al. Prognostic significance of free peritoneal tumor cells in the peritoneal cavity before and after neoadjuvant chemotherapy in patients with gastric carcinoma undergoing potentially curative resection. Ann Surg Oncol 2010;17(10):2733–9.

This study demonstrated changes in the positivity of peritoneal washings in patients with gastric cancer receiving neoadjuvant chemotherapy.

129. Anderson DN, Campbell S, Park KG. Accuracy of laparoscopic ultrasonography in the staging of upper gastrointestinal malignancy. Br J Surg 1997;84:580.

130. Finch MD, John TG, Garden OJ, et al. Laparoscopic ultrasonography for staging gastroesophageal cancer. Surgery 1997;121:10–7.

131. Richardson W, Stefanidis D, Mittal S, et al. SAGES guidelines for the use of laparoscopic ultrasound. Surg Endosc 2010;24(4):745–56.

132. Kwee RM, Kwee TC. Imaging in local staging of gastric cancer: a systematic review. J Clin Oncol 2007;25(15):2107–16.

133. Anzidei M, Napoli A, Zaccagna F, et al. Diagnostic performance of 64-MDCT and 1.5-T MRI with high-resolution sequences in the T staging of gastric cancer: a comparative analysis with histopathology. Radiol Med 2009;114(7):1065–79.

134. Wu LF, Wang BZ, Feng JL, et al. Preoperative TN staging of esophageal cancer: comparison of miniprobe ultrasonography, spiral CT and MRI. World J Gastroenterol 2003;9:219–24.

135. Herth F, Ernst A, Schulz M, et al. Endobronchial ultrasound reliably differentiates between airway infiltration and compression by tumor. Chest 2003;123(2):458–62.

136. Osugi H, Nishimura Y, Takemura M, et al. Bronchoscopic ultrasonography for staging supracarinal esophageal squamous cell carcinoma: impact on outcome. World J Surg 2003;27(5):590–4.

137. Wakamatsu T, Tsushima K, Yasuo M, et al. Usefulness of preoperative endobronchial ultrasound for airway invasion around the trachea: esophageal cancer and thyroid cancer. Respiration 2006;73(5):651–7.

138. Geh JI, Crellin AM, Glynne-Jones R. Preoperative chemoradiotherapy in oesophageal cancer. Br J Surg 2001;88:338–56.

139. Zhang X, Shen L, Li J, et al. A phase II trial of paclitaxel and cisplatin in patients with advanced squamous-cell carcinoma of the esophagus. Am J Clin Oncol 2008;31(1):29–33.

140. Ilson DH. Oesophageal cancer: new developments in systemic therapy. Cancer Treat Rev 2003;29:525–32.

141. Di Fiore F, Lecleire S, Pop D, et al. Baseline nutritional status is predictive of response to treatment and survival in patients treated by definitive chemoradiotherapy for a locally advanced esophageal cancer. Am J Gastroenterol 2007;102(11):2557–63.

142. Brown WA, Thomas J, Gotley D, et al. Use of oesophagogastroscopy to assess the response of oesophageal carcinoma to neoadjuvant therapy. Br J Surg 2004;91(2):199–204.

143. Jost C, Binek J, Schuller JC, et al. Endosonographic radial tumor thickness after neoadjuvant chemoradiation therapy to predict response and survival in patients with locally advanced esophageal cancer: a prospective multicenter phase II study by the Swiss Group for Clinical Cancer Research (SAKK 75/02). Gastrointest Endosc 2010;71(7):1114–21.

144. Jones DR, Parker LA, Detterbeck FC, et al. Inadequacy of computed tomography in assessing patients with esophageal carcinoma after induction chemoradiotherapy. Cancer 1999;85:1026–32.

145. Griffith JF, Chan AC, Chow LT, et al. Assessing chemotherapy response of squamous cell oesophageal carcinoma with spiral CT. Br J Radiol 1999;72:678–84.

146. Younes M, Lechago LV, Somoano JR. Wide expression of the human erythrocyte glucose transporter Glut1 in human cancers. Cancer Res 1996;56:1164–7.

147. Warburg O. On the origin of cancer cells. Science 1956;123:309–14.

148. Couper GW, McAteer D, Wallis F, et al. The detection of response to chemotherapy using positron emission tomography in patients with oesophageal and gastric cancer. Br J Surg 1998;85:1403–6.

149. Brucher BL, Weber W, Bauer M, et al. Neoadjuvant therapy of esophageal squamous cell carcinoma: response evaluation by positron emission tomography. Ann Surg 2001;233(3):300–9.

150. Weber WA, Ott K, Becker K, et al. Prediction of response to preoperative chemotherapy in adenocarcinomas of the esophagogastric junction by metabolic imaging. J Clin Oncol 2001;19(12):3058–65.

151. Kato H, Kuwano H, Nakajima M, et al. Usefulness of positron emission tomography for assessing the response of neoadjuvant chemoradiotherapy in patients with esophageal cancer. Am J Surg 2002;184(3):279–83.

152. Flamen P, Van Cutsem E, Lerut A, et al. Positron emission tomography for assessment of the response to induction radiochemotherapy in locally advanced oesophageal cancer. Ann Oncol 2002;13(3):361–8.

153. Downey RJ, Akhurst T, Ilson D, et al. Whole body 18FDG-PET and the response of esophageal cancer to induction therapy: results of a prospective trial. J Clin Oncol 2003;21(3):428–32.

154. Lordick F, Ott K, Krause BJ, et al. PET to assess early metabolic response and to guide treatment of adenocarcinoma of the oesophagogastric junction: the MUNICON phase II trial. Lancet Oncol 2007;8(9):797–805.

155. Boonstra JJ, Kok TC, Wijnhoven BP, et al. Chemotherapy followed by surgery versus surgery alone in patients with resectable oesophageal squamous cell carcinoma: long-term results of a randomised controlled trial. BMC Cancer 2011;11:181.

156. Kim TJ, Kim HY, Lee KW, et al. Multimodality assessment of esophageal cancer: preoperative staging and monitoring of response to therapy. Radiographics 2009;29(2):403–21.

157. Cerfolio RJ, Bryant AS, Ohja B, et al. The accuracy of endoscopic ultrasonography with fine-needle aspiration, integrated positron emission tomography with computed tomography, and computed tomography in restaging patients with esophageal cancer after neoadjuvant chemoradiotherapy. J Thorac Cardiovasc Surg 2005;129(6):1232–41.

158. Smithers BM, Couper GW, Watts N, et al. Positron emission tomography and pathological evidence of response to neoadjuvant therapy in adenocarcinoma of the oesophagus. Dis Esophagus 2008;21(2):151–8.

159. Schmidt M, Bollschweiler E, Dietlein M, et al. Mean and maximum standardized uptake values in [^{18}F]FDG-PET for assessment of histopathological response in oesophageal squamous cell carcinoma or adenocarcinoma after radiochemotherapy. Eur J Nucl Med Mol Imaging 2009;36(5):735–44.

160. Vallbohmer D, Holscher AH, Schneider PM, et al. [^{18}F]-Fluorodeoxyglucose-positron emission tomography for the assessment of histopathologic response and prognosis after completion of neoadjuvant chemotherapy in gastric cancer. J Surg Oncol 2010;102(2):135–40.

161. Kato H, Miyazaki T, Nakajima M, et al. Sentinel lymph nodes with technetium-99m colloidal rhenium sulfide in patients with esophageal carcinoma. Cancer 2003;98(5):932–9.

162. Lamb PJ, Griffin SM, Burt AD, et al. Sentinel node biopsy to evaluate the metastatic dissemination of oesophageal adenocarcinoma. Br J Surg 2005;92:60–7.

163. Kosugi S, Nakagawa S, Kanda T, et al. Radio-guided sentinel node mapping in patients with superficial esophageal carcinoma: feasibility study. Minim Invasive Ther Allied Technol 2007;16:181–6.

164. Takeuchi H, Fujii H, Ando N, et al. Validation study of radio-guided sentinel lymph node navigation in esophageal cancer. Ann Surg 2009;249:757–63.

165. Grotenhuis BA, Wijnhoven BP, van Marion R, et al. The sentinel node concept in adenocarcinomas of the distal esophagus and gastroesophageal junction. J Thorac Cardiovasc Surg 2009;138:608–12.

166. Dresner SM, Lamb PJ, Bennett MK, et al. The pattern of metastatic lymph node dissemination from adenocarcinoma of the esophagogastric junction. Surgery 2001;129:103–9.

167. Liu CG, Lu P, Lu Y, et al. Distribution of solitary lymph nodes in primary gastric cancer: a retrospective study and clinical implications. World J Gastroenterol 2007;13(35):4776–80.

168. Kunisaki C, Shimada H, Nomura M, et al. Distribution of lymph node metastasis in gastric carcinoma. Hepatogastroenterology 2006;53(69):468–72.

169. Bangor University. Cancer of the oesophagus or gastricus: new assessment of the technology of endosonography (Cognate). Available at http://www.bangor.ac.uk/imscar/cognate/trialsummary; [accessed 12.09.12].
The results of this multicentre randomised trial are awaited and should provide guidance on the current role of EUS.

4

Preoperative assessment and perioperative management in oesophageal and gastric surgery

Sheraz R. Markar
James Helman
Donald E. Low

Introduction

Perioperative management strategies have been shown to be important in postoperative outcome following oesophageal and gastric surgery.[1] Structured pre- and perioperative management has also been shown to have an important role in outcome from a number of other major surgical procedures.[2] The overriding principle of preoperative assessment is to identify comorbidities that may complicate the patient's operative intervention and perioperative recovery. Identification, recognition and treatment of these comorbidities allow the patient to be optimised prior to undergoing surgery in an effort to reduce the incidence of perioperative mortality and postoperative complications.

There is continual advancement in medical therapy and surgical technology for the treatment of oeophagogastric malignancy, including advances in chemotherapy, radiotherapy and endoscopic therapy. This increased diversity in therapeutic approach makes the decision regarding patient selection for surgical resection a complex interaction between patient (i.e. premorbid status) and disease characteristics (i.e. tumour stage). This range in available therapies increases the desirability of individualising the approach according to these issues.

Perioperative management is another critical factor that can have a significant impact upon clinical outcome following oesophagectomy or gastrectomy.[3] This includes selection of surgical and anaesthetic techniques, methodology of intraoperative monitoring, minimising blood losses and perioperative fluid management, as well as lung isolation techniques and intraoperative organ support. Thus, although surgical technique plays an important role in determining outcome following oesophagectomy and gastrectomy, it remains only one variable amongst many others that play a significant part.[4]

Recently the role of the multidisciplinary team has become increasingly important in the care of this complex cohort of patients. A collaborative approach fosters an open dialogue between surgeons, anaesthetists, oncologists, radiologists, cancer specialist as well as ward nurses, nutritionists, physiotherapists and critical care teams. This dialogue allows the patient to work with highly specialised medical professionals and ideally be included in validated clinical pathways, in order to provide a high-quality service and successful outcome.[5] In this chapter, we will review some of the governing principles of preoperative assessment and perioperative management in the context of oesophagogastric surgery, and examine recent developments in this field.

Physiological stress during the treatment of oesophagogastric malignancy

The multimodal nature of treatment of oesophagogastric malignancy imparts significant physiological stress. There are specific issues that can affect a patient's tolerance to treatment. These issues classically include cardiac and pulmonary reserve, renal function and any other conditions that limit patient mobility and the potential for patients complying with standardised postoperative goals. Clinical outcome following major surgery involves interplay between patient characteristics (e.g. comorbidities), disease characteristics (e.g. tumour stage, grade and cell type), choice of treatment modality (e.g. surgery, chemotherapy, radiotherapy or combination of several modalities) and postoperative recovery.[6,7] The results and interpretation of preoperative testing may affect a patient's treatment course at multiple levels. Thus the goal of preoperative assessment is to identify relevant risk factors in patients, in order to provide a tailored patient-centred approach to the management of oesophagogastric malignancy.

Surgical resection is one modality in the treatment of oesophagogastric malignancy and remains the most commonly applied approach in physiologically appropriate patients with early and locoregional cancer. Surgery does, however, involve a significant physiological challenge.[8] Prolonged operations with blood loss and fluid shifts, large thoracic and abdominal incisions, extensive lymph node and tissue dissection around vital organs, and the potential requirement for single lung ventilation are some of the intraoperative factors that can place significant strain upon the cardiorespiratory system of the patient undergoing surgery.[9] Adjunctive therapy, including chemo- and radiotherapy in selected patients, can also result in significant physiological impact.[10,11] Prediction of patients with sufficient reserve to undergo multimodality therapies is the most important factor when assigning a treatment approach.

Diagnosis

The diagnosis of gastro-oesophageal malignancy is based on a good clinical history and examination, with the utilisation of appropriate further investigations.

✔ Clinical assessment undertaken at primary care consultation must highlight important symptoms including dysphagia and odynophagia to trigger further investigation. Studies have shown that an under-appreciation of the importance of dysphagia in younger patients can lead to a delay in presentation and an advanced tumour stage, resulting in a poorer prognosis in younger patients.[12,13]

Standard staging investigations for oesophagogastric malignancy (Box 4.1) include endoscopy, endoscopic ultrasound (EUS), computerised tomography (CT) and positron emission tomography (PET) with or without staging laparoscopy (for oesophagogastric junctional, cardial or gastric tumours). Among the currently available staging modalities, EUS is considered the best for T stage and assessment of regional lymph nodes, whereas PET is the most accurate for the detection of distant nodal and metastatic spread.[14] Apart from being increasingly useful in initial staging of oesophageal cancer, [18F]fluorodeoxyglucose positron emission tomography (FDG-PET) scanning has been identified as a potential tool for assessing the therapeutic response after neoadjuvant therapy and detection of recurrent malignancy.[15,16]

Box 4.1 • Oesophagogastric cancer diagnostic and staging investigations

- Endoscopy
- Endoscopic ultrasound
- Computerised tomography
- Positron emission tomography
- Staging laparoscopy

It is the combination of the results of these investigations assessing tumour characteristics and further investigations to evaluate patient comorbidities that will guide decisions regarding suitable patient-centred treatment pathways.

Multidisciplinary team evaluation

Patients referred for specialist oesophagogastric treatment are reviewed and discussed by the multidisciplinary team (MDT). This consists of a lead clinician (often a surgeon or a medical specialist in oncology), medical and clinical oncologists, radiologist (may have an interest in interventional radiology), histopathologist, specialist nurses and MDT coordinators. Other members of the MDT may include gastroenterologists, dieticians, palliative care nurses, intensivists and anaesthetists. MDT discussion allows presentation of the radiological and histopathological findings in the context of patients' physical assessment, functional reserve, mental and nutritional status, and social support network.

The MDT has become the cornerstone of cancer treatment in order to provide an unbiased and evidence-based approach to treatment of malignancy. The role of the cancer specialist nurse is critical in providing a means of communication with the patient and family, in order to ascertain their expectations from treatment along with further information regarding social and support networks. In our centre this initial comprehensive interview takes place before travel to the speciality centre and is routinely recognised as valuable in patient satisfaction surveys. This initial communication includes providing specific information regarding the make-up of the care team, required investigations and potential treatment options. This also provides a contact person (key worker) within the clinical team for the patient and family.

✔ Centralisation of oesophagogastric cancer treatment has further improved the opportunities for informed multidisciplinary discussion through increasing specialisation and higher volume centres, resulting in improved clinical outcomes.[17,18] This has in turn led to increased recruitment to clinical trials, a process that has been further facilitated by the presence of clinical oncologists as part of the MDT discussion.

Neoadjuvant therapy

Patient assessment and selection in the appropriate clinical context is crucial given the increasing use of neoadjuvant therapies in the treatment of oesophageal malignancy. The treatment of gastro-oesophageal cancer is no longer as simple as ensuring a safe passage through oesophagectomy or gastrectomy. MDT discussion allows formulation of a plan based on evidence-based principles including surgery with or without neoadjuvant therapies, given the premorbid status of the patient and characteristics of the tumour. Assessment of physiological issues is important because although some patients may benefit from multimodality therapy, some will not be fit enough.

Radiotherapy

Several studies have demonstrated a survival benefit in the use of neoadjuvant chemoradiotherapy in oesophageal cancer.[19,20] Although this combination therapy has been shown to be effective, it may result in a significant physiological impact on the patient.[21] Changes in myocardial perfusion have been reported following chemoradiotherapy for oesophageal malignancy.[22] Hence it is important to identify patients with cardiac comorbidities and impaired preoperative cardiac testing that may be more at risk from resultant myocardial ischaemia. Respiratory reserve as measured by pulmonary function testing can also be adversely affected by the use of thoracic radiotherapy.[23] Some chemotherapeutic agents, including 5-fluorouracil and cisplatin, have a radiosensitising effect by decreasing the ability of DNA damage repair mechanisms, thus potentiating both therapeutic and toxic effects of radiotherapy.[24] This illustrates the importance of reassessment following completion of neoadjuvant therapy, prior to undertaking surgical resection of the gastro-oesophageal cancer. Timing of surgery around neoadjuvant chemoradiotherapy is also an important consideration as in our institution we would recommend surgery 4–6 weeks following the cessation of radiotherapy; however, surgery within 4–10 weeks would be acceptable.

Chemotherapy

Previous studies have shown a clear benefit to the use of adjunctive chemotherapy in the treatment of advanced stage oesophagogastric malignancy.[25] Chapter 9 will discuss in more detail the merits of chemotherapy in this disease. However, it is important to note that chemotherapeutic agents can cause significant side-effects, including vomiting, bleeding, malnutrition, compromised immunity, etc. Thus patients undergoing neoadjuvant chemotherapy must be re-evaluated from a physiological and immunological standpoint prior to undergoing surgical resection.

Nutrition

Nutritional assessment and optimisation is a cornerstone of good pre- and perioperative care in cancer surgery. Preoperative malnutrition and associated immunosuppression have been shown to be well correlated with septic complications and mortality following oesophageal cancer surgery.[26] The mechanism of malnutrition (Box 4.2) is often related to dysphagia, disease cachexia or neoadjuvant chemotherapy. Nutritional assessment should be a component of the MDT review.

The relative merits of enteral over parenteral methods of feeding in the malnourished patient have been the subject of debate for several years. The proposed benefits of enteral feeding include improved gut oxygenation, colonisation with gut flora serving to reduce septic complications and a reduced cost compared to parenteral feeding.[27] There are several potential approaches to enteral feeding (Box 4.3).

Box 4.2 • Definition of malnutrition

- Body mass index (BMI) <18.5 kg/m^2
- Unintentional weight loss of >10% within the last 3–6 months
- BMI <20 kg/m^2 and unintentional weight loss >5% within the last 3–6 months

Box 4.3 • Approaches to enteral feeding

- **Jejunal feeds:** nasojejunal tube, surgical or interventional radiologically placed jejunal tubes
- **Stomach feeds:** percutaneous gastrostomy (PEG) – not advisable due to potential compromise of the gastric conduit
- **Endoscopic removable temporary stents:**[28] self-expanding plastic (SEPS) or metal (SEMS) stents

Nasojejunal feeding is often poorly tolerated for long periods by patients and thus is not routinely used at our institution. Radiologically placed jejunal tubes also suffer from complications, including perforation of other abdominal viscera during placement and slippage. Thus we advocate surgical placement of feeding jejunal tubes either by an open or a laparoscopic approach. We often combine this procedure with other procedures such as subcutaneous port placement or diagnostic laparoscopy.

At the time of surgery many surgeons would advocate the routine placement of a feeding jejunostomy to ensure nutrition through the perioperative period and allow a more measured approach to reinstating oral nutrition. This can simplify discharge and avoid postoperative problems during the critical healing period, as in our patients jejunal tube feeding is initiated on postoperative day 1. It is important to emphasise that feeding jejunostomies can still be associated with complications in a proportion of cases,[28] which should be discussed with the patient prior to placement. In our own experience, we have found that placing a large 14Fr feeding tube decreases problems with tube obstructions.

Although percutaneous endoscopic gastrostomy (PEG) feeding provides a good method of nutritional supplementation, in oesophageal cancer patients it may compromise the gastric conduit used in surgery. In recent years the development of endoscopic stents has served as a well-tolerated treatment modality to bypass obstructing oesophageal lesions and allow oral enteral feeding either for preoperative optimisation or as a palliative measure. However, despite these benefits, fully covered oesophageal self-expanding metal stents (SEMS) are associated with an increased risk of migration (6–43.8%)[29] that may significantly impact upon the patient's nutritional status and surgical resection. Furthermore, many clinical oncologists are hesitant to use radiotherapy in a patient with an oesophageal metal stent. Thus the future of stents as a nutritional bridge during neoadjuvant therapy remains inconclusive, with further studies required.

The role of the dietician or nutritionist in optimising perioperative nutrition is important in ensuring that the short- and long-term nutritional requirements of these patients are met. Current practice suggests that most centres employ a dedicated specialised gastrointestinal dietician who will nutritionally assess patients daily in the postoperative period.

Preoperative assessment

In general terms, the most familiar and simple classification of preoperative physical status and risk is that of the American Society of Anesthesiologists (ASA) (Table 4.1). Although the correlation of ASA grade with perioperative risk has limitations, it does provide a useful global assessment tool and its use is universal and familiar. Several other clinical risk indices have been developed, including the Eastern Cooperative Oncology Group (ECOG) performance status, the Karnofsky performance scale index and the Charlson comorbidity index. ECOG performance status allows assessment of the effect of oesophagogastric cancer on the daily living abilities of the patient. The Karnofsky performance scale index allows patients to be classified by their functional impairment, in a similar manner to the ECOG score. The Charlson comorbidity index predicts the 10-year mortality for a patient who may have a range of comorbid conditions such as heart disease, AIDS or cancer (22 conditions in total). This index allows quantitative scoring of a patient's comorbidities and may provide a useful tool in the preoperative assessment.

Cardiac assessment (Box 4.4)

As described previously, oesophagectomy or gastrectomy places significant physiological stress upon the cardiovascular system. Up to 10% of patients undergoing oesophagectomy will have a significant cardiovascular complication.[30] Furthermore, with increasing oesophagogastric surgery being undertaken in the elderly population, accurate

Table 4.1 • The American Society of Anesthesiologists' assessment of physical status

Grade	Definition
ASA 1	Normal healthy patient
ASA 2	Patient with mild systemic disease
ASA 3	Patient with a severe systemic disease that limits activity but is not incapacitating
ASA 4	Patient with incapacitating disease that is a constant threat to life
ASA 5	Moribund patient not expected to survive 24 hours with or without surgery

Box 4.4 • Cardiac preoperative investigations

- **History** – including functional capacity
- **Electrocardiogram (ECG)** – identifies electric conductional abnormalities
- **Stress testing** – exercise, pharmacological, echocardiography or radioisotope investigation and cardiopulmonary exercise testing (CPX)

identification of patients at risk from cardiovascular complications (associated with ischaemia or dysrhythmia) can help guide treatment planning.

History

A thorough history and appropriate clinical examination will help identify major cardiovascular risk factors. These include ischaemic heart disease, valvular abnormalities, arrhythmias, heart failure, etc. Ischaemic heart disease has been identified as a crucial risk factor predicting severe complications following major surgery.[31] Identification of atrial or ventricular tachyarrhythmias can also help identify patients at risk for the most common postoperative complication, atrial fibrillation. Any pertinent findings will help guide further investigations that may be required, including a full cardiology assessment prior to undertaking major surgery.

Functional capacity

Exercise capacity provides a useful measure of functional cardiorespiratory reserve. Poor exercise tolerance correlates with an increased risk of perioperative complications that are independent of age and other patient characteristics.[32] However, the ability to climb a flight of stairs does not preclude a patient from having underlying cardiorespiratory disease, and prior to undertaking surgery the majority of oesophagogastric surgeons and most anaesthetists would advocate the use of further cardiac investigation in all elderly patients or patients with multiple risk factors. In the absence of an agreed protocol, exercise testing for oesophagogastric cancer surgery patients remains an important consideration during preoperative evaluation; however, it should not be used as the sole criterion for denying a patient an operation.

Investigations (Box 4.4)

Electrocardiogram (ECG)

ECG is the most basic objective cardiac assessment, usually as part of any preoperative work-up prior to major surgery. It remains a useful baseline test to identify electric conductional abnormalities within the heart that may indicate further structural abnormalities that warrant further investigations. Patients with no prior history of cardiac disease but with an abnormal ECG represent a group that must undergo a higher level of investigation and are potentially amenable to intervention and risk reduction prior to surgery.

Cardiopulmonary exercise testing (CPX)

The relative merit of cardiopulmonary exercise testing in the setting of oesophagogastric surgery remains controversial. Some surgeons propose the view that CPX testing is expensive, time-consuming and unreliable for the prediction of cardiorespiratory complications following oesophagectomy or gastrectomy. The literature on this subject also fails to resolve the debate. In a retrospective cohort study, Nagamatsu et al.[33] divided patients into two groups based on the presence or absence of cardiopulmonary complications. Nagamatsu et al. found significant differences between the two groups in their preoperative VO_{2max} ($P < 0.001$) and anaerobic threshold (AT; $P < 0.001$). In the follow-up to this study, Nagamatsu et al.[34] performed a retrospective study of CPX testing in 91 patients who underwent radical oesophagectomy with three-field lymphadenectomy. They found VO_{2max} closely correlated with the occurrence of postoperative cardiopulmonary complications. On the basis of their results, Nagamatsu et al. chose a minimally acceptable value of 800 mL/m^2 for the VO_{2max} for patients undergoing curative transthoracic oesophagectomy. Forshaw et al.[35] undertook a similar study to determine the usefulness of CPX testing before oesophagectomy in a cohort of 78 patients. The study demonstrated there was a significantly reduced VO_{2peak} ($P = 0.04$) and a non-significant trend towards a reduced AT ($P = 0.07$), in patients who developed postoperative cardiopulmonary complications following oesophagectomy. Areas under the curve for AT and VO_{2peak} were 0.63 and 0.62, respectively, suggesting that CPX testing did not perform well in predicting postoperative cardiopulmonary complications.

Stress testing

Cardiac stress testing is a well-validated non-invasive modality that has been shown to accurately predict patients at risk of cardiac complications following non-cardiac surgery.[36] In addition, stress testing has been shown to identify patients with inducible ischaemia that may benefit from preoperative beta-blockade.[37] Preoperative non-invasive stress testing has been recommended for patients with cardiac risk factors (Table 4.2) by the American College of Cardiology and American Heart Association guidelines.[38] Exercise-induced hypotension is a sign of possible ventricular impairment secondary to coronary artery disease and warrants

Table 4.2 • Clinical predictors of increased perioperative cardiovascular risk (myocardial infarction, heart failure, death)

Classification	Predictor
Major	Unstable coronary syndromes: • Acute or Recent MI with evidence of important ischaemic risk by clinical symptoms or non-invasive study • Unstable or severe angina (Canadian class III or IV) Decompensated heart failure Significant arrythmias: • High-grade atrioventricular block • Symptomatic ventricular arrhythmias in the presence of underlying heart disease • Supraventricular arrhythmias with uncontrolled ventricular rate Severe valvular disease
Intermediate	Mild angina pectoris (Canadian Class I or II) Previous myocardial infarction by history or pathological Q waves Compensated or prior heart failure Diabetes mellitus (particularly insulin dependent) Renal insufficiency
Minor	Advanced age Abnormal ECG (left ventricular hypertrophy, left bundle branch block, ST-T abnormalities) Rhythm other than sinus (e.g. atrial fibrillation) Low functional capacity (e.g. inability to climb one flight of stairs with a bag of groceries) History of stroke Uncontrolled systemic hypertension

further investigation with a coronary angiogram or myocardial perfusion imaging. Several exercise methods for cardiac stress testing exist, including stair climbing, treadmill and shuttle walk testing. Further investigation in patients who are unable to complete exercise testing due to reduced mobility secondary musculoskeletal disease may include pharmacological to stress testing. Commonly used pharmacological agents include adenosine, dipyridamole, dobutamine and propanolol. The choice of pharmacological drug used in stress testing usually depends upon potential drug interactions with other treatments and concomitant diseases. Cardiac stress echocardiography and radioisotope investigation (to measure cardiac perfusion) are also used to provide a more detailed cardiac assessment. The identification of reduced left ventricular ejection fraction by the latter modalities has been significantly associated with the development of cardiac complications following major surgery.[39]

Optimisation

Preoperative physical cardiopulmonary rehabilitation

Preoperative cardiopulmonary fitness has been shown to be well correlated with postoperative outcome following major surgery.[40] The use of intensive preoperative exercise has been shown to improve cardiopulmonary fitness prior to major surgery.[41] Although intensive preoperative exercise improves cardiopulmonary fitness, this short-term improvement has not been conclusively shown to correlate with postoperative outcome following major surgery and cancer resection.

Beta-blockade

ACC/AHA guidelines (2006) suggested that beta-blockers should be considered in all patients with an identifiable cardiac risk as determined by the presence of more than one clinical risk factor.[38] The hypothesis for this beneficial effect is that adrenergic beta-blockade slows the heart rate and as a result improves ischaemic ventricular dysfunction. Patients on long-term beta-blockade exhibit adrenergic hypersensitivity if the therapy is withdrawn and the intravenous route should be utilised until oral intake can be resumed. The cardioprotective effect of beta-blockers has been reported as persisting for up to 6 months following surgery, even after the cessation of therapy.[42] In order for beta-blockade therapy to be most effective, patients should be optimally blocked in the weeks preceding surgery and in the immediate postoperative period. Although not conclusively proven, it is believed that long-acting beta-blockers initiated before surgery are superior to shorter-acting agents.[38]

✔ The 2009 ACCF/AHA focused update on perioperative beta-blockade for non-cardiac surgery[43] states that beta-blockers titrated to heart rate and blood pressure are reasonable for patients in whom preoperative assessment identifies coronary artery disease or high cardiac risk, as defined by the presence of more than one clinical risk factor who are undergoing intermediate-risk surgery.[44] In addition, this update states: 'The usefulness of beta-blockers is uncertain for patients who are undergoing either intermediate-risk procedures or vascular surgery in whom preoperative assessment identifies a single clinical risk factor in the absence of coronary artery disease.'[45]

Other relevant cardiac medication

Statins

Current ACC/AHA guidelines on perioperative cardiovascular care recommend that patients should continue statin treatment throughout the perioperative period.[38] To date the evidence regarding the cardioprotective effects of statins in the perioperative period is controversial,[46] with no studies specifically in the setting of oesophagogastric surgery.

Anticoagulants

In performing oesophagogastric surgery on patients on anticoagulation, the major concern is when is it safe to perform surgery without increasing the risk of haemorrhage or increasing the risk of thromboembolism (e.g. venous, arterial) after discontinuing treatment.

Aspirin/clopidogrel

✔ Traditionally, patients are advised to stop aspirin or clopidogrel 7–10 days prior to undergoing major surgery. However, in the case of patients who have had a coronary stent placed within 6–12 months of oesophagogastric surgery, the advice of the American College of Chest Physicians is to continue aspirin or clopidogrel through the perioperative period,[47] which would be unacceptable to most oesophagogastric surgeons. Some surgeons are prepared to allow continuation of low-dose aspirin over the operative period but not clopidogrel.

Coronary stents include bare metal and drug-eluting stents, and their placement prior to surgery can significantly impact upon timing of surgical resection. Nuttall et al.[48] demonstrated an odds ratio of 3.6 for major cardiac events when surgery was performed within 30 days of bare metal stent placement, which was reduced to 1.6 when surgery was performed between 31 and 90 days. The available data suggest that 30 days should be the minimum interval between placement of a bare metal coronary stent and major non-cardiac surgery. Rabbits et al.[49] showed the risk of developing cardiac complications following drug-eluting stent placement is increased (6.4% vs. 3.3%) when surgery is performed within 365 days of stent placement. Thus it is clearly important to discuss the patient's perioperative plan with the consulting cardiologist prior to any percutaneous cardiac intervention or stent placement if a patient is being scheduled for major oesophagogastric surgery. The timing of when to restart anticoagulants is also a subject of debate, with little clear guidance currently present; however, in our institution we typically reinstitute aspirin on postoperative day 1 following oesophagectomy.

Warfarin

Patients on warfarin are typically told to stop this 4–5 days prior to undergoing major surgery, with the acquisition of an international normalised ratio (INR) assay on the day of surgery. Patients with mechanical heart valves, atrial fibrillation or venous thromboembolism should have an anticoagulation bridging plan with heparin for the perioperative period.[49] Patients who have recently sustained a venous thromboembolism should be considered for placement of temporary caval filters prior to radical surgery.

Pulmonary assessment

Oesophageal surgery has significant effects on pulmonary physiology that may predispose to complications. The incidence of postoperative pulmonary complications following oesophagogastric surgery ranges from 15.9% to 30%, with an associated increase in operative mortality.[50] Assessment of underlying pulmonary reserve is often recommended for identifying patients more likely to suffer from postoperative pulmonary problems, and then instituting effective aggressive preventative strategies including regular chest physiotherapy, early mobilisation and lung spirometry. For example, a patient with chronic obstructive pulmonary disease (COPD) and sputum retention should be identified as high risk preoperatively to allow the introduction of these preventative strategies early in the postoperative period; if not, this patient may require multiple therapeutic bronchoscopies in the postoperative period to treat mucus accumulation and lobar collapse.

History

A thorough history along with an appropriate examination will help identify pulmonary risk factors that will be important in the perioperative period. Risk factors for postoperative pulmonary complications include age, smoking status and physical activity levels.[51] Further pulmonary comorbidities that are important in the recovery following major surgery include COPD, asthma, pulmonary fibrosis or any further restrictive lung disease and previous pulmonary emboli. In the medication history it is important to specifically ask about the use of oral bronchodilator therapy that may be administered as a nebuliser in the postoperative period. Furthermore, the use of oral steroids will need consideration for cover with intravenous hydrocortisone during the perioperative period.

Investigations (Box 4.5)

Arterial blood gas (ABG)

Preoperative ABG sampling is commonly used in patients with pulmonary risk factors to gain an idea of baseline respiratory function. Patients with obstructive airway disease (COPD) may show evidence of carbon dioxide retention, which should be taken into account during the postoperative period. Patients with abnormal preoperative ABG results are more likely to suffer from postoperative pulmonary complications following major surgery.[52] Interpretation of ABG results in the context of clinical history and examination is important in ensuring optimal perioperative pulmonary care.

Chest X-ray (CXR)

Routine preoperative CXR is part of the work-up for most major surgical procedures. Results from a CXR are dependent upon interpretation by clinicians and subsequent action. Chronic disorders such as cardiomegaly and COPD can be detected in upto 65% of cases.[53] A preoperative CXR will elucidate obvious chest abnormalities; its greatest value may be as a comparison with postoperative films to act as a reference point.

Pulmonary function testing (PFT)

Preoperative PFT with spirometry in conjunction with clinical history and examination can be used to establish baseline lung function, evaluate dyspnoea, detect pulmonary disease, monitor effects of therapies used to treat respiratory disease, evaluate respiratory impairment and evaluate operative risk. Low forced expiratory volume in 1 second (FEV_1) or forced vital capacity (FVC) has been shown to be well correlated with postoperative pulmonary complications.[54] Abnormal PFT results will allow identification of patients at risk of postoperative pulmonary complications; this will enable targeted preventative strategies including chest physiotherapy, early mobilisation and lung spirometry to be employed in the perioperative period. However, routine pulmonary function testing can be time-consuming and expensive, and some surgeons would advocate a more measured approach, with PFTs being used in patients with pulmonary risk factors.

Box 4.5 • Pulmonary preoperative investigations

- **History** – including functional capacity
- **Arterial blood gas (ABG)** – gives a basic baseline respiratory function
- **Chest X-ray (CXR)** – identifies any obvious chest abnormalities
- **Pulmonary function testing (PFT)**

Optimisation

As discussed previously, the benefits of preoperative exercise or rehabilitation have been shown to improve cardiopulmonary fitness and postoperative outcome following major cancer resection. Identification of patients at risk from pulmonary complications may provide a justification for altering the method of surgical resection. Patients with very poor pulmonary function who previously would have been deemed unfit to undergo resection may benefit from a minimally invasive approach. Aggressive chest physiotherapy and early mobilisation may also help to reduce the incidence of pulmonary complications associated with oesophagogastric surgery in this cohort. There are several preoperative pulmonary risk factors that may be optimised in patients with impaired lung spirometry who are undergoing upper gastrointestinal surgery (Box 4.6).

Neurological assessment

History

Identification of patients with neurological risk factors is another crucial element of the preoperative global assessment. These risk factors include previous cerebrovascular accidents (CVAs),

Box 4.6 • Preoperative pulmonary risk-reduction strategies

- Cessation of cigarette smoking for a minimum of 8 weeks
- Aggressively treat airflow obstruction in patients with COPD or asthma
- Optimise haemoglobin concentration either with iron supplementation or transfusion if absolutely necessary
- Treat any respiratory tract infection with antibiotics, having first cultured the sputum
- Begin patient education regarding adequate exercise and lung expansion techniques with the assistance of a physiotherapist
- Encourage patient to lose weight if obese

transient ischaemic episodes (TIAs), epilepsy, dementia or cognitive decline and neuropsychiatric disorders. These factors can lead to severe neurological complications, including delirium, that may significantly impact upon postoperative recovery. The reported incidence of postoperative delirium following major surgery is highly variable, ranging from 9% to 53%, and more common in the elderly population.[55] Previous studies have also shown delirium to be significantly associated with a poor postoperative outcome following major surgery.[56] In our own institution delirium affects 9.2% of patients and is the second most common complication following oesophagectomy. Furthermore, delirium in our unit is associated with an increased incidence of postoperative pneumonia, pneumothorax, tracheal re-intubation, length of intensive care unit (ICU) and hospital stay, and increased overall cost.[57]

Investigations

Several risk factors for postoperative delirium have been identified previously, including age, dementia, functional impairment, depression, psychotropic drug use, increased comorbidity (cardiac, pulmonary, renal and neurological), laboratory abnormalities (electrolyte disturbance, anaemia and low albumin), preoperative visual impairment, hearing impairment, alcohol use, institutional residence and prior postoperative delirium. It is the accurate preoperative identification of these risk factors in vulnerable patients that will allow implementation of interventions to reduce delirium following major surgery.[58] Previous studies have attempted with variable success to produce risk scores that can be used to identify postoperative or hospitalised patients at risk from delirium.[59] Although creation and validation of these risk scores provides interesting academic points, often they are cumbersome and not designed for widespread clinical application. The presence of pre-existing dementia or cognitive impairment has been shown in a previous study[60] to have the strongest correlation with postoperative delirium. The Mini-Mental State Examination (MMSE) provides a means of a quick assessment of a patient's cognitive state at admission that may allow prediction of patients vulnerable to postoperative delirium.[60]

✔ The National Institute for Health and Clinical Excellence (NICE UK) has recently launched a new guideline that outlines several preventative strategies against delirium.[61] It describes the use of a multi-intervention package including assessment and modification of key clinical factors that may precipitate delirium.

Optimisation

The avoidance and treatment of postoperative delirium is a challenge, and thus prediction of vulnerable patients and employment of preventative strategies represent a more attractive option. More recent randomised trials have been aimed at designing multifaceted interventional programmes to prevent postoperative delirium, thus reducing length of hospital stay and mortality.[62] The most recent Cochrane review on 'Interventions for preventing delirium in hospitalised patients' highlighted the sparse nature of evidence regarding preventative measures against delirium. However, in the context of hip surgery there was a suggestion that proactive geriatric consultation and prophylactic low-dose haloperidol may reduce severity and duration of delirium episodes in vulnerable patients.[63] Specifically in the setting of oesophagectomy, bright light therapy or increased bright light exposure has been shown to be useful in reducing the incidence of postoperative delirium.[64]

Renal assessment

The presence of preoperative renal disease is a highly important factor that may impact upon postoperative outcome. This is illustrated by several risk scoring systems used to predict postoperative complications following major surgery, including renal disease as a variable, e.g Possum, APACHE II and Charlson scores. Due to improvements in perioperative care, patients with several medical comorbidities, including renal insufficiency, that previously may have been refused surgical intervention are now more likely to be considered for surgery. Thus the assessment and optimisation of preoperative renal disease will gain increasing importance due to the changing demographics of the population undergoing oesophagogastric surgery.

History

Patients may or may not be aware of pre-existing renal disease. However, in every elderly patient undergoing major surgery renal function should be assessed. Prior to the initiation of surgery, renal disease will influence many treatment modalities associated with oesophagogastric malignancy, including the use of certain medications, i.e. anti-inflammatory medications, radiological investigations, e.g. contrast use in CT scan, and neoadjuvant or adjuvant chemoradiotherapy.

Investigations

All patients undergoing major oesophagogastric surgery will have basic laboratory blood tests that should include markers of renal function, i.e. serum urea, creatinine and electrolytes. Together these results will identify the presence or absence of underlying renal insufficiency and the impact of this upon serum biochemistry and electrolyte disturbance.

✓ In the presence of previously undiagnosed severe renal impairment it would be prudent to investigate the aetiology to its conclusion, with renal imaging, e.g. ultrasound, MAG3 scan or renal biopsy. This is especially important when a conservative approach to fluid utilisation is considered in the perioperative period (see 'Fluid management' section below).

Optimisation

Previous studies have demonstrated that with good preoperative optimisation patients with impaired renal function can undergo gastrectomy with similar results to patients with a normal creatinine clearance.[65] Patients with severe renal impairment requiring dialysis are considered inappropriate surgical candidates for major oesophagogastric resection. Active involvement and consultation with a nephrologist will help guide perioperative management strategies, including fluid and electrolyte management, in this complex cohort of patients.

Anaesthetic technique

Thus far we have discussed a systems-based approach to preoperative assessment; in this next section we will move on to monitoring, assessment and control of intraoperative factors that may adversely affect outcome following oesophagogastric surgery.

Intraoperative monitoring

During major surgery traditionally, invasive adjuncts have formed the mainstay of intraoperative monitoring. More recently, anaesthetists are moving away from these invasive monitoring mechanisms, instead attempting to safely monitor a patient during major surgery using as minimally invasive monitoring mechanisms as possible without compromising safety. The aim of intraoperative monitoring should be to safely monitor patients' vital systems whilst they undergo a general anaesthetic for major surgery that can impact and attenuate the body's normal homeostatic mechanisms. Inadequate perfusion of the end-organs during major surgery not only increases the incidence of major complications, e.g. CVA, myocardial infarction and renal failure, but also may result in anastomotic or graft ischaemia and resultant leakage.

Cardiovascular system

Monitoring vital signs including heart rate and blood pressure can give clues as to a patient's intravascular volume, especially in challenging cases with significant blood loss. This monitoring can range from simple measures, including a blood pressure cuff and an oxygen saturation finger probe, to central venous lines and arterial lines. The advantages of central lines include venous access away from the operating field to allow anaesthetists to administer intravenous solutions without disturbing the operating procedure. These lines also allow monitoring of the central venous pressure, which can be used to guide fluid administration during the intra- and immediate postoperative period. These lines are not without complications, including infection, pneumothorax during insertion and venous thrombosis.

✓ We currently recommend the selective use of central lines in indicated cases with difficult venous access.

Arterial lines allow monitoring of the mean arterial pressure (MAP) to guide fluid administration during the intraoperative period. They also allow arterial blood to be sampled for blood gas analysis, to measure serum electrolytes, acid–base balance and lactate, that all give vital clues as to the status of vital organs. The complications of arterial lines include infection and thrombosis. Arterial lines do provide a useful intraoperative monitoring adjunct and we thus currently recommend their use in the majority of cases.

Renal system

From the measures described above, arterial blood gas monitoring allows measurement of serum electrolytes and lactate, both of which can indicate intraoperative renal impairment. The most common cause of renal impairment in a patient with no previous renal disease is renal hypoperfusion. Other causes include nephrotoxicity secondary to medication administered intraoperatively. Urinary catheterisation allows direct measurement of urinary output and an indirect measurement of renal function. This provides a less invasive approach to monitoring of renal function and is routinely used in all patients undergoing major oesophagogastric surgery.

Anaesthetic agents

✓ The effect of choice of anaesthetic agent upon inflammatory response and postoperative outcome following oesophagogastric surgery remains inconclusive.

Desflurane and sevoflurane have been shown to produce a reduced pulmonary inflammatory response and a decrease in the overall number of adverse events compared to propofol.[66] However, a more recent study suggested sevoflurane caused a greater inflammatory response than propofol during thoracic surgery.[67] These studies are limited by heterogeneity in patient demographics and comorbidities, along with duration of surgery and one-lung ventilation. Thus, although volatile anaesthetics produce dose- and time-dependent effects upon the inflammatory and immune systems, the nature of these effects in the setting of oesophagogastric surgery requires further investigation.

Airway management

Lung isolation techniques

Both gastric and oesophageal surgery can be performed in a patient intubated with a standard endotracheal tube. To allow intraoperative collapse of the right lung (during a two-stage transthoracic oesophagectomy), a left-sided double-lumen endobrochial tube is most commonly used (**Fig. 4.1**). It is crucial to ensure correct placement of the tube and recognise inadvertent upper lobe occlusion. Usually, endobrochial tube position is confirmed through auscultation of the chest and fibre-optic bronchoscopy.

Single lung ventilation (SLV) is commonly used in oesophageal surgery to facilitate dissection by operating surgeons by increasing the space available within the thoracic cavity. However, SLV has been shown to result in an inflammatory response, with the time period of SLV and surgical manipulation increasing alveolar injury and leucocyte recruitment in the dependent lung. During re-expansion of the collapsed lung, alveolar recruitment and reperfusion lung injury provide an additional source of lung injury.[68] Protective strategies aimed at reducing intraoperative lung injury include using small tidal volumes and positive end-expiratory pressure (PEEP) during SLV, and this has been shown to reduce the inflammatory response following oesophagectomy, improve lung function and result in early extubation.[69]

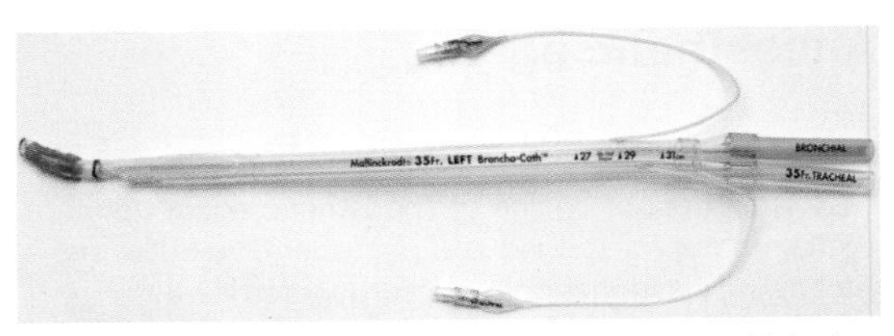

Figure 4.1 • Left-sided double-lumen endobronchial tube.

Endobronchial blockers (**Fig. 4.2**)

In some patients who are difficult to intubate in the presence of irregular dentition or limited temporomandibular joint movement, the use of a double-lumen endobronchial tube can be challenging due to its size. In this situation an endobronchial blocker passed fibre-optically through a single-lumen endotracheal tube may be beneficial to isolate the non-dependent lung. One important limitation to the routine use of endobronchial blockers is their tendency to migrate proximally or distally with mediastinal manipulation, resulting in sudden lung reinflation.

Timing of extubation

Immediate extubation following surgery has the advantage of giving the patient back control of their own respiratory system and allows them to begin their postoperative recovery immediately. In the past immediate extubation following major oesophagogastric surgery was not routinely considered. Furthermore, some patients with several respiratory comorbidities may require a measured approach to extubation. Patients with respiratory comorbidities are at greater risk from pulmonary complications and often require prolonged respiratory support.

✔ An operative approach that is individualised to patient and tumour characteristics, and based upon adhering to appropriate cancer principles with the minimising of blood loss and appropriate perioperative fluid administration, has allowed immediate extubation in up to 99.5% of cases following oesophagectomy.[70]

The benefits of early extubation have been clearly demonstrated, with reduced mortality and morbidity.[71] Early extubation has the additional benefit of reducing the requirement for postoperative ICU admission, instead allowing patients to be managed in a high-dependency setting and reducing overall cost. Postoperative extubation must be predicated on the basis of good pain control and is a prerequisite for early mobilisation.

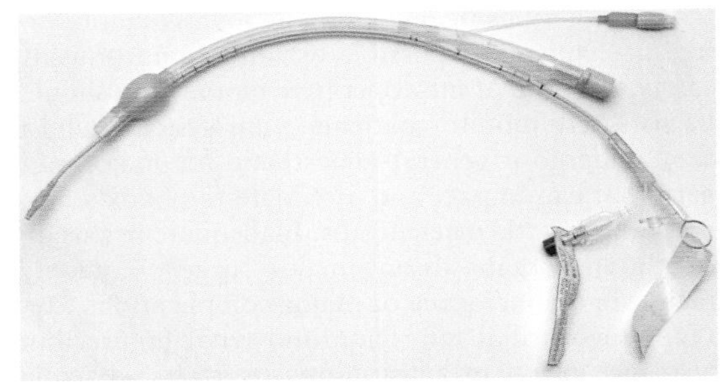

Figure 4.2 • Endobronchial blocker.

Fluid management

Perioperative fluid management involves a careful balance between maintaining perfusion pressure and oxygen delivery to vital organs and the newly fashioned anastomosis, and the prevention of excessive fluid accumulation that may delay recovery of gastrointestinal function, impair wound or anastomotic healing, and increase cardiac and respiratory complications.[72] Patients undergoing major oesophagogastric surgery have several sources of loss of fluid, including bowel preparation, dehydration secondary to tumour dysphagia, blood loss, insensible and nasogastric losses, wound exudation, urinary output, and evaporative fluid losses from open abdominal and chest cavities.

Recent publications have suggested that a more restrictive approach to fluid management during major surgery may be beneficial, with improved gastrointestinal recovery time and reduced respiratory complications.[73]

✔✔ Two studies have demonstrated the benefits associated with perioperative fluid restriction specifically in the setting of oesophagectomy.[74,75] Kita et al.[74] found that maintaining a central venous pressure of <5 mmHg and an adequate urinary output with intraoperative fluids administered at 4–5 mL/kg per hour resulted in reduced postoperative respiratory complications following oesophagectomy. Neal et al.[75] demonstrated a reduction in oesophagectomy-related morbidity by using a standardised multimodal management plan that included thoracic epidural analgesia, early extubation and avoidance of excessive intraoperative fluid administration.

Goal-directed fluid therapy includes minimising blood loss and maintaining haemodynamic stability, and this requires regular communication between surgeon and anaesthetic teams, i.e. during transhiatal dissection, where the blood pressure routinely decreases and anaesthetists typically respond by increasing fluid administration. In oesophagogastric surgery the monitoring of haemodynamic parameters is more challenging, as the most validated method remains oesophageal Doppler, the use of which is not possible in the context of oesophagectomy.[76] Other monitoring measures to allow goal-directed fluid administration include arterial lines to monitor arterial pressure variation and the FloTrach/Vigileo system (Edwards Lifesciences, Irvina, CA) to predict intravascular hypovolaemia.[77] Clear evidence and the optimal method for monitoring in goal-directed fluid therapy are yet to be determined; however, this approach to intraoperative fluid administration would appear to be beneficial in theory.

Postoperative analgesia

With inadequate postoperative pain relief patients are less likely to mobilise, take part in respiratory exercises and comply with standard postoperative goals. Hence the importance of good postoperative analgesia in the implementation and effectiveness of multimodality clinical pathways cannot be overstated.

Thoracic epidural analgesia for oesophagectomy has been shown to be a highly effective method of postoperative pain relief.[78] Furthermore, the proven benefits of thoracic epidural analgesia following oesophagectomy include earlier recovery of bowel function, reduced pulmonary complications and early extubation.[79] Further less well-validated benefits have been described, and these include reduced anastomotic leak and improved gastric conduit microcirculation.[80,81] However, aggressive epidural bolus dosing can reduce systolic arterial pressure and thus conduit perfusion. Measures to counteract this effect include changing rate of epidural and avoidance of bolusing, avoidance of hypovolaemia and the judicious use of vasopressor therapy.[82]

Epidural analgesia has been shown to be a highly effective method of reducing postoperative pain in gastrectomy.[83] Epidural analgesic therapies can vary between continuous infusions and patient-controlled analgesia (PCA). The advantages of the latter include subjective titration of a patient's pain and adequate treatment; however, usually a safety mechanism or lockout is in place to prevent the patient from overusing the PCA. Recent studies have suggested a combined regime of patient-controlled epidural analgesia during the day with a night-time infusion can help to reduce postoperative pain, and specifically pain associated with coughing, and provide a better sleep pattern.[84]

Other methods of effective postoperative analgesia following oesophagogastric surgery include intravenous patient-controlled analgesia and this is often the next line in the analgesic ladder following epidural analgesia. The main disadvantage of patient-controlled analgesia following major surgery is that it requires a well-orientated patient to be able to coordinate and administer their own pain relief. So in some situations the patient may not be able to do this, resulting in inadequate analgesia and increased risk of postoperative complications.

Extrapleural intercostal nerve blockade is another method of effective pain control following thoracotomy. An indwelling catheter may be left in the extrapleural space, most commonly during the operation, to allow the continuous infusion of local anaesthetic to the thoracotomy region. Extrapleural intercostal nerve blockade has been shown to be as effective as thoracic epidural analgesia in controlling thoracotomy-related pain and allowing recovery of pulmonary function in a randomised controlled trial.[85] Despite these benefits, extrapleural intercostal nerve blockade has yet to gain widespread acceptance, with thoracic epidural analgesia remaining the perceived gold standard for pain control following thoracotomy.

Oesophagogastric clinical pathways

The implementation of a clinical pathway for oesophagogastric cancer requires the personal commitment of all members of the care team and will impact a patient's treatment at virtually every stage; these individuals and teams should be involved in formulating and adapting the clinical pathway.

✔ Key players in the implementation of clinical pathways include:

- oesophagogastric cancer nurse specialist;
- oesophagogastric surgeons;
- anaesthetist;
- recovery room staff;
- pain service;
- ICU and ward nursing;
- physical therapy;
- dieticians;
- social service team;
- surgical trainees.

These pathways should be reassessed and updated every 24–36 months to allow continued re-evaluation of goals by the entire team and to look for areas in which outcomes can be improved over time. It is important to understand that clinical pathways are not limited to the postoperative period, but instead a good pathway will begin at the time of initial consultation and support a patient's journey and goals until treatment has been completed.

Preoperative

In our institution this process begins at the time of initial telephone interview between the patient and the oesophagogastric nurse specialist within 48 hours of referral. This telephone interview will include a review of the patient's past medical history, their current symptoms (swallowing and weight loss), current investigations, travel arrangements (accommodation), and an initial description of the process of preoperative work-up, surgery and postoperative recovery. This interaction allows specific planning to be made regarding what previous tests have been undertaken and what radiological examinations need to be obtained prior to the initial visit. In addition, specific plans are made to complete all staging and appropriate physiological tests within a specific time period (in our case 48 hours) around the initial trip to the oesophagogastric unit. At the initial visit careful history, examination and organisation of relevant clinical investigations as described previously in this chapter will provide an initial indication of physiological status. This physiological assessment is important in guiding all aspects of the patient's treatment for their oesophagogastric malignancy. In particular, it is important to be able to adapt the surgical approach according to both tumour location and patient physiology, i.e. in patients with severe coronary artery disease, arrhythmias or cardiomyopathy we typically utilise a right thoracic approach so as to minimise cardiac manipulation during oesophageal mobilisation. Following physiological investigations and tumour staging, all patients should be presented at a multidisciplinary tumour board (see 'Multidisciplinary team evaluation' section above) to allow an individually targeted goal-directed treatment plan to be formulated that takes into account both tumour and patient characteristics. A part of this MDT review will include reviewing suitability for enrolment in current clinical trials. The nutritional status of patients should also be discussed, with specific need for either feeding jejunostomy or removable self-expanding metal oesophageal stent (SEMS) being included in the final recommendation (see 'Nutrition' subsection above). At the MDT meeting, a plan is made regarding the timing of surgery in patients receiving neoadjuvant chemotherapy, but particularly chemoradiotherapy. Current recommendations indicate the optimum time for resection to be 4–6 weeks following completion of radiotherapy. Contact is maintained with the patient throughout neoadjuvant therapy by the oesophagogastric nurse specialist as well as post-treatment reassessments coordinated before surgery.

Intraoperative

Intraoperative aspects of the clinical pathway employed at our institution involve regular communication between the anaesthetic and operating teams. We routinely place a thoracic epidural in all of our patients undergoing oesophagectomy and liaise with the pain service to ensure their active involvement early in the postoperative period. During surgery we attempt to tailor the approach to minimise blood loss so as to reduce transfusion requirements. Over the past 6 years our median intraoperative blood loss has been 150 (50–400) mL during oesophagectomy with a median operative time of 416 (244–664) min. This has allowed us to adopt an increasingly conservative approach to intraoperative fluid utilisation (median 2700 (1250–7900) mL for oesophagectomies over the past 2 years); as described previously, this reduces gastrointestinal recovery time and pulmonary complications. Immediate extubation postoperatively allows immediate introduction of the postoperative goal-directed pathway to allow enhanced recovery following oesophagogastric surgery.

Postoperative

Postoperative care pathways allow the introduction of a targeted goal-directed approach to postoperative recovery following major oesophagogastric surgery. They provide a template for all medical personnel interacting with these patients, and can outline a goal-directed recovery for each patient. These pathways, once well established, can provide a framework for quality improvement and improving postoperative outcomes. Previous studies have demonstrated the effectiveness of these pathways in reducing postoperative mortality, pulmonary complications and length of hospital stay following oesophagectomy.[86,87] Involvement of the entire healthcare team in the design and implementation of these pathways will help ensure all team members are committed to achieving specific recovery goals.

A simple schematic for a postoperative care pathway is shown in Table 4.3. It is imperative that patients should be provided with this pathway and dietary expectations prior to undergoing surgery, as this will help to guide their expectations regarding their postoperative recovery. The use of specific pathways will help patients, families and their caregivers remain focused on a goal-orientated approach to recovery from major surgery. Through five revisions of our clinical care pathway over the past decade, we have seen our median length of hospital stay decrease from 10 to 8 days (median for past 2 years).

Table 4.3 • Clinical care pathway at Virginia Mason Medical Center 2011

Postoperative day	Aim or goal
Evening on day of surgery	• Sits up in bed • Maintain mean arterial pressure (MAP) >70 mmHg • Proton-pump inhibitor (PPI) initiated • Physiotherapy visit and introduction to incentive spirometry
Day 1	• Walks in the corridor in the morning prior to discharge from HDU, then 100–200 feet walks × 3 on day 1 • Discharge from or step down from ICU • Start jejunal tube feeding • Remove apical chest drain if no air leak
Day 2 onwards	• Walks 3–4 times per day ± physical therapy consult • Titrate epidural to facilitate mobilisation and maintain MAP >70 mmHg
Day 3, 4 or 5	• Chest drain 2 removed – depending on whether chest or cervical incision • Jejunal tube feeds increased to goal feeding
Day 4 or 5	• Gastrograffin/barium study to assess anastomosis and gastric emptying
Day 5 or 6	• Nasogastric tube removed • Discontinue epidural • Switch to oral or jejunostomy tube analgesics – all medications must be crushed or given as liquid down jejunostomy tube and PPI given orally. • Jejunal tube feeds moved to nocturnal feeding Dietary and home health consult • Limited oral liquid intake on discharge – 1 cup every 2 hours • No attempt to initiate solid diet prior to discharge • Dietary team provides specific directions regarding advancing oral intake over subsequent 3–4 weeks
Day 6 or 7	Planned discharge

Adapted from Low DE, Kunz S, Schembre D et al. Esophagectomy – it's not just about mortality any more: standardized perioperative clinical pathways improve outcomes in patients with esophageal cancer. J Gastrointest Surg 2007; 11:1395–402.

Key points

- The principle of preoperative assessment is to identify comorbidities, psychological and nutritional abnormalities that may complicate the patient's operative intervention and perioperative recovery.
- Several clinical risk indices have been utilised to assess operative risk, including ASA grade, Eastern Cooperative Oncology Group (ECOG) performance status, the Karnofsky performance scale index and the Charlson comorbidity index (CCI). CCI allows quantitative scoring of a patient's comorbidities and may provide a useful tool in the preoperative risk assessment.
- Poor exercise tolerance correlates with an increased risk of perioperative complications, which are independent of age and other patient characteristics. The use of intensive preoperative exercise has been shown to improve cardiopulmonary fitness prior to major surgery.
- Aggressive chest physiotherapy and early mobilisation may also help to reduce the incidence of pulmonary complications associated with oesophagogastric surgery in patients with respiratory risk factors.
- The multidisciplinary team (MDT) has become the cornerstone of standardising and coordinating cancer treatment. It is the appropriate venue for making specific recommendations regarding the overall treatment approach and the requirement for nutritional supplementation.
- Surgical and anaesthetic techniques, methodology of intraoperative monitoring, minimising blood losses and perioperative fluid management, as well as lung isolation techniques and intraoperative organ support, are all important perioperative factors that can influence clinical outcome following oesophagectomy or gastrectomy; producing basic platforms or pathways covering both surgery and anaesthesia perioperative standard work will help coordinate intraoperative care.
- Immediate extubation following surgery has the advantages of allowing the immediate initiation of postoperative protocols involving pain control, physiotherapy and early mobilisation.
- A more restrictive approach to fluid management during major surgery may be beneficial, with improved gastrointestinal recovery time and reduced respiratory complications. Goal-directed fluid therapy includes minimising blood loss and maintaining haemodynamic stability, and this requires regular communication between surgeon and anaesthetic teams.
- Thoracic epidural analgesia for oesophagectomy has been shown to be a highly effective method of postoperative pain relief. Furthermore, the proven benefits of thoracic epidural analgesia following oesophagectomy include earlier recovery of bowel function, reduced pulmonary complication and early extubation.
- Postoperative care pathways allow the introduction of a targeted goal-directed approach to postoperative recovery following major oesophagogastric surgery. They provide a template for all medical personnel interacting with these patients, and can outline a goal-directed recovery for each patient.
- The implementation of a clinical pathway for oesophagogastric cancer requires the personal commitment of all members of the care team and will affect a patient's treatment at virtually every stage; these individuals and teams should be involved in formulating and adapting the clinical pathway.
- Due to the increasing complexity of the work-up of patients undergoing oesophagogastric cancer surgery, the involvement of a nurse specialist is important to ensure appropriate liaison with the patient and planning of every stage of treatment.

References

1. Palmes D, Brüwer M, Bader FG, et al., German Advanced Surgical Treatment Study Group. Diagnostic evaluation, surgical technique, and perioperative management after esophagectomy: consensus statement of the German Advanced Surgical Treatment Study Group. Langenbecks Arch Surg 2011;396(6):857–66.
2. Troisi N, Dorigo W, Lo Sapio P, et al. Preoperative cardiac assessment in patients undergoing aortic surgery: analysis of factors affecting the cardiac outcomes. Ann Vasc Surg 2010;24(6):733–40.

3. Akutsu Y, Matsubara H. Perioperative management for the prevention of postoperative pneumonia with esophageal surgery. Ann Thorac Cardiovasc Surg 2009;15(5):280–5.
4. Whooley BP, Law S, Murthy SC, et al. Analysis of reduced death and complication rates after esophageal resection. Ann Surg 2001;233(3):338–44.
5. Adams R, Morgan M, Mukherjee S, et al. A prospective comparison of multidisciplinary treatment of oesophageal cancer with curative intent in a UK cancer. Eur J Surg Oncol 2007;33(3):307–13.
6. Law S, Wong KH, Kwok KF, et al. Predictive factors for postoperative pulmonary complications and mortality after esophagectomy for cancer. Ann Surg 2004;240:791–800.
7. Allum WH, Stenning SP, Bancewicz J, et al. Long-term results of a randomized trial of surgery with or without preoperative chemotherapy in esophageal cancer. J Clin Oncol 2009;27:5062–7.
8. Morita M, Egashira A, Yoshida R, et al. Esophagectomy in patients 80 years of age and older with carcinoma of the thoracic esophagus. J Gastroenterol 2008;43:345–51.
9. Kuppusamy MK, Chance FD, Helman JD, et al. Assessment of intra-operative haemodynamic changes associated with transhiatal and transthoracic oesophagectomy. Eur J Cardiothorac Surg 2010;38:665–8.
10. Wakui R, Yamashita H, Okuma K, et al. Esophageal cancer: definitive chemoradiotherapy for elderly patients. Dis Esophagus 2010;23:572–9.
11. Mak RH, Mamon HJ, Ryan DP, et al. Toxicity and outcomes after chemoradiation for esophageal cancer in patients age 75 or older. Dis Esophagus 2010;23:316–23.
12. Portale G, Peters JH, Hsieh CC, et al. Esophageal adenocarcinoma in patients ≤50 years old: delayed diagnosis and advanced disease at presentation. Am Surg 2004;70(11):954–9.
13. Patil PK, Patel SG, Mistry RC, et al. Cancer of the esophagus in young adults. J Surg Oncol 1992;50:179–82.
14. Omloo JM, Sloof GW, Boellaard R, et al. Importance of fluorodeoxyglucose-positron emission tomography (FDG-PET) and endoscopic ultrasonography parameters in predicting survival following surgery for esophageal cancer. Endoscopy 2008;40(6):464–71.
15. van Westreenen HL, Heeren PA, van Dullemen HM, et al. Positron emission tomography with F-18-fluorodeoxyglucose in a combined staging strategy of esophageal cancer prevents unnecessary surgical explorations. J Gastrointest Surg 2005;9(1):54–61.
16. Westerterp M, van Westreenen HL, Reitsma JB, et al. Esophageal cancer: CT, endoscopic US, and FDG PET for assessment of response to neoadjuvant therapy – systematic review. Radiology 2005;236(3):841–51.
17. Birkmeyer JD, Sun Y, Wong SL, et al. Hospital volume and late survival after cancer surgery. Ann Surg 2007;245:777–83.
18. Al-Sariria AA, David G, Willmott S, et al. Oesophagectomy practice and outcomes in England. Br J Surg 2007;94(5):585–91.
19. Van der Gaast A, van Hagen P, Hulshof M, et al. Effect of preoperative concurrent chemoradiotherapy on survival of patients with resectable esophageal or esophagogastric junction cancer: results from a multicenter randomized phase III study. Proc Am Soc Clin Oncol 2010;28(Suppl. 15):4004(abstr).
20. Lv J, Cao XF, Zhu B, et al. Long-term efficacy of perioperative chemoradiotherapy on esophageal squamous cell carcinoma. World J Gastroenterol 2010;16:1649–54.
21. Murthy SC, Rozas MS, Adelstein DJ, et al. Induction chemoradiotherapy increases pleural and pericardial complications after esophagectomy for cancer. J Thorac Oncol 2009;4:395–403.
22. Gayed I, Gohar S, Liao Z, et al. The clinical implications of myocardial perfusion abnormalities in patients with esophageal or lung cancer after chemoradiation therapy. Int J Cardiovasc Imaging 2009;25:487–95.
23. Cerfolio RJ, Talati A, Bryant AS. Changes in pulmonary function tests after neoadjuvant therapy predict postoperative complications. Ann Thorac Surg 2009;88:930–5.
24. Neuner G, Patel A, Suntharalingam M. Chemoradiotherapy for esophageal cancer. Gastrointest Cancer Res 2009;3:57–65.
25. Cunningham D, Allum WH, Stenning SP, et al. Perioperative chemotherapy versus surgery alone for resectable gastroesophageal cancer. N Engl J Med 2006;355:11–20.
26. Takagi K, Yamamori H, Morishima Y, et al. Preoperative immunosuppression: its relationship with high morbidity and mortality in patients receiving thoracic esophagectomy. Nutrition 2001;17(1):13–7.
27. Gabor S, Renner H, Matzi V, et al. Early enteral feeding compared with parenteral nutrition after oesophageal or oesophagogastric resection and reconstruction. Br J Nutr 2005;93(4):509–13.
28. Llaguna OH, Kim HJ, Deal AM, et al. Utilization and morbidity associated with placement of a feeding jejunostomy at the time of gastroesophageal resection. J Gastrointest Surg 2011;15(10):1663–9.
29. Pellen MG, Sabri S, Razack A, et al. Safety and efficacy of self-expanding removable metal esophageal stents during neoadjuvant chemotherapy for resectable esophagal cancer. Dis Esophagus 2012;25(1):48–53.
30. Griffin SM, Shaw IH, Dresner SM. Early complications after Ivor–Lewis subtotal esophagectomy with two-field lymphadenectomy. Risk factors and management. J Am Coll Surg 2002;194:285–97.

31. Eagle KA, Brundage BH, Chaitman BR, et al. Guidelines for perioperative cardiovascular evaluation for non-cardiac surgery. J Am Coll Cardiol 1996;27(4):910–48.

32. Allum WH, Blazeby JM, Griffin M, et al., on behalf of the Association of Upper Gastrointestinal Surgeons of Great Britain and Ireland, the British Society of Gastroenterology and the British Association of Surgical Oncology. Guidelines for the management of oesophageal and gastric cancer. Gut 2011;60:1449–72.

33. Nagamatsu Y, Yamana H, Fujita H, et al. The simultaneous evaluation of preoperative cardiopulmonary functions of oesophageal cancer patients in the analysis of expired gas with exercise testing. Nippon Kyoba Geka Gakkai Zasshi 1994;42:2037–40.

34. Nagamatsu Y, Ono H, Hiraki H, et al. Pre-operative screening test for lung cancer using the analysis of expired gas with exercise testing – principally VO_{2max}/m2. Nippon Kyobu Geka Gakkai Zasshi 1994;42(10):1910–5.

35. Forshaw MJ, Strauss DC, Davies AR, et al. Is cardiopulmonary exercise testing a useful test before esophagectomy? Ann Thorac Surg 2008;85:294–9.

36. Wijeysundera DN, Beattie WS, Austin PC, et al. Non-invasive cardiac stress testing before elective major non-cardiac surgery: population based cohort study. Br Med J 2010;340:b5526.

37. Poldermans D, Boersma E, Bax JJ, et al. The effect of bisoprolol on perioperative mortality and myocardial infarction in high-risk patients undergoing vascular surgery. N Engl J Med 1999;341:1789–94.

38. Fleisher LA, Beckman JA, Brown KA, et al. ACC/AHA 2006 guideline update on perioperative cardiovascular evaluation for noncardiac surgery: focused update on perioperative beta-blocker therapy: a report of the American College of Cardiology/American Heart Association Task Force on Practice Guidelines (Writing Committee to Update the 2002 Guidelines on Perioperative Cardiovascular Evaluation for Noncardiac Surgery) developed in collaboration with the American Society of Cardiovascular Anesthesiologists, Society for Cardiovascular Angiography and Interventions, and Society for Vascular Medicine and Biology. J Am Coll Cardiol 2006;47(11):2343–55.

39. Healy KO, Waksmonski CA, Altman RK, et al. Perioperative outcome and long-term mortality for heart failure patients undergoing intermediate- and high-risk non-cardiac surgery: impact of left ventricular ejection fraction. Congest Heart Fail 2010;16:45–9.

40. Lee JT, Chaloner EJ, Hollingsworth SJ. The role of cardiopulmonary fitness and its genetic influences on surgical outcomes. Br J Surg 2006;93(2):147–57.

41. Kothman E, Batterham AM, Owen SJ, et al. Effect of short-term exercise training on aerobic fitness in patients with abdominal aortic aneurysms: a pilot study. Br J Anaesth 2009;103(4):505–10.

42. Eichhorn EJ. Beta-blocker withdrawal: the song of Orpheus. Am Heart J 1999;138:387–9.

43. American College of Cardiology Foundation/American Heart Association Task Force on Practice Guidelines American Society of Echocardiography, et al. 2009 ACCF/AHA focused update on perioperative beta blockade incorporated into the ACC/AHA 2007 guidelines on perioperative cardiovascular evaluation and care for noncardiac surgery. J Am Coll Cardiol 2009;54:e13–118.

44. Dunkelgrun M, Boersma E, Schouten O, et al. Bisoprolol and fluvastatin for the reduction of perioperative cardiac mortality and myocardial infarction in intermediate-risk patients undergoing non-cardiovascular surgery: a randomized controlled trial (DECREASE IV). Ann Surg 2005;353:349–61.

45. Lindenauer PK, Pekow P, Wang K, et al. Perioperative beta-blocker therapy and mortality after major noncardiac surgery. N Engl J Med 2005;353:349–61.

46. Kapoor AS, Kanji H, Buckingham J, et al. Strength of evidence for perioperative use of statins to reduce cardiovascular risk: systematic review of controlled studies. Br Med J 2006;333:1149.

47. Douketis JD, Berger PB, Dunn AS, et al. The perioperative management of antithrombotic therapy: American College of Chest Physicians Evidence-Based Clinical Practice Guidelines (8th Edition). Chest 2008;133(Suppl. 6):299S–339S.

48. Nuttall GA, Brown MJ, Stombaugh JW, et al. Time and cardiac risk of surgery after bare-metal stent percutaneous coronary intervention. Anesthesiology 2008;109:588–95.

49. Rabbits JA, Nuttall GA, Brown MJ, et al. Cardiac risk of non-cardiac surgery after percutaneous coronary intervention with drug eluting stents. Anesthesiology 2008;109:596–604.

50. Avendano CE, Flume PA, Silvestri GA, et al. Pulmonary complications after oesophagectomy. Ann Thorac Surg 2002;73:922–6.

51. Quaseem A, Snow V, Itterman N, et al. Risk assessment and strategies to reduce perioperative pulmonary complications for patients undergoing noncardiothoracic surgery: a guideline from the American College of Physicians. Ann Intern Med 2006;144:575–80.

52. Poussel M, Nguyen Thi PL, Villemot JP, et al. Arterial oxygen partial pressure and cardiovascular surgery in elderly patients. Interact Cardiovasc Thorac Surg 2008;7:819–24.

53. Joo HS, Wong J, Naik VN, et al. The value of screening preoperative chest x-rays: a systematic review. Can J Anaesth 2005;52:568–74.

54. Bapoje SR, Whitaker JF, Schulz T, et al. Preoperative evaluation of the patient with pulmonary disease. Chest 2007;132:1637–45.

55. Mercantonio ER, Goldman L, Mangione CM, et al. A clinical prediction rule for delirium after elective noncardiac surgery. JAMA 1994;271:134–9.
56. Ganai S, Lee KF, Merrill A, et al. Adverse outcomes of geriatric patients undergoing abdominal surgery who are at high risk for delirium. Arch Surg 2007;142:1072–8.
57. Markar SR, Smith IA, Karthikesalingam A, et al. The Clinical and Economic Cost of Delirium Following Surgical Resection for Esophageal Malignancy. Ann Surg 2013 (Epub ahead of print)
58. Inouye SK, Bogardus Jr. ST, Charpentier PA, et al. A multicomponent intervention to prevent delirium in hospitalized older patients. N Engl J Med 1999;340:669–76.
59. O'Keeffe ST, Lavan JN. Predicting delirium in elderly patients: development and validation of a risk-stratification model. Age Ageing 1996;25:317–21.
60. Franco JG, Valencia C, Bernal C, et al. Relationship between cognitive status at admission and incident delirium in older medical inpatients. J Neuropsychiatr Clin Neurosci 2010;22:329–37.
61. O'Mahony R, Murthy L, Akunne A, et al., Guideline Development Group. Synopsis of National Institute for Health and Clinical Excellence guideline for prevention of delirium. Ann Intern Med 2011;154:746–51.
62. Mouchoux C, Rippert P, Duclos A, et al. Impact of a multifaceted program to prevent postoperative delirium in the elderly: the CONFUCIUS stepped wedge protocol. BMC Geriatr 2011;11:25.
63. Siddiqi N, Stockdale R, Britton AM, et al. Interventions for preventing delirium in hospitalized patients. Cochrane Database Syst Rev 2007;(2)CD005563.
64. Ono H, Taguchi T, Kido Y, et al. The usefulness of bright light therapy for patients after oesophagectomy. Intensive Crit Care Nurs 2011;27(3):158–66.
65. Mori S, Sawada T, Hamada K, et al. Gastrectomy for patients with gastric cancer and non-uremic renal failure. World J Gastroenterol 2007;13:4589–92.
66. Schilling T, Kozian A, Kretzchmar M, et al. Effects of propofol and desflurane anaesthesia on the alveolar inflammatory response to one-lung ventilation. Br J Anaesth 2007;99:369–75.
67. Abou-Elenain K. Study of the systemic and pulmonary oxidative stress status during exposure to propofol and sevoflurane anaesthesia during thoracic surgery. Eur J Anaesthesiol 2010;27:566–71.
68. Misthos P, Katsaragakis S, Milingos N, et al. Postresectional pulmonary oxidative stress in lung cancer patients. The role of one-lung ventilation. Eur J Cardiothorac Surg 2005;27:379–82.
69. Michelet P, D'Journo XB, Roch A, et al. Protective ventilation influences systemic inflammation after esophagectomy: a randomized controlled study. Anesthesiology 2006;105:911–9.
70. Low DE, Kunz S, Schembre D, et al. Esophagectomy – it's not just about mortality any more: standardized perioperative clinical pathways improve outcomes in patients with esophageal cancer. J Gastrointest Surg 2007;11:1395–402.
71. Chandrashekar MV, Irving M, Wayman J, et al. Immediate extubation and epidural analgesia allow safe management in a high-dependency unit after two-stage oesophagectomy. Results of eight years of experience in a specialized upper gastrointestinal unit in a district general hospital. Br J Anaesth 2003;90:474–9.
72. Brandstrup B, Tonnesen H, Beier-Holgersen R, et al. Effects of intravenous fluid restriction on postoperative complications: comparison of two perioperative fluid regimens: a randomized assessor-blinded multicenter trial. Ann Surg 2003;238:641–8.
73. Nisanevich V, Felsenstein I, Almogy G, et al. Effect of intraoperative fluid management on outcome after intraabdominal surgery. Anesthesiology 2005;103:25–32.
74. Kita T, Mammoto T, Kisis Y. Fluid management and postoperative respiratory disturbances in patients with transthoracic esophagectomy for carcinoma. J Clin Anesth 2002;14:252–6.
This is the first trial to demonstrate significantly reduced length of hospital stay with reduced intraoperative fluid administration specifically in the setting of oesophagectomy.
75. Neal JM, Wilcox RT, Allen HW, et al. Near-total esophagectomy: the influence of standardized multimodal management and intraoperative fluid restriction. Reg Anesth Pain Med 2003;28:328–34.
This trial demonstrated a significantly reduced incidence of pulmonary complication and earlier extubation associated with intraoperative fluid restriction.
76. Abbas SM, Hill AG. Systematic review of the literature for the use of oesophageal Doppler monitor for fluid replacement in major abdominal surgery. Anaesthesia 2008;63:44–51.
77. Kobayashi M, Koh M, Irinoda T, et al. Stroke volume variation as a predictor of intravascular volume depression and possible hypotension during the early postoperative period after esophagectomy. Ann Surg Oncol 2009;16:1371–7.
78. Rudin A, Flisberg P, Johansson J, et al. Thoracic epidural analgesia or intravenous morphine analgesia after thoracoabdominal esophagectomy: a prospective follow-up of 201 patients. J Cardiothorac Vasc Anesth 2005;19:350–7.
79. Popping DM, Elia N, Marret E, et al. Protective effects of epidural analgesia on pulmonary complications after abdominal and thoracic surgery: a meta-analysis. Arch Surg 2008;143:990–9.
80. Michelet P, D'Journo XB, Roch A, et al. Perioperative risk factors for anastomotic leakage after esophagectomy: influence of thoracic epidural analgesia. Chest 2005;128:3461–6.

81. Lazar G, Kaszaki J, Abraham S, et al. Thoracic epidural anesthesia improves the gastric microcirculation during experimental gastric tube formation. Surgery 2003;134:799–805.
82. Ng JM. Update of anesthetic management for esophagectomy. Curr Opin Anesth 2011;24:37–43.
83. Doi K, Yamanaka M, Shono A, et al. Preoperative epidural fentanyl reduces postoperative pain after upper abdominal surgery. J Anesth 2007;21:439–41.
84. Komatsu H, Matsumoto S, Mitsuhata H. Comparison of patient-controlled epidural analgesia with and without night-time infusion following gastrectomy. Br J Anaesth 2001;87:633–5.
85. Kaiser AM, Zollinger A, De Lorenzi D, et al. Prospective, randomized comparison of extrapleural versus epidural analgesia for postthoracotomy pain. Ann Thorac Surg 1998;66:367–72.
86. Munitiz V, Martinez-de-Haro LF, Ortiz A, et al. Effectiveness of a written clinical pathway for enhanced recovery after transthoracic (Ivor Lewis) oesophagectomy. Br J Surg 2010;97:714–8.
87. Cerfolio RJ, Bryant AS, Bass CS, et al. Fast tracking after Ivor Lewis esophagogastrectomy. Chest 2004;126:1187–94.

5

Surgery for cancer of the oesophagus

S. Michael Griffin
Richard G. Berrisford

Introduction

Oesophageal cancer is one of the most challenging conditions confronting the surgeon. Resection of the oesophagus requires surgical experience within chest, abdomen and neck. The approach, extent of resection and method of reconstruction require a versatile skillset to which minimally invasive skills may now be added. Oesophageal resection, even in the best of hands, carries the highest risk of morbidity of any operation, and the management of complications challenges the most experienced of surgeons. Not only is the complete resection of all disease often challenging, restoration of gastrointestinal continuity with a gastric or intestinal graft, maintaining an intact anastomosis, is an exacting discipline.

While treatment for cancer of the oesophagus is multidisciplinary, surgery is still the primary mode of therapy. In the UK, 70% of patients now present with adenocarcinoma of the lower oesophagus or gastro-oesophageal junction, which represent a different disease from the previously more common squamous carcinoma. This chapter discusses the surgical management of adenocarcinoma of the lower oesophagus and the cardia (Siewert types 1 and 2), which are frequently staged and treated as oesophageal cancers, but not subcardial tumours (Siewert type 3), which are described elsewhere (Chapter 7).

Unfortunately, the disease often presents late when increasing dysphagia has developed over several months. As a result of poor fitness or unresectable disease only 30–40% of patients are suitable for radical, potentially curative treatment, whilst the majority receive non-surgical therapies with the aim of palliation. Outcome is strongly stage dependent; whilst early tumours have excellent results with surgery alone, the majority with transmural or node-positive tumours benefit from multimodality therapy, combining surgery with neoadjuvant chemotherapy or chemoradiotherapy (Chapter 9). The multidisciplinary team must exercise judgment in the choice of the appropriate combination of therapies for each individual patient. This will depend on patient age, fitness, symptoms, prognosis and evidence base, as well as the overall stage and histopathology.

Surgical pathology

The vast majority of oesophageal neoplasms are epithelial in origin. Some arise from squamous mucosa, but most arise from metaplastic columnar epithelium, resulting in glandular carcinomas affecting the specialised epithelium in the lower oesophagus. Tumour site and histology are two crucial factors requiring assessment: tumours arising from different sites in the oesophagus vary in their behaviour.

Squamous cell carcinoma arising in the cervical and thoracic oesophagus and adenocarcinoma arising in the thoracic oesophagus and cardia differ in their mode of spread and response to therapeutic modalities. It is essential that the anatomical divisions of the oesophagus are described such that the different therapeutic surgical procedures adopted for tumours at each site can be understood (**Fig. 5.1**).

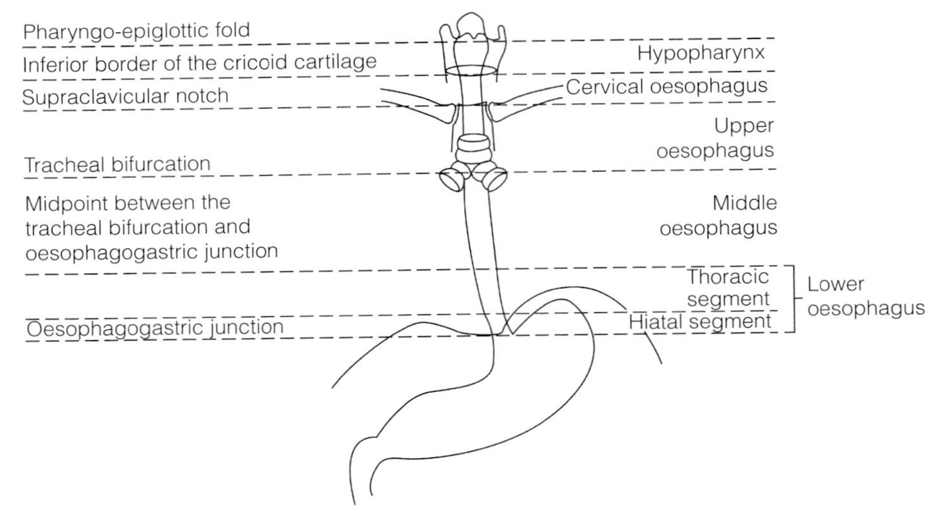

Figure 5.1 • Anatomical regions of the hypopharynx, oesophagus and gastric cardia.

Surgical anatomy

The oesophagus is a midline hollow viscus, starting at the cricopharyngeal sphincter at the level of the sixth cervical vertebra, entering the chest at the level of the suprasternal notch, traversing the posterior mediastinum and entering the abdomen through the oesophageal hiatus in the diaphragm to join the stomach at the cardia. It bears a close relationship to the trachea and pericardium in front and the vertebral column posteriorly. The vagus and its branches are in close proximity over its entire length. There is no serosal covering. The thoracic duct enters the posterior mediastinum through the aortic opening in the diaphragm. It lies on the bodies of the thoracic vertebrae posterolateral to the oesophagus and between the aorta and the azygos vein. The left atrium and the inferior pulmonary veins lie in intimate contact with the left wall of the lower third of the oesophagus.

The TNM classification (Version 7, released in 2009)[1] combines the salient features of the staging process. This classification has divided the oesophagus into discrete anatomical regions (Fig. 5.1) and is described in Chapter 2.

Hypopharynx and cervical oesophagus

The region between the level of the pharyngoepiglottic fold and the inferior border of the cricoid cartilage is known as the hypopharynx, that above as the oropharynx. The cervical oesophagus begins at the lower border of the cricoid cartilage and terminates at the level of the thoracic inlet or jugular notch. Surgical management of carcinomas in these regions differs from that of other parts of the oesophagus, because tumour extension in these two areas commonly overlaps. This is considered separately later in the chapter.

Upper oesophagus

The upper oesophagus extends from the level of the jugular notch and the carina (approximately 24 cm from incisors).

Middle oesophagus

The mid oesophagus extends from the tracheal bifurcation (approximately 24 cm from incisors) to the midpoint between the tracheal bifurcation and the oesophagogastric junction (approximately 32 cm from incisors).

Lower oesophagus

The lower oesophagus comprises both the lower thoracic oesophagus and the hiatal segment of the oesophagus. The latter segment is often termed the 'abdominal oesophagus'. The oesophagogastric junction is a somewhat nebulous term, and the anatomy depends on the differing viewpoints of surgeons, endoscopists, radiologists, pathologists and anatomists. It is further complicated by the presence or absence of a hiatal hernia and the presence or absence of a columnar-lined oesophagus.

Blood supply and lymphatic drainage

The blood supply is derived directly from the aorta in the form of oesophageal vessels together with branches adjacent to or from organs such as the pulmonary hilum, trachea, stomach and thyroid gland. The venous drainage is through tributaries draining into the azygos and hemiazygos system in the chest, via the thyroid veins in the neck and the left gastric vein in the upper abdomen.

The lymphatics of the oesophagus are distributed predominantly in the form of a submucosal plexus and a paraoesophageal plexus. Both plexuses receive lymph from all parts of the respective layers of the oesophageal wall. The plexuses communicate through penetrating vessels that traverse the longitudinal and circular muscle walls. The paraoesophageal plexus drains into the paraoesophageal lymph nodes, which are situated on the surface of the oesophagus, and also into perioesophageal lymph nodes, situated in close proximity to the oesophagus. Lymphatics also drain from the perioesophageal nodes to the lateral oesophageal nodes or directly from the paraoesophageal to the lateral oesophageal nodes, skipping the perioesophageal group[2] (Box 5.1).

Box 5.1 • Lymph nodes of the oesophagus

Paraoesophageal nodes (on the wall of the oesophagus)
Cervical (101)
Upper thoracic (105)
Middle thoracic (108)
Lower thoracic (110)

Perioesophageal nodes (in immediate apposition to the oesophagus)
Deep cervical (102)
Supraclavicular (104)
Paratracheal (106)
Tracheal bifurcation (107)
Para-aortic or posterior mediastinal (112)
Diaphragmatic (111)
Left gastric (7)
Lesser curvature (3)
Coeliac (9)
Right cardiac (1)
Left cardiac (2)

Lateral oesophageal nodes (located lateral to the oesophagus)
Lateral cervical (100)
Hilar (109)
Suprapyloric (5)
Subpyloric (6)
Common hepatic (8)
Greater curvature (4)

Preoperative surgical preparation

Meticulous preoperative evaluation to accurately stage the tumour and estimate surgical risk is a crucial prerequisite to successful surgical outcome in this disease (see also Chapters 3 and 4).

Nutritional support

Malnutrition is associated with loss of tissue function, leading to many potential complications during the postoperative period, such as wound breakdown, respiratory failure secondary to poor respiratory muscle function, deep vein thrombosis and infective complications.[3]

✔✔ The enteral route is preferred, as there is evidence that increased nosocomial infections occur when the gastrointestinal (GI) tract is not used for nutrition in the pre- and postoperative periods.[4]

Perioperative enteral nutrition with the addition of nutrients that can modulate the immune system, termed 'immunonutrition', has been proposed to further reduce postoperative complications and improve outcome.[5]

✔ The routine use of parenteral feeding (total parenteral nutrition, TPN) is contraindicated on general and immunological grounds and should be avoided in order to minimise nosocomial infections and associated sepsis.

Preoperative nutritional support

Patients who present with marked dysphagia are at particular risk of malnutrition and occasionally dehydration; they require urgent active management. In this situation, oesophageal dilatation is high risk, and can affect cure rates if perforation occurs. Stent placement makes dissection and operative decision-making more difficult and displacement can occur. Early feeding jejunostomy (laparoscopic or open) may be the most appropriate option if induction therapy is clearly indicated and primary resection cannot be expedited.

Placement of a feeding jejunostomy at the time of surgery is routine in many units. Although mortality related specifically to feeding jejunostomy is less than 1%,[6] it is not without morbidity, both in-hospital and longer term (from adhesions). Nevertheless, establishing enteral nutrition in patients with complications following oesophagectomy, when they are most catabolic septic and ill, is a major therapeutic problem and avoiding re-operation has significant advantages.

Routine preoperative and postoperative feeding by jejunostomy in every patient has yet to be proven efficacious on current evidence.[7] Furthermore, a recent randomised controlled study comparing standard perioperative nutrition with immunonutrition failed to demonstrate any clinical advantage.[7]

A variety of other routes of nutrition have been assessed, with a recent systematic review showing no strong direct evidence to support one particular route.[8] Nasojejunal and nasoduodenal tubes are associated with a significant rate of dislodgement.[8]

Respiratory care

Optimisation of respiratory function is vital in preventing serious pulmonary complications associated with prolonged surgery and thoracotomy (see Chapter 4). Smoking must be stopped as early as possible, ideally 6 weeks prior to surgery, with the aid of nicotine replacement. Preoperative physiotherapy with coughing exercises and effective use of the diaphragm by restoration of muscle strength through ambulation is encouraged. High-risk patients should also be provided with vigorous physiotherapy with or without bronchodilators prior to surgery. Orodental hygiene should be undertaken, removing any source of chronic sepsis that could disseminate infection to the tracheobronchial tree during intubation. Many surgeons advocate routine use of an incentive spirometer; they are inexpensive, and used properly they help to set goals for patients that can be measured, albeit indirectly.

Prophylactic low-molecular-weight heparin together with antithromboembolism stockings must be provided as soon as the patient comes into hospital to reduce the incidence of thromboembolic complications.

Mental preparation/communication

It is now well established that enhanced recovery programmes can result in better outcomes, reduced length of stay, savings in resources, and improved staffing environment. Elements of such programmes include: preoperative assessment, planning and preparation before admission, reducing the physical stress of the operation, using a structured, goal-oriented approach to recovery, and early mobilisation.

Patients and their families should be introduced to the hospital environment, including the intensive care unit if they are routinely sent there during recovery. They should understand what to expect will happen to them through their inpatient journey. A patient diary and information sheet can help them to follow their own progress and reduce uncertainty. Aspects of their pre- and postoperative management should be shared with them, including pain relief, oxygen and intravenous fluid administration, drains, tubes and nutrition. They should have been counselled prior to admission about their treatment options, paying particular attention to results, limitations and expectations of surgery. The counselling process is greatly enhanced by the involvement of a trained clinical nurse specialist in oesophagogastric cancer.

Detailed perioperative preparation and anaesthetic details are highlighted and explained in depth in Chapter 4.

Surgical objectives

Oesophagectomy for cancer should only be undertaken when a potentially curative R0 resection (complete removal of all macroscopic and microscopic cancer) is expected. Unlike colorectal carcinoma, there is no role for resection in the presence of proven distant metastases (e.g. liver), no matter how localised.

Survival is related to the stage of disease. Patients with stage I disease can expect a 5-year survival of greater than 80%,[9] emphasising the importance of early detection. Resection alone, therefore, must be the chosen method of therapy in fit patients with T1 tumours of the middle and lower thirds of the oesophagus. In stage III disease, surgery alone produces poor results with prolonged survival for only 10–20% of cases.[10] It appears that both neoadjuvant chemotherapy and radiotherapy provide a benefit for these patients.[11] Further randomised trials must be completed in order to outline the optimal therapeutic strategy.

Survival following surgical resection for all stages of tumour has improved over the past 20 years, with morbidity and mortality falling. The reasons for this are listed in Box 5.2 and were well described in the

Box 5.2 • Reasons for improved results for oesophageal resection

- Increase in specialist units
- Multidisciplinary approach
- Earlier diagnosis
- Better patient selection
- Improved perioperative management
- Enhanced recovery programmes

COG Guidance Report on Upper GI Cancers.[12] Many studies have confirmed that results parallel experience in managing this condition,[13] and poor results occur when experience is limited.[14,15] There is now overwhelming evidence to confirm the influence of surgeon case volume on the outcome of site-specific cancer surgery.[14–16] Centralisation of oesophagogastric resection in specialist units in the UK has provided sufficient caseload to support strong multidisciplinary teams. Other reasons for improved outcome include better patient selection, earlier diagnosis by open-access endoscopy, surveillance of Barrett's oesophagus, and improved preoperative, operative and postoperative management.

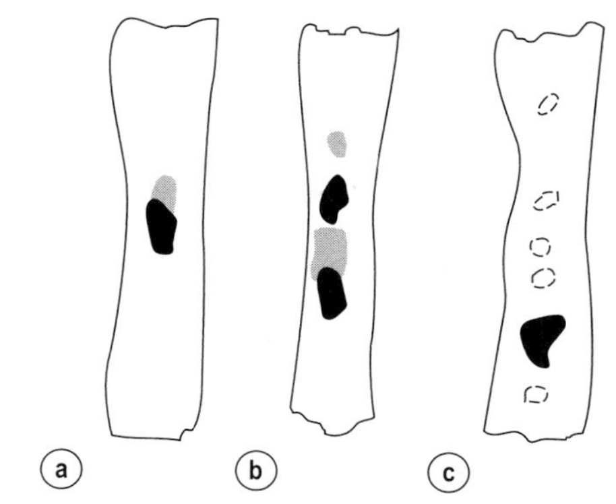

Figure 5.2 • **(a)** A single cancer. **(b)** Multifocal cancer. **(c)** Intramural lymphovascular spread. There is a high risk of positive resection margins in **(b)** and **(c)**. Shaded areas represent submucosal spread.

Principles of oesophagectomy

Resection of primary tumour

Oesophageal cancer spreads longitudinally in the submucosal lymphatics. It is crucial to obtain accurate information to guide the longitudinal resection margin through endoscopy and endoscopic ultrasound. It is still sometimes difficult to ascertain the length required for clear longitudinal margins, particularly in high lesions, making frozen section obligatory for some patients.

Rules on resection margins

The majority of authors favour a subtotal oesophagectomy to optimise longitudinal margins and take into account submucosal spread of both squamous and adenocarcinomas. There has been much debate around what length of macroscopically normal oesophagus to allow for complete resection margins. In squamous carcinoma this pertains especially to the proximal margin, whereas in adenocarcinoma the distal margin (gastric) is usually the greater concern. Skinner[17] advocated a minimum resection margin of 10 cm from the palpable edge of the tumour. However, this figure does not take into account the nature, location and pattern of occurrence of the primary cancer. Neither does it discriminate between in vivo margins and margins measured by the histopathologist after shrinkage has occurred during fixation.[18]

Primary tumours with multicentric lesions require more extensive longitudinal margins. In squamous cancers, three representative patterns of presentation are encountered (**Fig. 5.2**).[19] Failure to take these into account may explain high R1 rates (40%) when the oesophageal resection margin is limited to only 4 cm; compared to this, R1 was 17% when the margin was 10 cm. A 10-cm resection margin is a goal to attain in both directions *if this is possible.* In practice, this rule can rarely be achieved. A 10-cm margin either side of a 6-cm tumour would require an overall length of specimen exceeding that of the normal human oesophagus. It is the authors' opinion that when only a short resection margin can be obtained through the thoracic exposure, a cervical phase with near total oesophagectomy is advisable.

Adenocarcinoma of the lower oesophagus commonly infiltrates the gastric cardia, fundus and lesser curve. Extensive sleeve resection of the lesser curve and fundus with the formation of a tubular conduit is necessary to minimise positive distal resection margins. Other studies have demonstrated that patients with microscopically positive margins undergoing palliative resection died of other manifestations before clinical evidence of locoregional recurrence.[20,21] A tumour-free surgical margin is therefore not the only important factor to be considered in radical surgery. Nevertheless, it should remain the main goal of every operation.

A clear radial resection margin is equally important and is accepted as an independent prognostic factor for oesophageal cancer, with a definition of R1 being less than 1 mm clear margin.[22,23] The potential benefits of extended lymphadenectomy, discussed later, only pertain if the primary tumour has been completely excised (R0). Radical en-bloc resection techniques, outlined below in operative description, aim to produce a clear radial resection margin. Roder et al.[24] showed a statistically significant difference between R0 and R1 (microscopic residual disease) or R2 (macroscopic residual disease) resections for squamous cell carcinoma in a series of 204 resections with 5-year survival rates of 35% and <10%, respectively. Lerut et al.[25] demonstrated a 20% 5-year survival for R0 vs. zero 5-year survival for R1 and R2 resections in advanced stage III and stage IV adenocarcinomas and squamous cell carcinomas.

Resection of lymph nodes

Lymph node involvement is another independent variable for prognosis, in terms of both locoregional recurrence and survival. Patients with higher nodal burdens have worse outcomes after resection. The Worldwide Esophageal Cancer Collaboration has used pooled data from centres that have undertaken radical lymphadenectomy to report in detail the relationship between nodal involvement and survival.[26]

Nodal tiers

Lymph node tiers draining oesophageal cancer have been described according to the anatomy of the lymphatic drainage of the oesophagus.[2,27,28] The extent of lymphadenectomy associated with resection of these tiers is demonstrated in Box 5.1 and **Fig. 5.3.**

One-field lymphadenectomy describes removal of diaphragmatic, right and left paracardiac, lesser curvature, left gastric, coeliac, common hepatic and splenic artery nodes.

Two-field lymphadenectomy describes removal of para-aortic nodes (together with the thoracic duct), right and left pulmonary hilar, paraoesophageal nodes, subcarinal and right paratracheal nodes.

Three-field lymphadenectomy describes removal of the first and second fields along with a neck dissection clearing the brachiocephalic, deep lateral and external cervical nodes, as well as right and left recurrent nerve lymphatic chains (deep anterior cervical nodes).

The fields of nodal dissection should not be confused with the histopathological staging of nodal involvement (see Chapter 3, Table 3.3).

As for many other solid-organ tumours, controversy persists as to the value of lymphadenectomy in squamous and adenocarcinoma of the oesophagus.

In the past some authors felt that lymph node metastases were simply markers of systemic disease and their removal conferred no benefit.[23] Others contended that cure could be obtained in some patients with positive nodes by a radical lymphadenectomy with clear resection margins.[29] There has been increasing support for radical lymphadenectomy over the last 5 years.[30]

The rationale for lymphadenectomy

The arguments for formal radical lymphadenectomy are: optimal staging, improved locoregional control and improved cure rates. Formal radical lymphadenectomy goes hand in hand with radical en-bloc resection; for example, resection of the para-aortic nodes requires the plane of dissection to extend to the aortic adventitia. Negative resection margins (especially circumferential margins) go hand in hand with radical lymphadenectomy.

Optimal staging

Radical lymphadenectomy allows more accurate pathological staging.[25,31–32] TNM7 relies not only on the finding of positive lymph nodes, but on how many are found (N1, 1–2; N2, 3–6; N3, ≥7). Without an adequate lymphadenectomy, the patient is deprived of the most accurate prognosis available, and the patient's unit is deprived of a quality benchmark. Quality control is not possible as the baseline information, accurate pathological stage, is missing. If an inadequate lymphadenectomy is undertaken, survival will be worse than predicted for stage (the phenomenon of stage migration).

Locoregional tumour control

Locoregional tumour control is an important goal in treating oesophageal carcinoma; recurrent locoregional mediastinal disease can be very difficult to palliate. As Lerut et al. emphasise, long-term palliation is a significant benefit for those patients who are not cured by surgery.[25] It is impossible to separate potential benefits of radical lymphadenectomy from radical en-bloc resection, as already mentioned.

Radical en-bloc resection with lymphadenectomy has been associated with prolonged tumour-free survival; this is partly a result of consistently clear resection margins and partly a result of complete removal of involved nodes. Nodal and local tumour recurrence is less common after radical en-bloc resection in a number of retrospective series.[25,31,33–35] Single-institution comparative studies have also shown better survival.[36,37] Altorki et al. described a local recurrence rate of only 9.7% and a 33% 5-year survival for node-positive oesophageal cancer patients using a three-field lymphadenectomy and en-bloc resection.[38]

Locoregional recurrence may be further reduced by induction therapy, whether chemotherapy alone or chemoradiotherapy, with fewer positive nodes as well as an increase in R0 resection, consistent with improved disease-free and overall survival in some randomised trials.[39]

Improved cure rate

It is extremely difficult to demonstrate that radical lymphadenectomy improves cure rate in a conventional randomised controlled trial. Patients allocated to less than radical lymphadenectomy would be understaged, so no baseline would exist and the groups would not be comparable. Furthermore, most patients now have induction therapy that changes their nodal status during treatment. There are therefore very few randomised trials in the literature.[40–42]

Despite the limitations, there are indications from the Dutch trial,[40,43] comparing radical transthoracic

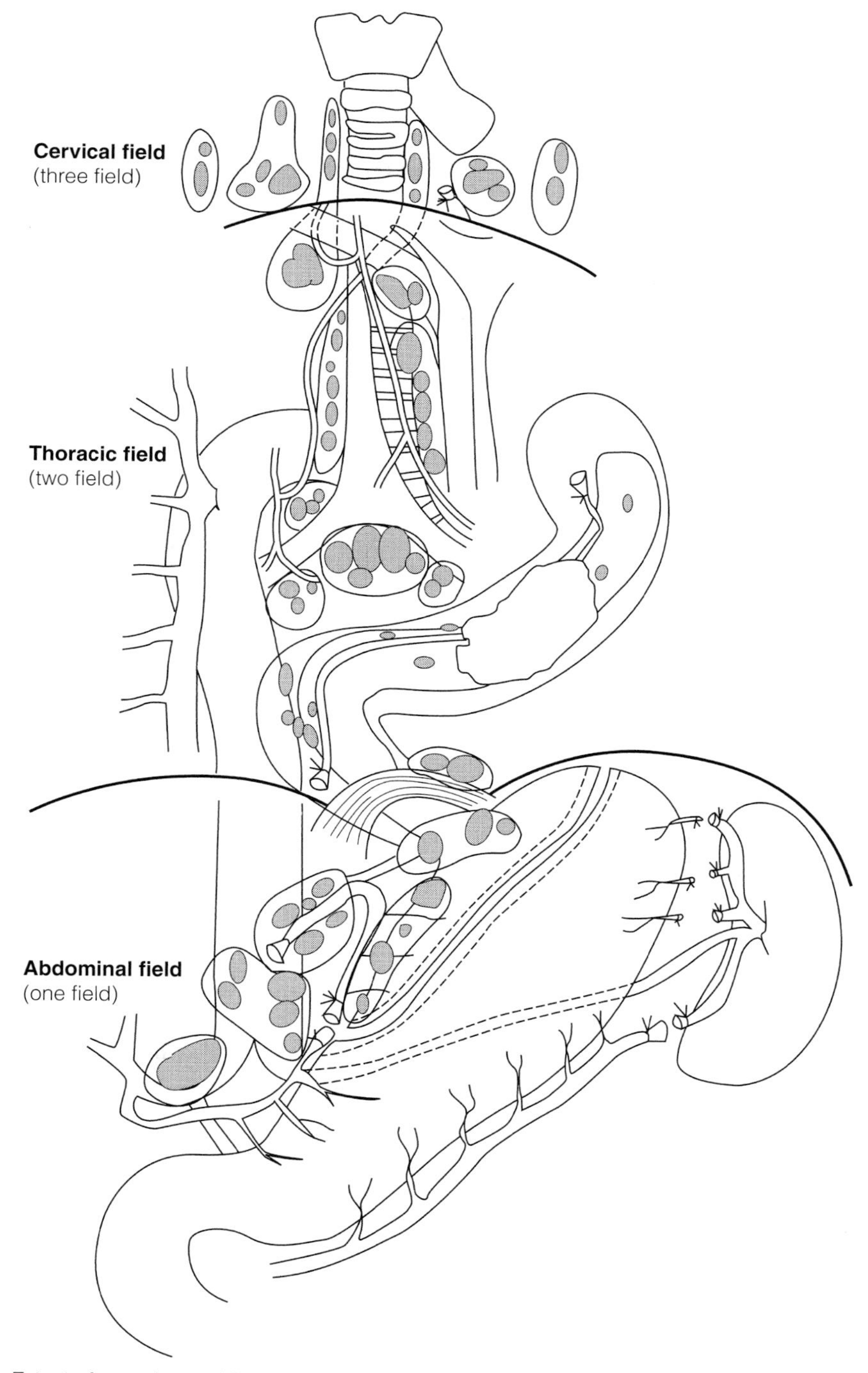

Figure 5.3 • Extent of resection and fields of lymph node dissection routinely carried out for cancer of the oesophagus.

and transhiatal resection, that patients with a limited number of positive nodes (1–8) had a significantly better survival following radical transthoracic oesophagectomy compared with less radical transhiatal resection. This group of patients would be expected to benefit from extended lymphadenectomy if it conferred survival advantage. Node-negative patients did well and those with a higher nodal burden did poorly, irrespective of the radicality of surgery (see **Fig. 5.4**). Another smaller,

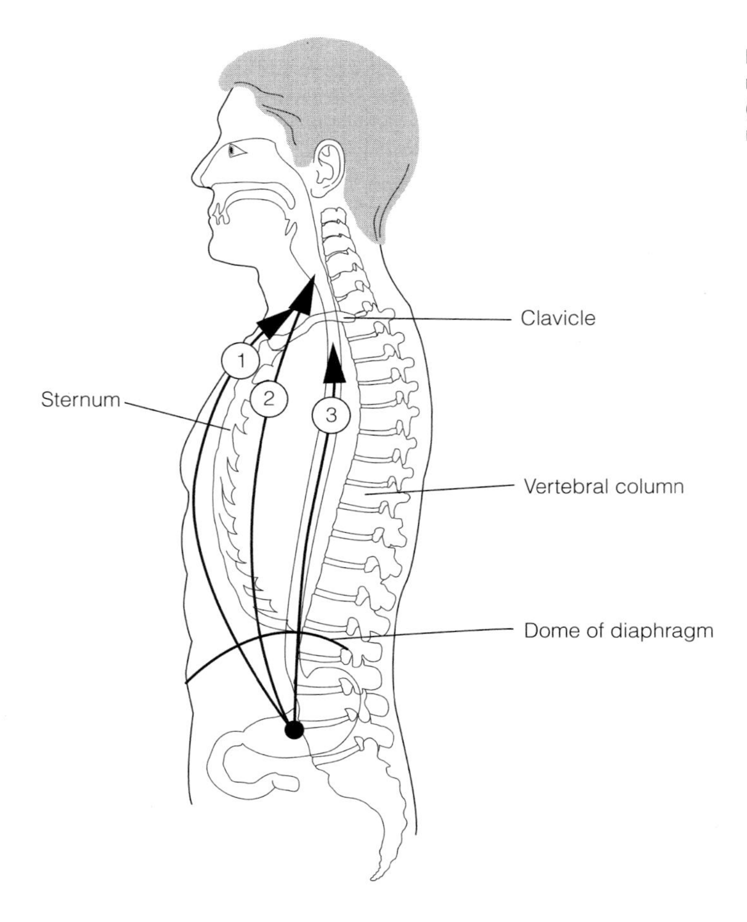

Figure 5.4 • Three routes of oesophageal reconstruction: (1) presternal route; (2) retrosternal route; (3) posterior mediastinal route.

retrospective comparison showed improved survival with radical en-bloc resection compared with transhiatal resection in patients with T3N1 disease with fewer than eight nodes involved.[44]

The role of radical lymphadenectomy in early-stage disease remains in question, and depends on the precise depth of invasion of the primary tumour.[40] There is some evidence that even patients with early-stage carcinoma, in whom a significant proportion can have nodal involvement, could benefit from extensive resection with lymphadenectomy.[45]

The most important recent evidence in support of radical lymphadenectomy comes from the Worldwide Esophageal Cancer Collaboration, who reported on their multi-institution international database comprising over 4600 resections for oesophageal cancer in patients who had not had induction therapy.[46] They showed that prognosis was highly dependent on the number of lymph nodes involved; patients with more than three nodes involved had a 50% likelihood of systemic disease and patients with more than eight nodes involved had almost 100% likelihood of systemic disease.[30,47]

Even more important was their finding that survival depended not only on how many nodes were involved, but also on how many were removed at resection.[47] The number of lymph nodes removed was the third strongest predictor of survival after depth of invasion and number of nodes involved. This finding has been corroborated in an analysis of the SEER (Surveillance, Epidemiology and End Results) database, both for oesophageal cancer[48] and gastric cancer.[49] It does appear from these data that the number of nodes resected has an effect on survival.

Harvested nodal counts of 23[47] and 30[48] have been suggested as the optimal number, with caveats given that this is a goal and not an expected target in all patients. The recommendation for adequate staging for TNM7 is a minimum of six nodes. The AJCC (American Joint Committee on Cancer Staging) suggest 18 lymph nodes as the minimum number for accurate staging.[50] The authors' view is that this is too low.

The role of the more extensive three-field dissection in oesophageal malignancy is less clear. Five-year survival rates showed no significant difference between two-field and three-field dissection for lower-third squamous tumours;[32] the same pertains to patients with adenocarcinoma of the lower oesophagus. Patients with cancer of the upper thoracic oesophagus (third field) may benefit from dissection in the neck.[24,38,51]

Summary

There is little justification for oesophagectomy to be performed with intent to cure without any attempt to clear the first level of lymph nodes. Patients with either squamous carcinoma or adenocarcinoma of the oesophagus affecting the upper, middle and lower regions have mediastinal lymph node metastases in over 70% of cases.[21,31,32,52] Over three-quarters of patients presenting with lower-third tumours have positive upper abdominal lymph nodes.[53] In order to perform a potentially curative resection for carcinoma in the middle and lower thirds, a dissection of abdominal and mediastinal lymph nodes is therefore essential.

✔ It is the authors' opinion that a radical en-bloc oesophagectomy with two-field lymph node dissection is the operation of choice for patients with mid and lower third oesophageal cancer and type I tumours of the oesophagogastric junction.

Method of reconstruction of the oesophagus

Route of reconstruction

After resection of the cervical, thoracic or abdominal oesophagus, one of three main paths can be used for reconstruction: presternal, retrosternal and posterior mediastinal (Fig. 5.4).

Presternal route

This route is mentioned for historic completeness. It is approximately 2 cm longer than the retrosternal route, which in turn is approximately 2 cm longer than the posterior mediastinal route. The only indication for using this route is in the situation of multiple previous reconstructions that have compromised the other two routes.

Retrosternal route (anterior mediastinal)

The potential space between the sternum and the anterior mediastinum is easily opened up through effective dissection. There is reported to be a lower incidence of cervical anastomotic dehiscence compared with that of the presternal route. Its major disadvantage stems from the unnatural position of the cervical oesophagus in front of the trachea, which can result in an unpleasant sensation on swallowing.

This route is used for reconstruction following emergency treatment of anastomotic dehiscence or the dehiscence of a gastric substitute that has caused posterior mediastinal sepsis. After incomplete resection (R1 and R2) there is some evidence that a retrosternal conduit would be preferable to the posterior mediastinal route.[54]

The retrosternal route is created by blunt finger dissection through the abdominal and cervical incisions and further developed by insertion of a malleable intestinal retractor. The tip of this instrument is passed up to the neck in direct contact with the back of the sternum. Care is taken not to deviate from the midline. The sternohyoid and sternothyroid muscles are divided in the neck and this allows the passage of the oesophageal substitute easily into the left or right side of the neck. If used for a colonic interposition graft, it is sometimes necessary to resect part of the manubrium/sternoclavicular joint to make room for the colonic graft and anastomosis.

Posterior mediastinal route

This route provides the shortest distance between the abdomen and the apex of the thorax and also the neck.

✔ The posterior mediastinal route is the preferred route of reconstruction in the primary surgical excision of oesophageal cancers.[54,55]

Gastric or colonic substitutes are easily passed through the posterior mediastinum after completion of the oesophageal dissection in the thorax. No attempt is made to close the pleura after this route of reconstruction.

Organ of reconstruction

Reconstruction with stomach

The method of reconstruction should be kept as simple as possible, to minimise complications. The oesophageal replacement is determined by the site of the primary lesion. The stomach is the preferred option as this organ is easy to prepare and involves only one anastomosis.

The patient is positioned supine and exposure obtained using an upper midline incision. There are five broad principles and practices that must be observed in the preparation of the stomach as an oesophageal substitute:

1. **The use of isoperistaltic stomach maintaining vascular supply.** The right gastroepiploic and the right gastric artery and veins are vital to the viability of the stomach when used as an oesophageal substitute. The greater omentum is opened and the entire course of the right

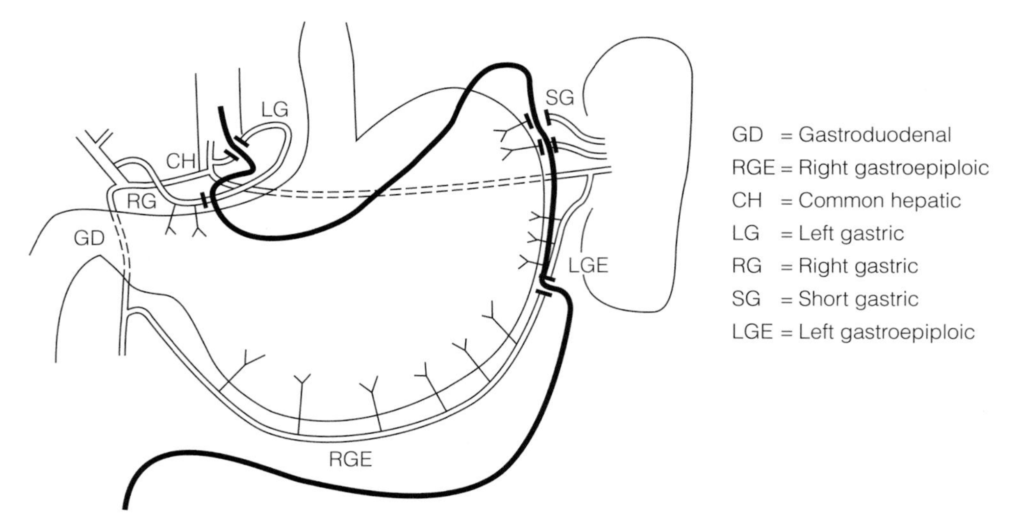

Figure 5.5 • Main arteries of the stomach and points of division of vessels and stomach for oesophageal substitution.

gastroepiploic artery is carefully identified and preserved. The vascular arcade is interrupted at the junction where the right gastroepiploic artery meets the left. The short gastric vessels are divided and ligated (**Fig. 5.5**).

2. **Excision of the lesser curvature.** Cancers of the lower two-thirds of the oesophagus require clearance of the lesser curve lymph nodes as well as the left gastric, common hepatic and proximal splenic artery lymph nodes. The left gastric artery should be ligated at its origin and resection of the proximal half of the lesser curvature of the stomach, including the cardia, is performed. The right gastric artery contributes to the maintenance of the gastric intramural vascular network and should be preserved if possible. Although the width of gastric conduit appeared not to impact on outcome in one study,[56] the authors recommend using a gastric tube of 5 cm width or greater to minimise the risk of ischaemia as described by Akiyama et al.[57] in the 1970s.
3. **Preservation of the intramural vascular arcade.** Extensive intramural arterial anastomoses between the vascular arcades of the lesser and greater curvatures exist. This has been well demonstrated by el-Eishi et al.[58] and Thomas et al.[59] This vascular network must be preserved during resection of the left gastric area of the lesser curvature and the cardia of the stomach. The extent of the resection of the lesser curvature is determined by a line connecting the highest point of the fundus (**Fig. 5.6**) and the lesser curvature at the junction of the right and left gastric arteries. This allows the removal of all potentially involved lymph nodes, yet preserves the arterial network to the fundus. There is no evidence that the trunk and descending branches of the left gastric artery running along the lesser curve need to be preserved and, from an oncological point of view, it is important that these are excised with the specimen. Care should be taken to ligate the short gastric vessels

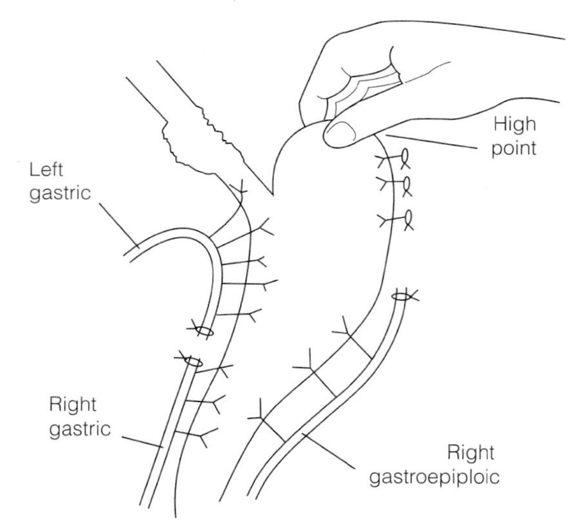

Figure 5.6 • The high point of the stomach.

away from the greater curvature of the stomach to avoid damage to the intramural network and to preserve the extramural vascular network as well. The right gastroepiploic artery provides an adequate blood flow to maintain vascularity in the region of the fundus, which is the area used for anastomosis.

4. **The high point of the stomach.** The stomach is a flexible and capacious organ; its high point is the logical and sensible place at which to fashion an anastomosis with the remaining oesophagus. It is easily identified by applying traction with the surgeon's fingers in an upward direction after all preparations have been completed. The stomach is transected as described previously (Fig. 5.6).
5. **Gastric drainage.** Pyloroplasty or pyloromyotomy after gastric reconstruction is contentious. There is some evidence that pyloroplasty reduces the incidence of gastric outlet obstruction.[60] As short-term complications of pyloroplasty are minimal, the authors routinely perform a pyloroplasty to prevent the life-threatening early complications of gastric stasis and aspiration as well as late vomiting and bloatedness.[46,61]

On occasions the upper anastomosis may need to be as high as the back of the tongue, so the following methods of stomach lengthening must be considered:

1. **Kocher manoeuvre.** This manoeuvre allows the distance between the first part of the duodenum and the hiatus to be reduced.
2. **Excision of the lesser curve of the stomach.** When the lesser curve of the stomach is unusually short, an increase in length of the gastric substitute can be obtained, by dividing the lesser curve between curved clamps, before its resection. If absolutely necessary, a tense right gastric artery may be sacrificed by division at the level of the pylorus.
3. **Incision of the serosa on the gastric wall.** Multiple incisions placed in the gastric serosa may lengthen the stomach. A longitudinal incision placed along the resection line allows this to occur. The indications for this procedure are extremely rare.

Reconstruction with colon

The principal indication for the use of colonic interposition is for tumours requiring an extensive oesophageal as well as gastric resection, although with thorough staging few of these patients are suitable for resection. A small proportion of patients presenting with oesophageal malignancy will have had a previous gastric resection for peptic ulcer disease, precluding the use of stomach as the oesophageal substitute. The numbers of patients such as this are diminishing. The choice of an oesophageal replacement under these circumstances lies between colon and jejunum. The colon is often recommended because of its advantage in having a greater capacity as a reservoir than the jejunum.

Rarely, colon may be used as a conduit after failed gastric interposition that has resulted in gastric necrosis. The disadvantage of colonic transposition is that the function of the conduit deteriorates over time and is therefore not as durable a substitute as the stomach in the long term.

Indications for colonic reconstruction (Box 5.3)

It is preferable to use the colon in an isoperistaltic fashion. Unfortunately the vascular pattern of the colon varies and careful selection of the correct vascular pedicle to ensure viability of the transverse colon is essential. Each case requires evaluation on its own merit because of variations in anatomy. Not infrequently, the marginal artery is found to be of insufficient calibre to maintain viability of the transposed colon. Although the vascular appearance determines the appropriate colonic segment for use in each individual, the two possibilities for effective use of isoperistaltic colon are: (a) transverse colon based on the left colic vessels; (b) right colon based on the middle colic vessels.

The disadvantage of transverse colon is that an abnormally narrow marginal artery may exist at the splenic flexure, compromising the blood supply of the proximal colonic segment. Preoperative assessment by angiography of the colonic vascular pathway has been suggested,[62] but careful intraoperative observation of the vascular anatomy with temporary occlusion of vessels before division is a simple manoeuvre that is effective in most cases.

Surgical technique

Preoperative mechanical bowel preparation is necessary, as is oral antibiotic cover to sterilise the bowel for 48 hours prior to surgery. The omentum is freed from the transverse colon and the hepatic and splenic flexures, while the entire colon is mobilised so that it can be placed outside the abdominal cavity for inspection of its vascular blood supply. Mobilising the sigmoid colon provides additional length so that

Box 5.3 • Indications for colonic reconstruction

- Previous gastric resection
- Tumours with extensive gastric involvement
- Failed gastric transposition

the transverse colon can be tunnelled into the chest, to reach the neck. The proximal colon should be divided and, after anastomosis to the oesophagus, placed on sufficient stretch to prevent redundancy within the chest or in the substernal area. The colon should then be anchored in the straightened position by sutures to the crural margin of the hiatus, although not circumferentially. Continuity of the large bowel is re-established by end-to-end anastomosis, which is conveniently performed before the colo-jejunostomy or colo-gastrostomy for anatomical reasons. An excellent technical description of the use of various segments of colon has been provided by DeMeester et al.[63] O'Sullivan and colleagues have described a useful refinement whereby resection of a short length of colon at either end of the chosen graft, leaving redundant mesentery, maximises blood supply at the critical points of the graft.[64]

Reconstruction with jejunum

Replacement of the lower oesophagus is accomplished using either a Roux-en-Y technique or by segmental interposition. Replacement of the upper oesophagus is accomplished by free jejunal transfer with microvascular anastomosis of the jejunal pedicle to neck vessels. It is sometimes possible to create a long loop for replacement of the entire thoracic oesophagus, particularly when the proximal jejunum has adapted after previous gastric surgery. The jejunum should be considered the third choice, after stomach and colon.

No specific measures are required to prepare the small bowel preoperatively other than to ensure that patients are not known to have small-bowel pathology. A loop of jejunum is identified in the upper segments within the first 25 cm after the duodenojejunal flexure. The typical jejunal vascular pattern of arterial arcades is encountered in this area, and the veins and arteries are close together but bifurcate at separate levels, making individual division of the veins and arteries essential. Transillumination of the mesentery helps to identify the jejunal vascular tree precisely. It is important to appreciate that, during the creation of a jejunal loop, it is the length of the free edge of the mesentery that will determine the length of the loop created rather than the length of the jejunum itself. The jejunum is usually longer than the mesentery and will therefore have a tendency to become redundant.

The technique of microvascular free jejunal transfer for reconstruction of the upper oesophagus is well described elsewhere.[65] The specific indications for such a reconstruction are usually after pharyngo-laryngectomy performed for carcinoma of the hypopharynx, postcricoid region and cervical oesophagus. The operation is usually performed with a radical neck dissection as part of the primary treatment programme or as palliative surgery following recurrence after radiotherapy.

Open surgical approaches to oesophagectomy

The preceding discussion has described the method and rationale underpinning the surgical objectives in treating oesophageal cancer. The aims of resecting the primary tumour together with the lymph nodes and oesophageal reconstruction must be achieved safely and effectively and with ease of access. The method of surgical approach to obtain these objectives must be considered in each individual case. The choice of the surgical approach is dependent on the tumour location, the extent of spread, the fitness, age and build of the individual patient.

Pharyngolaryngo-oesophagectomy for carcinoma of the hypopharynx and cervical oesophagus

Resection of squamous lesions in this area is achieved by removal of the larynx, the lower pharynx, cervical trachea, one or both lobes of the thyroid gland, and the cervical oesophagus. If the tumour is located in the hypopharynx only (postcricoid region), the thoracic oesophagus may be conserved and a free graft of jejunum transferred by microvascular anastomosis, as previously described. If tumour has extended to the lower part of the cervical oesophagus, a total pharyngolaryngo-oesophagectomy and gastric transposition, with immediate pharyngogastric reconstruction, is the treatment of choice.

The patient is placed in the supine position with the neck hyperextended; a U-shaped incision provides excellent access. It allows the construction of a permanent tracheostomy with ease and may be extended into a Y-shaped incision ready for a median sternotomy if required. The resection includes a radical lymph node dissection in the neck. The thyroid and parathyroid glands are also removed en bloc with the internal jugular vein and the deep internal cervical nodes. The common carotid artery, vagus nerve and the sympathetic trunk are carefully protected.

✔ Left thoracotomy was the standard approach until the 1960s, and although it provided excellent access to the lower oesophagus, exposure of the upper and middle thoracic oesophagus was restricted by the aortic arch. Two-phase right thoracotomy (initially described by Lewis and Tanner) is now accepted as the open approach of choice to the thoracic oesophagus.[32,61]

Two-phase subtotal oesophagectomy via a right thoracotomy for carcinomas of the middle and lower thirds of the oesophagus

The first phase is abdominal mobilisation of the stomach performed through an upper midline laparotomy incision. The second phase is mediastinal dissection and oesophageal resection through a right thoracotomy. The stomach is delivered into the chest and an anastomosis fashioned at the thoracic inlet.

The procedure begins with a laparotomy to assess the primary tumour and exclude the presence of distant metastases. During gastric mobilisation, described earlier, it is important that all posterior attachments of the stomach are divided, especially at the antrum, so that the distal stomach can slide up to the right crus without tension. The gastroepiploic arcade must be separated from the transverse mesocolon in the bloodless plane to mobilise attachments inferior to the pylorus. Some helpful steps include use of retractors fixed to the operating table (Omni-Tract, Omni-Tract® Surgical, Minnesota Scientific Inc., St Paul, MN, USA) and, where short gastric vessel access is difficult, placement of a pack behind the spleen to bring it forward.

The coeliac trunk (common hepatic and the roots of the splenic and left gastric arteries) is skeletonised by complete removal of the surrounding lymph nodes. The left gastric artery is divided and ligated at its origin.

The abdominal oesophagus is dissected from the hiatus, taking a cuff of hiatal muscle if the tumour is located here, beginning the dissection into the chest. Anteriorly, all tissue posterior to the pericardium is taken en bloc, making the dissection plane for the thoracic phase clear. The right and left pleura at this point at this point are entered and resected en bloc if they are going to resect the oesophagus within its partial pleural envelope. There must be sufficient room at the hiatus for the conduit to lie unimpeded, so sometimes partial division of the right crus of the diaphragm is necessary.[64]

The patient is then placed in the left lateral decubitus position and is held firmly in place by a moulding mattress. The operating table is broken to widen the intercostal space. The right arm is fixed on a padded armrest while the left is stretched out on an arm support.

The mediastinal phase is performed via a right posterolateral thoracotomy through the fourth or fifth intercostal space. There is a tendency to open the chest through too low an incision. It is essential to count the ribs by palpation under the scapula and to go no lower than the fifth intercostal space. In high tumours, such as middle-third squamous lesions, a suprazygous dissection is performed.

The superior mediastinal pleura is incised along the course of the right vagus nerve and is extended upwards towards the brachiocephalic and subclavian arteries. The right recurrent laryngeal nerve is preserved and meticulous dissection is then applied to the lymph node chain alongside it. The pleura is incised along the border of the superior vena cava and the right paratracheal lymph nodes located between the trachea and the vein are then dissected free. Care is taken not to dissect circumferentially around the trachea, as this may prejudice its blood supply. This supra-azygous dissection is not necessary for lower-third lesions.

Routine division and/or resection of the arch of the azygos vein is crucial for adequate exposure. The azygos vein marks the line of dissection caudally to the hiatus. The incision through the pleura is deepened to expose the adventitia on the descending aorta. The thoracic duct itself is rarely the site of metastases, except in extensive disease. There are, however, numerous lymph nodes scattered along the length of the duct in the para-aortic region. To remove these, an en-bloc resection together with the duct is necessary. The duct is easily identified after minimal sharp dissection in the inferior mediastinum on the adventitia of the right aspect of the descending thoracic aorta just above the hiatus. The duct is first ligated at this point and then at the proximal end after resection in the superior mediastinum, along the posterior border of the oesophagus. Chylothorax secondary to inadvertent and undetected damage to the thoracic duct is therefore prevented. Dissection continues on to the right pulmonary hilum, where there is almost always a small anthracotic lymph node. The right bronchial, subcarinal and left bronchial nodes are dissected. It is advisable to avoid monopolar diathermy in this region because of the vulnerability of the membranous part of both the trachea and bronchi.

The stomach is delivered into the chest and the specimen removed after careful sleeve resection of the lesser curvature, as previously described. The oesophagus is then transected high in the chest once sufficient gastric conduit length is confirmed. An oesophagogastric anastomosis is fashioned in the apex of the thorax. In addition to ensuring adequate resection margins, it is vital that the whole gastric conduit is within the thorax for a good functional outcome. If a lower anastomosis is fashioned, differences in abdominal and mediastinal pressure promote reflux and inhibit gastric emptying, resulting in troublesome symptoms and poor quality of life.

The chest is closed in layers with two intercostal drains on the right; a left intercostal drain is placed if the left pleura has been breached or resected.

Combined synchronous two-team oesophagectomy

Modification of the standard access for oesophagectomy has been described wherein mobilisation of the stomach and abdominal oesophagus proceeds synchronously with mobilisation of the thoracic oesophagus via a right anterolateral thoracotomy using a second operating team.[66,67] A reduction in operating and anaesthetic time was suggested as a possible reason for decreased operative morbidity and mortality rates in Hong Kong Chinese patients. Patients in the study had a lower incidence of pulmonary and cardiovascular disease than those with oesophageal cancer in the West.

✔ A comparison of the synchronous two-team approach with conventional two-stage subtotal oesophagectomy was performed in Western patients. Not only was there a higher incidence of complications and a higher mortality rate, but an adequate nodal dissection in larger, more obese patients was technically very difficult because of the limited surgical access.[68]

Three-phase subtotal oesophagectomy for tumours of the upper middle third of the oesophagus

Exposing and dividing the oesophagus in the neck certainly provides excellent access for anastomosis, although it does not allow resection of much more oesophagus than can be removed by the two-phase approach. This is because the cervical oesophagus is relatively short and it is difficult to perform an anastomosis unless a stump of oesophagus is left, hence the term subtotal oesophagectomy. McKeown[69] recommended cervical anastomosis on the grounds that a leak in the neck is less catastrophic than a thoracic leak. This is probably an overstatement and is now of less significance as overall true oesophageal anastomotic leakage is uncommon (ideally less than 5%). The three-phase operation takes longer to complete and is also associated with early postoperative difficulty in swallowing. This is probably because of the extensive proximal mobilisation of the cervical oesophagus. Proponents of the three-phase operation claim that a more complete oesophagectomy is achieved. If the tumour cannot be resected with an adequate proximal longitudinal margin then the three-phase technique ought to be employed.

The first phase of this operation is routine gastric mobilisation with dissection of the nodal groups, as described above. The second phase should mirror the dissection described in the preceding section, but adding the mobilisation of the oesophagus in the apex of the thorax. It is useful here to mobilise the cervical oesophagus from below and place a Penrose drain around it and leave it high in the root of the neck. This helps in the cervical dissection. The right thorax is closed and the patient turned supine once again. Through either a left- or right-sided cervical incision, the whole of the thoracic oesophagus can be removed and the stomach delivered into the neck and an oesophagogastrostomy fashioned. Operating time may be reduced by performing the thoracic phase first and then turning the patient supine for synchronous abdominal and neck phases.

Left-sided subtotal oesophagectomy for lower-third oesophageal cancers

A left-sided approach has been popular in the past for lower-third tumours, predominantly amongst thoracic surgeons, initially using a thoracotomy and phrenotomy, and later a thoraco-abdominal incision, crossing the costal arch.[70,71] Exposure is not adequate to perform a thorough abdominal lymphadenectomy without dividing the costal arch, and indeed at least one author has described a higher positive resection margin with the left thoracotomy approach.[72] A left-sided approach is absolutely contraindicated if the tumour is situated at or above the aortic arch as exposure of this part of the oesophagus is inadequate.

The left thoraco-abdominal approach is still appropriate for selected patients to resect tumours that have limited but significant involvement of the cardia[73] and for patients requiring extended total gastrectomy. A good operative description is given by Sundaresan.[70] It is important to use a circumferential incision to divide the diaphragm rather than a radial incision that denervates part of the left diaphragm. A paravertebral catheter can be used to provide good analgesia for this unilateral, single-dermatome incision.[74] The Japanese Clinical Oncology Group trial has shown that, for proximal gastric cancer, the left thoraco-abdominal approach has a higher complication rate and no survival benefit compared to the alternative transhiatal approach to gastrectomy.[75]

Transhiatal oesophagectomy for upper- and lower-third tumours of the oesophagus

Controversy still exists about the role of oesophagectomy without thoracotomy in oesophageal cancer surgery. Proponents of the technique argue that outcome is dependent on the stage at presentation rather than the operative technique employed. Opponents claim improvements in survival for some undergoing radical en-bloc resection.[25,35] The original technique was a blind procedure, defying the fundamental principle that surgery should always be carried out under direct vision.[76–78] Nevertheless, refinements to the technique have been made and the operation has developed and gained many advocates.[79] Orringer et al. have published a series of over 2000 transhiatal resections that demonstrates an improvement in outcomes over 30 years with refinements of technique.[80] Data on resection margins and lymph node harvest are not supplied. When questioned about the absence of radical lymphadenectomy in these patients, Dr Orringer gave the caveat that if nodal disease is suspected by postneoadjuvant staging, he would opt for a transthoracic approach with formal lymphadenectomy.[80] The issue of routine radical lymphadenectomy has been discussed earlier in this chapter.

A modified technique of transhiatal oesophagectomy under direct vision has been described[81] using a modification of the transhiatal technique described by Pinotti.[81] Almost the entire procedure is undertaken under direct vision, ensuring adequate local clearance by avoiding direct contact with the tumour, and the anastomosis performed in the neck as a combined synchronous operation. The authors demonstrated no evidence of proximal or distal resection margin involvement with the tumour and an acceptable morbidity and mortality.

Details of the surgical procedure are clearly described elsewhere.[82] At present there are selected indications for transhiatal oesophagectomy:

- **Carcinoma of the hypopharynx and cervical oesophagus.** If the tumour is localised the incidence of mediastinal metastases is low. In this situation oesophagectomy without thoracotomy can be safely performed by blunt dissection. Radical neck dissection with pharyngolaryngo-oesophagectomy is carried out at the same time and reconstruction fashioned using the stomach through the posterior mediastinal route.
- **Intraepithelial squamous carcinoma of the oesophagus.** These tumours rarely disseminate via the lymphatics.[19] With substantial progress in endoscopic techniques using epithelial dye staining and endoscopic ultrasonography, early tumours can be more accurately staged. When tumour penetration is confined to the epithelial layer, resection by transhiatal oesophagectomy is entirely feasible (Chapter 6).
- **Patients with high-grade dysplasia within a Barrett segment,** in whom endoscopic mucosal resection and/or radiofrequency ablation is not an option, in the absence of invasion or nodal disease.

The debate will continue over which operative procedure is most appropriate for the treatment of lower-third oesophageal carcinoma. Randomised studies have rarely been performed and no clear survival advantage has emerged for any particular operative technique.

✔✔ Four randomised controlled trials comparing the transhiatal approach with the transthoracic approach have been published.[40,41,83,84] These have failed to demonstrate significant differences between the two approaches.

The strongest evidence so far comes from the Dutch trial,[40,43] which included 220 patients with adenocarcinoma of the middle and lower oesophagus. Significantly more nodes were dissected in the thoracic approach, but pulmonary complications were also greater. Significance was reached for an increased survival in the radical transthoracic approach, which continued with long-term data. Interestingly, patients with lower oesophageal tumours (Siewert type 1) and those with a low burden (1–8 nodes) of nodal disease appeared to benefit from extended transthoracic oesophagectomy, as discussed earlier in the chapter.

Minimally invasive surgical approaches to oesophagectomy

During the last 20 years, much progress has been made in attempting to reduce the morbidity of open surgery by the introduction of minimal access procedures across all surgical specialties. Surgical access undoubtedly adds to the trauma of oesophagectomy, but it is still unclear by how much. Whatever approach is taken, the extensive dissection involved in radical en-bloc oesophagectomy is still a very significant physiological challenge. The additional mental stress that oesophagectomy and a cancer diagnosis places on the patient still means that oesophagectomy is a challenging ordeal for the perioperative and postoperative period regardless of approach.

It is entirely appropriate that much energy has been invested in the search for the 'holy grail' of a radical oesophageal resection that can be undertaken with minimum trauma of access. However, outcomes from series of minimal access procedures must be comparable with the best outcomes from open surgery. Low and colleagues report a consecutive series of 340 patients, with an anastomotic leak rate of 3.4% and an in-hospital mortality of 0.3%, outcomes with which few if any minimally invasive series can compare. However, there were a variety of open procedures used by Low and colleagues, the majority being left thoraco-abdominal.[85]

Minimally invasive three-stage procedures

The first publications from Luketich et al.[86,87] describing the total minimally invasive thoracoscopic, laparoscopic oesophagectomy with cervical anastomosis held out the potential of being the minimal access approach for some time. The procedure was technically challenging, even if a mini-laparotomy was added for gastric tube formation,[88] and the learning curve was steep. For many surgeons who do not routinely perform a cervical anastomosis for lower-third tumour excision, adopting this operation would add, in their view, unnecessary complexity and risk. It was not worth adopting a three-stage approach to avoid the technical challenge of a minimally invasive intrathoracic anastomosis.

Despite enormous interest in the procedure, few centres other than Pittsburgh have published their results.[88–93] Some authors reported significant anastomotic leak rates[87,88] and highlighted an increased conduit necrosis rate.[89] This was of sufficient concern that attempts were made by two centres to improve gastric conduit vascularity through ischaemic conditioning,[94–96] although there are no randomised studies to show this to be effective. Non-randomised comparative studies from single institutions suggested that the three-stage total minimally invasive procedure had equivalent but not better outcomes than open surgery.[92–94] A multicentre feasibility study (Eastern Cooperative Oncology Group ECOG 2202) comprising 106 patients in 16 institutions suggests that short-term outcomes are acceptable.[97]

To the authors' knowledge only one multicentre randomised controlled trial, comparing three-stage minimally invasive oesophagectomy with open surgery, has been conducted and recently published (TIME trial).[98]

Minimally invasive two-stage procedures

It is significant that Luketich and colleagues describe a change in practice, away from a cervical phase, favouring a minimally invasive two-stage laparoscopic, thoracoscopic procedure with a minithoracotomy, first reported in 2006.[99] Levy and colleagues report disadvantages with the cervical phase including recurrent nerve injury, perturbations in pharyngeal transit and swallowing dysfunction even in the absence of overt recurrent laryngeal nerve injury.[100] Thoracoscopic, laparoscopic two-stage oesophagectomy has become their preferred approach, but they caution a steep learning curve and emphasise the critical importance of appropriate thoracic port placement. There are few large series of this procedure, and no randomised studies on which to recommend this approach.

Minimally invasive hybrid procedures

There are two main hybrid approaches that are commonly undertaken. The first is a three-stage procedure with a thoracoscopic oesophageal mobilisation combined with an open abdominal phase and a cervical anastomosis. Smithers et al. have published series of this procedure in a non-randomised comparison with totally minimally invasive oesophagectomy.[92] The advantage of this approach is extracorporeal gastric conduit formation together with manual passing of the conduit through the mediastinum to the neck, avoiding traction injury, carefully presenting the conduit to the neck. Disadvantages are those of a cervical phase mentioned above as well as the need for an epidural for analgesia.

The second hybrid procedure is a two-stage approach with a laparoscopic abdominal phase and an open thoracic phase. There are few series of this approach published, but a prospective randomised trial (MIRO trial) has been completed at the time of writing, awaiting publication of early outcomes.[101] The potential advantages of this approach are, again, extracorporeal gastric conduit formation, ideal conditions for performing an anastomosis and gentle handling of the conduit within the chest. Another advantage is that an epidural catheter can be avoided if a paravertebral catheter is used for analgesia.[102,103]

While we do not have robust evidence to recommend minimal access approaches to oesophagectomy in favour of open procedures at the time of writing, there is evidence that Health Related Quality of Life appears to be well preserved, at least in the early postoperative period, in particular with total minimally invasive approaches,[104] although this may be a short-lived advantage, with one series reporting significantly more delayed gastric emptying.[90]

Overview of minimally invasive approaches

The many individual series of hybrid or totally minimally invasive resection have been reviewed collectively,[46,58–61] showing no advantage, or a relatively small advantage of a minimally invasive approach. There may be better evidence in the near future from prospective randomised trials,[98,101] but in the absence of this quality of evidence, the authors' opinion is that totally minimally invasive and hybrid approaches to oesophagectomy have yet to prove themselves superior to open surgery.[105]

Current practice

Mamidanna et al.[106] have recently published HES (Hospital Episode Statistics) data showing that, of the 7502 oesophageal resections undertaken in England between April 2005 and March 2010, 15.5% were performed with a minimally invasive component. This has risen to 24.7% for the year 2009–10, a fourfold increase over the decade. These procedures were not uniformly distributed amongst surgeons or trusts. The authors examined whether there were differences in short-term outcome between minimally invasive and open procedures.

There was no difference in 30-day mortality (4.0% for minimally invasive approaches, 4.3% for open), 30-day postoperative morbidity (38% for minimally invasive approaches, 39.2% for open) or hospital readmissions (13.1% for minimally invasive approaches, 13.0% for open). There was little difference in length of stay, but in view of the population size, there was a slightly shorter length of stay for minimally invasive approaches. There was a significantly higher re-intervention rate (unplanned procedures within 30 days) for minimally invasive approaches (21.0% vs. 17.6%, $P=0.06$) including a higher re-operation rate (8.8% vs. 5.6%, $P<0.001$). Re-intervention was associated with increased morbidity. The odds ratio for re-intervention increased with each study year. Those resections that involved thoracoscopy and laparoscopy had twice the re-intervention rate of hybrid procedures where only thoracoscopy or laparoscopy was involved.

Rice and Blackstone[107] raise significant questions about minimally invasive approaches to oesophagectomy that arise from this study and list them in their editorial.

Technique of anastomosis

Meticulous technique is essential in minimising the risk of leakage after oesophageal anastomosis, which is still associated with a significant mortality. The surgical principles relating to anastomoses are universal. Emphasis is placed on:

- adequate blood supply;
- absence of tension;
- accurate approximation of epithelial edges;
- precise layer-to-layer suturing with primary healing.

One-, two- and three-layer anastomoses have been described, but no conclusive randomised controlled studies have been reported. A two-layer oesophagogastric anastomosis is advocated by Akiyama,[19] who emphasises the absence of a serosal layer, which he believes would reinforce strength at the anastomotic site. He therefore advocates a carefully preserved adventitia, which provides sufficient strength to support sutures.

Stapling devices have been developed for ease of introduction and application, with a low-profile head that permits a larger-diameter anvil to be introduced into the oesophageal stump. A larger-diameter anastomosis is thereby fashioned, reducing the rate of benign anastomotic stricture formation, most commonly seen with a staple ring diameter of 25 mm or less.[9,52,108] The staple head can now also be inserted transorally, allowing a double-staple technique, similar to that in colorectal surgery, to be used.

Anastomotic leakage is more frequent in the neck than the chest, although the related mortality rates have not been shown to differ between these anastomotic sites.[109] Leakage rate does not depend on suture material or the technical modalities used to perform the anastomosis. Indeed, there is no evidence that the overall decrease in anastomotic complications is related to the use of a specific conduit approach or route of reconstruction; it is more likely due to progress made in general perioperative management.[110]

The semi-mechanical anastomosis, with a side-to-side configuration, a linear stapled posterior wall and a hand-sewn anterior wall has been described by Collard et al.[111] and by Orringer et al.[112] with an associated reduction in cervical anastomotic leak rate and long-term stricture rate. However, the majority of these anastomoses have been performed during transhiatal oesophagectomy for lower-third tumours, so that sufficient length of cervical oesophagus could be left without compromising resection margins. The authors would caution against this anastomosis if the purpose of the cervical dissection is primarily proximal clearance; in this situation a high anastomosis using interrupted sutures to a short cervical oesophagus allows more proximal clearance. The authors have many years' experience of wrapping the anastomosis with transposed omentum.

✔ No significant difference has been demonstrated between leakage rates using hand-sewn and mechanical anastomoses.[110]

Postoperative management

A detailed account of immediate postoperative care after oesophageal cancer surgery is described in Chapter 4, and a summary is given in Boxes 5.4 and 5.5. Meticulous attention to the maintenance of fluid balance and respiratory care is essential in the immediate postoperative period. Adequate pain control via a thoracic epidural and physiotherapy are crucial. It is the authors' routine practice to enterally feed patients undergoing oesophagectomy in the postoperative period, commencing feeding via jejunostomy early postoperatively. Early mobilisation as part of an enhanced recovery programme is important in preventing venous thrombosis and pulmonary embolus. It also enhances ventilation, clearance of sputum and early bowel movement. Removal of the chest drains by the fifth postoperative day helps in mobilisation, especially once free oral fluids have recommenced.

Box 5.4 • Routine postoperative measures

- Fluid balance
- Intensive physiotherapy
- Analgesia
- Antithromboembolic measures
- Nutrition

Box 5.5 • Routine sequence of events after extubation

1. 25 mL water/hour from day 1
2. Four times daily intensive physiotherapy from days 1 to 4
3. Antibiotics days 0–2
4. Mobilisation at day 1
5. Nasogastric suction for days 1–5
6. Chest drains removed on days 5 and 6

The role of routine postoperative radiological imaging of the oesophageal anastomosis has become clearer. There is no evidence that the routine use of contrast radiology is of any value in patients who are asymptomatic in the postoperative phase.[113,114] Patients who are clinically well should be started on oral feeding, while video endoscopy or contrast radiology should be reserved for patients showing signs of sepsis, pleural effusion or haemodynamic instability. Non-ionic contrast media may pick up gross leaks, but if no leak is shown should be followed up by barium investigations or an endoscopy to exclude a small leak.

Routine nasogastric decompression is continued for 5 days until gastrointestinal activity is restored. Patients are allowed 25 mL of water every hour soon after extubation. Subcutaneous low-dose heparin is administered routinely until and after the patient is discharged for a further 4 weeks. Chest physiotherapy is commenced in intensive care and continued 4-hourly for the first 3 days. Prophylactic antibiotics are commenced on the morning of surgery and continued for two postoperative doses. All patients should be counselled by the surgeon, an oesophageal cancer nurse specialist and a dietician prior to discharge.

Postoperative complications

Postoperative complications may be subdivided into those that are common to any major surgical procedure in an elderly population and those specific to oesophageal resection. The complication rate of oesophageal surgery is relatively high, in the region of 30–40%. Some studies have found increased morbidity rates following neoadjuvant therapy, particularly respiratory problems after chemoradiotherapy. This seems to be further compounded with salvage oesophagectomy after definitive chemoradiotherapy for squamous carcinoma.[115] Early recognition of complications and rapid proactive management are essential to achieve good results for all patients. It has been proposed that postoperative complications are not only associated with poor early outcome, but also, possibly through immunosuppression, with early death from cancer recurrence.[116]

General complications

These complications (see also Chapter 4) may be minimised by improved preoperative patient evaluation. Respiratory complications constitute the largest proportion of this group. Pain is the major contributor to decreased ventilation and atelectasis, which leads to bronchopneumonia and respiratory failure. Extensive lymphadenectomy can cause poor lymphatic drainage of the pulmonary alveoli, leading to parenchymal fluid retention and a consequent acute pulmonary oedema. Significant respiratory complications occur in approximately 24% of cases following subtotal oesophagectomy.[117]

Thromboembolic complications are not uncommon in malignant disease in the elderly. Myocardial ischaemia and cerebral vascular episodes are specific to the age group undergoing surgery and are precipitated by hypoxia, hypotension and underlying vascular occlusive disease.

Major haemorrhage is uncommon and as a result of meticulous technique and the use of new techniques, such as the ultrasonic scalpel during gastric mobilisation, routine blood loss is less than 500 mL, with only a small minority of patients requiring transfusion. Secondary haemorrhage is also rare and is almost always associated with a mediastinal infection from a specific complication such as an anastomotic leakage. The value of minimisation of surgical blood loss should not be underestimated. Perioperative blood transfusion is a significant predictor of decreased overall survival.[118]

Specific complications

The second group of complications following oesophageal surgery for cancer is specific to the procedure.

Anastomotic leakage and leakage from the gastric conduit

Anastomotic leakage is influenced by a variety of factors, including cancer hypermetabolism, malnutrition, anastomotic vascular deficit, anastomotic tension and surgical technique. The incidence of anastomotic leakage has decreased significantly over the last 10 years and rates of well under 5% should be expected.[110,113,119]

Early disruption (within 48–72 hours) is the result of a technical error. If early disruption is confirmed and the general condition of the patient is good, then the patient should be re-explored for correction of the technical fault.

✔ High-definition upper gastrointestinal endoscopy is important in diagnosis and particularly the identification of any conduit necrosis.[113]

Total gastric necrosis can, rarely, occur with catastrophic consequences. This complication must be diagnosed early by high-resolution endoscopy, resuscitation given immediately and the patient returned to theatre for the formation of a cervical oesophagostomy and closing of the viable component of the gastric remnant. The establishment of a feeding jejunostomy is essential if not already in place. At a later date when the patient has stabilised, a colonic interposition is used to restore intestinal continuity. Later disruptions manifest themselves between the fifth and tenth postoperative days and are due to ischaemia of the tissues or tension on the anastomotic line. For leaks from the oesophagogastric anastomosis operative intervention is likely to be hazardous and possibly detrimental. Intensive non-operative treatment with nasogastric suction, radiologically guided chest and mediastinal drainage, therapeutic antibiotic regimens and early enteral nutrition via a jejunostomy are all essential. Late anastomotic leakage should not result in a high mortality if it is aggressively managed.

✔ The authors would strongly urge against the insertion of self-expandable stents in this situation as they prevent adequate drainage of sepsis, are prone to migrate, and may ultimately erode into surrounding structures.

Dehiscence of the gastric resection line is rare but requires re-exploration as the extent of leakage is frequently large.[113]

Chylothorax

The thoracic duct can often be damaged during mobilisation of advanced oesophageal cancers, whether via a right thoracotomy or through the transhiatal route. A comprehensive review reports chylothorax occurring in up to 10% of patients after blunt transhiatal oesophagectomy.[120] An incidence of 2–3% during open resection is commonly reported.[121] Accidental damage to the thoracic duct can be prevented by identification during dissection, as previously described, and ligating the duct low in the inferior mediastinum on the right lateral aspect of the descending thoracic aorta. Chylothorax usually presents in the first 7 days after surgery, when the patient has commenced oral intake, or jejunostomy feeds, especially of fat-containing nutrients. A massive increase in chest drainage occurs, that if left untreated results in malnutrition and significant immune suppression, with a markedly reduced CD4 count, from the subsequent white cell loss. It is difficult to predict whether a chylous leak will spontaneously heal despite attempts to quantify the size of the leak.[122] Immediate re-exploration is therefore recommended for major leaks, as the damaged thoracic duct is usually easily identified, following a bolus of cream, at the time of re-exploration.[121] Leaks of less than 500 mL/day may resolve with enteral feeding using medium-chain triglycerides. Prolonged total parenteral nutrition has been used but patients who rapidly become malnourished are prone to nosocomial infections and frequently require a long hospital stay. Prophylactic antibiotic cover with co-trimoxazole for *Pneumocystis* is essential for the lymphopenic patient.[123] On rare occasions, chylothorax can be resistant to treatment, whether re-exploration or conservative therapy. This is often due to abnormal lymph anatomy around the hiatus. The author has documented up to three large ducts in the posterior mediastinum in such patients. Pleuroperitoneal shunting has resulted in successful outcomes in resistant chylous leaks. This allows reabsorption of chyle and prevents the sequelae of immune suppression.

Recurrent laryngeal palsy

The incidence of recurrent laryngeal palsy has increased over recent years due to the increase of cervical oesophagogastric anastomoses. It is extremely rare when the anastomosis is constructed in the apex of the chest via the thoracotomy route for subtotal oesophagectomy. If the palsy is transient but unilateral, the opposite cord may well compensate. If the palsy is permanent, Teflon injection of the cord or a formal thyroplasty can restore adequate voice volume and a satisfactory cough.[124]

Gastric outlet obstruction

Gastric outlet obstruction is prevented by the routine use of a pyloroplasty or a pyloromyotomy. Emptying problems are kept at a minimum when the anastomosis is in the apex of the thorax. Procedures that leave part of the stomach as an abdominal organ and part of the stomach as a thoracic organ predispose to duodeno-gastro-oesophageal reflux. Prokinetic agents such as low-dose erythromycin can improve gastric emptying and minimise these complications. Dumping syndrome after oesophagogastric reconstruction is relatively common but usually resolves in the 12 months following surgery. It is adequately treated by the avoidance of high carbohydrate loads.

Duodeno-gastro-oesophageal reflux

Acid or alkaline reflux is common[125,126] and, although it may be controlled by motility agents and acid suppressants, can be troublesome. There is some evidence that performing a modified fundoplication as an antireflux manoeuvre at the time of oesophagectomy is effective in controlling post-oesophagectomy reflux in the majority of patients.[127]

Benign anastomotic stricture

These strictures are not uncommon but usually respond to a single dilatation performed with the flexible video endoscope under image intensification and sedation.[9]

Overall results of single-modality resectional therapy

Overall results of surgical therapy in oesophageal cancer can be analysed in terms of hospital mortality and patient survival. Assessment of quality of life (patient-related outcomes) as an outcome measure is essential as there is increasing evidence relating it to overall survival.[128] The fact that it takes 9 months for quality of life to recover following surgery illustrates the scale of trauma that oesophagectomy produces. Very few new data have become available on single-modality surgery for oesophageal cancer. Increasingly, published results include patients subjected to multimodality treatments.

Hospital mortality

Although individual units have achieved considerably better results, three comprehensive reviews during the last two decades shed some light on trends in both hospital mortality and overall survival.[8,129,130]

✔ The review of Jamieson et al.[130] confirmed that the average hospital mortality rate following oesophagectomy had continued to decrease, from 28% (1953–1978), to 13% (1980–1988), to 8.8% (1990–2000).

This may be attributed to improvements in anaesthesia, surgical technique, perioperative care, and the specialisation and centralisation of oesophageal cancer services. No evidence has been provided to relate tumour biology to mortality rate following oesophageal resection and there is no difference in mortality rates between resections for squamous cell carcinoma and adenocarcinoma. Overall mortality rates in many series can be confusing because of variations in definitions. 'In-hospital' and not 30-day mortality rates should be quoted in all papers, but unfortunately this continues not to be the case. Series from specialist centres in the last few years cite operative hospital mortality rates of less than 5%.[31,51,113] This includes a huge series of over 20 000 oesophagectomies from China.[131] There is no longer any place for the occasional oesophagectomist in the management of this disease. There is clearly still further room for improvement as data from a large multicentre UK audit recently reported mortality rates of over 10%.[132]

Comparisons of hospital mortality rates for different resection techniques reveal only minor differences. In the review by Muller et al.,[119] the lowest mortality rate was for transhiatal oesophagectomy, with a median figure of 8%. These data, however, are not strictly comparable because transhiatal resection was the most recent surgical development and therefore benefited from the experience of recent advances in perioperative care.

✔✔ Nevertheless, preoperative risk analysis using a J composite scoring system to predict operative risk managed to show a decrease in mortality in a large series from 9.4% to 1.6%.[16] No overall difference was noted in the randomised controlled trial of transthoracic versus transhiatal approaches in the Dutch study.

Rigorous preoperative assessment will continue to reduce hospital mortality from this major thoraco-abdominal operation (see Chapter 4).

Survival figures

In a review of the 1980s, Muller et al. found that 56% of all resected patients survived the first postoperative year, 34% the second, 25% the third, 21% the fourth and 20% the fifth year after resection. It was depressing to note that these figures were very similar to those collected by Earlam and Cunha Melo, revealing that despite improved hospital mortality, the overall long-term prognosis had remained unchanged. No differences in the 5-year survival rates were noted between different techniques of resection but en-bloc resections showed a significantly better long-term prognosis.[28,77] Data from the Dutch trial[40] revealed 5-year survival was 36% and 34% after transhiatal and transthoracic resection, respectively. There is some evidence to suggest that adenocarcinomas tend to fare worse than squamous lesions, although this may simply reflect the more advanced stage at which these lesions tend to present.[72] With increasing numbers of early tumours being diagnosed on surveillance programmes for Barrett's oesophagus, this hypothesis will be tested. The primary determinants of overall outcome appear to be the stage of the tumour and the cell type.

Trying to identify improvements in overall survival for adenocarcinoma over time from surgery alone is difficult because of the now widespread use of neoadjuvant treatment for locally advanced disease. Over the past decade the continued reporting of results combining both adenocarcinoma and squamous cell cancers has made interpretation even more confounding. Most recent 'surgery-alone' series reflect operations for very early disease that would not allow for comparisons with the earlier publications. However, as discussed earlier there are data from the Dutch trial that revealed 5-year survival for adenocarcinoma was 34% and 36% after transhiatal and transthoracic resection, respectively.[40] The long-term results of the OEO2 study showed that for adenocarcinoma the unimodality surgery patients had a 5-year survival of 17.6%.[133] A population-based study from Sweden evaluated survival with resection alone from 1997 to 2005: the 5-year survival for adenocarcinoma was 28.3% for the 2001–2005 cohort.[134] The Worldwide Esophageal Cancer Collaboration (WECC) data included surgery-alone patients from several decades and produced separate survival curves for adenocarcinoma and squamous cancer.[135] Five-year survival for adenocarcinoma was approximately 80% for TNM7 stages 0 and 1A, approximately 64% for stage 1B, 50% for 2A, 40% for 2B and 25% for 3A.[135]

Overall survival is therefore strongly stage dependent. There are many case series describing stage-specific survival but there has been no systematic review of these reports. The authors' published results confirm a greater than 90% 5-year survival for stage 0 and stage 1 disease. For stage 2a, 2b and stage 3 disease, 5-year survival is 60%, 19% and 15% respectively.[31] Other specialist units have achieved similar results with resection and two-field lymphadenectomy as unimodality therapy.[17,31,38,40,41,45,51] The poor outcome for patients with node-positive disease has led to multimodality therapy becoming the standard of care for these patients. A recent meta-analysis demonstrated a greater 2-year survival benefit for both neoadjuvant chemoradiotherapy and chemotherapy, although the standardisation of the staging investigations and surgical resection has been questioned in many of these trials[115] (see Chapter 9).

Summary and future research

The main areas of progress and interest in surgery for oesophageal cancer have been the introduction of a multidisciplinary approach, improved disease staging, the development of new surgical and endoscopic techniques for the management of early tumours including minimally invasive oesophagectomy, and the introduction of multimodality therapy for locally advanced disease. The future of oesophageal cancer surgery will be based on procedures tailored to the individual patient. Certain patients with early adenocarcinoma may initially undergo endoscopic resection to identify those requiring a formal oesophagectomy. These patients may undergo sentinel node mapping[53] such that patients potentially can be spared radical node dissection. Patients with locally advanced adenocarcinoma, particularly those with a low burden of nodal disease, will be targeted with increasingly effective multimodality regimens including, based on the Dutch trial, a radical en-bloc oesophagectomy with two-field lymph node dissection. Neoadjuvant regimes should be tailored, possibly by genetic profiling, to determine the best therapeutic strategy for each patient. Despite all this, significant improvements in long-term outcome for oesophageal cancer will only be achieved if focus is placed on earlier detection of what continues to be a very aggressive disease.

Key points

- The overall results of surgical resection for all stages of tumour have improved over the past 20 years.
- Meticulous preoperative evaluation and estimation of surgical risk is a prerequisite to successful surgical outcome in this disease.
- There is now overwhelming evidence to confirm the influence of surgeon case volume on the outcome of site-specific cancer surgery.
- Enteral feeding is preferred over parenteral feeding (TPN) for nutritional support.
- Subtotal oesophagectomy should be carried out in patients with tumours of the middle and lower oesophagus to make allowance for intramural submucosal spread of squamous and adenocarcinomas.
- The stomach is the preferred conduit for oesophageal reconstruction.

- Two-phase oesophagectomy with two-field lymphadenectomy is recommended for lower oesophageal adenocarcinoma, particularly those with a low nodal burden.
- Multimodality therapy including high-quality surgery should be considered for patients with>T2 N0 tumours.
- Outcome is strongly stage dependent – the focus must be on early detection.

References

1. Sobin LH, Gospodarowicz MK, Witteking Ch. TNM classification of malignant tumours. 7th ed. Oxford: Wiley-Blackwell; 2009.
2. Japanese Society for Oesophageal Diseases. Guidelines for the clinical and pathological studies on carcinoma of the oesophagus. Part 1: clinical classification. Jpn J Surg 1976;6:64–78.
3. Tetteroo GW, Wagenvoort JH, Castelein A, et al. Selective decontamination to reduce Gram-negative colonisation and infections after oesophageal resection. Lancet 1990;335(8691):704–7.
4. Moore FA, Feliciano DV, Andrassy RJ, et al. Early enteral feeding, compared with parenteral, reduces postoperative septic complications. The results of a meta-analysis. Ann Surg 1992;216(2):172–83.
   This meta-analysis emphasises the benefits of enteral feeding in the perioperative period.
5. Gianotti L, Braga M, Nespoli L, et al. A randomized controlled trial of preoperative oral supplementation with a specialized diet in patients with gastrointestinal cancer [see comment]. Gastroenterology 2002;122(7):1763–70.
6. Couper G. Jejunostomy after oesophagectomy: a review of evidence and current practice. Proc Nutr Soc 2011;70:316–20.
7. Sultan J, Griffin SM, Di Franco F, et al. Randomized clinical trial of omega-3 fatty acid-supplemented enteral nutrition versus standard enteral nutrition in patients undergoing oesophagogastric cancer surgery. Br J Surg 2012;99(3):346–55.
8. Markides GA, Alkhaffaf B, Vickers J. Nutritional access routes following oesophagectomy – a systematic review. Eur J Clin Nutr 2011;65:565–73.
9. Griffin SM, Woods SD, Chan A, et al. Early and late surgical complications of subtotal oesophagectomy for squamous carcinoma of the oesophagus. J R Coll Surg Edinb 1991;36(3):170–3.
10. Lerut T. Oesophageal carcinoma – past and present studies. Eur J Surg Oncol 1996;22(4):317–23.
11. Gebski V, Burmeister B, Smithers BM, et al. Survival benefits from neoadjuvant chemoradiotherapy or chemotherapy in oesophageal carcinoma: a meta-analysis. Lancet Oncol 2007;8(3):226–34.
12. Department of Health. In: Guidance on commissioning cancer services. Improving outcomes in uppergastrointestinal cancers. The manual. London: NHS Executive; 2001.
13. Sutton DN, Wayman J, Griffin SM. Learning curve for oesophageal cancer surgery. Br J Surg 1998;85(10):1399–402.
14. Finlayson EV, Goodney PP, Birkmeyer JD, et al. Hospital volume and operative mortality in cancer surgery: a national study. Arch Surg 2003;138(7):721–6.
15. Kuo EY, Chang Y, Wright CD, et al. Impact of hospital volume on clinical and economic outcomes for esophagectomy. Ann Thorac Surg 2001;72(4):1118–24.
16. Begg CB, Cramer LD, Hoskins WJ, et al. Impact of hospital volume on operative mortality for major cancer surgery [see comment]. JAMA 1998;280(20):1747–51.
17. Skinner DB. En bloc resection for neoplasms of the esophagus and cardia. J Thorac Cardiovasc Surg 1983;85(1):59–71.
18. Siu KF, Cheung HC, Wong J, et al. Shrinkage of the esophagus after resection for carcinoma. Ann Surg 1986;203(2):173–6.
19. Akiyama H. Surgery for cancer of the oesophagus. Baltimore: Williams & Wilkins; 1990.
20. Mandard AM, Chasle J, Marnay J, et al. Autopsy findings in 111 cases of esophageal cancer. Cancer 1981;48(2):329–35.
21. Sons HU, Borchard F. Cancer of the distal esophagus and cardia. Incidence, tumorous infiltration, and metastatic spread. Ann Surg 1986;203(2):188–95.
22. Dexter SP, Sue-Ling H, McMahon MJ, et al. Circumferential resection margin involvement: an independent predictor of survival following surgery for oesophageal cancer. Gut 2001;48(5):667–70.
23. Pultrum BB, Honing J, Smit JK, et al. A critical appraisal of circumferential resection margins in esophageal carcinoma. Ann Surg Oncol 2010;17:812–20.
24. Roder JD, Busch R, Stein HJ, et al. Ratio of invaded to removed lymph nodes as a predictor of survival in squamous cell carcinoma of the oesophagus. Br J Surg 1994;81(3):410–3.
25. Lerut T, De Leyn P, Coosemans W, et al. Surgical strategies in esophageal carcinoma with emphasis on radical lymphadenectomy. Ann Surg 1992;216(5):583–90.
    This important publication sets out the evidence for radical en-bloc resection with lymphadenectomy, demonstrating a reduction in operative mortality during the previous decade and excellent survival in relatively advanced disease.

26. Rice TW, Rusch VW, Apperson-Hansen C, et al. Worldwide esophageal cancer collaboration. Dis Esophagus 2009;22:1–8.

27. Sato T, Sacamoto K. Illustrations and photographs of surgical oesophageal anatomy, specially prepared for lymph node dissection. In: Sato T, Sacamoto K, editors. Colour atlas of surgical anatomy for oesophageal cancer. Toyko: Springer; 1992. p. 25–90.

28. Tanabe G, Baba M, Kuroshima K, et al. Clinical evaluation of the esophageal lymph flow system based on RI uptake of dissected regional lymph nodes following lymphoscintigraphy [in Japanese]. Nippon Geka Gakkai Zasshi 1986;87(3):315–23.

29. Orringer MB, Marshall B, Iannettoni MD. Transhiatal esophagectomy for benign and malignant esophageal disease. World J Surg 2001;25(2):196–203.

30. Peyre CG, Hagen JA, DeMeester SR, et al. Predicting systemic disease in patients with esophageal cancer after esophagectomy: a multinational study on the significance of the number of involved lymph nodes. Ann Surg 2008;248:979–85.

31. Dresner SM, Griffin SM. Pattern of recurrence following radical oesophagectomy with two-field lymphadenectomy. Br J Surg 2000;87(10):1426–33.

32. Akiyama H, Tsurumaru M, Udagawa H, et al. Radical lymph node dissection for cancer of the thoracic esophagus. Ann Surg 1994;220(3):364–73.

33. Hagen JA, DeMeester SR, Peters JH, et al. Curative resection for esophageal adenocarcinoma: analysis of 100 en bloc esophagectomies. Ann Surg 2001;234:520–30.

34. Sihvo EI, Luostarinen ME, Salo JA. Fate of patients with adenocarcinoma of the esophagus and the esophagogastric junction: a population-based analysis. Am J Gastroenterol 2004;99:419–24.

35. Clark GW, Peters JH, Ireland AP, et al. Nodal metastasis and sites of recurrence after en bloc esophagectomy for adenocarcinoma. Ann Thorac Surg 1994;58(3):646–54.

36. Altorki NK, Girardi L, Skinner DB. En bloc esophagectomy improves survival for stage III esophageal cancer. J Thorac Cardiovasc Surg 1997;114:948–55.

37. Hagen JA, Peters JH, DeMeester TR. Superiority of extended en bloc esophagogastrectomy for carcinoma of the lower esophagus and cardia. J Thorac Cardiovasc Surg 1993;106:850–8.

38. Altorki N, Kent M, Ferrara C, et al. Three-field lymph node dissection for squamous cell and adenocarcinoma of the esophagus. Ann Surg 2002;236(2):177–83.

39. Cunningham D, Allum WH, Stenning SP. MAGIC Trial Participants. Perioperative chemotherapy versus surgery alone for resectable gastroesophageal cancer. N Engl J Med 2006;355:11–20.

40. Hulscher JB, van Sandick JW, de Boer AG, et al. Extended transthoracic resection compared with limited transhiatal resection for adenocarcinoma of the esophagus. N Engl J Med 2002;347(21):1662–9.
This trial suggests that both techniques are safe but that there is lower morbidity in the transhiatal group and a trend to longer survival in the extended transthoracic groups.

41. Goldminc M, Maddern G, Le Prise E, et al. Oesophagectomy by a transhiatal approach or thoracotomy: a prospective randomized trial. Br J Surg 1993;80(3):367–70.

42. Kato H, Watanabe H, Tachimori Y, et al. Evaluation of neck lymph node dissection for thoracic esophageal carcinoma. Ann Thorac Surg 1991;51(6):931–5.

43. Omloo JM, Lagarde SM, Hulscher JB, et al. Extended transthoracic resection compared with limited transhiatal resection for adenocarcinoma of the mid/distal esophagus: five-year survival of a randomized clinical trial. Ann Surg 2007;246:992–1000.

44. Johansson J, DeMeester TR, Hagen JA, et al. En bloc vs transhiatal esophagectomy for stage T3 N1 adenocarcinoma of the distal esophagus. Arch Surg 2004;139:627–31.

45. Kato H, Tachimori Y, Mizobuchi S, et al. Cervical, mediastinal, and abdominal lymph node dissection (three-field dissection) for superficial carcinoma of the thoracic esophagus. Cancer 1993;72(10):2879–82.

46. Law S, Cheung MC, Fok M, et al. Pyloroplasty and pyloromyotomy in gastric replacement of the esophagus after esophagectomy: a randomized controlled trial. J Am Coll Surg 1997;184(6):630–6.

47. Peyre CG, Hagen JA, DeMeester SR, et al. The number of lymph nodes removed predicts survival in esophageal cancer: an international study on the impact of extent of surgical resection. Ann Surg 2008;248:549–56.

48. Schwarz RE, Smith DD. Clinical impact of lymphadenectomy extent in resectable esophageal cancer. J Gastrointest Surg 2007;11:1384–93.

49. Smith DD, Schwarz RR, Schwarz RE. Impact of total lymph node count on staging and survival after gastrectomy for gastric cancer: data from a large US-population database. J Clin Oncol 2005;23:7114–24.

50. Rizk N, Venkatraman E, Park B, et al. The prognostic importance of the number of involved lymph nodes in esophageal cancer: implications for revisions of the American Joint Committee on Cancer staging system. J Thorac Cardiovasc Surg 2006;132:1374–81.

51. Lerut T, Coosemans W, De Leyn P, et al. Is there a role for radical esophagectomy. Eur J Cardiothorac Surg 1999;16(Suppl. 1):S44–7.

52. Siewert JR, Roder JD. Lymphadenectomy in oesophageal cancer surgery. Dis Esophagus 1992;2:91–7.
53. Lamb PJ, Griffin SM, Burt AD, et al. Sentinel node biopsy to evaluate the metastatic dissemination of oesophageal adenocarcinoma. Br J Surg 2005;92(1):60–7.
54. Gawad KA, Hosch SB, Bumann D, et al. How important is the route of reconstruction after esophagectomy: a prospective randomized study. Am J Gastroenterol 1999;94(6):1490–6.
55. Bartels H, Thorban S, Siewert JR. Anterior versus posterior reconstruction after transhiatal oesophagectomy: a randomized controlled trial. Br J Surg 1993;80(9):1141–4.
These trials confirm that the mediastinal route is the preferred route for reconstruction after curative resection.
56. Tabira Y, Sakaguchi T, Kuhara H, et al. The width of a gastric tube has no impact on outcome after esophagectomy. Am J Surg 2004;187(3):417–21.
57. Akiyama H, Miyazono H, Tsurumaru M, et al. Use of the stomach as an esophageal substitute. Ann Surg 1978;188:606–10.
58. el-Eishi HI, Ayoub SF, el-Khalek MA. The arterial supply of the human stomach. Acta Anat (Basel) 1973;86(3):565–80.
59. Thomas DM, Langford RM, Russell RC, et al. The anatomical basis for gastric mobilization in total oesophagectomy. Br J Surg 1979;66(4):230–3.
60. Khan OA, Manners J, Rengarajan A, et al. Does pyloroplasty following esophagectomy improve early clinical outcomes? Interact Cardiovasc Thorac Surg 2007;6(2):247–50.
61. Cheung HC, Siu KF, Wong J. Is pyloroplasty necessary in esophageal replacement by stomach? A prospective, randomized controlled trial. Surgery 1987;102(1):19–24.
62. Ventemiglia R, Khalil KG, Frazier OH, et al. The role of preoperative mesenteric arteriography in colon interposition. J Thorac Cardiovasc Surg 1977;74(1):98–104.
63. DeMeester TR, Johansson KE, Franze I, et al. Indications, surgical technique, and long-term functional results of colon interposition or bypass. Ann Surg 1988;208(4):460–74.
64. Maguire D, Collins C, O'Sullivan GC. How I do it – Replacement of the oesophagus with colon interposition graft based on the inferior mesenteric vascular system. Eur J Surg Oncol 2001;27:314–5.
65. Sasaki TM, Baker HW, McConnell DB, et al. Free jejunal graft reconstruction after extensive head and neck surgery. Am J Surg 1980;139(5):650–3.
66. Nanson EM. Synchronous combined abdominothoracocervical (oesophagectomy). Aust N Z J Surg 1975;45(4):340–8.
67. Chung SC, Griffin SM, Wood SD, et al. Two team synchronous esophagectomy. Surg Gynecol Obstet 1990;170(1):68–9.
68. Hayes N, Shaw IH, Raimes SA, et al. Comparison of conventional Lewis–Tanner two-stage oesophagectomy with the synchronous two-team approach. Br J Surg 1995;82(3):426.
This small randomised trial demonstrated higher complication and mortality rates in Western patients operated on by the synchronous technique.
69. McKeown KC. The surgical treatment of carcinoma of the oesophagus. A review of the results in 478 cases. J R Coll Surg Edinb 1985;30(1):1–14.
70. Sundaresan S. Left thoracoabdominal incision. Operat Tech Thorac Cardiovasc Surg 2003;8:71–85.
71. Matthews HR, Steel A. Left-sided subtotal oesophagectomy for carcinoma. Br J Surg 1987;74(12):1115–7.
72. Molina JE, Lawton BR, Myers WO, et al. Esophagogastrectomy for adenocarcinoma of the cardia. Ten years' experience and current approach. Ann Surg 1982;195(2):146–51.
73. Forshaw MJ, Gossage JA, Ockrim J, et al. Left thoracoabdominal esophagogastrectomy: still a valid operation for carcinoma of the distal esophagus and esophagogastric junction. Dis Esophagus 2006;19(5):340–5.
74. Kelly FE, Murdoch JA, Sanders DJ, et al. Continuous paravertebral block for thoraco-abdominal oesophageal surgery. Anaesthesia 2005;60:98–9.
75. Sasako M, Sano T, Yamamoto S, et al. Left thoracoabdominal approach versus abdominal–transhiatal approach for gastric cancer of the cardia or sub-cardia: a randomised controlled trial. Lancet Oncol 2006;7(8):644–51.
76. Le Quesne LP, Ranger D. Pharyngolaryngectomy, with immediate pharyngogastric anastomosis. Br J Surg 1966;53(2):105–9.
77. Turner GG. Excision of thoracic oesophagus for carcinoma with construction of an extra thoracic gullet. Lancet 1933;1:1315–6.
78. Ong GB. Carcinoma of the hypo-pharynx and cervical oesophagus. In: Smith RE, editor. Progress in clinical surgery. London: J & A Churchill; 1969. p. 155–78.
79. Orringer MB, Sloan H. Esophagectomy without thoracotomy. J Thorac Cardiovasc Surg 1978;76(5):643–54.
80. Orringer MB, Marshall B, Chang AC, et al. Two thousand transhiatal esophagectomies: changing trends, lessons learned. Ann Surg 2007;246:363–72.
81. Alderson D, Courtney SP, Kennedy RH. Radical transhiatal oesophagectomy under direct vision Br J Surg 1994;81:404–7.
82. Pinotti HW. A new approach to the thoracic esophagus by the abdominal transdiaphragmatic route. Langenbecks Arch Chir 1983;359(4):229–35.
83. Chu KM, Law SY, Fok M, et al. A prospective randomized comparison of transhiatal and transthoracic resection for lower-third esophageal carcinoma. Am J Surg 1997;174(3):320–4.

84. Jacobi CA, Zieren HU, Muller JM, et al. Surgical therapy of esophageal carcinoma: the influence of surgical approach and esophageal resection on cardiopulmonary function. Eur J Cardiothorac Surg 1997;11(1):32–7.

These two small randomised studies failed to demonstrate differences in cardiopulmonary complications between the transhiatal and transthoracic approaches.

85. Low DE, Kunz S, Schembre D, et al. Esophagectomy – it's not just about mortality anymore: standardized perioperative clinical pathways improve outcomes in patients with esophageal cancer. J Gastrointest Surg 2007;11:1395–402.

86. Luketich JD, Schauer PR, Christie NA, et al. Minimally invasive esophagectomy. Ann Thorac Surg 2000;70:906–11.

87. Luketich JD, velo-Rivera M, Buenaventura PO, et al. Minimally invasive esophagectomy: outcomes in 222 patients. Ann Surg 2003;238:486–94.

88. Palanivelu C, Prakash A, Senthilkumar R, et al. Minimally invasive esophagectomy: thoracoscopic mobilization of the esophagus and mediastinal lymphadenectomy in prone position – experience of 130 patients. J Am Coll Surg 2006;203:7–16.

89. Berrisford RG, Wajed SA, Sanders D, et al. Short term outcomes following total minimally invasive oesophagectomy. Br J Surg 2008;95:602–10.

90. Nafteux P, Moons J, Coosemans W, et al. Minimally invasive oesophagectomy: a valuable alternative to open oesophagectomy for the treatment of early oesophageal and gastro-oesophageal junction carcinoma. Eur J Cardiothorac Surg 2011;40(6): 1455–64.

91. Nguyen NT, Hinojosa MW, Smith BR, et al. Minimally invasive esophagectomy: lessons learned from 104 operations. Ann Surg 2008;248: 1081–91.

92. Smithers BM, Gotley DC, Martin I, et al. Comparison of the outcomes between open and minimally invasive esophagectomy. Ann Surg 2007;245:232–40.

93. Zingg U, McQuinn A, DiValentino D, et al. Minimally invasive versus open esophagectomy for patients with esophageal cancer. Ann Thorac Surg 2009;87:911–9.

94. Berrisford RG, Veeramootoo D, Parameswaran R, et al. Laparoscopic ischaemic conditioning of the stomach may reduce gastric-conduit morbidity following total minimally invasive oesophagectomy. Eur J Cardiothorac Surg 2009;36:888–93.

95. Nguyen NT, Nguyen XM, Reavis KM, et al. Minimally invasive esophagectomy with and without gastric ischemic conditioning. Surg Endosc 2012;26(6):1637–41.

96. Nguyen NT, Longoria M, Sabio A, et al. Preoperative laparoscopic ligation of the left gastric vessels in preparation for esophagectomy. Ann Thorac Surg 2006;81:2318–20.

97. Luketich J, Pennathur A, Catalano PJ, et al. Results of a phase II multicenter study of minimally invasive esophagectomy (Eastern Cooperative Oncology Group Study E2202). J Clin Oncol ASCO Annual Meeting Proceedings 2009;27:4516.

98. Biere SS, Maas KW, Bonavina L, et al. Traditional invasive vs. minimally invasive esophagectomy: a multi-center, randomized trial (TIME-trial). BMC Surg 2011;11:2.

99. Bizekis C, Kent MS, Luketich JD, et al. Initial experience with minimally invasive Ivor Lewis esophagectomy. Ann Thorac Surg 2006;82:402–6.

100. Levy RM, Wizorek J, Shende M, et al. Laparoscopic and thoracoscopic esophagectomy. Adv Surg 2010;44:101–16.

101. Briez N, Piessen G, Bonnetain F, et al. Open versus laparoscopically-assisted oesophagectomy for cancer: a multicentre randomised controlled phase III trial – the MIRO trial. BMC Cancer 2011;11:310.

102. Berrisford RG, Sabanathan SS, Mearns AJ, et al. Pulmonary complications after lung resection: the effect of continuous extrapleural intercostal nerve block. Eur J Cardiothorac Surg 1990;4:407–10.

103. Sabanathan S, Mearns AJ, Bickford Smith PJ, et al. Efficacy of continuous extrapleural intercostal nerve block on post-thoracotomy pain and pulmonary mechanics. Br J Surg 1990;77:221–5.

104. Parameswaran R, Blazeby JM, Hughes R, et al. Health-related quality of life after minimally invasive oesophagectomy. Br J Surg 2010;97:525–31.

105. Berrisford RG. Editorial comment: Totally minimally invasive three-stage oesophagectomy – an achievable goal or a step too far? Eur J Cardiothorac Surg 2011;40:1464–5.

106. Mamidanna R, Bottle A, Aylin P, et al. Short-term outcomes following open versus minimally invasive esophagectomy for cancer in England: a population-based national study. Ann Surg 2012;255:197–203.

107. Rice TW, Blackstone EH. Minimally invasive versus open esophagectomy for cancer: more questions than answers. Ann Surg 2012;255:204–5.

108. Dresner SM, Lamb PJ, Wayman J, et al. Benign anastomotic stricture following transthoracic subtotal oesophagectomy and stapled oesophago-gastrostomy: risk factors and management. Br J Surg 2000;87(3):362–73.

109. Egberts JH, Schniewind B, Bestmann B, et al. Impact of the site of anastomosis after oncologic esophagectomy on quality of life – a prospective, longitudinal outcome study. Ann Surg Oncol 2008;15(2):566–75.

110. Lerut T, Coosemans W, Decker G, et al. Anastomotic complications after esophagectomy. Dig Surg 2002;19(2):92–8.

111. Collard JM, Romagnoli R, Goncette L, et al. Terminalized semimechanical side-to-side suture

technique for cervical esophagogastrostomy. Ann Thorac Surg 1998;65:814–7.

112. Orringer MB, Marshall B, Iannettoni MD. Eliminating the cervical esophagogastric anastomotic leak with a side-to-side stapled anastomosis. J Thorac Cardiovasc Surg 2000;119:277–88.

113. Griffin SM, Lamb PJ, Dresner SM, et al. Diagnosis and management of a mediastinal leak following radical oesophagectomy. Br J Surg 2001;88(10):1346–51.

114. Lamb PJ, Griffin SM, Chandrashekar MV, et al. Prospective study of routine contrast radiology after total gastrectomy. Br J Surg 2004;91(8):1015–9.

115. Smithers BM, Cullinan M, Thomas JM, et al. Outcomes from salvage esophagectomy post definitive chemoradiotherapy compared with resection following preoperative neoadjuvant chemoradiotherapy. Dis Esophagus 2007;20(6):471–7.

116. Lagarde SM, de Boer JD, ten Kate FJ, et al. Postoperative complications after esophagectomy for adenocarcinoma of the esophagus are related to timing of death due to recurrence. Ann Surg 2008;247(1):71–6.

117. Tandon S, Batchelor A, Bullock R, et al. Peri-operative risk factors for acute lung injury after elective oesophagectomy. Br J Anaesth 2001;86(5):633–8.

118. Dresner SM, Lamb PJ, Shenfine J, et al. Prognostic significance of peri-operative blood transfusion following radical resection for oesophageal carcinoma. Eur J Surg Oncol 2000;26(5):492–7.

119. Muller JM, Erasmi H, Stelzner M, et al. Surgical therapy of oesophageal carcinoma. Br J Surg 1990;77(8):845–57.

120. Wemyss-Holden SA, Launois B, Maddern GJ. Management of thoracic duct injuries after oesophagectomy. Br J Surg 2001;88(11):1442–8.

121. Merigliano S, Molena D, Ruol A, et al. Chylothorax complicating esophagectomy for cancer: a plea for early thoracic duct ligation. J Thorac Cardiovasc Surg 2000;119(3):453–7.

122. Dugue L, Sauvanet A, Farges O, et al. Output of chyle as an indicator of treatment for chylothorax complicating oesophagectomy. Br J Surg 1998;85(8):1147–9.

123. Thaker H, Snow MH, Spickett G, et al. *Pneumocystis carinii* pneumonia after thoracic duct ligation and leakage. Clin Infect Dis 2001;33(11):E129–31.

124. Griffin SM, Chung SC, van Hasselt CA, et al. Late swallowing and aspiration problems after esophagectomy for cancer: malignant infiltration of the recurrent laryngeal nerves and its management. Surgery 1992;112(3):533–5.

125. Dresner SM, Griffin SM, Wayman J, et al. Human model of duodenogastro-oesophageal reflux in the development of Barrett's metaplasia. Br J Surg 2003;90(9):1120–8.

126. Aly A, Jamieson GG. Reflux after oesophagectomy. Br J Surg 2004;91(2):137–41.

127. Aly A, Jamieson GG, Pyragius M, et al. Antireflux anastomosis following oesophagectomy. Aust N Z J Surg 2004;74(6):434–8.

128. Blazeby JM, Brookes ST, Alderson D. The prognostic value of quality of life scores during treatment for oesophageal cancer. Gut 2001;49(2):227–30.

129. Earlam R, Cunha-Melo JR. Oesophageal squamous cell carcinoma: I. A critical review of surgery. Br J Surg 1980;67(6):381–90.

130. Jamieson GG, Mathew G, Ludemann R, et al. Postoperative mortality following oesophagectomy and problems in reporting its rate. Br J Surg 2004;91(8):943–7.

131. Liu JF, Wang QZ, Ping YM, et al. Complications after esophagectomy for cancer: 53-year experience with 20,796 patients. World J Surg 2008;32(3):395–400.

132. McCulloch P, Ward J, Tekkis PP. Mortality and morbidity in gastro-oesophageal cancer surgery: initial results of ASCOT multicentre prospective cohort study. Br Med J 2003;327(7425):1192–7.

133. Allum WH, Stenning SP, Bancewicz J, et al. Long-term results of a randomized trial of surgery with or without preoperative chemotherapy in esophageal cancer. J Clin Oncol 2009;27(30):5062–7.

134. Rutegard M, Charonis K, Lu Y, et al. Population-based esophageal cancer survival after resection without neoadjuvant therapy: an update. Surgery 2012;152(5):903–10.

135. Rice TW, Rusch VW, Ishwaran H, et al. Cancer of the esophagus and esophagogastric junction: data-driven staging for the seventh edition of the American Joint Committee on Cancer/International Union Against Cancer Cancer Staging Manuals. Cancer 2010;116(16):3763–73.

6

Treatment of early oesophageal cancer

B. Mark Smithers
Iain Thomson

Introduction

The prevalence of early oesophageal cancer is increasing due to the rising incidence of adenocarcinoma (AC) in the West, persistent high incidence of squamous cell carcinoma (SCC) in the East, along with improving methods of endoscopic diagnosis and surveillance strategies identifying high-risk changes in the mucosa. The management of early oesophageal cancer is in a process of evolution due to the improvement in endoscopic techniques to sample, remove and ablate oesophageal mucosa, leading to potentially fewer patients requiring an oesophagectomy.

Definition of early oesophageal cancer and relevant pathology

A cancer in the oesophagus is considered 'early' if it is contained within the superficial components of the epithelial lining and there is no lymph node involvement. Using the latest American Joint Committee on Cancer (AJCC) staging criteria, for both SCC and AC, this would include oesophageal cancer diagnosed at stages 0 or IA.[1] Stage 0 includes Tis or high-grade dysplasia (HGD) of the epithelium. This had previously been called carcinoma in situ.[2] Stage I relates to the depth of invasion into the oesophageal wall with no lymph nodes involved. This stage includes cancers that are T1–2. However, the pathological stage can only be diagnosed after the resection of the oesophagus. The deeper the invasion into the mucosa and submucosa, the higher the incidence of nodal metastasis, so that a clear definition of the T stage is vital when assessing a patient thought to have an 'early' oesophageal cancer.

The T stage can be subclassified into cancer that is restricted to the mucosa, T1a, and to the submucosa, T1b. Within the mucosa (T1a) the invasion can be subclassified into cancers confined to the epithelium (m1), the lamina propria (m2) and the muscularis mucosae (m3).[1] Patients with Barrett's oesophagus may have duplication of the muscularis mucosae but they are still m3 so long as the muscularis mucosae has not been breached. Cancers infiltrating into the submucosa (T1b) may be subclassified into sm1 (inner third), sm2 (middle third) and sm3 (outer third)[1] (**Fig. 6.1**).

The relevance of subclassification relates to the risk of lymphatic invasion. The lymphatic network in the oesophagus is concentrated in the submucosa; however, there are lymphatic channels in the lamina propria. From studies of patients that have had a resection for T1 cancer it is clear that there is a higher risk of nodal involvement if it invades to T1b level compared with T1a cancers.[3–17] There are subtle differences between patients with AC and SCC. HGD in Barrett's epithelium and in squamous epithelium as well as AC or SCC involving m1 do not have nodal disease.[3–5,10,11,13,17] AC invading to m2 and m3 do not have lymph node metastasis.[3–6,8]

However, for patients with SCC to the m2 level, there have been reports of patients with positive lymph nodes found in 3.3%[9] and 5.6%,[17] although this is not clear as others have reported no evidence

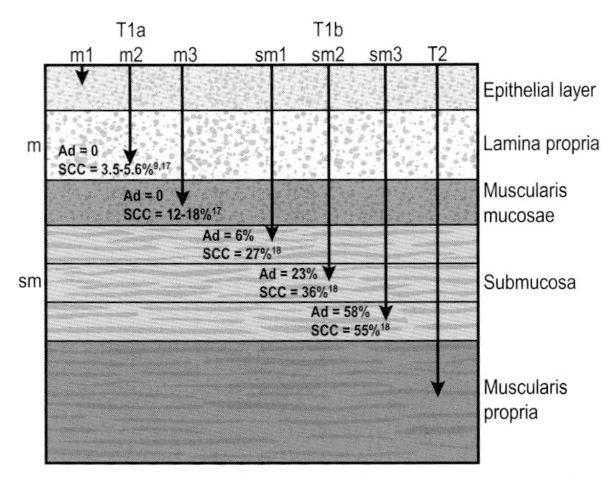

Figure 6.1 • Anatomical layers of the oesophagus with risk of lymph node involvement. Ad, adenocarcinoma.

of positive nodes at this level.[10–15] If the tumour extends to m3, the node-positive rate has been reported to be 18% in a large single-centre series[17] and 12.2% in a review of 1740 patients with early SCC.[9] The histological finding of lymphatic invasion in association with m3 invasion has been shown to increase the risk of positive lymph nodes[11,17] from 10% to 42%.[17]

For either AC or SCC invading the submucosa (T1b), the potential for nodal metastasis increases from sm1 to sm3.[18] A review of articles from 1980 to 2009 reported an overall lymph node-positive rate of 37%, with the incidence higher for SCC (45%) than AC (26%). For sm1 disease, the presence of lymphatic invasion on histology increases the risk of positive lymph nodes from 11% to 65%.[11] The incidence of node positivity was higher in patients with SCC compared with AC at sm1 (27% vs. 6%) and sm2 (36% vs. 23%) levels, but the same at sm3 (55% vs. 58%).[18] The implication may be that SCC is more biologically aggressive at presentation.

✔ For mucosal disease (T1a), patients with HGD or AC are suitable for endoscopic therapy if the disease can be cleared. Patients with squamous HGD and SCC with invasion to m1 and m2 disease are suitable for endoscopic therapy. Given the operative morbidity and mortality and effect on quality of life of an oesophagectomy, the role of endoscopic therapy for SCC invading to the m3 level, without associated lymphatic invasion, is not clear and will relate to patient factors when considering treatment options.

For patients with T1b cancers the optimal oncological therapy is an oesophagectomy with a systematic lymphadenectomy. There may be 'low-risk' sm1 patients with AC that might be considered for endoscopic therapies but it is not so clear for patients with SCC. The 'low-risk' AC is a patient with a well-differentiated cancer with no evidence of lymphovascular invasion.[5,8] One report of 85 patients with T1 AC analysed four subgroups with differing nodal involvement and prognosis. Patients with T1a disease had no nodes and 100% disease-specific survival (DSS). Those with T1b cancers were split into three groups: well differentiated and no lymphatic/vascular invasion (LVI) – 4% nodal involvement, 85% 5-year DSS; poorly differentiated and no LVI – 22% nodal involvement, 65% 5-year DSS; and any cancer with LVI – 46% nodal involvement, 40% 5-year DSS.[5]

The reason for the difference between histological subtypes is not clear but explanations include: fewer lymphatic channels in the lamina propria in the lower oesophagus (where AC occurs[7]) and SCC is more biologically aggressive at an earlier stage.[18]

Investigations

The patient will have had a biopsy reporting either HGD or invasive carcinoma in either the squamous epithelium or Barrett's glandular epithelium.

Endoscopic assessment

Barrett's neoplasia

Patients with the diagnosis of HGD or intramucosal carcinoma in Barrett's epithelium should have the endoscopy repeated according to a protocol of four quadrant biopsies 1 cm apart and targeted biopsies of macroscopically suspect lesions.[19] The pathology should be reviewed by two independent experienced gastrointestinal pathologists to confirm the diagnosis.

Squamous neoplasia

Patients with a diagnosis of HGD in squamous epithelium or suspected early invasive carcinoma should have the endoscopy repeated to clearly establish the extent of the disease process. The use of Lugol's iodine staining is recommended to allow targeted biopsies of the non-stained areas.[20] Knowledge of the extent of the mucosal change is important when planning treatment as very long segments may only be treated with oesophagectomy. If endoscopic therapy is to be considered, the non-stained areas outline the targets for endoscopic resection or ablation.

Endoscopic mucosal resection (EMR)

This is the removal of the mucosa and a varying degree of submucosa. In patients with HGD or suspected intramucosal carcinoma (IMC) this is the most accurate and definitive method of confirming the histology and defining the T stage of abnormal mucosa or any mucosal lesion.[21,22] Endoscopic mucosal resection offers better T staging than endoscopic ultrasonography (EUS) and computed tomography (CT) scanning,[23] and will alter the histological grade or the local T stage of mucosal neoplasia in up to 48% of patients,[24] thereby potentially influencing the management (**Fig. 6.2**).

Patients with squamous epithelial neoplasia can have abnormailites targeted with EMR. A study of 51 patients who had an EMR for squamous HGD reported 31% to be m2/3, with over a third of these lesions being flat such that they were unrecognisable from HGD alone.[25] This also stresses the need for extensive mapping biopsies of squamous epithelial neoplasia, using Lugol's iodine, if endoscopic therapies are to be considered.

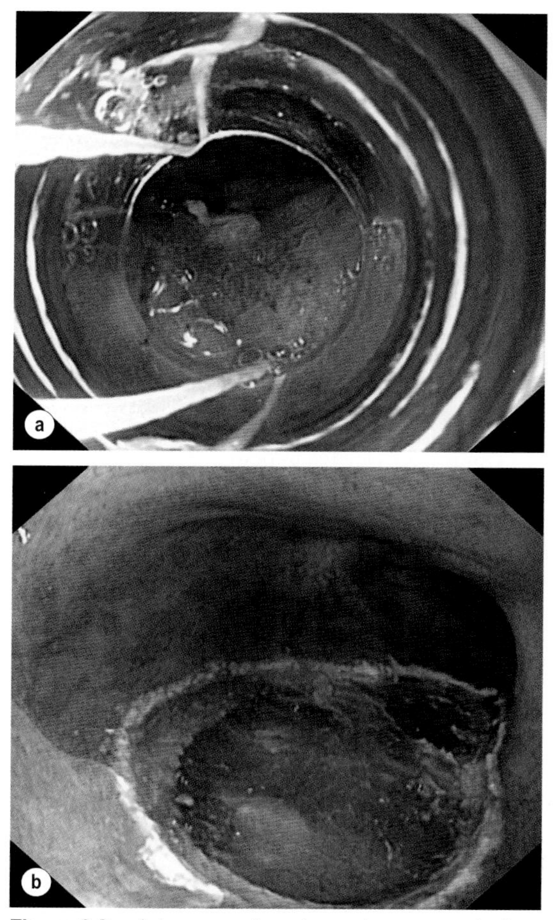

Figure 6.2 • Intramucosal carcinoma in a segment of Barrett's epithelium before **(a)** and after **(b)** endoscopic mucosal resection.

Endoscopic submucosal dissection (ESD)

This technique is widely used in Asia, notably by the Japanese, for definitive treatment of patients with superficial gastric cancer. It has been used for squamous neoplasia because it entails a formal dissection in the submucosal plane to remove a complete segment of mucosa and submucosa. The advantage is that the whole abnormal segment of oesophagus may be removed en bloc[26,27] and there is less likelihood of margins being involved when compared with EMR in the tubular oesophagus.[26,28]

Imaging

The accuracy of differentiating the layers of the mucosa has been reported to be 85–100% with the use of the higher frequency (15 and 20 MHz) miniprobes;[29] however, the numbers are small and these are expert centres. In general practice this differentiation is not good enough to stratify patients to allow decisions relating to endoscopic therapy and oesophagectomy.[6] It may be the value of EUS will be for examination of the local lymph nodes and, if considered suspicious, achieving confirmation with fine-needle aspiration.[29] When the tumour is considered to be invasive there is a role for anatomical imaging with CT scanning and functional imaging with positron emission tomography (PET) for formal staging.[30]

✔ Endoscopic mucosal resection of defined mucosal abnormalities offers the most sensitive method of obtaining a T stage for early oesophageal neoplasia.

Management of early oesophageal cancer

The definitive management of an invasive oesophageal cancer is the complete eradication of the primary lesion with a margin of normal epithelium along with the draining lymph nodes. Patients with HGD in Barrett's oesophagus may have an associated carcinoma and patients with superfical SCC of the oesophagus have a higher potential for lymph node involvement, making surgical resection the definitive therapy for these patients. Oesophagectomy remains the gold standard and any other therapy must be carefully assessed using resection as the benchmark. However, in selected patients, it is reasonable to consider endoscopic therapies or radiotherapy with or without chemotherapy.

Oesophageal resection

The clear advantage of complete removal of the disease process provided by an oesophageal resection must be weighed against the potential mortality and morbidity of the procedure.

In a review from 2007 of 29 series of patients having a resection for Barrett's HGD, it was reported that cancer was found in the specimen in 37% of cases with 60% of this group (22% of the total) invading beyond the mucosa.[31] They reported no downward trend in this incidence in recent years. This review consists of a number of older series where patients were not likely to have had a systematic approach to biopsy of the Barrett's mucosa, and none of the patients underwent an EMR of abnormal mucosa, which would offer a better histological assessment with improved T staging. The factors that have been reported to be associated with a co-existing cancer in HGD are a visible lesion, ulceration and HGD at multiple levels.[32,33] The potential for an unexpected finding of an invasive cancer is now lower than previously reported.

For patients confirmed to have squamous dysplasia the potential for the development of an invasive cancer increases with time. For low-grade intraepithelial neoplasia (LGIN), the risk at 3.5 and 13.5 years has been reported as 5% and 24%, respectively, for moderate-grade intraepithelial neoplasia (MGIN) 27% and 50%, respectively, and for high-grade intraepithelial neoplasia (HGIN) 65% and 74%, respectively.[34] Definitive treatment should be directed towards HGD with careful observation in patients with lower levels of dysplasia.

Although patients with HGD do not have an invasive cancer the risk is removed completely with an oesophagectomy. In the short term the potential for short-term cancer mortality is very low, so it is important that the surgical outcomes are optimal. In the last decade operative mortality for oesophageal resection in high-volume centres has been reported to be 2–4%, with rates of 0–1% when the resection was for HGD or IMC.[31,35] The long-term disease-specific survival (DSS) following an oesophagectomy for HGD should be 100% and for early invasive oesophageal cancer (stage I) for AC 80–90%[7,36] and SCC 3-year survival of 85%[37] and 5-year DSS of 53–77%[38,39] have been reported.

Because of the associated high morbidity, mortality and effects on the quality of life, alternatives to a traditional oesophagectomy and lymphadenectomy have been explored. For lesser procedures to be successful a degree of predictability of the lymph node drainage is necessary. For stage I disease, in one study, patients with AC had the majority of positive nodes below the tracheal bifurcation, locally associated with the primary cancer in all but 2%. For SCC the nodal site was not predicable, with the positive nodes widely distributed in the chest and upper abdomen.[7]

Thus, for early AC this had led to groups attempting variations from a major resection. Two variations described for patients with Barrett's HGD and IMC are a limited resection of the oesophagogastric junction[40] and vagal-sparing oesophagectomy.[41] The resection of the oesophagogastric junction with jejunal interposition (Merendino operation) is performed using a transabdominal approach, with splitting of the oesophageal hiatus. The dissection can be carried out, through the hiatus, to the level of the tracheal bifurcation incorporating a lower mediastinal and upper abdominal lymphadenectomy with or without preservation of the vagal innervation of the distal stomach. Following resection of the distal oesophagus, cardia and proximal stomach, the gastrointestinal continuity is restored by means of interposition of an isoperistaltic pedicled jejunal loop to prevent postoperative reflux.[40] The outcome of over 100 procedures for early Barrett's cancer reported similar outcomes in terms of long-term survival compared with a radical oesophagectomy. The advantages were lower peri- and postoperative morbidity, and a good postoperative quality of life. The procedure has been reported to be technically challenging and requires attention to detail to achieve good long-term functional results.[40]

Vagal-sparing oesophagectomy (VSO) has recently been popularised for HGD and T1a adenocarcinoma of the lower oesophagus. Reconstruction is via the use of a gastric tube or colon pull-up. The authors report a reduction in side-effects attributed to the vagal resection that occurs with a more aggressive resection.[41] The operative mortality has been reported to be 2% with major complications in 35% of patients, but there was a reduction, but not abolition, of diarrhoea and dumping symptoms.[41]

Alternative approaches are the transhiatal approach and minimally invasive approaches to an oesophageal resection. The transhiatal approach has been reported to reduce respiratory complications compared with an open oesophagectomy.[42,43] Although suitable for AC the transhiatal approach does not address the issue of the unpredictable lymphatic drainage of SCC, so that a systematic lymphadenectomy should be performed with the benefits of an upper and cervical mediastinal lymphadenectomy being weighed against the added morbidity.[7,10,44]

Minimally invasive approaches to oesophagectomy will allow resection of the primary cancer and a lymphadenectomy. Reports suggest there may be a reduction in respiratory complications when the chest and abdominal components are performed using minimally invasive approaches.[45–47]

The approach has also been described allowing a dissection of the mediastinum, as required for SCC.[48]

Oesophagectomy does have an effect on the quality of life of patients. There have been reports that claim the long-term functional outcomes from a resection are at least equivalent to the general population.[49,50] However, despite their conclusions there are patients that have significant gastro-oesophageal reflux (59–68%), dysphagia (38%), dumping (15%), diarrhoea (55%) and bloating (45%).[49,50] Others have confirmed the higher incidences of functional symptoms such as dumping syndrome, bloat, reflux and diarrhoea, which do not settle in the long term.[51]

✔ Resection offers the most definitive treatment aimed at cure for early oesophageal neoplasia. The disease and the associated high-risk mucosa are eradicated completely without the need for long-term surveillance. However, this approach has a defined potential for mortality with unpredictable effects on short- and long-term quality of life.

Endoscopic therapy

The recent trend is for patients with localised neoplasia, confined to the mucosa, to be managed endoscopically. The techniques involve resection of a segment of mucosa and a variable amount of submucosa or ablation of the diseased segment, or a combination of both. To be acceptable the endoscopic therapy must completely remove or eradicate the neoplastic epithelium. Also, the risk of residual positive lymph nodes should be zero or very low.

Endoscopic mucosal resection

Aside from diagnosis and T-stage assessment this technique may be therapeutic, removing the lesion completely. The techniques used for this procedure result in piecemeal segments of mucosa and submucosa being removed. Techniques such as 'inject, suck and cut'(endoscopic resection cap, ER-cap) and 'band and snare' (endoscopic resection multiband mucosectomy, ER-MBM) are used, and have been shown to provide the pathologist with equivalent and adequate depths of mucosa and submucosa.[52] A randomised study assessing the two techniques has shown that ER-cap produces specimens of larger diameter but with equivalent amount of submucosa. ER-MBM was quicker, less costly and had a similar safety profile.[53] Short segments of neoplastic epithelium (Barrett's or squamous) can be completely removed in up to 80–94% of patients.[54] The recurrence rate increases with the length of follow-up because the treatment may not deal with all the Barrett's epithelium, some of which may not be visible.[3] When EMR alone is used to eradicate the Barrett's segment the complete eradication rate may reach 97%, but the incidence of stricture increases up to 37%.[55] It is likely the optimal use of EMR will be in combination with Barrett's ablative techniques. The technique has been shown to be safe, with a low incidence of complications such as bleeding (0–1.5%), perforation (0.3–0.5%) and stricture formation if segmental regions are treated (7–9%).

For squamous epithelial neoplasia the results from EMR are similar to Barrett's neoplasia, with rates of recurrence reported to be 10–26%.[26,56,57] When examining the recurrence rate in association with depth of invasion, the incidence has been reported to be 13–18% in lesions that are m1/2.[57]

Endoscopic submucosal dissection (ESD)

This is a technically demanding procedure and, aside from the risk of perforation, there is a higher incidence of stricture formation when compared with EMR because of the deeper resection plane and larger segments removed. This technique has not been readily taken up in the West for the management of Barrett's neoplasia, although there have been European reports of the technique being used for SCC.[56,58] The potential for recurrence of the squamous neoplasia, after ESD, is low at 1–2%.[26,59] Bleeding occurs in 10% in larger series; however, this is typically dealt with during the procedure or in the first 24 hours. Perforation occurs in 4–10% and is typically treated with endoscopic clips. Because of the length of segments removed, the stricture rate can be high (6–26%).[59]

Mucosal ablation

Accepting that EMR and ESD target the high-risk lesions, allowing complete histological assessment, the high-risk mucosa should then be removed or ablated. The technique offering the most promise for mucosal ablation is radiofrequency ablation (RFA), with other options that include photodynamic therapy (PDT) and argon plasma coagulation (APC). PDT is very intensive and only performed in specialist units, so that it has essentially been replaced by APC and RFA. PDT offers a durable remission with replacement by squamous epithelium in 50–80% of patients[60] and a risk of recurrence of the HGD in up to 8% of patients.[61] The stricture rate can be as high as 36%.[61]

APC will eradicate the superficial mucosa to a variable depth, allowing complete eradication in 38–99% of patients, with recurrence of 3–16%.[62–64] APC has a better ablation rate when compared with PDT.[65] For each technique, it is not unusual for the patient to require repeat therapy. Both techniques carry a risk of the development of subsquamous Barrett's (buried Barrett's) under the regenerated squamous epithelium, reported to be around 20%.[65] This entity has the potential for malignant transformation.[66]

RFA is a balloon-based radiofrequency device that will ablate the mucosal layer of the tubular oesophagus to a defined depth. There is also a device that will treat distinct residual patches of Barrett's mucosa. The potential for complete eradication has been reported to be 90% in HGD, 80% in Barrett's dysplasia and 54% for intestinal metaplasia.[67] Residual disease is typically seen as small islands or tongues and can be treated separately. Complete eradication cannot be guaranteed, with newly detected metaplasia at 1 year, seen in up to 26% with 8.5% reported to have dysplasia.[68] The stricture rate was 0.4% and the incidence of buried glands much lower than with the other techniques.[67] A recent randomised trial comparing stepwise EMR and RFA demonstrated comparable response rates, with fewer sessions and less morbidity in the RFA group.[69]

There are very few data available relating to the use of RFA for squamous neoplasia. In a study of 29 patients with dysplasia (18), HGD (10) and SCC m1 (1) treated with RFA, after a single treatment at 3 months the complete response rate (CR) was 86%. At 12 months, with further RFA treatments, the CR was 83% (14% low-grade dysplasia).[70] For both histological entities, it is likely that there may be a role for EMR followed by RFA in selected patients.

Results from endoscopic therapy for early oesophageal cancer

Adenocarcinoma

For HGD or IMC/T1a carcinoma in Barrett's epithelium, the group in Weisbaden, Germany, assess 80 patients and treat 60–70 with endoscopic therapy per year.[71] They report complete resection rates of 97%. The median follow-up period was 64 months and there was a metachronous lesion in 21%. The higher risk for recurrence is in patients who have piecemeal resection, long-segment Barrett's, no ablation of the Barrett's (PDT performed selectively), multifocal neoplasia and time to complete removal of the identified lesion of more than 10 months. Importantly, this group highlight the need to intensively follow patients. Surgery was required in 3.7% because of failure of endoscopic therapy to clear the disease.[71] Others have reported the development of a new metachronous cancer following ablative therapy to occur in 6–20%.[72,73]

In a review of studies assessing the role of Barrett's ablation (no RFA) compared with patients observed with HGD, the long-term cancer risk was reduced by ablation but not abolished. After ablation the risk of malignant change was 16.66/1000 patient-years compared with 65.8/1000 patient-years for observation. The frequency of recurrence of intestinal metaplasia was 0–68%.[74] In a small study of 31 patients, using RFA following EMR, it was possible to eradicate the high-risk mucosa in patients with early AC (16), HGD (12) or LGD (3). At median 21 months, all dysplasia was eradicated with a 9% stricture rate.[75]

Two studies of institutional comparisons between endoscopic therapy (ET) and resection for HGD and/or IMC have shown no mortality for either treatment, with little to no morbidity for ET but early morbidity rates around 39% in the resection group.[73,76] Equivalent cancer-specific survivals were reported. However, a new metachronous primary neoplastic lesion occurred in 20%[73] and 12%[76] of the endotherapy groups. These were usually treated endoscopically. There has been one case-controlled comparative study assessing oesophagectomy compared with EMR and ablation in patients with intramucosal adenocarcinoma (T1a).[77] The resection group had a median follow-up of 4 years with no tumour recurrence. The major complication rate was 32% and 90-day mortality 2.6%. Following endoscopic therapy there was no major morbidity or mortality, and 6.6% of patients needed further local therapy during the median follow-up time of 3.7 months.[77]

The use of EMR has been reported in a cohort of 21 patients having endoscopic therapy for 'low-risk' T1b adenocarcinoma. Low risk was defined as: invasion of the upper sm1; absence of lymphatic/vascular invasion; grade I/II; polypoid or flat lesion (not ulcerated). APC was used for Barrett's ablation in 73%. At a median follow-up of 62 months there was an initial 90% complete resection rate with 28% recurrence of metachronous carcinoma. There were no tumour-related deaths. For this subset of patients one needs to consider this treatment as experimental and more suitable for patients not considered to be surgical candidates until more data are available.[78]

Squamous cell carcinoma

The majority of the studies are from Japan using EMR or ESD.[9,26,27,59] There is one series of ESD from Italy[58] and one from Germany using EMR.[56] A study assessing EMR in 351 patients reported a 5-year disease-free survival of 98%. At a median follow-up of 9 months the local recurrence rate was 2% in patients with m1/2 disease, 7% with m3/sm1 and 7% with sm2/3. The only patients who developed metastasis had sm1/2 disease.[79] The largest single-centre series has 300 patients with m1–3 (m3 15%) disease, in whom 184 had EMR and

116 ESD.[26] A positive margin was seen in 3% who had ESD and 22% who had an EMR. However, the stricture rate was 17% for ESD compared with 9% who had an EMR. Local recurrence was 10% after EMR in patients that had a piecemeal resection. Recurrence may also manifest as recurrent nodes or systemic disease. This is more likely to occur in patients who had lesions that were m3 or submucosal treated with EMR or ESD.[27,56,59]

✔ Endoscopic therapy is a suitable alternative to resection of the oesophagus for intramucosal oesophageal cancer that can be removed completely. However, there will be a recurrence of the neoplasia that is reduced but not eradicated when the surrounding high-risk mucosa is removed or ablated. Thus, it is essential that the patient undergo careful and vigilant endoscopic follow-up. For submucosal disease there will be very few patients for whom endoscopic therapy is a suitable treatment unless they are not fit for surgery or refuse resection.

Definitive radiotherapy with or without chemotherapy

Most often this modality is offered when patients are unfit for resection or refuse an operation. In patients with invasive SCC (stage II/III), there is evidence from randomised trials for the use of definitive chemoradiation (CRT)[80] over radiation (RT) alone and for definitive chemoradiation as replacement for resection alone.[81] For adenocarcinoma, there are no data from randomised trials for the use of definitive radiation with or without chemotherapy. For adenocarcinoma the evidence is extrapolated from the histological responses that may occur in the primary tumour in phase II and III trials of neoadjuvant therapy followed by resection of the oesophagus.[82]

A Cochrane analysis of CRT compared with RT alone reports the value of CRT to be a reduction in local persistence/recurrence of 12%.[83] Assessing local control of disease following definitive CRT for stage I disease, two studies from Japan report initial complete responses of 93%[84] and 87%.[85] The incidence of recurrence after CRT has been reported to be 20–30%.[38,84] Salvage may be possible with EMR or resection.[38,84] The more recent studies examining outcomes from CRT in patients with stage I SCC have reported 3-year DSS of 85%,[37] 4-year DSS of 80%[86] and 5-year DSS of 77%[84] and 76%.[38] The 5-year DSS survival for T1a was 84% compared with 50% for patients who were T1b.[38]

There has been one institutional study that has compared the outcomes from CRT with a three-field oesophagectomy for stage I SCC with definitive CRT.[37] Resection or definitive CRT was offered to patients who had clinical stage I disease, who were not considered candidates for endoscopic therapy (disease >5 cm and more than two-thirds of the circumference). There was a bias towards CRT for the elderly and longer lesions. In the 54 patients who had CRT there was a complete endoscopic response in 53. Local recurrence occurred in 21%. Primary resection had a complication rate of 34%, some very serious. The 1- and 3-year disease-specific survivals were 98.1% and 88.75%, respectively, for CRT and 97.4% and 85.5%, respectively, for oesophagectomy. Adjusting for age, sex and tumour size, the hazard ratio for CRT for overall survival was 0.95 (95% confidence interval 0.37–2.47).[37]

✔ In Japan the current recommendations are:[87]

- m1–2; m3/sm1 (without LVI): EMR/ESD if unwilling or unfit for resection;
- sm2/3: resection with CRT an alternative option.

As previously stated, the data relating to the use of radiation for early adenocarcinoma of the oesophagus are not clear. Thus, this modality is an option for patients not suitable for surgery but who are considered suitable candidates for a definitive therapy. This is particularly the case if the patient is considered to be high risk for residual primary disease or localised lymph node metastasis. As such, the guidelines used for SCC as stated above would appear reasonable. However, for both histological subtypes, it is yet to be proven that the addition of chemotherapy to patients having treatment for T1a and sm1 disease without LVI is worthwhile, given the potential increase in the side-effect profile.

Role of a multidisciplinary team

Patients with early oesophageal neoplasia including HGD, stage O and stage I disease have a potential for cure of their disease. The long-term results from the endoscopic therapies are not known. Patients and those treating them must commit to a diligent protocol of regular follow-up endoscopy accepting that this approach, although low in morbidity, is not absolutely proven as a cancer therapy. An operative death is a disaster but equally a death from metastatic AC or SCC in a patient who had endoscopic therapy for a potentially curable disease is also a disaster. Because of the evidence for multimodality therapy for locally advanced therapy, patient management decisions are now typically made in a multidisciplinary environment, including the surgeon, radiation oncologist and medical oncologist. Thus, for early oesophageal cancer the management discussions should include an interventional endoscopist, allowing all the alternatives to surgery to be considered in the same multidisciplinary, collaborative environment. It is clear that improved oesophagectomy outcomes occur in specialist high-volume centres; however, the technical expertise of the surgeon is only one component in the operative and cancer outcomes for these patients. For endoscopic therapies, it is likely that the better neoplasia eradication figures and procedural outcomes will occur in centres that have a specific interest in this problem, with specialist interventional endoscopists who have strict follow-up endoscopy protocols in a multidisciplinary clinical environment.

Conclusion

The choice of management with operative versus non-operative therapy for early oesophageal cancer has improved in the last decade. In appropriately selected patients with HGD and intramucosal cancer, endoscopic therapy is increasingly the treatment of choice as it has the potential to achieve the same curative effect as surgery, with minimal invasiveness and low complication rates. Surgery remains the definitive choice for complicated, extensive HGD, SCC in situ, deep mucosal SCC and any cancer with submucosal infiltration. There is a role for definitive radiotherapy, possibly chemotherapy, in selected patients with SCC and possibly adenocarcinoma, where surgery is not an option. Multidisciplinary assessment and planning are important to achieve optimal outcomes.

Key points

- Early oesophageal cancer may be glandular in origin (Barrett's oesophagus) or squamous in origin and includes malignant involvement of the oesophageal mucosa and submucosa.
- High-grade intraepithelial neoplasia or high-grade dysplasia in the mucosa is equivalent to carcinoma in situ for both squamous and glandular epithelium.
- The risk of lymph node involvement relates to the depth of invasion into the mucosa and submucosa, with the risk being higher for squamous neoplasia involving the mucosa compared with adenocarcinoma in Barrett's oesophagus.
- Endoscopic resection of high-grade intraepithelial neoplasia or intramucosal carcinoma offers improved local staging and in selected cases may be therapeutic/curative, avoiding oesophageal resection.
- Endoscopic ablation of residual neoplastic epithelium using radiofrequency ablation (RFA) should be considered in patients who have had endoscopic resection of Barrett's high-grade dysplasia or intramucosal carcinoma. The role of RFA for residual squamous intraepithelial neoplasia is not clear.
- Long-term intensive endoscopic surveillance is required following endoscopic treatment for early oesophageal neoplasia.
- Oesophagectomy with lymphadenectomy is the definitive treatment for oesophageal cancer invading into the submucosa and in patients in whom the mucosal neoplasia cannot be adequately treated endoscopically.
- For early squamous cell carcinoma, definitive radiotherapy with concurrent chemotherapy is an alternative to oesophagectomy. The results are not as clear for early oesophageal adenocarcinoma.

References

1. Edge SB, Byrd DR, Compton CC, et al., editors. AJCC cancer staging manual. 7th ed. New York: Springer; 2009.
2. Rice TW, Blackstone EH, Rusch VW. 7th edition of the AJCC Cancer Staging Manual: esophagus and esophagogastric junction. Ann Surg Oncol 2010;17(7):1721–4.
3. Larghi A, Lightdale CJ, Memeo L, et al. EUS followed by EMR for staging of high-grade dysplasia and early cancer in Barrett's esophagus. Gastrointest Endosc 2005;62(1):16–23.
4. Buskens CJ, Westerterp M, Lagarde SM, et al. Prediction of appropriateness of local endoscopic treatment for high-grade dysplasia and early adenocarcinoma by EUS and histopathologic features. Gastrointest Endosc 2004;60(5):703–10.
5. Barbour AP, Jones M, Brown I, et al. Risk stratification for early esophageal adenocarcinoma: analysis of lymphatic spread and prognostic factors. Ann Surg Oncol 2010;17(9):2494–502.
6. Griffin SM, Burt AD, Jennings NA. Lymph node metastasis in early esophageal adenocarcinoma. Ann Surg 2011;254(5):731–7.

7. Stein HJ, Feith M, Bruecher BL, et al. Early esophageal cancer: pattern of lymphatic spread and prognostic factors for long-term survival after surgical resection. Ann Surg 2005;242(4):566–75.

8. Sepesi B, Watson TJ, Zhou D, et al. Are endoscopic therapies appropriate for superficial submucosal esophageal adenocarcinoma? An analysis of esophagectomy specimens. J Am Coll Surg 2010;210(4):418–27.

9. Kodama M, Kakegawa T. Treatment of superficial cancer of the esophagus: a summary of responses to a questionnaire on superficial cancer of the esophagus in Japan. Surgery 1998;123(4):432–9.

10. Fujita H, Sueyoshi S, Yamana H, et al. Optimum treatment strategy for superficial esophageal cancer: endoscopic mucosal resection versus radical esophagectomy. World J Surg 2001;25(4):424–31.

11. Tajima Y, Nakanishi Y, Ochiai A, et al. Histopathologic findings predicting lymph node metastasis and prognosis of patients with superficial esophageal carcinoma: analysis of 240 surgically resected tumors. Cancer 2000;88(6):1285–93.

12. Hölscher AH, Bollschweiler E, Schröder W, et al. Prognostic impact of upper, middle, and lower third mucosal or submucosal infiltration in early esophageal cancer. Ann Surg 2011;254(5):802–8.

13. Endo M, Yoshino K, Kawano T, et al. Clinicopathologic analysis of lymph node metastasis in surgically resected superficial cancer of the thoracic esophagus. Dis Esophagus 2000;13(2):125–9.

14. Shimada H, Nabeya Y, Matsubara H, et al. Prediction of lymph node status in patients with superficial esophageal carcinoma: analysis of 160 surgically resected cancers. Am J Surg 2006;191(2):250–4.

15. Tachibana M, Hirahara N, Kinugasa S, et al. Clinicopathologic features of superficial esophageal cancer: results of consecutive 100 patients. Ann Surg Oncol 2008;15(1):104–16.

16. Noguchi H, Naomoto Y, Kondo H, et al. Evaluation of endoscopic mucosal resection for superficial esophageal carcinoma. Surg Laparosc Endosc Percutan Tech 2000;10(6):343–50.

17. Eguchi T, Nakanishi Y, Shimoda T, et al. Histopathological criteria for additional treatment after endoscopic mucosal resection for esophageal cancer: analysis of 464 surgically resected cases. Mod Pathol 2006;19(3):475–80.

18. Gockel I, Sgourakis G, Lyros O, et al. Risk of lymph node metastasis in submucosal esophageal cancer: a review of surgically resected patients. Expert Rev Gastroenterol Hepatol 2011;5(3):371–84.

19. Sampliner RE. Updated guidelines for the diagnosis, surveillance, and therapy of Barrett's esophagus. Am J Gastroenterol 2002;97(8):1888–95.

20. Mori M, Adachi Y, Matsushima T, et al. Lugol staining pattern and histology of esophageal lesions. Am J Gastroenterol 1993;88(5):701–5.

21. DeMeester SR. New options for the therapy of Barrett's high-grade dysplasia and intramucosal adenocarcinoma: endoscopic mucosal resection and ablation versus vagal-sparing esophagectomy. Ann Thorac Surg 2008;85(2):S747–50.

22. Stein HJ, Feith M. Surgical strategies for early esophageal adenocarcinoma. Best Pract Res Clin Gastroenterol 2005;19(6):927–40.

23. Pech O, May A, Gunter E, et al. The impact of endoscopic ultrasound and computed tomography on the TNM staging of early cancer in Barrett's esophagus. Am J Gastroenterol 2006;101(10):2223–9.

24. Moss A, Bourke MJ, Hourigan LF, et al. Endoscopic resection for Barrett's high-grade dysplasia and early esophageal adenocarcinoma: an essential staging procedure with long-term therapeutic benefit. Am J Gastroenterol 2010;105(6):1276–83.

25. Shimizu Y, Kato M, Yamamoto J, et al. Histologic results of EMR for esophageal lesions diagnosed as high-grade intraepithelial squamous neoplasia by endoscopic biopsy. Gastrointest Endosc 2006;63(1):16–21.

26. Takahashi H, Arimura Y, Masao H, et al. Endoscopic submucosal dissection is superior to conventional endoscopic resection as a curative treatment for early squamous cell carcinoma of the esophagus (with video). Gastrointest Endosc 2010;72(2):255–64, 264.e1–2

27. Ono S, Fujishiro M, Niimi K, et al. Long-term outcomes of endoscopic submucosal dissection for superficial esophageal squamous cell neoplasms. Gastrointest Endosc 2009;70(5):860–6.

28. Saito Y, Takisawa H, Suzuki H, et al. Endoscopic submucosal dissection of recurrent or residual superficial esophageal cancer after chemoradiotherapy. Gastrointest Endosc 2008;67(2):355–9.

29. Lightdale CJ, Kulkarni KG. Role of endoscopic ultrasonography in the staging and follow-up of esophageal cancer. J Clin Oncol 2005;23(20):4483–9.

30. Liberale G, Van Laethem JL, Gay F, et al. The role of PET scan in the preoperative management of oesophageal cancer. Eur J Surg Oncol 2004;30(9):942–7.

31. Williams VA, Watson TJ, Herbella FA, et al. Esophagectomy for high grade dysplasia is safe, curative, and results in good alimentary outcome. J Gastrointest Surg 2007;11(12):1589–97.

32. Tharavej C, Hagen JA, Peters JH, et al. Predictive factors of coexisting cancer in Barrett's high-grade dysplasia. Surg Endosc 2006;20(3):439–43.

33. Portale G, Peters JH, Hsieh CC, et al. Can clinical and endoscopic findings accurately predict early-stage adenocarcinoma? Surg Endosc 2006;20(2):294–7.

34. Wang GQ, Abnet CC, Shen Q, et al. Histological precursors of oesophageal squamous cell carcinoma: results from a 13 year prospective follow up study in a high risk population. Gut 2005;54(2):187–92.

35. Low DE. Update on staging and surgical treatment options for esophageal cancer. J Gastrointest Surg 2011;15(5):719–29.
36. Nigro JJ, Hagen JA, DeMeester TR, et al. Occult esophageal adenocarcinoma: extent of disease and implications for effective therapy. Ann Surg 1999;230(3):433–40.
37. Yamamoto S, Ishihara R, Motoori M, et al. Comparison between definitive chemoradiotherapy and esophagectomy in patients with clinical stage I esophageal squamous cell carcinoma. Am J Gastroenterol 2011;106(6):1048–54.
38. Yamada K, Murakami M, Okamoto Y, et al. Treatment results of chemoradiotherapy for clinical stage I (T1N0M0) esophageal carcinoma. Int J Radiat Oncol Biol Phys 2006;64(4):1106–11.
39. Igaki H, Kato H, Tachimori Y, et al. Clinicopathologic characteristics and survival of patients with clinical Stage I squamous cell carcinomas of the thoracic esophagus treated with three-field lymph node dissection. Eur J Cardiothorac Surg 2001;20(6):1089–94.
40. Stein HJ, Hutter J, Feith M, et al. Limited surgical resection and jejunal interposition for early adenocarcinoma of the distal esophagus. Semin Thorac Cardiovasc Surg 2007;19(1):72–8.
41. Peyre CG, DeMeester SR, Rizzetto C, et al. Vagal-sparing esophagectomy: the ideal operation for intramucosal adenocarcinoma and Barrett with high-grade dysplasia. Ann Surg 2007;246(4):665–74.
42. Hulscher JB, Tijssen JG, Obertop H, et al. Transthoracic versus transhiatal resection for carcinoma of the esophagus: a meta-analysis. Ann Thorac Surg 2001;72(1):306–13.
43. Hulscher JB, van Sandick JW, de Boer AG, et al. Extended transthoracic resection compared with limited transhiatal resection for adenocarcinoma of the esophagus. N Engl J Med 2002;347(21):1662–9.
44. Matsubara T, Ueda M, Abe T, et al. Unique distribution patterns of metastatic lymph nodes in patients with superficial carcinoma of the thoracic oesophagus. Br J Surg 1999;86(5):669–73.
45. Luketich JD, Alvelo-Rivera M, Buenaventura PO, et al. Minimally invasive esophagectomy: outcomes in 222 patients. Ann Surg 2003;238(4):486–95.
46. Palanivelu C, Prakash A, Senthilkumar R, et al. Minimally invasive esophagectomy: thoracoscopic mobilization of the esophagus and mediastinal lymphadenectomy in prone position – experience of 130 patients. J Am Coll Surg 2006;203(1):7–16.
47. Smithers BM, Gotley DC, Martin I, et al. Comparison of the outcomes between open and minimally invasive esophagectomy. Ann Surg 2007;245(2):232–40.
48. Itami A, Watanabe G, Tanaka E, et al. Multimedia article. Upper mediastinal lymph node dissection for esophageal cancer through a thoracoscopic approach. Surg Endosc 2008;22(12):2741.
49. Headrick JR, Nichols 3rd. FC, Miller DL, et al. High-grade esophageal dysplasia: long-term survival and quality of life after esophagectomy. Ann Thorac Surg 2002;73(6):1697–703.
50. Chang LC, Oelschlager BK, Quiroga E, et al. Long-term outcome of esophagectomy for high-grade dysplasia or cancer found during surveillance for Barrett's esophagus. J Gastrointest Surg 2006;10(3):341–6.
51. Moraca RJ, Low DE. Outcomes and health-related quality of life after esophagectomy for high-grade dysplasia and intramucosal cancer. Arch Surg 2006;141(6):545–51.
52. Abrams JA, Fedi P, Vakiani E, et al. Depth of resection using two different endoscopic mucosal resection techniques. Endoscopy 2008;40(5):395–9.
53. Pouw RE, van Vilsteren FG, Peters FP, et al. Randomized trial on endoscopic resection-cap versus multiband mucosectomy for piecemeal endoscopic resection of early Barrett's neoplasia. Gastrointest Endosc 2011;74(1):35–43.
54. Peters FP, Kara MA, Rosmolen WD, et al. Stepwise radical endoscopic resection is effective for complete removal of Barrett's esophagus with early neoplasia: a prospective study. Am J Gastroenterol 2006;101(7):1449–57.
55. Chennat J, Konda VJ, Ross AS, et al. Complete Barrett's eradication endoscopic mucosal resection: an effective treatment modality for high-grade dysplasia and intramucosal carcinoma – an American single-center experience. Am J Gastroenterol 2009;104(11):2684–92.
56. Pech O, Gossner L, May A, et al. Endoscopic resection of superficial esophageal squamous-cell carcinomas: Western experience. Am J Gastroenterol 2004;99(7):1226–32.
57. Esaki M, Matsumoto T, Hirakawa K, et al. Risk factors for local recurrence of superficial esophageal cancer after treatment by endoscopic mucosal resection. Endoscopy 2007;39(1):41–5.
58. Repici A, Hassan C, Carlino A, et al. Endoscopic submucosal dissection in patients with early esophageal squamous cell carcinoma: results from a prospective Western series. Gastrointest Endosc 2010;71(4):715–21.
59. Fujishiro M, Yahagi N, Kakushima N, et al. Endoscopic submucosal dissection of esophageal squamous cell neoplasms. Clin Gastroenterol Hepatol 2006;4(6):688–94.
60. Ackroyd R, Brown NJ, Davis MF, et al. Photodynamic therapy for dysplastic Barrett's oesophagus: a prospective, double blind, randomised, placebo controlled trial. Gut 2000;47(5):612–7.
61. Overholt BF, Wang KK, Burdick JS, et al. Five-year efficacy and safety of photodynamic therapy with Photofrin in Barrett's high-grade dysplasia. Gastrointest Endosc 2007;66(3):460–8.
62. Attwood SE, Lewis CJ, Caplin S, et al. Argon beam plasma coagulation as therapy for high-grade dysplasia in Barrett's esophagus. Clin Gastroenterol Hepatol 2003;1(4):258–63.

63. Ragunath K, Krasner N, Raman VS, et al. Endoscopic ablation of dysplastic Barrett's oesophagus comparing argon plasma coagulation and photodynamic therapy: a randomized prospective trial assessing efficacy and cost-effectiveness. Scand J Gastroenterol 2005;40(7):750–8.
64. Madisch A, Miehlke S, Bayerdorffer E, et al. Long-term follow-up after complete ablation of Barrett's esophagus with argon plasma coagulation. World J Gastroenterol 2005;11(8):1182–6.
65. Kelty CJ, Ackroyd R, Brown NJ, et al. Endoscopic ablation of Barrett's oesophagus: a randomized-controlled trial of photodynamic therapy vs. argon plasma coagulation. Aliment Pharmacol Ther 2004;20(11–12):1289–96.
66. Mino-Kenudson M, Ban S, Ohana M, et al. Buried dysplasia and early adenocarcinoma arising in Barrett esophagus after porfimer-photodynamic therapy. Am J Surg Pathol 2007;31(3):403–9.
67. Ganz RA, Overholt BF, Sharma VK, et al. Circumferential ablation of Barrett's esophagus that contains high-grade dysplasia: a U.S. Multicenter Registry. Gastrointest Endosc 2008;68(1):35–40.
68. Vaccaro BJ, Gonzalez S, Poneros JM, et al. Detection of intestinal metaplasia after successful eradication of Barrett's esophagus with radiofrequency ablation. Dig Dis Sci 2011;56(7):1996–2000.
69. van Vilsteren FG, Pouw RE, Seewald S, et al. Stepwise radical endoscopic resection versus radiofrequency ablation for Barrett's oesophagus with high-grade dysplasia or early cancer: a multicentre randomised trial. Gut 2011;60(6):765–73.
70. Bergman JJ, Zhang YM, He S, et al. Outcomes from a prospective trial of endoscopic radiofrequency ablation of early squamous cell neoplasia of the esophagus. Gastrointest Endosc 2011;74(6):1181–90.
71. Pech O, Behrens A, May A, et al. Long-term results and risk factor analysis for recurrence after curative endoscopic therapy in 349 patients with high-grade intraepithelial neoplasia and mucosal adenocarcinoma in Barrett's oesophagus. Gut 2008;57(9):1200–6.
72. Das A, Singh V, Fleischer DE, et al. A comparison of endoscopic treatment and surgery in early esophageal cancer: an analysis of surveillance epidemiology and end results data. Am J Gastroenterol 2008;103(6):1340–5.
73. Zehetner J, DeMeester SR, Hagen JA, et al. Endoscopic resection and ablation versus esophagectomy for high-grade dysplasia and intramucosal adenocarcinoma. J Thorac Cardiovasc Surg 2011;141(1):39–47.
74. Wani S, Puli SR, Shaheen NJ, et al. Esophageal adenocarcinoma in Barrett's esophagus after endoscopic ablative therapy: a meta-analysis and systematic review. Am J Gastroenterol 2009;104(2):502–13.
75. Pouw RE, Gondrie JJ, Sondermeijer CM, et al. Eradication of Barrett esophagus with early neoplasia by radiofrequency ablation, with or without endoscopic resection. J Gastrointest Surg 2008;12(10):1627–37.
76. Prasad GA, Wu TT, Wigle DA, et al. Endoscopic and surgical treatment of mucosal (T1a) esophageal adenocarcinoma in Barrett's esophagus. Gastroenterology 2009;137(3):815–23.
77. Pech O, Bollschweiler E, Manner H, et al. Comparison between endoscopic and surgical resection of mucosal esophageal adenocarcinoma in Barrett's esophagus at two high-volume centers. Ann Surg 2011;254(1):67–72.
78. Manner H, May A, Pech O, et al. Early Barrett's carcinoma with "low-risk" submucosal invasion: long-term results of endoscopic resection with a curative intent. Am J Gastroenterol 2008;103(10):2589–97.
79. Shimizu Y, Tsukagoshi H, Fujita M, et al. Long-term outcome after endoscopic mucosal resection in patients with esophageal squamous cell carcinoma invading the muscularis mucosae or deeper. Gastrointest Endosc 2002;56(3):387–90.
80. Herskovic A, Martz K, al-Sarraf M, et al. Combined chemotherapy and radiotherapy compared with radiotherapy alone in patients with cancer of the esophagus. N Engl J Med 1992;326(24):1593–8.
81. Chiu PW, Chan AC, Leung SF, et al. Multicenter prospective randomized trial comparing standard esophagectomy with chemoradiotherapy for treatment of squamous esophageal cancer: early results from the Chinese University Research Group for Esophageal Cancer (CURE). J Gastrointest Surg 2005;9(6):794–802.
82. Geh JI, Crellin AM, Glynne-Jones R. Preoperative (neoadjuvant) chemoradiotherapy in oesophageal cancer. Br J Surg 2001;88(3):338–56.
83. Wong R, Malthaner R. Combined chemotherapy and radiotherapy (without surgery) compared with radiotherapy alone in localized carcinoma of the esophagus. Cochrane Database Syst Rev 2006;(1)CD002092.
84. Ura T, Muro K, Shimada Y, et al. Definitive chemoradiotherapy may be standard treatment option in clinical stage I esophageal cancer. Proc Am Soc Clin Oncol 2004;22(317S)abstr 4017.
85. Kato H, Sato A, Fukuda H, et al. A phase II trial of chemoradiotherapy for stage I esophageal squamous cell carcinoma: Japan Clinical Oncology Group Study (JCOG9708). Jpn J Clin Oncol 2009;39(10):638–43.
86. Kato H, Tachimori Y, Watanabe H, et al. Superficial esophageal carcinoma. Surgical treatment and the results. Cancer 1990;66(11):2319–23.
87. Shitara K, Muro K. Chemoradiotherapy for treatment of esophageal cancer in Japan: current status and perspectives. Gastrointest Cancer Res 2009;3(2):66–72.

7

Surgery for cancer of the stomach

Takeshi Sano

Introduction

There seem to be two different worlds for surgeons who confront gastric cancer. In Japan and Korea, where nearly half of the tumours are T1, 'advanced gastric cancer' usually means non-early tumours that are still potentially curable by radical surgery. Surgeons have developed minimally invasive techniques for T1 tumours and perform meticulous extended dissection for 'advanced' cancers. In the rest of the world, where patients present with much more advanced disease, the chance of cure by surgery is limited and surgeons' best efforts are often not rewarded. Furthermore, the prevalence of a new disease called oesophageal adenocarcinoma has increased significantly in Western countries, almost overtaking distal gastric cancer, which is rapidly decreasing. Under the circumstances, surgeons in different parts of the world naturally have different strategies and standards to confront the disease. However, the ideal treatment for a patient with gastric cancer, wherever the diagnosis is given, ought to be the same as long as the disease is the same.

This chapter provides a Japanese perspective on surgery for gastric cancer from an international viewpoint, with the goal that surgeons in different circumstances select the best available treatment towards the same goal.

Modes of spread and areas of potential failure after gastric cancer surgery

Gastric cancer arises in the mucosa and seldom metastasises until it penetrates the muscularis mucosae. The submucosal layer has numerous lymphatic and venous capillaries through which cancer cells spread, first to the lymph nodes and subsequently to the liver. Once the tumour penetrates the serosa, peritoneal dissemination becomes common. The depth of tumour invasion (T-stage) is an important prognostic factor itself, and is closely correlated to all patterns of metastasis.

A rational approach to surgery for gastric cancer requires an understanding of the modes of spread of this cancer and how it recurs after surgery. This knowledge is essential to define the aims and limitations of radical surgery.

In addition, it should be noted that the patterns of failure after gastric cancer surgery have been variously reported using similar classifications but with different definitions. An example is shown in Table 7.1: hepatic and lymph node recurrences are categorised as distant and local failure respectively in the Dutch D1/D2 trial,[1,2] but as regional failure in the Intergroup 0116 study.[3]

Metastatic pathway

Lymphatic spread

Lymphatic spread is the most common mode of dissemination in gastric cancer. Lymph node metastasis is histologically proven in 10% of T1 tumours, and the rate increases as the invasion deepens, up to 80% of T4a tumours.[4,5]

The lymphatic drainage system from the stomach has been well demonstrated in lymphography studies (**Fig. 7.1**). Unlike other parts of the digestive tract, the stomach has multidimensional mesenteries that

Table 7.1 • Different definitions of patterns of failure in the Dutch and American trials on gastric cancer surgery

Pattern of failure	Dutch D1/D2 trial[1,2]	US Intergroup 0116[3]
Local	Gastric bed, anastomosis, regional lymph nodes	Gastric bed, anastomosis, residual stomach
Regional	Peritoneal carcinomatosa	Liver, lymph nodes, peritoneal carcinomatosa
Distant	Liver, lung, ovary and other organs	Outside the peritoneal cavity

contain dense lymphatic networks. Cancer cells can flow out of the stomach through any of these routes and by way of the nearby perigastric nodes, to reach the nodes around the coeliac artery. They then enter the para-aortic nodes and finally flow into the thoracic duct and systemic circulation. Systemic metastasis can occur via this route. In particular, bone marrow carcinomatosis occurs most frequently in cases with extensive nodal disease.[6,7]

The stomach has the largest number of 'regional lymph nodes' of any organ in the human body. After a total gastrectomy with D2 lymphadenectomy, more than 40 lymph nodes can usually be collected with careful retrieval. Of the malignant tumours listed in the UICC/TNM classification,[8] stomach cancer requires the largest number of nodes to be removed as a minimal requirement to allow a pN0 diagnosis (16 nodes) and the largest number of positive nodes for the highest N category (pN3b, 16 or more positive nodes).This suggests that lymphatic metastasis from gastric cancer may remain in the dense lymphatic filters for some time and that patients with nodal metastasis can still be cured by adequate dissection.

Peritoneal spread

Peritoneal metastasis is the most common type of failure after radical surgery for gastric cancer.[9] Once the tumour penetrates the serosal surface (T4a), cancer cells may be scattered in the peritoneal space. They can be implanted in the gastric bed or any part of the peritoneal cavity and subsequently cause intestinal obstruction or ascites. Peritoneal metastasis is much more common in diffuse-type cancers than the intestinal type[10] and later causes peritonitis carcinomatosa, a characteristic recurrent pattern of gastric cancer, which is relatively uncommon in colorectal adenocarcinomas that are mostly of the intestinal type.

Peritoneal lavage cytology is a sensitive test for this metastasis. Almost all patients with positive cytology subsequently develop peritoneal recurrence even after macroscopically curative surgery. In the UICC/TNM 7th edition,[8] positive cytology ('cy+') has been included in the definition of pM1.

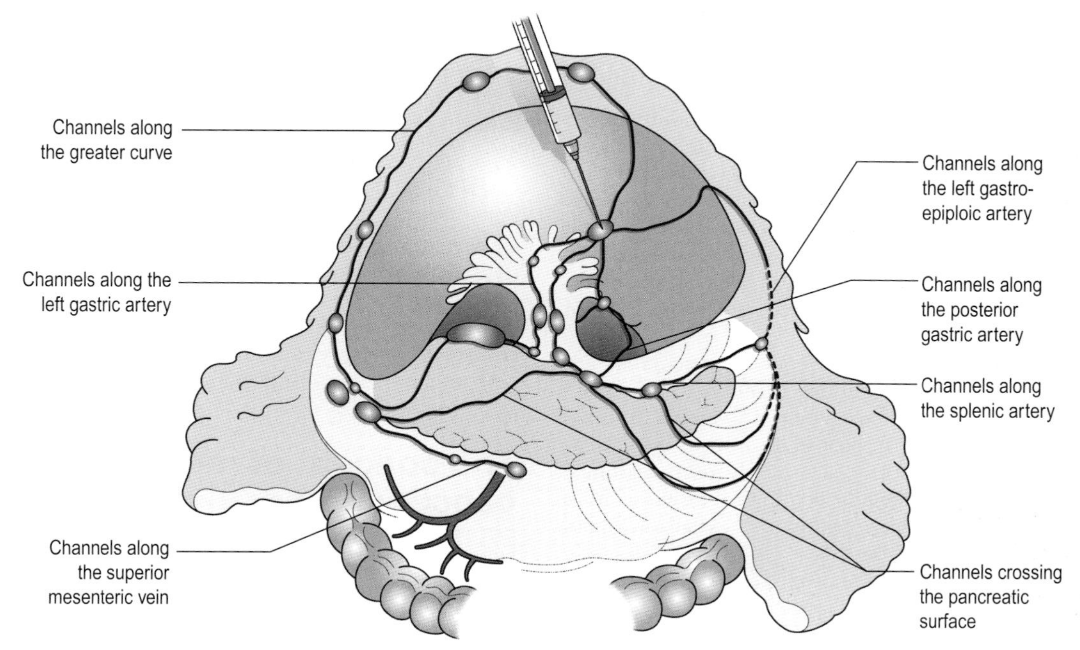

Figure 7.1 • Lymphography of the stomach. Courtesy of K. Maruyama.

In general, surgery has no curative role in treating this mode of spread. However, in some exceptional cases where a small number of peritoneal metastases exist in the upper abdomen but peritoneal cytology is negative, complete removal of these visible nodules may bring cure.

Peritoneal metastasis is refractory to systemic chemotherapy. Intraperitoneal chemotherapy with or without hyperthermia is being vigorously tested in various centres. Some promising results have been reported,[11] but the evidence is not yet compelling.

Haematogenous spread

Liver metastasis is relatively uncommon at the time of diagnosis of gastric cancer, but is commonly seen as a part of systemic failure. In the 15-year follow-up report of the Dutch D1/D2 trial, liver metastasis was found, either as the sole site or with other sites in 102 of 319 deaths with recurrence.[12] It occurs predominantly in intestinal-type tumours. Unlike in colorectal cancer, liver metastasis from gastric cancer is usually multiple and associated with other modes of spread. Resection is rarely indicated and, even if it is carried out, the prognosis is poor.

Metastasis by uncertain pathway

Lung, bone or other distant metastases are relatively rare at the time of diagnosis and appear as a part of systemic dissemination at the terminal stage. These may be regarded as haematogenous spread, but as many such cases lack liver metastasis, the initial route of spread may be the lymphatic–caval system mentioned above rather than the venous portal–caval route.

Ovarian metastasis (Krukenberg tumour) may occur especially from diffuse-type tumours, including signet-ring cell carcinoma. It is not uncommon for patients, to present with ovarian tumours, and histological proof of signet-ring cells in the resected ovary leads to the diagnosis of gastric cancer. Ovarian metastasis may occur as part of peritoneal spread, but considering the absence of peritoneal disease in some cases and usual association with lymphatic involvement, it may be considered as a special form of lymphatic spread.

Retroperitoneal spread frequently occurs in advanced diffuse-type tumours. It causes urinary tract obstruction and/or 'frozen pelvis' symptoms. This is usually considered as part of peritoneal dissemination, but it may occur as a purely retroperitoneal disease without visible or cytological disease within the peritoneal cavity. Lymphatic extension again may be responsible for this.

Direct extension

Gastric cancer penetrating the serosa sometimes extends to the adjacent organs or structures. When the operation is potentially curative, these may be excised en bloc with the stomach. It is of note that, in a considerable proportion of apparent T4b cases, pathological assessment shows only inflammatory adhesion without direct tumour invasion.[13]

Intraoperative spillage

Surgery itself can be a cause of cancer spread, especially in terms of peritoneal dissemination. A T4a tumour penetrating the gastric serosa without visible or cytological peritoneal disease sometimes recurs in the peritoneal cavity after potentially curative surgery. There are two possible explanations for this: (1) cancer cells had already been implanted but the cytology test was not sensitive enough; (2) there were no free cancer cells before surgery, but operative manipulation caused cancer cell spillage from the tumour surface.

Even serosa-negative tumours can recur in the peritoneal cavity after surgery. These cases are usually associated with lymph node metastasis. A possible explanation for this is that during lymph node dissection lymphatic channels were broken and cancer cells in the lymph nodes spilled out. This was proven in a unique study from Korea,[14] though it has not been confirmed whether these spilled cells are implanted and grow.

These intraoperative spillages of cancer cells might be prevented by careful non-touch isolation techniques and/or by use of clips or vessel-sealing devices. However, the simplest means to prevent cancer cell implantation during surgery will be peritoneal wash with a large volume of saline before abdominal closure. A small-scale randomised study showed a significant survival benefit of extensive intraoperative peritoneal lavage (EIPL) in gastric cancer patients with positive cytology.[15]

Summary

Of the four patterns of spread of gastric cancer (lymphatic, peritoneal, haematogenous and direct), lymphatic metastasis occurs at the earliest stage and this can lead to other types of metastases. Surgical control of this spread at an early phase of the disease may prevent subsequent systemic failure.

The concept of radical gastric cancer surgery

Surgery plays an essential role in the curative treatment of gastric cancer. Although radical surgery has been attempted in many centres worldwide, it is Japanese surgeons who have been at the forefront of the practice of radical gastric resection and lymphadenectomy.

Gastric cancer surgery in Japan

The incidence of gastric cancer in Japan is among the highest in the world. Approximately 100 000 new cases are diagnosed every year, accounting for 11% of all cases in the world.[16] The age-standardised incidence, however, has been rapidly decreasing as in other countries in the world, probably due to the decreasing infection of *Helicobacter pylori*. The peak incidence was in the 1950s (male 71, female 37 per 10^5 population), the time when the mass screening programme was planned and the basic style of radical D2 gastrectomy was proposed (for reference, the incidences in 2010 were 12.4 and 7.1 respectively).

The Japanese Research Society for Gastric Cancer (JRSGC) was founded in 1962 and the nationwide registry started using a new documentation system, the General Rules for Gastric Cancer in Surgery and Pathology. This just preceded the UICC's publication of the TNM classification for gastric cancer.

The General Rules (the English name was later changed to the Japanese Classification of Gastric Carcinoma) played a key role in the standardisation of surgery and pathology for gastric cancer in Japan. Detailed clinicopathological information, especially on lymph node metastasis, was prospectively collected from a large number of institutions and the optimal extent of lymphadenectomy was eagerly sought. The concept of 'lymph node groups' was established and the dissection of group 1 and 2 nodal stations was proposed as the standard radical surgery, which Japanese surgeons almost blindly accepted and followed.

This concept has never been tested in a randomised trial in Japan. As D2 gastrectomy is safely performed with good results in the country, Japanese surgeons think it unethical even to plan a trial in which half of the patients should undergo surgery that they consider inferior (D1).

Development of gastric cancer surgery in the West

The Japanese documentation system and excellent treatment results influenced the Western concept of radical surgery for gastric cancer. Some surgeons visited Japanese institutions to convince themselves of the feasibility and efficacy of the technique and have successfully reproduced the results in the West.[17,18] However, most non-specialist surgeons could not overcome their scepticism and were reluctant to practise this aggressive surgery in their patients. An important obstacle is the difficulty in directly comparing the results between Japan and the West due to the following two issues.

Different staging systems

The UICC and the AJCC unified their TNM staging system in their fourth edition in 1985. The N category in that edition was defined according to the anatomical location of the involved lymph nodes: metastasis in the perigastric nodes within 3 cm of the primary tumour was staged as N1, metastasis in the other perigastric nodes and those along the named branches of the coeliac artery as N2. Although the Japanese definitions of nodal groups 1 and 2 were different, as detailed later, the basic concept of the two systems was similar in that the anatomical location of the involved lymph nodes determined the N category. Thus, the treatment results of tumours staged by the two different systems were able to be compared, neglecting minor differences.

In 1997 the UICC/AJCC adopted the numerical N category in the fifth edition, and the Japanese classification and the TNM classification became totally distinct systems. The Japanese results were able to be expressed using the new TNM system because the number of positive nodes in each case was also recorded, but the reverse was impossible because the anatomical data were no longer available in the West. Japanese surgeons and pathologists continued to use their system as the primary staging method, thus sticking to the surgical significance of lymph node anatomy, and they use the TNM system only when they write English papers. On the other hand, Western surgeons' interest in lymphadenectomy may have diminished because the N category was determined regardless of the extent of lymphadenectomy.

Different disease hypotheses

A hypothesis that gastric cancer in the West may be a different disease to that in Japan prevails and prevents positive discussion to advance optimal treatment for gastric cancer patients on a global level. In the studies biologically analysing and comparing surgical specimens, no evidence has been shown to support the hypothesis.[19,20] The following are the currently discussed differences.

Proximal location

It has been repeatedly highlighted that Western gastric cancers are predominantly located in the proximal stomach while Japanese tumours are found mostly in the distal stomach. This might suggest that these are different diseases. However, this needs careful consideration.

Adenocarcinoma of the lower oesophagus and the oesophagogastric junction is one of the most rapidly increasing malignant tumours in the West, especially among white males.[21] This trend, together with the rapid decrease of distal gastric cancers, makes it plausible that Western gastric cancer arises mostly in the proximal stomach. However, the lower oesophageal adenocarcinoma is a new, distinct disease with a different aetiology and contrasting patient backgrounds,[22] and therefore should be considered separately from 'classical' gastric cancer. In the three large-scale Western surgical trials, the Dutch D1/D2,[1] the British MRC D1/D2[23] and United States INT0116 studies,[3] the proportion of proximal third tumours was 10.3%, 30.5% and 19.5% respectively, and was not significantly different from that (19.1%) in the Japanese D2/D3 study[24] (**Fig. 7.2**). This suggests that, as far as surgically targeted gastric cancers are concerned, tumour location is not largely different between the West and Japan. The apparent predominance of proximal tumours in the West may be a simple reflection of the mixture of different diseases, i.e. increasing oesophageal and decreasing gastric adenocarcinomas.

Patient factor

Western patients with gastric cancer are on average 10 years older, much more likely to be obese and more frequently have comorbidities, especially of cardiovascular diseases, than their Japanese counterparts.[25] Although this does not mean that the disease is different, it certainly affects surgical process and outcomes. In particular, obesity hampers the completion of extended lymphadenectomy for gastric cancer, even in specialist Japanese centres. It has been shown to be an independent risk factor for postoperative morbidity.[26]

Role of radical surgery in Western practice

Due to the decreased incidence and the technically demanding therapeutic requirements, gastric cancer in the West is today considered as a disease that should be treated in specialist centres. Several studies have shown relationships between the hospital/surgeon volume of gastric cancer treatment and operative mortality.[27] Given the accelerated 'proximal shift' of the disease and the increasing surgical risks in Western patients, the trend of centralisation will further progress.

> ✔ Although solid evidence of extended lymphadenectomy is yet to be established, D2 gastrectomy without splenectomy or pancreatectomy was officially recommended by the European Society of Medical Oncology in 2009.[28] The NCCN guidelines for gastric cancer in the USA also recommend D2 for potentially curable gastric cancer with the condition that experienced surgeons perform it in specialist cancer centres.[29] However, as the possible benefit of this extensive surgery could be easily offset by the increased mortality, careful selection of patients is important even in specialist centres. There is an increasing move towards tailoring operations, taking not only the stage of the disease but also patient-related factors into account.

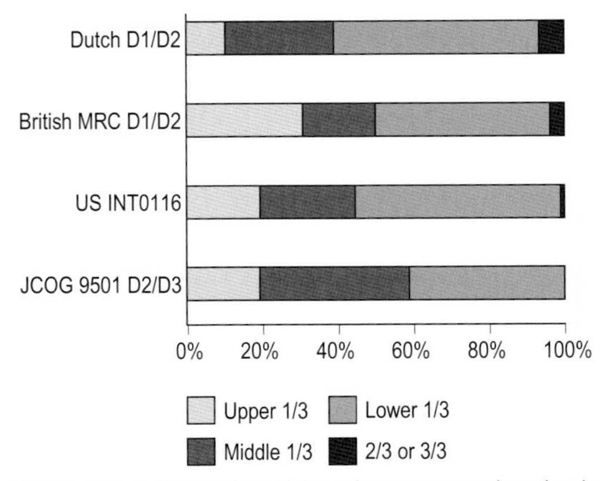

Figure 7.2 • Proportion of the primary tumour location in prospective trials of gastric cancer surgery.

Summary

There are large differences between Japan and the West in incidence, staging system, tumour location and patient factors. Consequently, the concept of radical surgery has developed separately in Japan and the West. Today in the West, gastric cancer is considered as a disease to be treated by specialists, preferably with D2 lymphadenectomy without splenectomy.

Principles of radical gastric cancer surgery

Extent of gastric resection

The primary objective of gastric cancer surgery is to adequately excise the primary lesion with clear longitudinal and circumferential margins. Selection of gastrectomy depends on the tumour location and the mode of infiltration in the stomach wall. Preoperative diagnosis should focus on this, and careful assessment of lateral tumour spread is indispensable.

Resection margins

Proximal resection margin is the main determinant in selecting a total or distal gastrectomy. During surgery for T2 or deeper tumours, the resection line should be determined with a sufficient margin from the palpable edge of the tumour. A 5-cm margin has traditionally been recommended.[30] In some guidelines, even 8 cm is recommended for diffuse-type tumours,[31] but this would necessitate most tumours of the gastric body requiring a total gastrectomy or oesophagogastrectomy.

✔ According to Japanese treatment guidelines,[32] a 5-cm margin is recommended for tumours showing an infiltrative growth pattern with indistinct borders or diffuse-type histology, but 3 cm is usually sufficient for those showing an expansive growth pattern with grossly distinct borders, for which the histology is most frequently of the intestinal type.

For gastric cancers invading the oesophagus, a 5-cm margin is not necessarily required, but frozen section examination of the resection line is desirable to ensure an R0 resection.

In cT1 tumours, lateral mucosal extension should be preoperatively detected or excluded by stepwise biopsy, and placing clips on the negative border is helpful to accurately resect impalpable lesions.

Type of gastrectomy

Common types of gastrectomy for gastric cancer are as follows.

Total gastrectomy

This involves removal of the whole stomach including the cardia (oesophagogastric junction) and the pylorus. It is indicated for tumours arising at or invading the proximal stomach.

Distal (subtotal) gastrectomy

This involves removal of the stomach including the pylorus but preserving the cardia. Two-thirds or more of the stomach is usually removed for gastric cancer. It is indicated for middle or lower third tumours with sufficient resection margins mentioned above.

Proximal gastrectomy

This involves removal of the stomach including the cardia but preserving the pylorus. It is indicated for proximal tumours with or without oesophageal invasion, where more than half of the distal stomach can be preserved.

Other resections for T1 tumours

Pylorus-preserving gastrectomy (PPG) is indicated for T1 tumours in the gastric body having negligible possibility of metastasis to the peripyloric lymph nodes. About a 3-cm pyloric cuff with the right gastric artery is preserved.

Segmental gastrectomy is a circumferential resection of a small part of the stomach preserving the cardia and pylorus. Local resection is a non-circumferential resection of the stomach wall. These resections are not considered as a standard cancer treatment and may be indicated for small T1 tumours in patients with high operative risks.

Total gastrectomy 'de principe' for distal cancers

Some European surgeons have argued that all cancers of the stomach, even those in the distal third, should be treated by total gastrectomy. This principle is based on the experience of frequent involvement of proximal resection margin and consequent anastomotic local recurrence. Theoretically, total gastrectomy ensures more certain negative margins and sufficient lymphadenectomy. In addition, the possible occurrence of multicentric cancer in the gastric stump can be prevented. On the other hand, total gastrectomy is associated with a higher operative morbidity and mortality, increased risk of long-term nutritional problems and impaired quality of life as compared to distal gastrectomy.

✔✔ Randomised trials comparing total and distal gastrectomies in distal gastric cancer failed to show the survival benefit for total gastrectomy.[33]

The policy of total gastrectomy de principe should be abandoned for the following reasons:

1. Provided the rules on safe margins of resection listed above are adhered to, a positive proximal resection margin is rare. If the margins are still positive, this usually indicates an aggressive and extensive malignancy and the resection line involvement will not be a major determinant of prognosis.
2. The lymph nodes that can be removed only by total gastrectomy, station nos. 2 (left cardia), 4sa (upper greater curve), 10 (splenic hilum) and 11d (distal splenic artery), are seldom involved in distal gastric cancers. If they are involved, again this indicates an aggressive malignancy and extended surgery would not alter survival outcome.
3. The incidence of second primary cancer in the gastric stump is low. Long-term surveillance by endoscopy may detect a new lesion that can be removed by endoscopic submucosal dissection.

Lymphadenectomy

Lymph node metastasis is the most common mode of spread in gastric cancer. Histological nodal metastasis has been proven in 80% of T4a/T4b tumours, and even T1 tumours have a 10% probability of lymph node metastasis (T1a 3%, T1b 18%).[4,5] Unlike hepatic and other distant metastases, lymph node metastasis from gastric cancer can be surgically removed for potential cure as long as it is confined to the regional area.The optimal extent of lymphadenectomy, however, has been controversial.

Lymph node groups in the former Japanese classifications

Japanese surgeons and pathologists have extensively investigated the distribution of lymph node metastasis. They have recorded it using standardised anatomical station numbers (**Fig. 7.3**). They then classified the stations into three groups, basically according to the incidence of metastasis (N groups 1–3). As the pattern of lymph node metastasis varies with the location of the primary tumour, N groups 1–3 were separately defined depending on the primary tumour location. These numbers of nodal groups were also used to express the grade of nodal disease (N1–3) and the extent of lymphadenectomy (D1–3), e.g. cancer with metastasis to a node in the second group was designated as N2, and complete dissection of up to the second group nodes was defined as D2.

Since its first edition published in 1962, the Japanese Classification of Gastric Carcinoma (JCGC) has undergone periodic revisions, and each time the definitions of the lymph node groups have been slightly modified. The Dutch and MRC D1/D2 trials were conducted using the N and D ('R' at that time) definitions of the 11th edition of the JCGC[34] (Table 7.2), while the Taipei D1/D3 trial[35] and the Japanese D2/D3 trial[24] used the 12th edition,[36] in which the lymph nodes were grouped from N1 to N4. In the 13th edition,[37] the nodal grouping was completed, with four groups (N1–3 and 'M') in five categories of the primary tumour location (Table 7.3). This definition was based on the 'dissection efficiency index' of each lymph node station,[38] calculated using the incidence of metastasis and survival data of a large number of patients. As compared to the 11th edition, D2 lymphadenectomy defined in the 13th edition required more extensive dissection, e.g. for distal third tumours, station nos. 11p, 12a and 14v were included as N2 nodes.

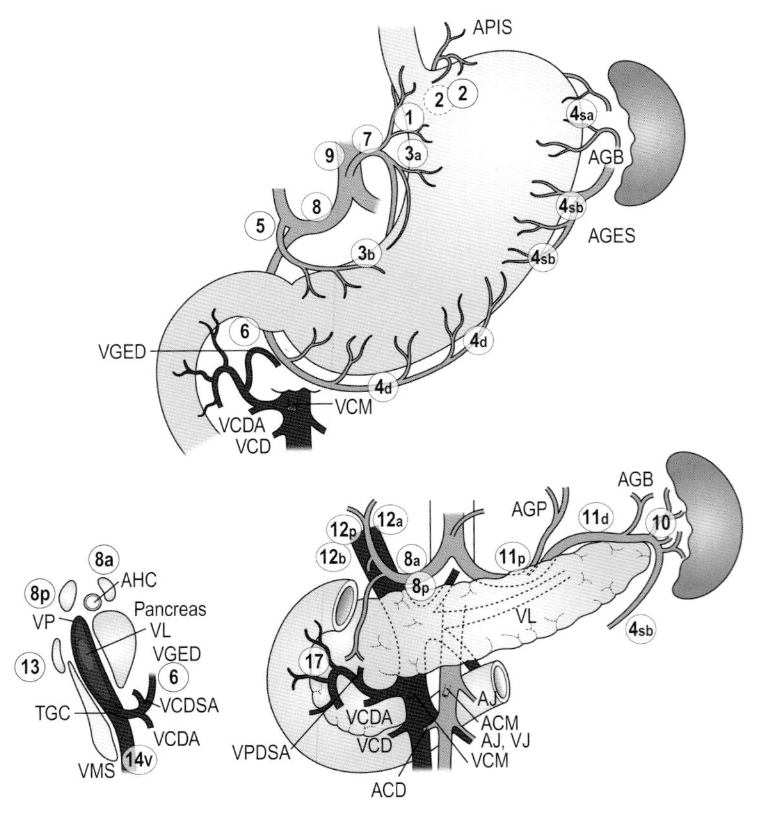

Figure 7.3 • Station numbers of lymph nodes around the stomach. Modified from the Japanese classification of gastric carcinoma, 3rd English edn.[39] ACM, A. colica media; AGB, Aa. gastrica breves; AGES, A. gastroepiploica sinistra; AHC, A. hepatica communis; AJ, A. jejunalis; APIS, A. phrenic inferior sinistra; TGC, truncus gastrocolicus; VCD, V. colica dextra; VCDA, V. colica dextra accessoria; VCM: V. colica media; VGED, V. vastroepiploica dextra; VJ:V. jejunalis; VL, V. lienalis; VMS, V. mesenterica superior; VP, V. portae; VPDSA, V. pancreaticoduodenalis inferior anterior.

Table 7.2 • Lymph node groups used in the Dutch and MRC D1/D2 trials (Japanese classification, 11th edn)

	Location			
	AMC, MAC, MCA, CMA	A, AM	MA, M, MC	C, CM
Group 1 (N1)	1, 2, 3, 4, 5, 6	3, 4, 5, 6	3, 4, 5, 6, 1	1, 2, 3, 4s
Group 2 (N2)	7, 8, 9, 10, 11	7, 8, 9, 1	2†, 7, 8, 9, 10†, 11	4d‡, 7, 8, 9, 10, 11, 5*, 6*
Group 3 (N3)	12, 13, 14, 110*, 111*	2*, 10*, 11, 12, 13, 14	12, 13, 14	12, 13, 14, 110*, 111*

A, lower third; M, middle third; C, upper third.
*Resection or non-resection of these nodes does not affect the D number.
†These nodes should be excised if the primary tumour site is the MC. If the primary tumour site is MA or M, removal is optional.
‡In proximal gastrectomy, non-resection of these nodes does not affect the D number.

Table 7.3 • Lymph node grouping in the 13th edition of the Japanese classification

	LMU/MUL MLU/UML	LD/L	LM/M/ML	MU/UM	U	+E
No. 1	1	2	1	1	1	
No. 2	1	M	3	1	1	
No. 3	1	1	1	1	1	
No. 4sa	1	M	3	1	1	
No. 4sb	1	3	1	1	1	
No. 4d	1	1	1	1	2	
No. 5	1	1	1	1	3	
No. 6	1	1	1	1	3	
No. 7	2	2	2	2	2	
No. 8a	2	2	2	2	2	
No. 8b	3	3	3	3	3	
No. 9	2	2	2	2	2	
No. 10	2	M	3	2	2	
No. 11p	2	2	2	2	2	
No. 11d	2	M	3	2	2	
No. 12a	2	2	2	2	3	
No. 12bp	3	3	3	3	3	
No. 13	3	3	3	M	M	
No. 14v	2	2	3	3	M	
No. 14a	M	M	M	M	M	
No. 15	M	M	M	M	M	
No. 16a1	M	M	M	M	M	
No. 16a2, b1	3	3	3	3	3	
No. 16b2	M	M	M	M	M	
No. 17	M	M	M	M	M	
No. 18	M	M	M	M	M	
No. 19	3	M	M	3	3	2
No. 20	3	M	M	3	3	1
No. 110	M	M	M	M	M	3
No. 111	M	M	M	M	M	3
No. 112	M	M	M	M	M	3

Tumour location: L, lower third, M, middle third; U, upper third; +E, oesophageal invasion. Lymph node category: 'M', distant metastasis.

Outside Japan, it is widely believed that Japanese N1 nodes are perigastric and N2 nodes are those along the coeliac artery and its branches. Although this expression roughly reflects the nodal groups, it is apparently incorrect in terms of the original concept of grouping based on the primary tumour location. The misunderstanding seems to be due to the over-complicated definitions of the JCGC. In the latest 14th edition (third English edition[39]), the traditional nodal grouping system has been abandoned, and the simplified 'D' has been defined according to the type of gastrectomy (**Fig. 7.4**).

New definition of lymphadenectomy

The new 'D' definitions in the Japanese Treatment Guidelines[32] are simple, practical and mostly compatible with those in the 13th edition, with only

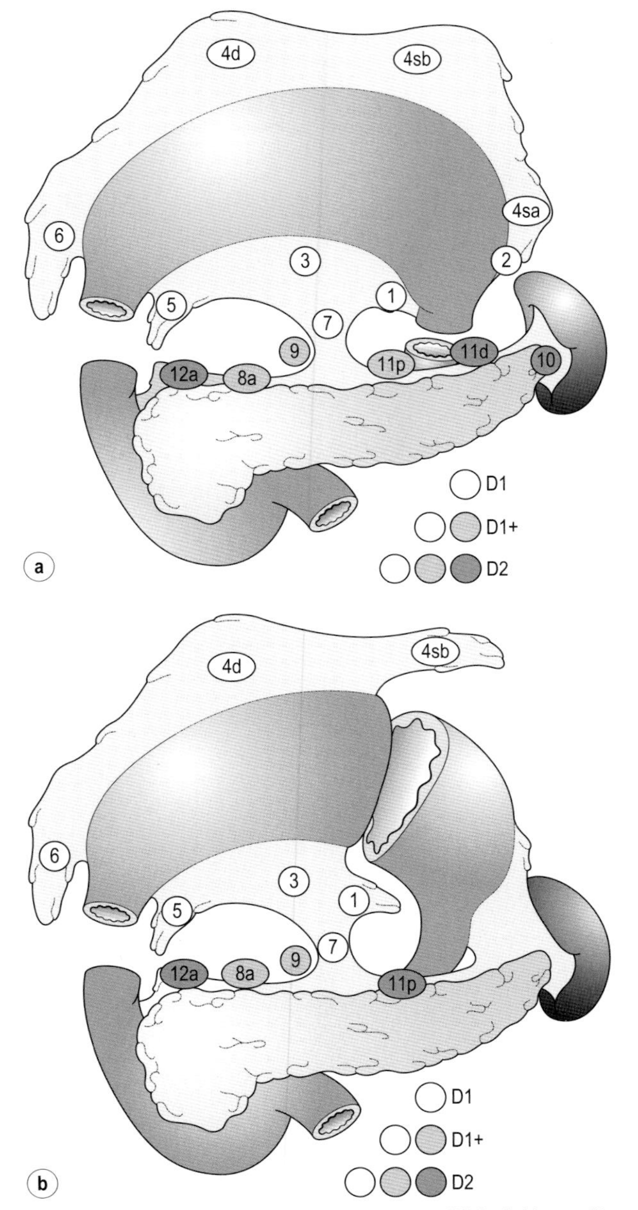

Figure 7.4 • (a) Definitions of lymphadenectomy (D) in total gastrectomy. **(b)** Definitions of lymphadenectomy (D) in distal gastrectomy. Modified from Japanese gastric cancer treatment guidelines 2010 (ver. 3).[32]

some exceptions. D1, D1+ and D2 (D3 is no longer included) are defined for the two major types of gastrectomy, total and distal, regardless of the tumour location. It should be noted that the lymph nodes along the left gastric artery (no. 7), which used to be classified as N2 for tumours in any location, are now included in the D1 category for any type of gastrectomy. This is based not only on the previously mentioned efficacy index analysis, but also on the view that surgery for gastric carcinoma should as a minimum include the division of the left gastric artery at its origin.

✔ The JGCA recommends that non-early, potentially curable gastric cancer should be treated by D2 lymphadenectomy. D1 or D1+ should be considered as an option for T1 tumours. In a poor-risk patient or under circumstances where D2 cannot be safely performed, D1+ can be a substitute for D2.

D2 lymphadenectomy – evidence

D2 lymphadenectomy is the gold standard for potentially curable advanced gastric cancer in Japan and Korea, while general surgeons in the West have been reluctant to adopt this radical approach.

In Japan, the benefits of D2 over less extensive dissections have never been tested in a randomised study. Instead, D2 was compared with more extensive surgery, D2 plus para-aortic nodal dissection (PAND), in a well-designed, multicentre randomised controlled trial (RCT).[24] This confirmed that D2 and D2+PAND were performed with low operative mortality (0.8%) by specialist surgeons,[40] but failed to show a survival benefit of PAND. They have abandoned this super-extended lymphadenectomy as a means of prophylaxis, but they still never consider that D2 may not be superior to D1. A single institutional RCT in Taipei showed a significant survival benefit of D2/3 over D1,[35] and this is so far the only RCT that showed superiority of extended lymphadenectomy for gastric cancer.

✔✔ In the West, where D0/D1 was the standard, D2 was tested as an experimental treatment in two large RCTs.[1,23] In both trials, D2 was associated with higher morbidity and mortality than D1, and no significant survival benefit of D2 was shown.

In these trials, total gastrectomy in the D2 arm was performed with pancreatosplenectomy, which caused high morbidity and mortality. Despite these negative results for D2, the Dutch group continued the follow-up of the patients for 15 years and finally published remarkable results.[12] They compared the recurrence of gastric cancer in both arms on the basis of autopsy findings and found a significantly lower rate of gastric cancer death in D2 than in D1 patients. They concluded the study by stating that D2 should be performed as potentially curative surgery for gastric cancer.

✔ There are several non-randomised observational studies in Europe that suggest benefits of extended lymphadenectomy, and today the guidelines officially recommend D2 lymphadenectomy without splenectomy by experienced surgeons.[28]

Number of lymph nodes and extent of lymphadenectomy

In the Western literature, the definition of extent of lymphadenectomy for gastric cancer is often ambiguous. The number of retrieved lymph nodes is sometimes used as a surrogate for 'D', e.g. extended lymphadenectomy means retrieval of 25 or more nodes.[41] This is a useful method to retrospectively assess the volume of lymphadenectomy in a gastrectomy where anatomical information of dissected lymph nodes is unavailable.

Generally the more extensive the surgery is, the more lymph nodes are retrieved. However, the number of retrieved nodes in a gastrectomy specimen is influenced by other factors as well:

1. **Who picked up the nodes from which condition of the specimen for what goal.** More nodes are retrieved when a surgeon tries to pick up as many nodes as possible in a fresh specimen than when a pathologist picks up swollen nodes from a formalin-fixed specimen up to the minimal requirement number.
2. **Disease stage.** In advanced disease with multiple lymph node metastases, the nodes are hard and easily recognised, even if they are small.
3. **Patient factor.** In obese patients, the lymph nodes are not easily recognised.

✔ Thus, it should be kept in mind that the number of retrieved lymph nodes is a combination of the surgery and pathological handling, and does not necessarily reflect the extent of lymphadenectomy. Surgeons should plan and perform lymphadenectomy according to anatomical extent rather than to fulfil an aim of removing 25 or more nodes.

Bursectomy

Bursectomy is the complete removal of the lesser sac (omental bursa) that consists of the lesser/greater omenta, the anterior sheet of the transverse mesocolon and the pancreatic sheath. It is performed in potentially curative gastrectomy for T4a tumours penetrating the serosa of the posterior gastric body with the aim of removing possible cancer seeding inside the bursa.

Its impact on survival is yet to be established, but it does increase morbidity related to pancreatic fistula, and it is no longer a standard procedure even in Japan. A small RCT suggested its survival benefits[42] and a new RCT recruiting 1000 patients is active in Japan.

Splenectomy

Embryologically the spleen and the body of the pancreas arise in the dorsal mesentery of the foregut, sharing the vessels and lymphatics with the stomach, and in gastric cancer surgery these two may be removed together with the stomach as a total mesogastric excision. Indeed, a total gastrectomy with distal pancreatectomy and splenectomy (DP+S) enables complete en bloc resection without touching or incising the tumour of the stomach.

On the other hand, all clinical studies have shown that splenectomy or DP+S significantly increases operative morbidity and in the West, mortality, without obvious survival benefit.[43–45] Today splenectomy or DP+S for gastric cancer is avoided in most countries. However, this needs some consideration.

Proximal gastric cancer may metastasise to the splenic hilar nodes (no. 10) via the gastrosplenic ligament (no. 4sa) and/or the left gastroepiploic lymphatics (no. 4sb). The incidence of no. 10 metastasis increases up to 25–30% when the tumour invades the greater curvature of the upper gastric body.[38] These can be completely cleared by splenectomy, and up to 25% of the patients having positive no. 10 nodes survive more than 5 years. Total gastrectomy with splenectomy can be performed by specialist surgeons without increasing mortality.[40] In this situation the author advocates gastrectomy with splenectomy.

Although a number of observational studies have demonstrated a lack of survival benefit or even a negative prognostic effect of splenectomy,[43,44] these are all heavily biased, retrospective comparisons and cannot advocate spleen preservation. Medium-sized RCTs were conducted in Chile[46] (*N*=187) and Korea[47] (*N*=207) to compare total gastrectomy (TG) and TG+splenectomy (TGS). In both studies, TGS did not increase operative mortality by experienced surgeons, and although the 5-year survival rate of TGS was higher than that of TG, the difference was not statistically significant. They concluded that splenectomy was not justified. These are negative studies, but are still unconvincing.

In a multicentre RCT conducted in Japan,[48] 503 patients with proximal gastric cancer were randomised to receive TG or TGS during a curative operation, and are currently being followed up until the final survival analysis with complete 5-year results, which is scheduled in 2014. The TGS showed higher operative morbidity (23.6%) than TG (16.7%), but similar mortality (0.4% vs. 0.8%).[49]

In the meantime, the JGCA treatment guidelines recommend splenectomy in a curative total gastrectomy for a T2–T4 tumour invading the greater curvature.[32]

A spleen-preserving no. 10 dissection is feasible in thin patients. It is, however, technically demanding, and thorough anatomical knowledge of the splenic vessels is essential.

Distal pancreatectomy

Distal pancreatectomy and splenectomy (DP+S) used to be a part of D2 gastrectomy for proximal gastric cancer regardless of the presence or absence of pancreatic invasion of the tumour, and actually was performed in the Dutch and British D1/D2 trials.[1,23] The aim of the routine use of this aggressive procedure was complete dissection of the lymph nodes along the splenic artery (nos. 11p and 11d) and those in the splenic hilum (no. 10).

However, DP+S is associated with high operative morbidity including pancreatic leakage and abscess formation, even in specialist Japanese centres.[50] Since the technique of complete dissection of no. 11 nodes without pancreatectomy has been established,[51] DP+S is currently indicated only for tumours directly invading the pancreas.

It is of note that pathological assessment in apparent T4b cases shows that the adhesion to the other organ is often inflammatory rather than neoplastic.[13] In order to avoid unnecessary DP+S in ambiguous cases, it may be worthwhile surgically separating the adhesion without DP+S, paying special attention not to injure the pancreatic parenchyma.

Extended resections

The goal of surgery for potentially curable gastric cancer is to achieve R0 resection by standard gastrectomy with sufficient resection margin and adequate lymphadenectomy. Some tumours may exceed this range but still be resectable. In such cases, extended resection should be considered.

En bloc resection of involved adjacent organs

Proximal gastric cancer may invade the distal pancreas, necessitating pancreatosplenectomy as discussed above. Middle to distal third gastric cancer may invade and penetrate the transverse mesocolon. When the invasion involves major colic vessels then partial colectomy may be necessary for en bloc resection.

When a distal tumour invades the pancreatic head or extends to the duodenum for a long distance intramurally, a pancreatoduodenectomy may enable en bloc tumour resection. However, this operation is rarely indicated because such tumours are frequently associated with other non-curative factors such as peritoneal disease. Although some case series from high-volume centres suggest survival benefit in R0 resection, the selection criteria are difficult to define.[52]

Tumours penetrating the anterior wall of the stomach may invade the lateral segment of the liver, and can usually be removed by partial liver excision without segmentectomy.

Extended lymphadenectomy

✔✔ The role of extended lymphadenectomy exceeding D2 is ambiguous. Prophylactic para-aortic nodal dissection did not improve the survival of standard D2 in a large-scale Japanese RCT[24] and has been abandoned in Japan.

An Italian group of surgeons are still performing this surgery, aimed at improving the prognosis of patients.[53]

The retropancreatic lymph nodes (no. 13) are not regional nodes of gastric cancer and the prognosis of patients with positive no. 13 nodes is extremely poor. However, for distal tumours invading the duodenum, no. 13 nodes are considered as regional nodes according to the TNM rules, and indeed some patients with a pyloric cancer invading the duodenum survive after dissection of positive no. 13 nodes.[54]

Resection of liver metastases

Unlike for colorectal cancer, liver resection for gastric cancer is rarely indicated. In the literature, only some case series from Japanese high-volume centres suggest possible survival benefit in selected cases.[55,56] In Koga et al.'s study,[56] for example, of 5520 patients who underwent gastric cancer surgery during a 20-year period, 121 (2.2%) had synchronous liver metastases and 126 (2.3%) developed metachronous ones, and only 42 patients underwent liver resection, of whom eight had survived more than 5 years at the time of analysis. In these reports, the authors' proposals for selection criteria of liver resection are not consistent. They mostly agree that liver resection should be considered for solitary liver tumours without other non-curative factors.

Summary

Radical surgery for gastric cancer consists of a gastric resection with adequate margins and systematic lymphadenectomy. Total gastrectomy 'de principe' should be abandoned. The Japanese Association has totally renovated and simplified the definition of D2, which has the potential to be the world standard. More extended surgery including combined resections of the involved organs shows no evidence of improving survival, but may become necessary for R0 resection on an individual case basis.

Technique of gastric resection with D2 lymphadenectomy

Incision

An upper midline incision is used for resection of non-cardia gastric cancer. For a bulky proximal tumour, especially in an obese patient, an inverted T-shaped or a bilateral subcostal incision is useful.

For a proximal gastric cancer invading the oesophagus, either transhiatal (TH) or left thoracoabdominal (LTA) approach is selected. LTA provides excellent exposure of the paracardiac area and lower mediastinum, but is associated with an increased morbidity. A Japanese randomised trial compared TH and LTA for Siewert type 2 and 3 gastric cancer invading the oesophagus within 3 cm and showed no survival improvement but increased morbidity in LTA approach.[57]

Intraoperative staging

The sensitivity and specificity of diagnostic imaging to stage gastric cancer is not sufficient to allow preoperative selection of optimal treatments. Surgical exploration or staging laparoscopy provides information on the T and M categories, especially on peritoneal metastasis. However, even by careful intraoperative palpation and inspection, lymph node metastasis cannot be accurately staged. Sentinel node diagnosis is not yet reliable due to the complicated lymphatic network around the stomach.

Therefore, for radical gastrectomy, a systematic lymphadenectomy should always be considered unless the tumour is diagnosed as T1.

Procedure of D2 lymphadenectomy

Distal gastrectomy

Kocherisation

Mobilisation of the duodenum facilitates a safe and smooth procedure for the subsequent infrapyloric lymphadenectomy. The assistant should hold the descending portion of the duodenum to stretch the parietal peritoneum. The peritoneum close to the duodenum should be incised and the incision extended along the duodenum. The assistant should then 'roll up' the duodenum and proceed to the back of the pancreatic head, staying close to the posterior pancreatic fascia, and mobilise the pancreatic head. The para-aortic area should be palpated and, if suspicious nodes exist, they should be sampled.

Omentectomy

Though omentectomy is not necessarily a part of D2 dissection, it is usually performed for T3/T4 tumours to remove possible tumour spread into the omenta. The omentum is removed from the right side of the transverse colon and the duodenum. It is then dissected along the transverse colon toward the lower pole of the spleen.

When omentectomy is omitted in D2 gastrectomy, the incision line of the omentum should be at least 3 cm away from the right gastroepiploic arcade so that the no. 4d lymph nodes along the arcade are completely dissected.

Division of left gastroepiploic vessels

At the lower splenic hilum and the pancreatic tail, the left gastroepiploic artery (LGEA) arises from the end of the splenic artery, sometimes as a branch of the lower polar splenic artery. The LGEA and the vein of the same name should be ligated and then cut. As the lymph nodes along the LGEA (no. 4sb) are rarely metastatic from distal gastric tumours, the dissection does not have to include the trunk of this artery. However, tumours in the gastric body, especially those located on the greater curvature, may metastasise to the splenic hilar nodes (no. 10) via no. 4sb. The LGEA should be dissected at the origin in these cases.

On the greater curve of the stomach, there is usually some avascular area between the first branch of the LGEA and the short gastric arteries, and this will be a landmark of the upper limit of dissection in distal gastrectomy.

Infrapyloric node dissection (no. 6)

In distal gastric cancers, a precise dissection of no. 6 lymph nodes is essential because they are most frequently involved and the dissection of positive nodes can still bring cure.

The (second) assistant should hold the transverse colon and gently stretch the mesocolon. The middle colic vein should be identified and pursued, to the approach of the gastrocolic venous junction point (**Fig. 7.5**). Identify the accessory right colic vein (ARCV), right gastroepiploic vein (RGEV), gastrocolic trunk and the anterior superior pancreaticoduodenal vein (ASPDV). The middle colic vein usually drains directly into the superior mesenteric vein (SMV).

The RGEV should be ligated and cut prior to its junction with the ASPDV. A small vein draining from the pancreas to the RGEV should be carefully cauterised. When no. 6 nodes are grossly metastatic, dissection of the nodes in front of the SMV (no. 14v) should be considered.

Then, the gastric antrum should be pulled up and the gastroduodenal artery (GDA) identified between the duodenum and the pancreas. The GDA is exposed distally as far as the origin of the right gastroepiploic artery (RGEA) (**Fig. 7.6**). The infrapyloric artery arises either from the GDA or from the RGEA. The RGEA and the infrapyloric artery should be ligated and cut together or separately at their origin.

The GDA should be pursued proximally to its origin from the common hepatic artery (CHA). A large, flat lymph node (no. 8a) usually covers the CHA. The peritoneum covering this node at its right edge is opened and the surface of the CHA exposed. Using this procedure, no. 5 (suprapyloric) and no. 8a nodes are separated. A gauze is placed to the right of the no. 8a node, which will serve as a landmark of the correct layer in the subsequent suprapyloric dissection.

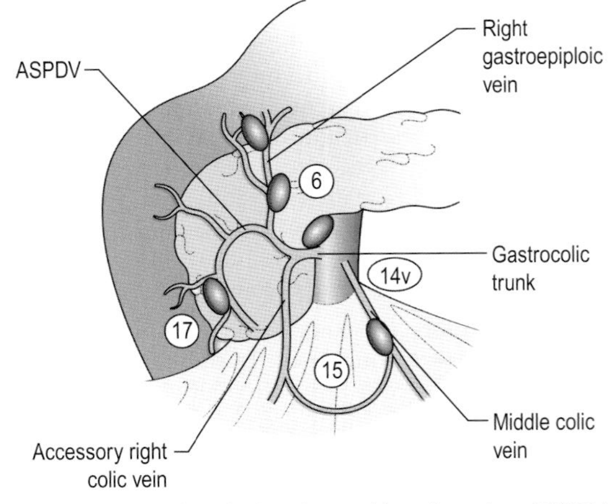

Figure 7.5 • Infrapyloric veins and lymph nodes. ASPDV, anterior superior pancreaticoduodenal vein.

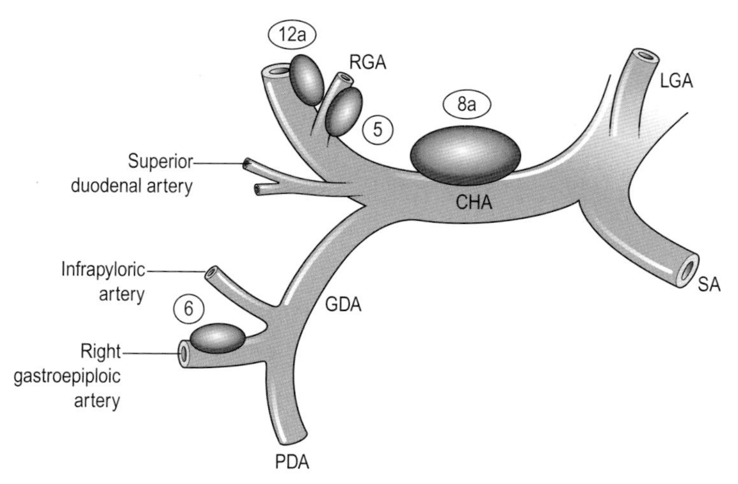

Figure 7.6 • Branches of the common hepatic artery and lymph node numbers. CHA, common hepatic artery; GDA, gastroduodenal artery; LGA, left gastric artery; PDA, pancreaticoduodenal artery; RGA, right gastric artery; SA, splenic artery.

Suprapyloric nodes dissection (no. 5) and transection of the duodenum

The assistant pulls down the pylorus and the duodenum to stretch the suprapyloric area. The right gastric artery (RGA) and the superior duodenal arteries (SDAs) are identified and the serosa between them incised. The previously placed gauze is encountered, protecting the GDA and CHA.

The SDA arising from the GDA and/or the proper hepatic artery (PHA) is cut. The origin of the RGA and the right gastric vein that runs just close to the artery and drains into the portal vein is then exposed. The RGA and vein together are ligated and cut to dissect no. 5 nodes. The anterior peritoneum of the hepatoduodenal ligament is removed to expose the PHA for subsequent no. 12a dissection.

The duodenum is transected using a linear stapler, and the staple line sutured with seromuscular stitches.

Exposure of the oesophageal hiatus

The assistant pulls down the stomach to stretch the lesser omentum. It is incised close to the liver, and the incision extended toward the right cardia. The accessory left hepatic artery is sometimes encountered and can be dissected. If it is large and replaces the proper left hepatic artery then it should be preserved. In this case, the division of the left gastric artery needs special attention, as described later.

At the upper end of the lesser omentum, the peritoneum covering the right diaphragmatic crus is excised to enter the oesophageal hiatus. The crus is exposed towards the coeliac artery, which will be helpful for later dissection around the coeliac axis.

Dissection of the upper border of the pancreas (nos. 8a, 9, 11p and 12a)

This is the core of D2 lymphadenectomy. The nerve tissue surrounding the major arteries in this area does not have to be removed in lymphadenectomy for gastric cancer because the lymphatic tissue between the nerve and the arterial adventitia is sparse and the perineural infiltration at this level is very rare.

The assistant should gently pull down the pancreas and expose the field of dissection. The peritoneal covering is incised along the upper border of the pancreas and the vascular structures (CHA, splenic artery (SpA), left gastric vein (LGV), etc.) broadly identified. The lymphadenectomy should be started at the no. 8a nodes that have already been exposed. There are small vessels between no. 8a nodes and the pancreatic parenchyma, which may require ligature or coagulation. The surface of the CHA should be exposed towards the coeliac axis until the root of the SpA appears. The LGV often drains to the splenic vein across the CHA, and is ligated and cut.

Then a change of direction is necessary and the CHA should be exposed towards the hepatoduodunal ligament. The lymph nodes are dissected along the PHA (no. 12a), exposing the left side of the portal vein.

The dissection then turns back towards the coeliac artery behind the CHA. The LGV draining to the portal vein is most frequently encountered at this point and is ligated and cut. The lymph nodes on the right side of the coeliac artery are then dissected.

The bifurcation of the coeliac artery (to the CHA and SpA) is identified, and the anterior surface of the coeliac artery is exposed until the left gastric artery (LGA) appears, surrounded by thick nerve fibres.The LGA sometimes arises very close to the aorta. The LGA is ligated (usually double) and cut at the origin. The surface of the diaphragmatic crus exposed previously is encountered, and the dissection of no. 9 lymph nodes is completed by removing lymphatic tissue in this area.

The left side of the coeliac artery is not easy to expose because, unlike the right side that can be accessed directly from the free peritoneal surface, the left side is covered by complicated fusion of the retropancreatic fascia and the parietal peritoneum.

When the accessory left hepatic artery arising from the LGA is to be preserved, the LGA should not be ligated but dissected at the origin, which exposes its trunk longitudinally until the origin of the 'proper' LGAs (usually two) appear. These are ligated and dissected to leave the arterial arcade from the coeliac artery to the left liver exposed.

The SpA originating from the coeliac artery immediately passes behind the pancreas, then reappears on the upper border of the pancreas and winds towards the spleen (**Fig. 7.7**). The left side of the coeliac artery and the proximal part of the SpA are dissected. In distal gastrectomy for distal tumours, dissection around the proximal 4–5 cm of the artery is sufficient. Note that there are lymphatic channels from the infrapyloric no. 6 area to the splenic artery nodes crossing the surface of the pancreas, and the no. 11p nodes often have metastases from pyloric tumors (Fig. 7.1).

Dissection of the upper lesser curvature nodes (nos. 1 and 3a)

The lymph nodes along the lesser curve (no. 3) are most frequently involved with tumours of the gastric body, and therefore complete removal is essential. The assistant should pull down the stomach. The lesser omental surface is lifted and incised close to the gastric wall, and then peeled away towards the cardia. The anterior trunk of the vagal nerve is cut and the left cardia nodes (no. 1) dissected. The posterior vagal trunk is then cut and the stomach reflected. Complete the no. 1 and 3 dissection by removing the lymphatics on the posterior aspect of the cardia.

Total gastrectomy

Most aspects of D2 lymphadenectomy in total gastrectomy are common to those in distal gastrectomy. Additional procedures are as follows.

Dissection of the upper greater curvature nodes (nos. 2 and 4sa)

Following the division of the LGEA at its origin, the upper stomach is raised to inspect the splenic hilum from inside the lesser sac. The wall of the left bottom of the lesser sac is the dorsal gastric mesentery, which connects the upper greater curve of the stomach, the spleen, and the pancreatic body and tail. The gastrosplenic ligament is part of the dorsal mesentery.

The winding SpA and its terminal branches are broadly identified. The gastrosplenic ligament should be held and kept tense. The ligament is dissected close to the spleen, dividing the short gastric vessels towards the superior pole of the spleen. The peritoneal fusion at the back of the gastric fundus is then incised and the upper stomach mobilised from the abdominal wall.

The left paracardiac area has arterial supply from either the oesophagocardiac branch of the left subphrenic artery or the left cardiac branch of the LGA.

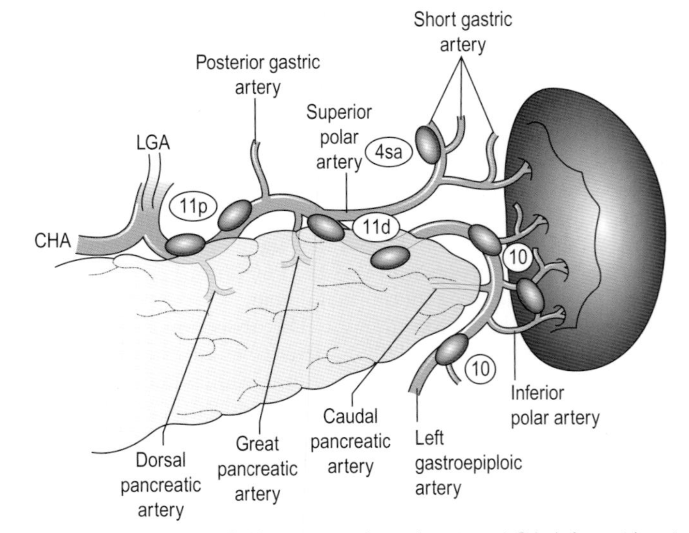

Figure 7.7 • Splenic artery and its branches. CHA, common hepatic artery; LGA, left gastric artery.

Lymphatic flow from this area can directly reach the left para-aortic network.

Dissection along the distal splenic artery (no. 11d) and splenic hilum (no. 10)

Following the 11p dissection, the procedure is continued along the SpA towards the spleen. The winding SpA gives off several branches to both the pancreas and the stomach (Fig. 7.7). The great pancreatic artery, though not so large as its name suggests, is an important blood supply to the pancreatic tail. The caudal pancreatic artery arises near the splenic hilum. These pancreatic branches are preserved.

The remaining dorsal mesentery connects the posterior aspect of the upper stomach and the splenic artery and vein, and includes the posterior gastric artery and vein. This artery usually arises in the middle of the SpA and nourishes the dorsal part of the cardia. It should be ligated and cut at the root. Cancers in the upper stomach, especially those located on the posterior wall, frequently metastasise to the SpA nodes through the lymphatic channels in this mesentery.

The dissection is sometimes dangerous owing to kinking of the artery. Appropriate traction by the second assistant is particularly helpful.

Splenectomy

Splenectomy is required when the tumour invades the tail of the pancreas and/or splenic hilum without other non-curative factors. It may also be indicated for complete dissection of no. 10 lymph nodes in tumours invading the greater curvature of the proximal stomach.

Mobilisation of the pancreas and spleen is started at the lower border of the pancreas. The bottom of the anterior sheet of the mesocolon is incised close to the pancreas. Several vessels arising from the pancreas to the anterior mesocolon (posterior epiploic arteries) should be cut.

The pancreatic body is lifted and entered behind the pancreas, leaving the retropancreatic fusion fascia to the retroperitoneal space. This is continued towards the spleen until the pancreatic tail is lifted. If the proper layer is entered, no vessels are encountered in this procedure.

The assistant should pull down the left kidney. The pancreatic tail is pulled up with the lower pole of the spleen. Then the parietal peritoneum behind the spleen can be visualised from its medial aspect. It is then incised and the spleen mobilised. This incision is continued towards the cardia, mobilising the whole dorsal mesentery from Gerota's fascia covering the kidney and left adrenal gland.

When the pancreas and spleen have been totally mobilised, the surgeon moves to the left side of the patient to continue the procedure.

The assistant should hold the reversed spleen. Holding the tail of the pancreas in the left hand, the lymph nodes are dissected along the distal SpA. The SpA is double ligated and cut, then the vein, and the spleen removed from the pancreas.

When the pancreas is also removed for tumour invasion, the SpA is ligated and dissected as close to the root as possible. Then the vein is ligated and cut close to the resection line, and the pancreas transected.

Summary

✔ D2 lymphadenectomy is a systematic, standardised, technically demanding procedure that necessitates thorough knowledge of the anatomy of major gastric arteries and veins.

Modified surgery for early gastric cancer

Lymph node metastasis from early gastric cancer

In undertaking D2 lymphadenectomy, almost all regional lymph nodes that may contain metastases are removed. In T1 tumours (early gastric cancer, EGC), lymph node metastasis is infrequent (about 10%) and mostly limited to the perigastric nodes.

✔ Therefore, when the clinical diagnosis of EGC is reliable, D2 lymphadenectomy is not necessary, and the extent of gastric resection can also be reduced.

There is a clear correlation between the depth of tumour invasion and the incidence of lymph node metastasis in gastric cancer. This is true between any two adjacent T categories, and even in the same T1 category, mucosal (T1a) and submucosal (T1b) tumours show clearly different chances of metastasis. However, the reported incidence of lymph node metastasis from pT1 tumours has not been consistent.[5,58] This is probably due to differences in the pathological process. In Japan the sectioning method of gastric cancer has been standardised by the Japanese Classification of Gastric Carcinomas,[39] and all lesions in the surgically resected specimens are sectioned at 5-mm intervals. With sectioning at wider intervals, or with only one or two central sectioning, the deepest invasion of a lesion can be overlooked and the T category would be under-staged. Then a group of tumours diagnosed as T1a may include some deeper ones having a greater chance of lymph node metastasis and the 'incidence of lymph node metastasis from T1a' will be reported as higher. With sectioning at smaller intervals, deeper invasion may be detected in a tumour and a diagnosis of deeper T category is given, resulting in a lower incidence of metastasis in more strictly staged T1a tumours.

On the other hand, lymph node retrieval and the sectioning method of the nodes will also change the results. By meticulous retrieval and multiple sectioning, the chance of detection of metastasis increases (by 20% according to one report[59]) and the incidence of metastasis in T1 tumours is reported as higher.

Considering these possibilities, the incidence of lymph node metastasis is broadly estimated to be 3% and 20% from T1a and T1b tumours respectively. It should be noted that once the tumour invades the proper muscle layer, the incidence increases up to 50%.[38]

Limited lymphadenectomy

The Japanese treatment guidelines define D1 and D1+ lymphadenectomy for tumours clinically diagnosed as T1. Since most metastasis from T1 is limited to the perigastric nodes and no. 7 and 8a nodes, D1 is sufficient to remove all possibly positive nodes. The problem is that the preoperative diagnosis of T1 is not always accurate: even for endoscopists who have diagnosed more than 100 ECGs, more than 10% of tumours they diagnose as T1 are pathologically T2 or deeper.[60] Surgeons should always bear this in mind and be ready to perform D2 whenever deeper invasion is suspected during surgery.

Pylorus-preserving gastrectomy (PPG) (**Fig. 7.8**)

PPG was originally developed as surgery for peptic ulcer disease,[61] but due to its excellent functional results it is currently applied for selected cases of EGC. A short cuff (usually 3 cm) of the pyloric antrum is preserved together with the pyloric branch of the anterior vagal nerve and the infrapyloric artery. The upper gastric remnant should be large enough to function as a reservoir. For these restrictions, the dissection of no. 1 and 5 nodes is incomplete compared to standard distal gastrectomy. Therefore, PPG is indicated for middle gastric tumours that have very low possibility of metastasis to these nodes, i.e. clinical T1N0 in the middle portion of the stomach with the distal tumour border at least 4 cm proximal to the pylorus.

The quality of life after PPG is superior to that after distal gastrectomy. Low incidence of early and late dumping syndromes, low incidence of iron-deficiency anaemia and less body weight loss are reported.[62,63] These are attributable to less rapid gastric emptying and prolonged acid contact of dietary iron. On the other hand, some patients suffer from early satiety and reflux due to malfunction of the pylorus and/or too small gastric remnant.

With careful selection of the cases, the oncological results are excellent and not at all inferior to standard distal gastrectomy.

Local tumour resection based on sentinel lymph node diagnosis

If the sentinel lymph nodes from a small gastric cancer are accurately detected and their negativity can be confirmed, gastrectomy can be omitted and local tumour resection is sufficient for cure. However, the lymphatic network surrounding the stomach is very complex and accurate identification of the sentinel nodes is not easy. Several prospective studies have failed to detect the 'lymph nodes that first receive metastasis'.[64] At present, this strategy still remains investigational.

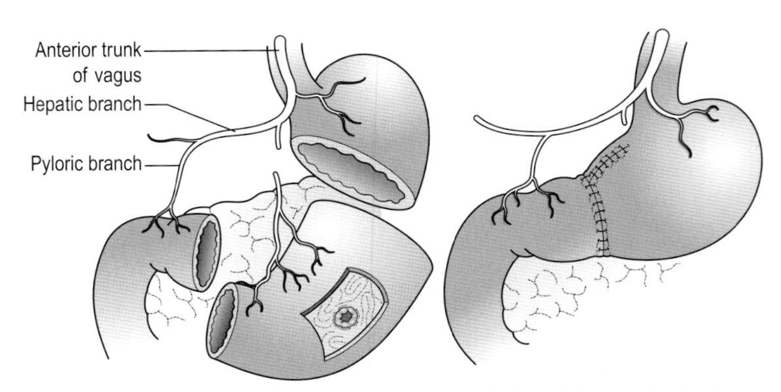

Figure 7.8 • Pylorus-preserving gastrectomy for early gastric cancer in the middle gastric body.

Summary

- ✔ Various less invasive or function-preserving surgeries have been developed for early cancers with good results. Indications for these treatments should be strictly confined to early cancers so as not to lose the chance of cure.

Reconstruction after gastric resection

A number of reconstruction methods have been proposed for gastrectomy. Each has advantages and disadvantages, and should be selected according to surgical and oncological conditions in each patient. The following points should be considered in selection:

1. **Safety of surgery.** In gastrectomy for advanced tumours (curative or palliative) or for patients having high operative risk, any procedure after removal of the tumour should be simple and safe, so as not to prolong the surgical time or increase the postoperative complications.
2. **Possible local recurrence.** In locally advanced tumours with wide serosal involvement and/or apparent nodal metastasis, gastric bed recurrence should be prepared for and a reconstruction with the least risk of obstruction should be selected.
3. **Long-term quality of life.** In gastrectomy with a high probability of cure, a reconstruction to maximise quality of life should be selected. Reflux of bile and alkaline duodenal juices into the oesophagus should be prevented. At the same time, long-term nutritional status should be considered.

Reconstruction after distal gastrectomy (Fig. 7.9)

While Roux-en-Y (R-Y) and Billroth II (B-II) reconstructions are widely used, Billroth I gastroduodenostomy (B-I) is also frequently employed in Eastern Asia.

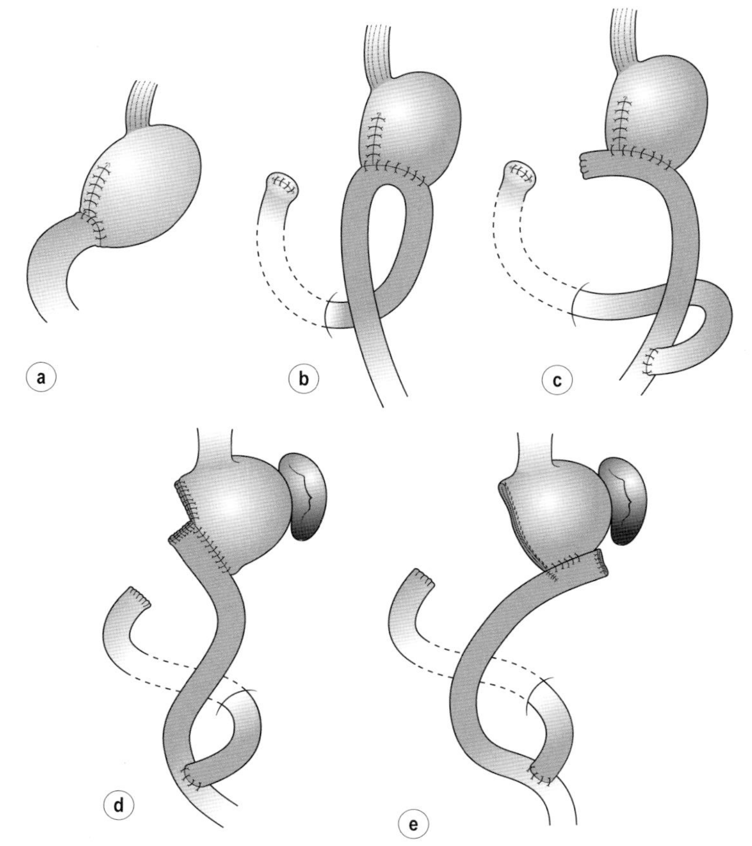

Figure 7.9 • Reconstructions after distal gastrectomy. **(a)** Billroth I. **(b)** Billroth II isoperistaltic. **(c)** Roux-en-Y. **(d)** Roux-en-Y (hand-sewing). **(e)** Roux-en-Y (stapler).

✔✔ Several RCTs and case series comparing these methods have been published with inconsistent results. A recent meta-analysis suggests that R-Y shows some clinical advantages over the other two methods.[65]

Roux-en-Y

Indication

Advantages of R-Y over B-I are absence of duodenal juice reflux, safe anastomosis with very low leak rate, and low risk of obstruction at gastric bed recurrence. Weak points include loss of easy endoscopic access to the duodenal papilla and possible nutritional problems due to non-physiological food passage, though no clear evidence has proven this. R-Y procedure involves jejunum and this may cause adhesive obstruction or internal hernia in the future. So-called 'Roux-en-Y syndrome', characterised by chronic abdominal pain and nausea that are aggravated by meals and associated with malnutrition, used to be reported mainly after ulcer surgery, but has not been observed as a serious problem lately.

R-Y reconstruction is applicable for most distal gastrectomies. The following are particularly good indications:

1. tumours involving the gastric body for which the remnant stomach after resection is small;
2. patients who suffer from reflux esophagitis before surgery;
3. patients with high operative risks for whom anastomotic leak must be prevented;
4. locally advanced disease with high risk of gastric bed recurrence.

In special patients with biliary tract problems or duodenal pathological conditions that require endoscopic access or follow-up, B-I reconstruction might be considered.

Procedure

The duodenum is transected using a linear-type stapler and many surgeons add covering seromuscular stitches. The jejunum 20–30 cm distal to the Treiz ligament is divided and the jejunal limb is pulled up either via the ante- or retrocolic route. In T4a/T4b tumours that have a significant risk of local recurrence involving the mesocolon, the antecolic route is preferred. Gastrojejunostomy is achieved either by stapler or hand-sewing; different anastomotic sites and jejunal directions are selected accordingly (Fig. 7.9d,e). The jejunojejunostomy is made 40 cm distal to the gastrojejunostomy. The mesentery holes are closed to prevent internal hernia.

When the retrocolic route is selected, the gastrojejunostomy site should be pulled down below the mesocolon and be fixed to it to prevent torsion or obstruction of the jejunal limb in the narrow space above the mesocolon.

Billroth I

Indication and procedure

Advantages of B-I over R-Y are physiological food passage, simple anastomosis without jejunal manipulation, and preserved endoscopic access to the duodenal papilla. B-I is useful for distal tumours at an early stage for which a relatively large proximal stomach can be preserved and recurrence is not thought likely. Weak points of B-I are duodenal juice reflux, possible anastomotic leak and possible obstruction at recurrence. Thus, B-I should be avoided in cases with high operative risks, small remnant stomach, preoperative presence of oesophageal reflux or locally advanced disease.

Gastroduodenostomy is made either by hand-sewing or using a circular stapler. When the anastomotic tension is high, Kocher's mobilisation of the duodenum is useful to reduce it.

Reconstruction after total gastrectomy (Fig. 7.10)

R-Y is the standard reconstruction after total gastrectomy. It is simple, safe and gives relatively good functional results. Weak points are early satiety due to lack of reservoir and consequent long-term malnutrition. Careful dietetic surveillance and education is essential.

Roux-en-Y

Indication

There is virtually no contraindication for R-Y. In rare cases where endoscopic access to the duodenum needs to be maintained for biliary tract problems, a jejunoduodenostomy is added at about 30–40 cm from oesophagojejunostomy (double-tract R-Y, Fig. 7.10b).

Procedure

The jejunum is transected 20–30 cm from the Treiz ligament. Either the ante- or retrocolic route is selected according to the criteria mentioned in the section on distal gastrectomy. The retrocolic pathway provides the shortest route and the least tension on the limb mesentery, especially in obese patients with a large omental residue.

Jejunal vessels are carefully prepared so that the mesentery tension is reduced, preserving the blood supply to the anastomotic site.

Oesophagojejunostomy is undertaken using a circular stapler. A 25-mm anvil is applicable in most

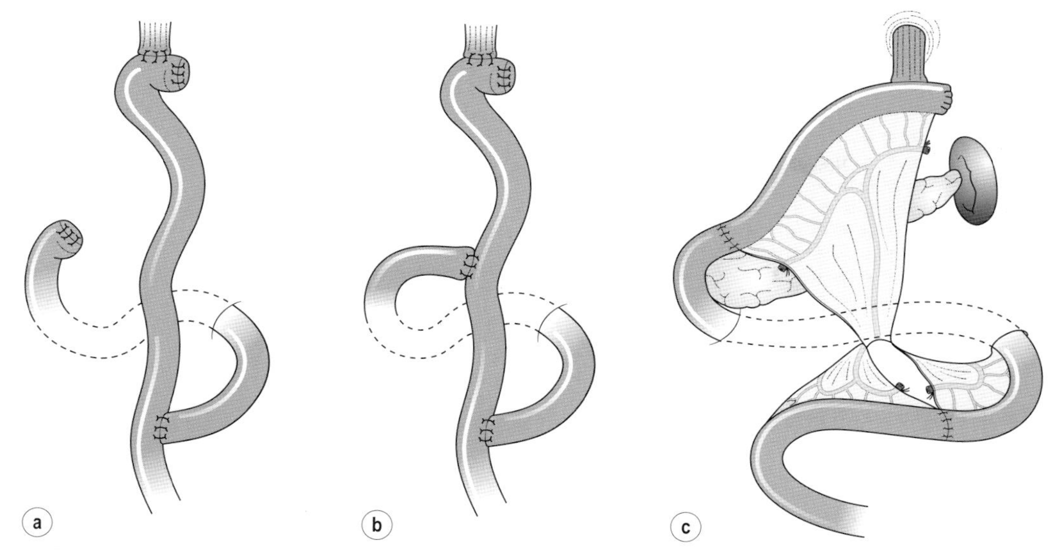

Figure 7.10 • Reconstructions after total gastrectomy. **(a)** Roux-en-Y. **(b)** Double tract Roux-en-Y. **(c)** Jejunal interposition.

cases. A larger size can be selected in patients with large oesophagus and jejunum.

Jejunojejunostomy is performed 40–50 cm below the oesophageal anastomosis. A shorter limb may cause reflux and a longer one may be disadvantageous from a nutritional viewpoint. In the double tract method, jejunojejunostomy is made 20 cm distal to the jejunoduodenostomy.

Jejunal interposition

This method is employed to maintain the physiological food passage to the duodenum.

> ✔ However, there is no solid evidence that this reconstruction has long-term nutritional advantage over standard R-Y.

The length of the interposed jejunum can be shorter (20–30 cm) than the jejunal limb in R-Y, probably because the jejunal juice can flow down the natural route without reflux.

Pouch formation

Various operations were devised to increase the reservoir capacity of the jejunum, with inconsistent results: some patients eat remarkably well but some others suffer from severe stasis or regurgitation.

Pouch formation does not significantly increase morbidity or extend the operation time, while patients with pouch have better food intake and improved quality of life. The technique is expected to be standardised in the near future.

> ✔✔ The pouch technique has been improved, and a recent meta-analysis of 13 RCTs comparing R-Y or jejunal interposition with and without pouch showed some clinical advantages for a pouch reconstruction.[66]

Reconstruction after proximal gastrectomy (Fig. 7.11)

Jejunal interposition

Indication

The original method was described by Merendino and Dillard in 1955 for reflux disease.[67] The interposed isoperistaltic jejunum prevents gastric juice reflux to the oesophagus, and strangely anastomotic ulcers do not appear. This reconstruction method is applicable to proximal gastrectomy for small tumours of the oesophagogastric junction in which resection of the oesophagus and stomach can be minimal. Note that even a short segment of the interposed jejunum could cause early dumping syndrome due to rapid food inflow.

Procedure

A short segment jejunum (10–15 cm) is used and anastomosed to the anterior wall[68] (Fig. 7.11). Pyloroplasty is usually made. It is not necessary when the anterior trunk and the hepatic branch of the vagal nerve are preserved.

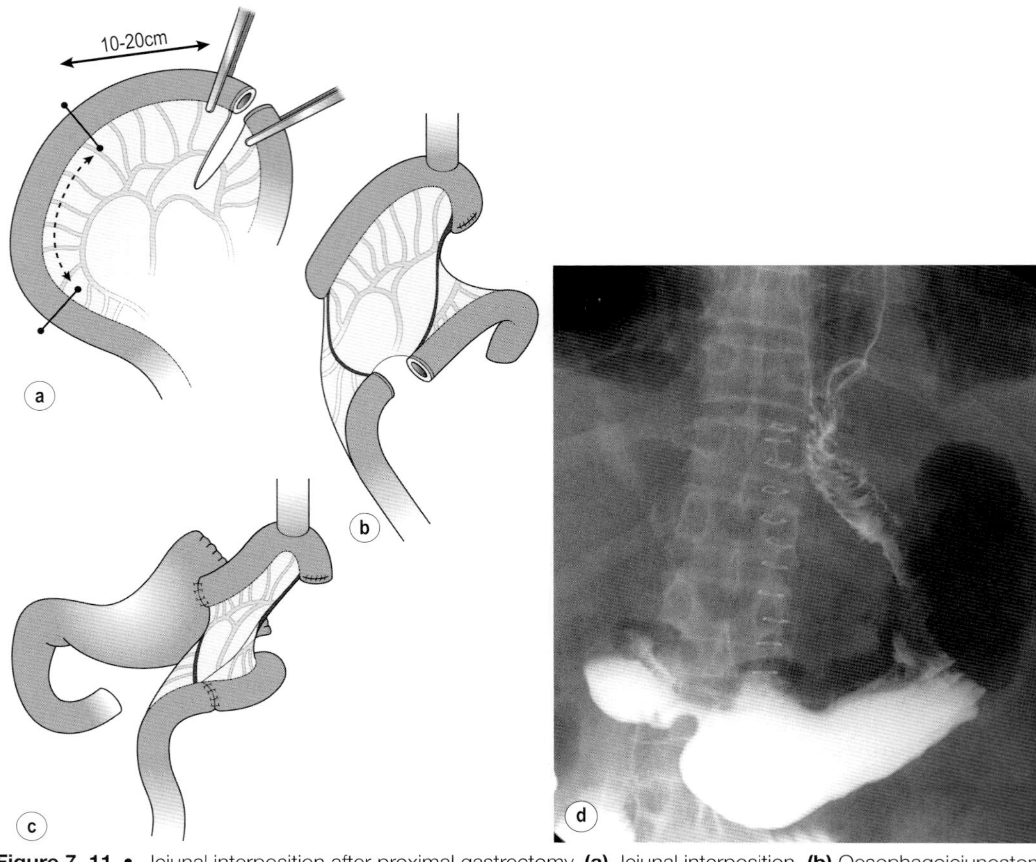

Figure 7. 11 • Jejunal interposition after proximal gastrectomy. **(a)** Jejunal interposition. **(b)** Oesophagojejunostomy. **(c)** Jejunogastrostomy. **(d)** Post operative Gastrografin swallow. Modified from Katai H, Sano T, Fukagawa T et al. Prospective study of proximal gastrectomy for early gastric cancer in the upper third of the stomach. Br J Surg 2003; 90:850–3.

Oesophagogastrostomy

Indication

Although this is a simple and safe reconstruction after proximal gastrectomy, some patients suffer from severe reflux oesophagitis and cannot quit medication. This is indicated for proximal gastrectomy in which the abdominal oesophagus is preserved. Reconstruction after lower oesophagectomy using a gastric tube is described in Chapter 5.

Procedure

Oesophagogastrostomy is performed on the anterior wall of the remnant stomach, usually using a circular stapler. A hand-sewing method is not very difficult, and the soft opening of the anastomosis instead of the fixed ring of the stapler seems to function as a protector for the reflux. Many surgeons add some extra stitches between the oesophagus and the stomach to prevent reflux.

Summary

✔ There is no single best reconstruction method after gastrectomy. Priority should be given to safety for poor risk patients, and to function for those with high possibility of cure. Roux-en-Y, following both distal and total gastrectomy, could be the first choice. Pouch formation seems to improve quality of life, and its procedure is expected to be standardised.

Early postoperative complications

Two major complications after gastrectomy for cancer are anastomotic leak and pancreatic fistula. They cause abdominal abscess, peritonitis, sepsis or massive haemorrhage. Complications are more common in total gastrectomy and extended lymphadenectomy than in distal gastrectomy and limited lymphadenectomy respectively. Most prospective studies have shown that splenectomy and distal pancreatectomy significantly increase postoperative morbidity and mortality. Close management by experienced surgeons, especially for pancreatic fistula, is essential to avoid mortality.

Use of prophylactic drains after gastrectomy is controversial. There is no evidence that drains decrease postoperative complications or death.[69] Distal gastrectomy without intraoperative problems usually needs no drains. However, in total gastrectomy or extended D2 dissection along the upper border of the distal pancreas, a suction drain along the pancreas gives useful information on pancreatic fistula or early anastomotic leak.

Anastomotic leak

Most anastomotic leaks after gastrectomy occur at the oesophagojejunostomy. Possible causes are tissue ischaemia or tension on the anastomotic line. These should be avoided by careful preparation of the jejunal loop. Correct usage of the anastomotic circular stapler is also important. Covering stiches are usually unnecessary, but should be used when the continuity of the 'doughnut' of the resected oesophagus or jejunum is incomplete.

Early anastomotic leak occurring within 72 hours would be life threatening without proper management. It may present as septic episodes or contaminated drain discharge. Contrast swallow (Gastrografin) should be done whenever a leak is suspected. Drainage is crucial to treat anastomotic leakage. When a prophylactic drain has been appropriately placed and the leak is minor without evidence of local diffusion, a conservative treatment with fasting and adequate nutrition will suffice. When there is no drain or septic signs are evident, re-operation is strongly advised. Anastomotic failure can be repaired in some early cases, or at worst a drain can be placed close to the leak site. In either case, a feeding jejunostomy should be constructed.

The management of a delayed leak is controversial. Usually drains have already been removed and meals are started. The patient may have some difficulty in swallowing and, though perhaps being afebrile, blood tests suggest continuous inflammation. When a contrast study reveals only a minor leak, fasting and adequate nutrition will be sufficient. A naso-intestinal tube placed beyond the jejunojejunostomy may be useful for enteral feeding. If the patient is septic, a drain must be placed. Contrast-enhanced computed tomography will be helpful whether the intervention is achieved surgically or radiologically. Surgery at this point is technically difficult due to severe adhesions in the upper abdomen, but should be carried out when the abdominal infection is diffuse.

Duodenal stump leak

A properly stapled duodenal stump rarely leaks. However, stump leak occurs when the duodenal tissue is damaged or becomes ischaemic. There is no evidence that covering stiches reduce leak, but some surgeons use them. Duodenal stump leak may also occur when the intraduodenal pressure increases due to afferent limb obstruction or possibly unusually strong peristalsis.

A prophylactic drain that is placed near the stump gives good information. If its discharge contains bile, it is an indication for immediate re-operation. Re-closure of the stump is usually very difficult due to tissue inflammation. If there is a major defect, a Foley-type catheter can be placed in the duodenum with a plan to form a controlled fistula. When the leak is from a pinhole on the staple line, a suction drain is placed close to it and retrograde insertion of a duodenal decompression tube from the jejunum should be considered. Feeding jejunostomy is useful not only for nutrition but also for returning the suctioned duodenal content to the intestine. With good duodenal decompression, enteral feeding does not have to be stopped or reduced.

Pancreatic fistula

After D2 lymphadenectomy, pancreatic leak may occur even without pancreatectomy. It is more common when the pancreatic capsule has been removed as a part of bursectomy or the pancreas has been mobilised for splenectomy. Placement of a prophylactic suction drain along the upper border of the pancreas is recommended in these operations. Increased amylase content in the drain fluid on the first or second postoperative day is a useful marker to predict later development of pancreatic fistula. The fluid containing high amylase usually takes on a dark red (wine) colour. Suction drainage is also useful to prevent diffusion of pancreatic fluid and localise the fistula.

When the tail of the pancreas is resected, pancreatic leak is more common and drain placement is strongly recommended. A suction tube should be placed close to the stump via the shortest percutaneous route.

It is controversial as to whether the use of somatostatin analogues prevents pancreatic fistula. RCTs for pancreatic surgery showed inconsistent results, and meta-analyses did not support a positive effect.[70] No RCT has been conducted on this subject in gastrectomy.

When pancreatic leak occurs, the management should concentrate on prevention of infection and abscess control. Adequate drainage is essential and radiological intervention should be considered. Abscess drainage takes time and may require frequent adjustments of the drain tip. When the abscess is localised and surrounded by a solid wall, saline irrigation of the cavity will enhance healing.

Haemorrhage

Haemorrhage within the first few hours of surgery should be treated by early re-laparotomy. It must be remembered that drains can occlude with blood clot and the clinical suspicion of bleeding in a haemodynamically unstable patient is a sufficient indication to operate.

Secondary haemorrhage caused by intra-abdominal infection following anastomotic leak and/or pancreatic fistula is truly life threatening. A poorly drained abscess causes pseudo-aneurysm of a major artery (most frequently the splenic artery)and then causes massive haemorrhage. In the stage of pseudo-aneurysm, a small amount of bleeding may precede massive haemorrhage, which must not be overlooked. Immediate radiological intervention may detect an unruptured pseudo-aneurysm that can be embolised. Once massive bleeding occurs, immediate angiography again should first be considered because it not only provides the chance of embolisation but can also identify the bleeding point. In immediate re-laparotomy, the bleeding artery is sometimes difficult to identify or reach due to severe adhesion and/or inflammation.

Postsplenectomy infections

There is increasing evidence that splenectomy predisposes the patient to an increased risk of bacterial infections in both the early postoperative period and probably for the remainder of their life. Immediate prophylaxis with twice daily oral penicillin is now recommended for patients of all ages. The patient should also be immunised with vaccines against pneumococci, meningococcus and *Haemophilus influenzae*. If the splenectomy has been planned as part of a radical procedure these vaccines are most effective if administered preoperatively. The patient should have an annual influenza vaccine and an updated pneumococcal vaccine about every 3 years.

Late sequelae and complications

Side-effects and postprandial sequelae

No gastrectomised patient can eat in the same way he or she used to eat, at least during the first few postoperative months. Good dietary advice is essential and patients should understand what their stomach used to do and how they can cope with their status without part or all of their stomach. The author usually explains this as follows: 'The stomach has three major functions:(1) it stores the food that has been swallowed; (2) it digests and dilutes it; and (3) it slowly pushes it out to the duodenum (taking many hours after a greasy meal). These functions help the small bowel to effectively absorb nutrients. When the stomach has been removed, it is necessary to change eating habits to help the small intestine to work as before: chew well, take time to have the next bite, and have frequent small meals.'

Patients should also be able to accept that their stomach will never come back, and that the lost stomach functions are compensated not by medicine but by an appropriate eating style. Additional specific advice from a dietician will help further.

Early dumping syndrome

Early dumping syndrome appears within 30 minutes after a meal, or even during a meal. The rapid filling of the proximal small intestine with hypertonic food leads to rapid movement of fluid from the extracellular fluid compartment into the gut, and also triggers a complex neurohumoral response. This produces various gastrointestinal and cardiovascular symptoms such as palpitation, bloating, cramping, diarrheoa and nausea, requiring some patients to lie down for an hour after each meal. Most patients with early dumping syndrome can be treated by appropriate dietary adaptation. In severe cases, however, quality of life is restricted and malnutrition can occur rapidly. Careful management involving an experienced dietician should be considered.

Late dumping syndrome or reactive hypoglycaemic attacks

Late dumping syndrome appears 2–3 hours after a meal, and is characterised by faintness, severe hunger, dizziness and cold sweating, which are symptoms of hypoglycaemia. Rapid inflow of carbohydrate to the jejunum causes oxyhyperglycaemia, which induces hyperinsulinemia followed by hypoglycemia. Glucagon-like peptide-1 (GLP-1) secreted from the proximal jejunal mucosa is thought to play some role in this hypersecretion of insulin.

Dietary adaptation is again the main treatment for late dumping syndrome. Patients are advised to decrease the carbohydrate load in their main meals and to take small amounts of carbohydrate between main meals. Those with frequent attacks should carry dextrose tablets to eat at the first sign of symptoms.

In a large-scale investigation into dumping syndrome after gastrectomy (N=1153),[71] early dumping syndrome was more commonly experienced than late dumping syndrome (68% vs. 38%) and the incidence varied according to the type of gastrectomy but not the postoperative period. Early and late dumping syndromes have different aetiologies and appear independently. During follow-up, a careful history should be taken and appropriate dietary advice should be given.

Nutritional problems

Gastrectomy may cause deficits of specific nutrients. Of the three major nutrients, fat absorption particularly decreases because mixing with duodenal contents (bile acid, pancreatic lipase) and jejunal absorption become insufficient. Patients with fat malabsorption complain of steatorrhoea, which can be treated with pancreatic enzyme supplements.

Vitamin B_{12}

Vitamin B_{12} binds to intrinsic factor secreted by the parietal cells of the stomach and is absorbed in the ileum. After total gastrectomy, patients absorb no vitamin B_{12}, and body stores are gradually depleted resulting in megaloblastic anaemia, although this may take up to 24 months to become clinically apparent. All patients after total gastrectomy should receive 1 mg of hydroxycobalamin intramuscularly every 3 months for life.

Vitamin D

Absorption of fat-soluble vitamins (A, D, E, K) may decrease in patients with fat malabsorption. Of these, vitamin D malabsorption is clinically important, particularly in postmenopausal women. Combined with decreased calcium absorption after gastrectomy, it leads to metabolic bone disorders from 2 years after surgery. It is recommended that postmenopausal women and all patients over 70 should take an oral calcium and vitamin D supplement for life after a total gastrectomy.

Iron

Iron absorption occurs predominantly in the duodenum and upper jejunum. In the presence of gastric acid, ferric iron (Fe^{3+}) in foodstuffs is deoxidised to easily absorbable ferrous iron (Fe^{2+}). Iron absorption may be reduced after gastric resection due to decreased acid and rapid food passage in the intestine. Iron-deficiency anaemia is common, and oral iron supplement is useful.

Key points

- Lymphatic spread is the most common mode of dissemination in gastric cancer.
- Among the four patterns of spread of gastric cancer (lymphatic, peritoneal, haematogenous and direct), lymphatic metastasis occurs at the earliest stage and this can lead to other types of metastases. Surgical control of this spread at an early phase of the disease may prevent later systemic failure and patients can still be cured by adequate dissection.
- Peritoneal metastasis is the most common type of failure after radical surgery for gastric cancer. Peritoneal metastasis is much more common in diffuse-type cancers than the intestinal type.
- Surgery itself can be a cause of cancer spread, especially in terms of peritoneal dissemination. Even serosa-negative tumours can recur in the peritoneal cavity after surgery. These cases are usually associated with lymph node metastasis. Adherence to the principles of good surgical cancer practice reduces the risk of spread.
- There is an increasing move towards tailoring gastric cancer operations, taking not only the stage of the disease but also patient-related factors into account.
- According to the Japanese treatment guidelines a 5-cm resection margin is recommended for tumours showing an infiltrative growth pattern with indistinct borders or diffuse-type histology, but 3 cm is usually sufficient for those showing an expansive growth pattern with grossly distinct borders, the histology of which is most frequently the intestinal type.
- Randomised trials comparing total and distal gastrectomy in distal gastric cancer failed to show any survival benefit for total gastrectomy (known as total gastrectomy de principe).
- The Japanese Gastric Cancer Association (JGCA) recommends that non-early, potentially curable gastric cancer should be treated by D2 lymphadenectomy. D1 or D1+ should be considered as an

option for T1 tumours. In a poor-risk patient or under circumstances where D2 cannot be safely performed, D1+ can be a substitute for D2.

- Although solid evidence of extended lymphadenectomy is yet to be established, D2 gastrectomy without splenectomy or pancreatectomy has been officially recommended by the European Society of Medical Oncology in 2009.
- The number of lymph nodes retrieved is a combination of the surgery and pathological handling, and does not necessarily reflect the extent of lymphadenectomy. Surgeons should plan and perform lymphadenectomy according to anatomical extent rather than to fulfil an aim of removing 25 or more nodes.
- All clinical studies have shown that splenectomy or distal pancreatectomy plus splenectomy (DP+S) significantly increases operative morbidity and in the West, mortality, without obvious survival benefit.
- The JGCA treatment guidelines recommend splenectomy in a curative total gastrectomy for a T2–T4 tumour invading the greater curvature because of the high incidence of involved nodes in the splenic hilum.
- DP+S is associated with high operative morbidity, including pancreatic leakage and abscess formation, even in specialist Japanese centres. It is currently indicated only for tumours directly invading the pancreas.
- The role of extended lymphadenectomy exceeding D2 is ambiguous. Prophylactic para-aortic nodal dissection did not improve the survival over standard D2 in a large-scale Japanese RCT and has now been abandoned in Japan.
- Several RCTs and case series comparing Billroth I, Billroth II and Roux-en-Y (R-Y) reconstruction after distal gastrectomy have been published with inconsistent results. A recent meta-analysis suggests that R-Y shows some clinical advantages over the other two methods.
- R-Y is the standard reconstruction after total gastrectomy. A recent meta-analysis of 13 RCTs comparing R-Y or jejunal interposition with and without pouch showed some clinical advantages of pouch reconstruction.
- Complications are more common in total gastrectomy and extended lymphadenectomy than in distal gastrectomy and limited lymphadenectomy respectively. Most prospective studies have shown that splenectomy and distal pancreatectomy significantly increase postoperative morbidity and mortality.

References

1. Bonenkamp JJ, Songun I, Hermans J, et al. Randomised comparison of morbidity after D1 and D2 dissection for gastric cancer in 996 Dutch patients. Lancet 1995;345(8952):745–8.
2. Dikken JL, Jansen EP, Cats A, et al. Impact of the extent of surgery and postoperative chemoradiotherapy on recurrence patterns in gastric cancer. J Clin Oncol 2010;28:2430–6.
3. Macdonald JS, Smalley SR, Benedetti J, et al. Chemoradiotherapy after surgery compared with surgery alone for adenocarcinoma of the stomach or gastroesophageal junction. N Engl J Med 2001;345:725–30.
4. Maruyama K, Gunven P, Okabayashi K, et al. Lymph node metastases of gastric cancer. General pattern in 1931 patients. Ann Surg 1989;210:596–602.
5. Gotoda T, Yanagisawa A, Sasako M, et al. Incidence of lymph node metastasis from early gastric cancer: estimation with a large number of cases at two large centers. Gastric Cancer 2000;3:219–25.
   Detailed analysis of 5265 early gastric cancers that provided the grounds of expanded indications for endoscopic submucosal dissection.
6. Yoshikawa K, Kitaoka H. Bone metastasis of gastric cancer. Surg Today 1983;13:173–6.
7. Kobayashi M, Okabayashi T, Sano T, et al. Metastatic bone cancer as a recurrence of early gastric cancer: characteristics and possible mechanisms. World J Gastroenterol 2005;11:5587–91.
8. Sobin L, Gospodarowicz M, Wittekind C, editors. TNM classification of malignant tumours. 7th ed International Union Against Cancer; 2009.
9. Yoo CH, Noh SH, Shin DW, et al. Recurrence following curative resection for gastric carcinoma. Br J Surg 2000;87:236–42.

10. Marrelli D, Roviello F, de Mazoni G, et al. Different patterns of recurrence in gastric cancer depending on Lauren's histological type: longitudinal study. World J Surg 2002;26:1160–5.

11. Ishigami H, Kitayama J, Kaisaki S, et al. Phse II study of weekly intravenous and Intraperitoneal paclitaxel combined with S-1 for advanced gastric cancer with peritoneal metastasis. Ann Oncol 2010;21:67–70.

12. Songun I, Putter H, Kranenbarg EMK, et al. Surgical treatment of gastric cancer; 15-year follow-up results of the randomized nationwide Dutch D1D2 trial. Lancet Oncol 2010;11:439–49.
Long-term follow-up of an RCT finally showed significantly fewer gastric cancer deaths after D2 dissection.

13. Martin RC, Jaques DP, Brennan MF, et al. Extended local resection for advanced gastric cancer: increased survival versus increased morbidity. Ann Surg 2002;236:159–65.

14. Han TS, Kong SH, Lee HJ, et al. Dissemination of free cancer cells from the gastric lumen and from perigastric lymphovascular pedicles during radical gastric cancer surgery. Ann Surg Oncol 2011;18:2818–25.

15. Kuramoto M, Shimada S, Ikeshima S, et al. Extensive intraoperative peritoneal lavage as a standard prophylactic strategy for peritoneal recurrence in patients with gastric carcinoma. Ann Surg 2009;250:242–6.
A small-scale RCT showed that extensive peritoneal lavage before closure reduced peritoneal recurrence.

16. Ferlay J, Shin HR, Bray F, et al. Estimates of worldwide burden of cancer in 2008: GLOBOCAN 2008. Int J Cancer 2010;127:2893–917.

17. Sue-Ling HM, Johnston D, Martin IG, et al. Gastric cancer: a curable disease in Britain. Br Med J 1993;307:591–6.

18. McCulloch P. How I do it: D2 gastrectomy. Eur J Surg Oncol 2002;28:738–43.

19. McCulloch PG, Ochiai A, O'Dowd GM, et al. Comparison of the molecular genetics of c-erb-B2 and p53 expression in stomach cancer in Britain and Japan. Cancer 1995;75:920–5.

20. Livingstone JI, Yasui W, Tahara E, et al. Are Japanese and European gastric cancer the same biological entity? An immunohistochemical study. Br J Cancer 1995;72:976–80.

21. Pohl H, Welch G. The role of overdiagnosis and reclassification in the marked increase of esophageal adenocarcinoma incidence. J Natl Cancer Inst 2005;97:142–6.

22. DeMeester SR. Adenocarcinoma of the esophagus and cardia: a review of the disease and its treatment. Ann Surg Oncol 2005;13:12–30.

23. Cuschieri A, Fayers P, Fielding J, et al. Postoperative morbidity and mortality after D1 and D2 resections for gastric cancer: preliminary results of the MRC randomised controlled surgical trial The Surgical Cooperative Group. Lancet 1996;347:995–9.

24. Sasako M, Sano T, Yamamoto S, et al. D2 lymphadenectomy alone or with para-aortic nodal dissection for gastric cancer. N Engl J Med 2008;139:453–62.

25. Davis PA, Sano T. The difference in gastric cancer between Japan, USA and Europe: What are the facts? What are the suggestions? Crit Rev Oncol Hematol 2001;40:77–94.

26. Tsujinaka T, Sasako M, Yamamoto S, et al. Influence of overweight on surgical complications for gastric cancer: results from a randomized control trial comparing D2 and extended para-aortic D3 lymphadenectomy (JCOG9501). Ann Surg Oncol 2007;14:355–61.

27. Birkmeyer JD, Siewers AE, Finlayson EVA, et al. Hospital volume and surgical mortality in the United States. N Engl J Med 2002;346:1128–37.

28. Jackson C, Cunningham D, Oliveira J. Gastric cancer: ESMO clinical recommendations for diagnosis, treatment and follow-up. Ann Oncol 2009;20(S4):iv34–6.

29. NCCN Clinical Practice Guidelines in Oncology. http://www.nccn.org/professionals/physician_gls/f_guidelines.asp

30. Hornig D, Hermanek P, Gall FP. The significance of the extent of proximal margins on clearance in gastric cancer surgery. Scand J Gastroenterol 1977;22(Suppl. 133):69–71.

31. Moehler M, Al-Batran SE, Andus T, et al. German S3-guideline "Diagnosis and treatment of esophagogastric cancer" [in German]. Z Gastroenterol 2011;49:461–531.

32. Japanese Gastric Cancer Association. Japanese gastric cancer treatment guidelines 2010 (ver. 3). Gastric Cancer 2011;14:113–23.
The JGCA totally renewed the concept of D2 lymphadenectomy.

33. Bozzetti F, Marubini E, Bonfanti G, et al. Subtotal versus total gastrectomy for gastric cancer: five-year survival rates in a multicenter randomized Italian trial. Italian Gastrointestinal Tumor Study Group. Ann Surg 1999;230:170–8.

34. Japanese Research Society for Gastric Cancer. The general rules for the gastric cancer study in surgery and pathology. Jpn J Surg 1981;11:127–38.

35. Wu CW, Hsiung CA, Lo SS, et al. Nodal dissection for patients with gastric cancer: a randomized controlled trial. Lancet Oncol 2006;7:309–15.

36. Japanese Gastric Cancer Association. Japanese classifications of gastric carcinoma. 1st English ed. Tokyo: Kanehara; 1995.

37. Japanese Gastric Cancer Association. Japanese classification of gastric carcinoma, 2nd English edn. Gastric Cancer 1998;1:8–24.

38. Sasako M, McCulloch P, Kinoshita T, et al. New method to evaluate the therapeutic value of lymph node dissection for gastric cancer. Br J Surg 1995;82:346–51.
A new concept to evaluated lymphadenectomy was proposed based on the incidence of metastasis and survival of patients with positive nodes.
39. Japanese Gastric Cancer Association. Japanese classification of gastric carcinoma, 3rd English edn. Gastric Cancer 2011;14:101–12.
40. Sano T, Sasako M, Yamamoto S, et al. Gastric cancer surgery: morbidity and mortality results from a prospective randomized controlled trial comparing D2 and extended para-aortic lymphadenectomy – Japan Clinical Oncology Group Study 9501. J Clin Oncol 2004;22:2767–73.
41. Siewert JR, Böttcher K, Stein HJ, et al. Relevant prognostic factors in gastric cancer: ten-year results of the German Gastric Cancer Study. Ann Surg 1998;228:449–61.
42. Fujita J, Kurokawa Y, Sugimoto T, et al. Survival benefit of bursectomy in patients with resectable gastric cancer: interim analysis results of a randomized controlled trial. Gastric Cancer 2012;15:42–8.
43. Griffith JP, Sue-Ling HM, Martin I, et al. Preservation of the spleen improves survival after radical surgery for gastric cancer. Gut 1995;36:684–90.
44. Wanebo HJ, Kennedy BJ, Winchester DP, et al. Role of splenectomy in gastric cancer surgery: adverse effect of elective splenectomy on long-term survival. J Am Coll Surg 1997;185:177–84.
45. Maehara Y, Moriguchi S, Yoshida M, et al. Splenectomy does not correlate with length of survival in patients undergoing curative total gastrectomy for gastric carcinoma Univariate and multivariate analyses. Cancer 1991;67:3006–9.
46. Csendes A, Burdiles P, Rojas J, et al. A prospective randomized study comparing D2 total gastrectomy versus D2 total gastrectomy plus splenectomy in 187 patients with gastric carcinoma. Surgery 2002;131:401–7.
47. Yu W, Choi GS, Chung HY. Randomized clinical trial of splenectomy versus splenic preservation in patients with proximal gastric cancer. Br J Surg 2006;93:559–63.
48. Sano T, Yamamoto S, Sasako M. Randomized controlled trial to evaluate splenectomy in total gastrectomy for proximal gastric carcinoma: Japan Clinical Oncology Group study JCOG 0110-MF. Jpn J Clin Oncol 2002;32:363–4.
49. Sano T, Sasako M, Shibata T, et al. Randomized controlled trial to evaluate splenectomy in total gastrectomy for proximal gastric carcinoma (JCOG0110): analyses of operative morbidity, operation time, and blood loss. J Clin Oncol 2010;28(Suppl.):15s, abstr 4020.
50. Kodera Y, Sasako M, Yamamoto S, et al. Identification of risk factors for the development of complications following extended and superextended lymphadenectomies for gastric cancer. Br J Surg 2005;92:1103–9.
51. Maruyama K, Sasako M, Kinoshita T, et al. Pancreas-preserving total gastrectomy for proximal gastric cancer. World J Surg 1995;19:532–6.
52. Roberts P, Seevaratnam R, Cardoso R, et al. Systematic review of pancreaticoduodenectomy for locally advanced gastric cancer. Gastric Cancer 2012;15(Suppl. 1):S108–15.
53. Roviello F, Pedrazzani C, Marrelli D, et al. Super-extended (D3) lymphadenectomy in advanced gastric cancer. Eur J Surg Oncol 2010;36:439–46.
54. Tokunaga M, Ohyama S, Hiki N, et al. Therapeutic value of lymph node dissection in advanced gastric cancer with macroscopic duodenum invasion: is the posterior pancreatic head lymph node dissection beneficial? Ann Surg Oncol 2009;16:1241–6.
55. Sakamoto Y, Sano T, Shimada K, et al. Favorable indications for hepatectomy in patients with liver metastasis from gastric cancer. J Surg Oncol 2007;95:534–9.
56. Koga R, Yamamoto J, Ohyama S, et al. Liver resection for metastatic gastric cancer: experience with 42 patients including eight long-term survivors. Jpn J Clin Oncol 2007;37:836–42.
57. Sasako M., Sano T., Yamamoto S., et al. Left thoracoabdominal approach versus abdominal-transhiatal approach for cardia or subcardia cancer: a randomised controlled trial. Lancet Oncol 2006;7:644–51.
58. Hayes N, Karat D, Scott DJ, et al. Radical lymphadenectomy in the management of early gastric cancer. Br J Surg 1996;83:1421–3.
59. Natsugoe S, Aikou T, Shimada M, et al. Occult lymph node metastasis in gastric cancer with submucosal invasion. Surg Today 1994;24(10):870–5.
60. Choi J, Kim SG, Im JP, et al. Endoscopic prediction of tumor invasiondepth in early gastric cancer. Gastrointest Endosc 2011;73:917–27.
61. Maki T, Shiratori T, Hatafuku T, et al. Pylorus-preserving gastrectomy as an improved operation for gastric ulcer. Surgery 1967;61:838–42.
62. Nunobe S, Sasako M, Saka M, et al. Symptom evaluation of long-term postoperative outcomes after pylorus-preserving gastrectomy for early gastric cancer. Gastric Cancer 2007;10:167–72.
63. Tomikawa M, Korenaga D, Akahoshi T, et al. Quality of life after laparoscopy-assisted pylorus-preserving gastrectomy: an evaluation using a questionnaire mailed to the patients. Surg Today 2012;42(7):625–32.
64. Isozaki H, Kimura T, Tanaka N, et al. An assessment of the feasibility of sentinel lymph node-guided surgery for gastric cancer. Gastric Cancer 2004;7:149–53.
65. Zong L, Chen P. Billroth I vs. Billroth II vs. Roux-en-Y following distal gastrectomy: a meta-analysis based on 15 studies. Hepatogastroenterology 2011;58:1413–24.

66. Gertler R, Rosenberg R, Feith M, et al. Pouch vs. no pouch following total gastrectomy: meta-analysis and systematic review. Am J Gastroenterol 2009;104:2838–51.
A meta-analysis showed clinical benefits of pouch formation after total gastrectomy.

67. Merendino KA, Dillard DH. The concept of sphincter substitution by and interposed jejunal segment for anatomic and physiologic abnormalities at the esophagogastric junction: with special reference to reflux esophagitis, cardiospasm and esophageal varices. Ann Surg 1955;142:486–509.

68. Katai H, Sano T, Fukagawa T, et al. Prospective study of proximal gastrectomy for early gastric cancer in the upper third of the stomach. Br J Surg 2003;90:850–3.

69. Kim J, Lee J, Hyung WJ, et al. Gastric cancer surgery without drains: a prospective randomized trial. J Gastrointest Surg 2004;8:727–32.
A high-volume single institutional RCT showed that routine use of drain is not necessary after D2 gastrectomy.

70. Zeng Q, Zhang Q, Han S, et al. Efficacy of somatostatin and its analogues in prevention of postoperative complications after pancreaticoduodenectomy: a meta-analysis of randomized controlled trials. Pancreas 2008;36:18–25.

71. Mine S, Sano T, Tsutsumi K, et al. Large-scale investigation into dumping syndrome after gastrectomy for gastric cancer. J Am Coll Surg 2010;211:628–36.
Direct questionnaire to 1153 gastrectomised patients with various postoperative periods revealed actual conditions of dumping syndrome.

8

Endoscopic and surgical treatment of early gastric cancer

Joost Rothbarth
Arjun D. Koch
J. Jan B. van Lanschot

Introduction

Definition of early gastric cancer

Early gastric cancer (EGC) is defined as a tumour that is limited to the mucosal or submucosal layers (T1 cancer) and by definition absence of invasion into the proper muscle layer. This is irrespective of the presence of lymph node metastasis.[1]

Risk and development of early gastric cancer

The incidence of gastric cancer has steadily declined over many decades, yet it remains worldwide one of the most common malignancies. Most gastric cancers arise as a result of lifelong colonisation with *Helicobacter pylori*, inducing chronic active gastritis. An abundance of research over the past 20 years has yielded endoscopic and non-invasive methods to recognise both this infection and the various stages of the cascade leading from chronic gastritis via atrophic gastritis, intestinal metaplasia and dysplasia to early and advanced gastric cancer. Cohort studies with these methods have revealed the cancer risks associated with each premalignant condition, and showed that these risks increase with each subsequent stage of the cascade.[2] These advances have led to common identification of patients with dysplasia and early cancer of the stomach, a development which likely will be further enhanced by the recent introduction of a guideline for surveillance of patients with intestinal metaplasia and dysplasia of the stomach,[3] in particular when present in both antrum and corpus.[4] This chapter deals with the management of early gastric cancer.

Classification of early gastric cancer

Early gastric cancer usually arises in a mucosa that has undergone atrophic and metaplastic changes. These are recognisable with modern high-definition endoscopic equipment, in particular when combined with additional image enhancement techniques such as narrow-band imaging (NBI). Against this background, most EGCs amenable for endoscopic resection can be recognised by experienced endoscopists.[5] Complete staging and classification of EGCs is usually done in three steps. The first step is a pre-interventional endoscopic staging determining depth of tumour infiltration (with or without endoscopic ultrasonography) combined with histopathological sampling. The second step is the actual endoscopic resection, where the most valuable information is gathered from the submucosal lifting properties of the lesions. The third step is the final histopathological staging of the resected lesion.

Endoscopic appearance

Experienced endoscopists performing endoscopic mucosal resections (EMRs) or endoscopic submucosal dissections (ESDs) are trained to recognise and delineate early neoplasia, which includes assessment of invasion depth and thus the endoscopic resectability of the lesion. EGCs are classified by their endoscopic appearance according to the Paris classification (**Fig. 8.1**).[1] Superficial lesions are classified as either protruding (Paris 0-I), elevated (0-IIa), depressed (0-IIc) or excavated and often ulcerated lesions (0-III). Lesions that have both elevated and depressed components are classified into two groups: depressed lesions in which most of the surface is depressed and there is elevation in a portion of the peripheral ring are classified as 0-IIc+IIa, while elevated lesions with a central depression encircled by the elevated ring at the periphery are called 0-IIa+IIc. The combined patterns of excavation and depression are called 0-III+IIc or 0-IIc+III, depending on the relative surface area of the ulcer and of the depressed area. The classification helps to predict the extent of invasion into the submucosal layer and thus the choice between endoscopic or surgical treatment (Table 8.1). For instance, true protruding lesions in the stomach demonstrate a 57% relative frequency of submucosal invasion, whereas non-protruding, non-excavated lesions demonstrate submucosal invasion in frequencies between 20% and 40%. In excavated lesions, often the proper muscle layer is already involved. Although the exact percentage of involvement of the proper muscle layer is not reported in the literature, this number comes close to 100% and the Paris 0-III excavated types of lesions are usually not resectable by endoscopic means.

Additional characteristics that predict submucosal or deeper invasion are larger tumour size (>30 mm), presence of discoloration (remarkable redness) and ulceration.[5] Lesions that are confined to the mucosa tend to move over the peristaltic waves, whereas peristaltic waves seem to curve around tumours that have invaded the proper muscle layer. The latter provides a strong argument against endoscopic resection.

In most EMR and ESD techniques, submucosal injection of fluid is used to lift the early cancer from the proper muscle layer. This method has three major benefits: (i) it provides information on invasion depth and thus endoscopic resectability; (ii) it facilitates endoscopic resection; and (iii) it provides a safety fluid cushion for resecting the superficial lesion without damaging the deeper layers when using snares, knives or electrocautery.[6]

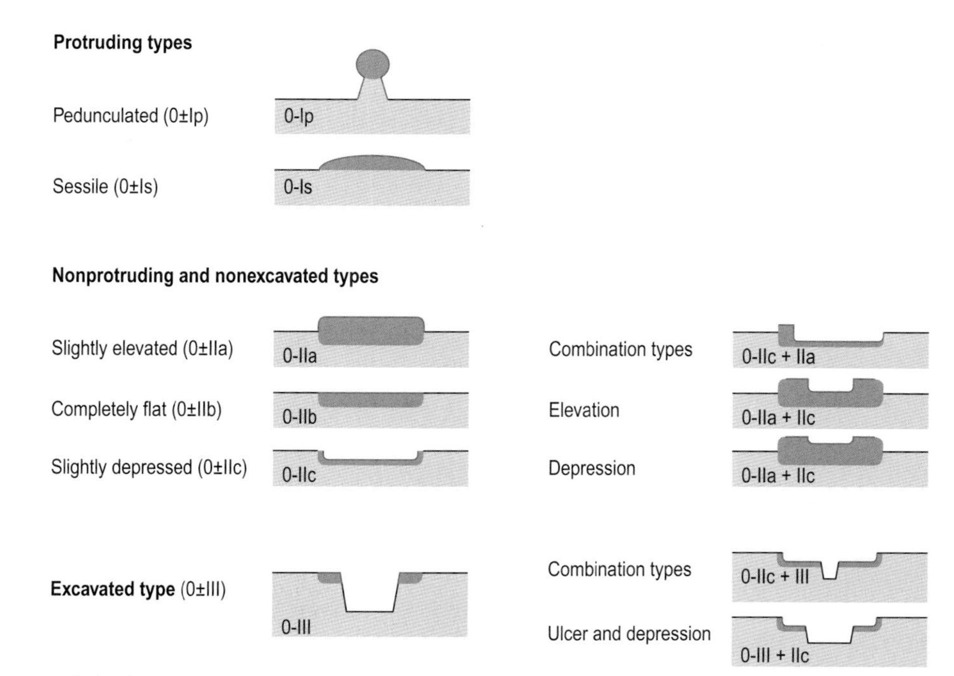

Figure 8.1 • Paris classification. Endoscopic appearance of superficial neoplastic lesions.

Table 8.1 • Paris classification of type 0 superficial lesions

Macroscopic appearance	Paris classification	Relative frequency of submucosal invasion in gastric lesions
Protruding	0-I	57%
Pedunculated	0-Ip	
Sessile	0-Is	
Non-protruding and non-excavated		
Slightly elevated	0-IIa	29%
Completely flat	0-IIb	20%
Slightly depressed	0-IIc	40%
Elevated and depressed types	0-IIa+IIc	
	0-IIc+IIa	
Excavated		
Ulcer	0-III	–
Excavated and depressed types	0-IIc+III	
	0-III+IIc	

The amount of lifting provides information on the invasion depth of the lesion. Mucosal or superficial submucosal lesions usually demonstrate complete lifting (m–sm1), whereas the lesions that infiltrate into the deeper submucosal layers often lift incompletely (sm2–sm3). A non-lifting sign most often represents invasion deeper than sm3.[6]

Lymph node metastasis

Endoscopic staging before resection does provide useful information on the prediction of lymph node metastasis. Differentiation grade can be assessed through simple biopsy. A large retrospective study from Japan assessed the occurrence of lymph node metastasis in 5265 patients who had undergone gastrectomy with lymph node dissection for early gastric cancer.[7] All specimens were reassessed for macroscopic appearance, size, ulceration, invasion depth and extent of submucosal invasion, differentiation grade and lymphovascular involvement.

The results are summarised in Table 8.2 and define the criteria for EMR and ESD.[7,8]

✓✓ It turned out that depressed or ulcerated lesions, larger than 30 mm in size, of the undifferentiated histological type or with lymphovascular involvement, were associated with an increased risk of nodal metastases (7.3%). In contrast, none of the differentiated EGCs less than 30 mm in size, regardless of ulceration, were associated with lymph node metastases. None of the differentiated lesions without ulceration were associated with nodal metastases regardless of the size of the lesion and none of the undifferentiated lesions without ulceration, less than 20 mm in size, were associated with positive lymph nodes. The results of this study provided the necessary evidence to widen the indications for endoscopic resections of EGCs.[7]

Endosonography

The role of endosonography remains debatable in EGCs. Endosonography lacks sufficient diagnostic accuracy in discriminating T1 from T2 lesions. The combined results of large recent studies show a diagnostic accuracy for T3 and T4 tumours

Table 8.2 • Criteria for EMR and ESD, according to the proposed guidelines

Depth	Mucosal cancer				Submucosal cancer	
	No ulcer		Ulcer		SM1	SM2
Differentiation	≤20 mm	>20 mm	≤30 mm	>30 mm	≤30 mm	Any size
Good/moderate	EMR	ESD	ESD	S	ESD	S
Poor/undifferentiated	CS	S	S	S	S	S

CS, consider surgery; EMR, suitable for endoscopic mucosal resections; ESD, suitable for endoscopic submucosal dissection; S, surgery.

of 88–100%, with 64–85% accuracy for T2 lesions and 75–82% accuracy for T1 tumours.[9,10] T1 lesions are often overstaged, probably because of submucosal fibrosis, connective tissue hyperplasia or ulceration. Diagnostic accuracy can be improved using mini-probes; however, complete assessment of larger lesions is difficult and bears the risk of underestimating the deepest invasion when parts of the lesion are missed and subsequently not assessed.[11] Many endoscopists rely, for these reasons, on endoscopic assessment alone followed by histopathological assessment of the resected specimen. A German study demonstrated a similar diagnostic accuracy of 83.4% and 79.6% using either high-resolution endoscopy or endosonography, respectively, in assessing infiltration depth in early neoplasia in the oesophagus.[12] The authors believe the same applies for early neoplasia in the stomach.

✔ Conventional endoscopic assessment of depth of infiltration in EGC has a similar accuracy compared to endosonography. For this reason, most highly experienced interventional endoscopists rely on endoscopic assessment and do not routinely perform endosonography before proceeding to EMR or ESD.[12]

Revised Vienna classification

Large discrepancies between Western and Japanese pathologists in the diagnostic criteria for adenoma, dysplasia and carcinoma in the gastrointestinal tract have led to considerable problems in the comparison between Western and Japanese data. This led to a consensus meeting in 1998 in Vienna, ultimately resulting in the Vienna classification of gastrointestinal epithelial neoplasia and the revised Vienna classification in 2002.[13] This classification allows not only for a more universal nomenclature of gastrointestinal epithelial neoplasia but also corresponds more properly with clinical management. The revised Vienna classification is shown in Table 8.3.

Endoscopic treatment

Endoscopic mucosal resection

The basic principle of what is nowadays termed endoscopic mucosal resection (EMR) is the removal of a mucosal lesion by resecting it from its deeper layers using a snare instrument. This method does not allow for lesions larger than 2 cm to be removed en bloc.[14] Larger lesions can be removed by EMR, but only in a piecemeal fashion. The technique is fundamentally different from ESD, where the submucosal layer is carefully and stepwise dissected. Using EMR, early neoplasia is often lifted from the proper muscle layer before resection using different solutions of saline for submucosal injection.[15–17] The lesions can then be sucked into a cap that is placed at the tip of the endoscope with a snare preloaded on to the rim of the cap. After sucking the lesion into the cap, the snare is pulled. The content of the snare is then resected using high-frequency current. An alternative resection method that is frequently used is the so-called 'band-and-cut' method. A lesion is sucked into a modified multiband ligator. By ligating the mucosa bearing the lesion, a pseudopolyp is created that can be resected using a snare. This multiple band mucosectomy allows for larger segments of neoplasia to be completely resected.[18] This method is increasingly used in larger Barrett's segments but is also applicable in the cardia and the antrum of the stomach.

Table 8.3 • The revised Vienna classification of gastrointestinal epithelial neoplasia

Category	Diagnosis	Clinical management
1	Negative for neoplasia	Optional follow-up
2	Indefinite for neoplasia	Endoscopic follow-up
3	Mucosal low-grade neoplasia	Endoscopic resection or follow-up
	Low-grade dysplasia	
	Low-grade adenoma	
4	Mucosal high grade neoplasia	Endoscopic or local surgical resection
4.1	High-grade adenoma/dysplasia	
4.2	Non-invasive carcinoma (carcinoma in situ)	
4.3	Suspicious for invasive carcinoma	
4.4	Intramucosal carcinoma	
5	Submucosal invasion by carcinoma	Surgical resection

Endoscopic submucosal dissection

Endoscopic submucosal dissection (ESD) was originally developed in Japan for the local treatment of superficial EGC limited to the mucosal layer or with a minimal invasion of the submucosal layer. The main goal of submucosal dissection is to retrieve the lesion en bloc for histopathological staging and to minimise the chance for local recurrence. ESD is performed in several steps. First, the lesion is delineated by placing circumferential dots using electrocautery around the lesion with a few millimetres of free margin. The lesion is then lifted from the proper muscle layer by submucosal injection in the same fashion as in EMR.[15–17] The solutions used are often stained with either indigo carmine or methylene blue. This dye will colour the submucosal layer and facilitate recognition of the separate layers and blood vessels. After lifting the lesion a circumferential incision of the mucosal layer is made, placing the markers just inside the circumferential cut. From this point onwards the submucosal layer is carefully dissected from the muscle layer, often with additional submucosal injections. In **Fig. 8.2** an example of a Paris 0-IIa+IIc is shown, which is subsequently removed by ESD. Different speciality knives have been developed for ESD. A breakthrough in ESD was the development of the insulated tip (IT) knife in 1996.[14] This is a speciality endoscopic knife with an insulated tip. An insulated small ceramic sphere is mounted on the top of a high-frequency needle knife, allowing safe and easy incision and separation of the mucosal and submucosal layers. Subsequently, the design of the original IT knife has been further adapted leading, for example, to the IT-2 knife, the hook knife, the flex knife, the triangular tip (TT) knife and the hybrid knife, the latter combining radiofrequency with a water-jet application.[19] This novel technique combines radiofrequency with a distance-dependent water-jet application, allowing for easier and safer submucosal lifting and cutting in ESD.[20,21]

Complete resections

The aim of both EMR and ESD is to strive for complete resection of the neoplastic lesion.

In theory, using the ESD technique, lesions of all sizes can be removed. However, attempts at curative resection are limited by a number of anatomical factors that relate to the primary lesion. These factors are related to the relative frequencies of lymph node metastasis, as described earlier in this chapter. Larger lesions, poorer differentiation or deeper penetration in the submucosal layer are associated

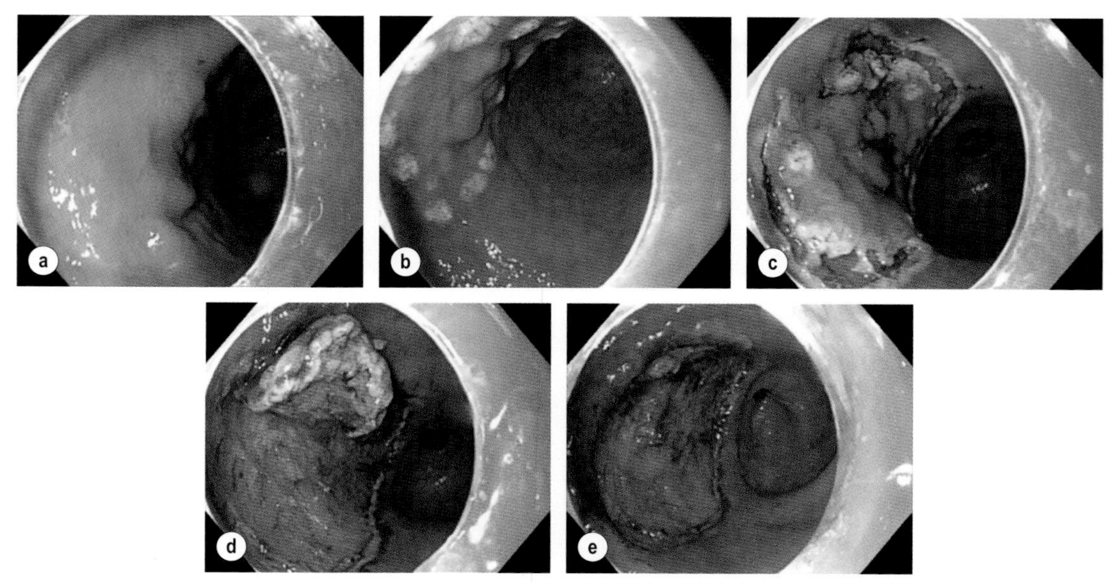

Figure 8.2 • Early gastric cancer removed by ESD. **(a)** A Paris 0-IIc+IIa early gastric cancer located in the antrum. **(b–e)** Markings are placed around the lesion **(b)** and after submucosal lifting and circumferential incision **(c)**, the lesion is stepwise dissected **(d)** and finally fully removed **(e)**. Histopathological assessment demonstrated a well-differentiated adenocarcinoma confined to the mucosal layer with a maximum extent into the muscularis mucosae and tumour-free resection margins.

✔✔ In the endoscopic treatment for early gastric cancer conventional EMR has been proven to be inferior to ESD, especially when it comes to lesions larger than 20mm or with ulceration. Piecemeal resection of these lesions leads to lower rates of complete resection and higher local recurrence rates up to 26%, even when histopathology of piecemeal fragments suggested complete resection. Even en bloc EMRs of lesions smaller than 20mm resulted in no more than a 45% margin-free resection rate, where ESD was clearly superior with an 87% margin-free resection rate.[14] Lesions up to 10mm can be removed either by EMR or ESD, with a comparable recurrence-free rate.[22]

with a rapidly increasing incidence of lymph node metastases.

Routinely, after endoscopic resection, the resected specimens are stretched and pinned on cork or paraffin and sent for pathological assessment. This final staging step by the pathologist should provide the necessary information on (i) quantitative criteria (lateral margins, deeper margins, maximum extent of submucosal invasion) and (ii) qualitative criteria (differentiation grade, lymphovascular involvement), which correspond with the risk of lymph node metastasis.[7,8] This ultimate information is pivotal for further management. It mandates additional surgery or allows for a surveillance policy. Because of an approximately 14% chance of metachronous gastric cancer over a 5-year period[23] and possible remnant neoplastic tissue, surveillance is usually carried out after endoscopic resection at 6-month intervals during the first year, followed by annual surveillance thereafter. Early detection of metachronous neoplasia can be treated by repeated endoscopic resection.

Complications of endoscopic resections

Endoscopic treatment is now accepted worldwide for early gastrointestinal neoplasia as it replaces the need for major surgery associated with considerable morbidity and mortality. Endoscopic treatment is also superior in terms of post-procedural functional results. The obvious example is the avoidance of gastrectomy by endoscopic resection of an early neoplastic lesion.

However, these novel endoscopic techniques also come with a risk of complications, ranging from bleeding and perforation to post-treatment strictures and, potentially, leading to considerable morbidity and even mortality.

Most bleeding complications occur during the procedures and can be dealt with instantly. Superficial bleeding vessels are identified and treated either by using coagulation, adrenaline injections or clips. Delayed bleeding also occurs and might necessitate subsequent re-intervention. A large prospective study found no risk factors for bleeding besides the presence of a gastric malignancy itself.[24]

In expert hands, perforations occur during EMR and ESD in about 0.2% and 1–4% of cases, respectively. A recent European study reported a 20% perforation rate after ESD at a tertiary referral centre.[25] This study clearly demonstrates a difference in expertise in some Western referral centres compared to Japanese and Korean expert centres. This is mostly due to a much lower incidence of EGCs in the Western world, resulting in an insufficient exposure to this type of pathology and resection techniques. Recently, a panel of European experts has attempted to set standards for quality criteria for ESD in European countries.[26] Perforations can lead to pneumoperitoneum and in severe cases to generalised peritonitis. Usually, perforations are recognised immediately during the procedure and endoscopic management is possible and frequently adequate.[27] Closure with clips is a safe treatment option together with nasogastric drainage and fasting.[28] Recently, in a small case series the use of the over-the-scope clip (OTSC) was described for closure of perforations in a clinical setting.[29] The OTSC device is a promising novel technique with a reported closure success rate of 92%.

Strictures after EMR and ESD occur mainly in the more narrow parts of the gastrointestinal tract such as the oesophagus, gastric cardia and pyloric region. Stricture formation is more frequent with circumferential resections or large size perimeters and is induced through ulcer scar healing. These strictures are often relatively easy to treat with balloon dilation, with the exception of strictures after circumferential ESD, which can prove quite difficult to treat because of severe scar fibrosis.

✔ In expert hands, perforations occur during EMR and ESD in about 0.2% and 1–4% of cases, respectively. Immediate endoscopic closure with clips is a safe treatment option in combination with nasogastric drainage and oral fasting.[28]

Surgical resection

As described in Chapter 7, the type of gastrectomy and extent of lymphadenectomy for EGC depend on the location of the tumour. In general, a total gastrectomy is performed for tumours in the middle and upper third of the stomach and a distal gastrectomy for tumours in the distal third.

Unfortunately, these extensive resections are associated with substantial postoperative short- and long-term complications and impaired quality of life. The low recurrence rates and high 5-year survival rates of EGC have led to the development of less extensive resections with a potentially improved postoperative quality of life and a comparable excellent long-term survival. In Japan and Korea proximal gastrectomy for EGC in the upper third of the stomach and pylorus-preserving gastrectomy (PPG) for EGC in the middle portion of the stomach are well-accepted procedures. Segmental or local gastric resections with or without lymphadenectomy have been described for gastric tumours, but still have to be considered experimental.

Proximal gastrectomy

Total gastrectomy with D1 or D2 lymphadenectomy is still the standard treatment for tumours in the upper third of the stomach. This type of resection is associated with the postgastrectomy syndrome, including dumping, epigastric pain, diarrhoea, hypoglycaemia, malnutrition and anaemia. As nodal metastases in the distal gastric lymph nodes (stations 5 and 6) are rare in EGC of the proximal stomach, less extensive resections have been proposed. Proximal gastrectomy (**Fig. 8.3a**) was developed as an alternative to total gastrectomy in order to reduce the long-term postoperative problems without compromising the oncological outcome. In proximal gastrectomy the proximal half of the stomach is resected, including a D1 or D1+ lymphadenectomy.[30] Several techniques for surgical reconstruction after proximal gastrectomy have been described, including reconstruction by jejunal interposition and a gastric tube (**Fig. 8.3b,c**), but the optimal method remains controversial.

As could be expected due to the relatively high incidence of EGC in the East, most studies on proximal gastrectomy are from Japan and Korea,[31–35] while data from Western countries are scarce.[36] Several studies have shown that proximal gastrectomy for upper EGC is a safe procedure with comparable 5-year survival rates.[31–34,36] However, conflicting data have been reported on the long-term complications and quality of life. Some studies showed an improved clinical outcome after proximal gastrectomy with oesophagogastrostomy or jejunal interposition, while others report a markedly higher complication rate including anastomotic stenosis and reflux oesophagitis.[32–35] Therefore, further evaluation on this type of gastric resection for proximal EGC is needed. As yet, randomised data are not available.

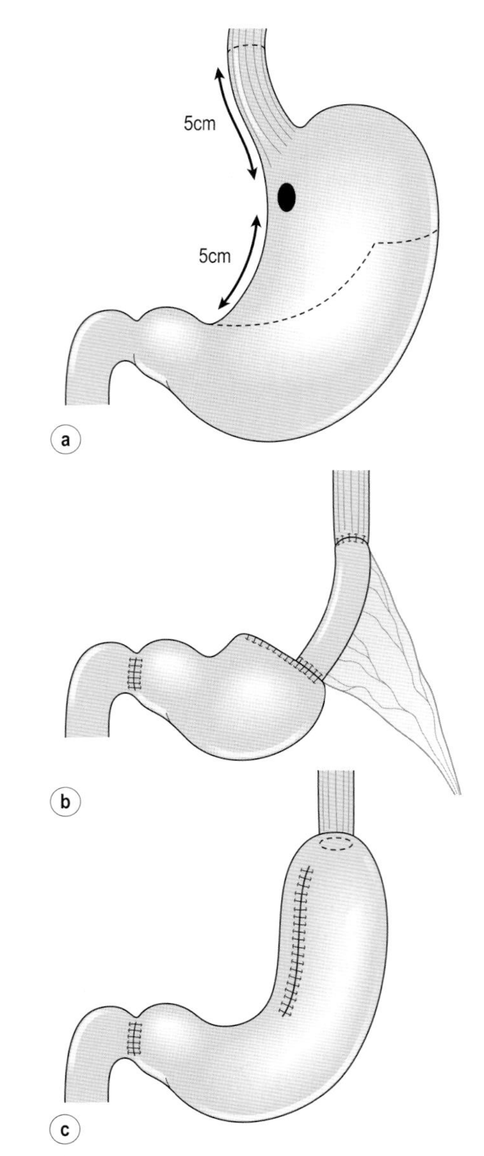

Figure 8.3 • Proximal gastrectomy **(a)**, with reconstruction by jejunal interposition **(b)** or gastric tube **(c)**.

Pylorus-preserving gastrectomy

PPG is a function-preserving procedure initially described for the treatment of peptic ulcer disease[37] (**Fig. 8.4**). For patients with EGC, favourable functional results have been reported with PPG compared to conventional distal gastrectomy. PPG is feasible for early tumours in the middle third of the stomach with the distal border at least 4 cm proximal to the pylorus. In PPG a distal gastrectomy is performed with preservation of the pylorus and both the right

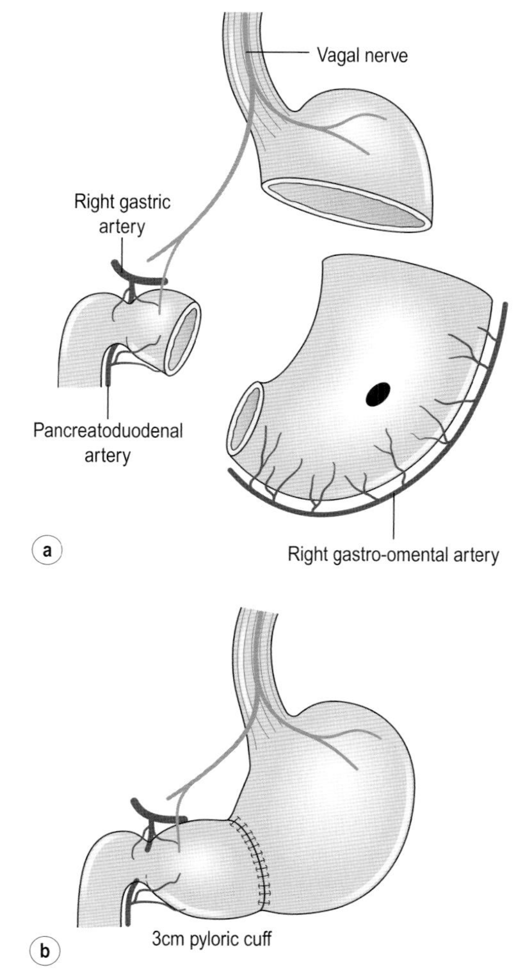

Figure 8.4 • Pylorus-preserving gastrectomy.

gastric artery and the pyloric branch of the vagal nerve, followed by a stomach-to-stomach anastomosis.[38] As a result, it is assumed that the pyloric function remains intact, preventing gastrointestinal symptoms such as dumping syndrome, epigastric fullness, reflux oesophagitis, bile regurgitation and cholelithiasis.[39] In contrast to conventional distal or total gastrectomy, the suprapyloric (second-tier) lymph nodes are not resected in PPG. In EGC this is probably justified as 80–90% of EGCs are negative for lymph node metastases and the vast majority of positive lymph nodes are located in the first-tier lymph nodes only. Retrospective data of a Japanese database of 3646 T1 tumours located in the middle third of the stomach showed only 0.2% metastases to the pyloric lymph nodes.[40] High 5-year survival rates up to 98% are reported after PPG with modified D2 lymph node dissection in patients with clinically diagnosed mucosal or submucosal gastric cancer (cT1) without lymph node metastases (cN0).[41] Similar to studies on proximal gastrectomy, most data on PPG are derived from studies done in Japan and Korea. In Western countries PPG is still considered investigational.

Local (or wedge) segmental resection

Local or wedge resection involves removal of only the tumour including the nearby lymph nodes and primary closure of the stomach (**Fig. 8.5**). In a segmental resection a limited segment between the lesser and the greater curvature of the stomach is resected including the nearby lymph nodes and a formal gastro-gastrostomy is performed (**Fig. 8.6**). Local and segmental gastric resections for (early) gastric cancer have the obvious potential advantage of a better functional postoperative outcome, because digestive and reservoir functions of the stomach are mostly preserved. Several small studies show superior results on nutritional status and the occurrence of dumping and reflux oesophagitis after local or segmental resection, compared to a total or distal gastrectomy.[42–45] These procedures can be safely performed in EGC with favourable features that cannot be resected by EMR or ESD for technical reasons. As mentioned before, the likelihood of lymph node metastases in these patients is very low and local or segmental resection with a limited lymphadenectomy seems justified.

For EGC with unfavourable features local or segmental resection with only limited lymphadenectomy is still investigational. In these patients the risk of lymph node metastases and local recurrence is relatively high and no clear evidence exists that similar recurrence and survival rates can be achieved compared to standard gastric resections. Intraoperative investigation of lymph nodes for tumour metastases by sentinel lymph node biopsy (SLNB) may lead to

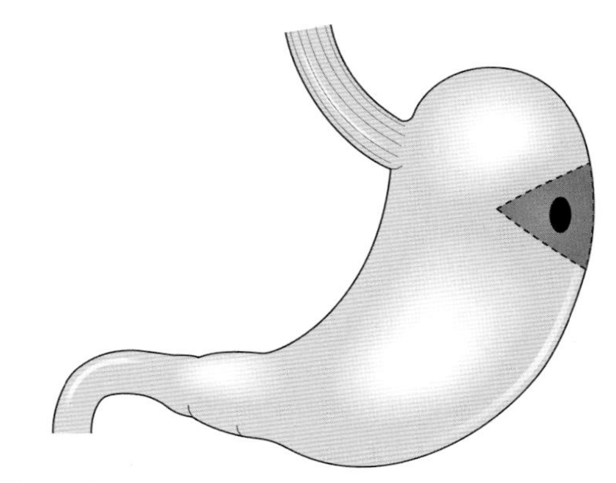

Figure 8.5 • Local or wedge gastric resection.

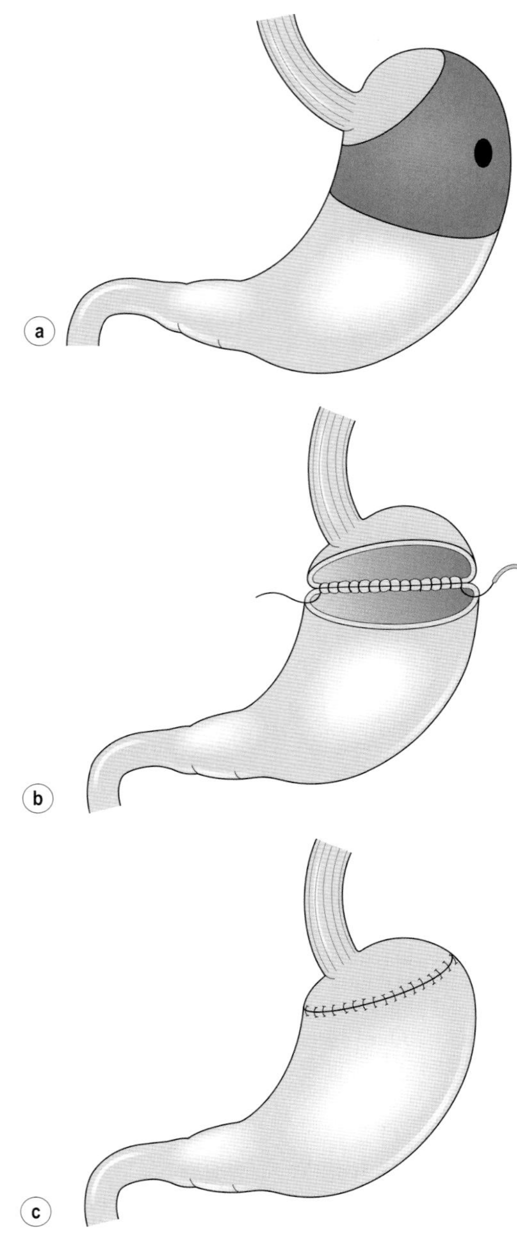

Figure 8.6 • Segmental gastric resection.

a better selection of patients eligible for a local or segmental resection, as will be discussed later.

Minimally invasive surgery

Over the past decade there has been a notable trend towards laparoscopic or laparoscopically assisted surgery for EGC, especially in Japan and Korea. The role of laparoscopy in gastric cancer is less clear in Western countries. Minimally invasive surgery has the obvious advantage of less postoperative pain for the patient, a faster recovery and better cosmetic results. In laparoscopic gastric cancer surgery the discussion has been mainly focused on whether the oncological outcome is comparable to open surgery.

Several large Japanese and Korean randomised controlled trials (RCTs) on laparoscopic versus open surgery have been conducted.

✔✔ A meta-analysis of six RCTs that included a total of 629 patients with EGC reported decreased blood loss, less postoperative early morbidity and a decreased but adequate number of harvested lymph nodes in laparoscopic surgery. Mortality and time to oral intake were similar.[46] A retrospective multicentre study[47] including 1294 patients with EGC and a single-centre retrospective study[48] with 601 patients with EGC showed similar short-term morbidity and mortality compared to open gastrectomy. Also, 5-year disease-free and overall survival rates were comparable to open surgery.

Some smaller studies from Europe and the USA showed similar results.[49,50] Thus, laparoscopic gastric resection for EGC is a technically safe procedure and seems to be justified for selected patients. However, results from RCTs will have to prove the oncological safety of laparoscopic gastrectomy.

Recently, natural orifice transluminal endoscopic surgery (NOTES) has been proposed as a new technique for the treatment of EGC. One study has reported the feasibility of a combined NOTES and laparoscopic resection of EGC in 14 patients.[51] Further studies have to define whether there is a role for NOTES in the treatment of EGC.

Lymphadenectomy

In gastric cancer, lymph node status is one of the crucial prognostic factors,[52] and the type of resection and the extent of lymphadenectomy are largely based on the likelihood of lymph node metastases to first- and second-tier lymph nodes. However, in parallel with many other tumours it is still debatable whether (extended) lymphadenectomy in gastric cancer really leads to improved survival.[53]

As mentioned at the beginning of this chapter, mucosal and submucosal tumours with favourable features (Table 8.2)[8] can be safely treated by EMR or ESD. This is based on the fact that these tumours have a very low risk of lymphatic dissemination. EGCs with unfavourable tumour characteristics harbour a high risk of lymph node metastases and are not amenable for endoscopic treatment. For these patients a gastric resection with lymphadenectomy is indicated. As discussed in Chapter 7, the extent of lymph node dissection in gastric cancer remains controversial. The discussion is mainly focused on the adequacy of a limited D1 lymphadenectomy versus the necessity of extended D2 or even D3 lymphadenectomy. In general, surgeons in Western countries tend to perform a more limited lymphadenectomy (D1), while surgeons in Japan and Korea perform a more extended lymphadenectomy (D2). The rationale for extended lymphadenectomy is improved staging, enhanced locoregional control and improved survival. The clearance of possible metastatic nodes in the region outside the perigastric nodes is presumed to have an impact on overall survival rates.

✔✔ However, two large randomised trials from the Netherlands and the UK comparing D1 and D2 dissection have not demonstrated that an improved overall survival or decreased relapse rate can be obtained by D2 dissection, while morbidity and mortality are increased.[54–56] A meta-analysis of the two randomised trials did show a possible survival benefit for serosa positive tumours (T3+)[54,55] and 10-year survival results from the Dutch Gastric Cancer Trial showed only a trend towards survival benefit in a subgroup of patients with N2 disease.[56]

In Taiwan an RCT was performed comparing D1 with D3 lymphadenectomy; in the extended arm a level 3 lymph node dissection (hepatoduodenal ligament, retropancreatic region and superior mesenteric vein lymph nodes) and an optional hemipancreatosplenectomy were performed. This trial demonstrated an overall survival benefit in favour of a D3 lymphadenectomy, with 5-year overall survival rates of 59.5% versus 53.6%.[57] These data suggest that extended (D2) lymphadenectomy can result in survival benefit for patients with advanced gastric cancer.

The optimal extent of lymph node dissection for EGC remains controversial. The incidence of lymph node metastases for mucosal EGC is only 2–4%, but increases to up to 45% in mucosal tumours with unfavourable features such as depressed or ulcerated lesions, tumours larger than 30 mm in size, tumours with undifferentiated histological type or with lymphovascular involvement.[7,58] Most patients with mucosal EGC are safely treated by EMR or ESD without lymphadenectomy (Table 8.2). In submucosal EGC lymph node metastases are found in approximately 20%, with a wide range from 10% to 64%.[59–61] In addition, approximately 5% of lymph node metastases from submucosal EGC are located in second-tier lymph nodes (mainly node stations 7, 8a and 9).[62,63] Because of the relatively high risk of lymph node metastases in submucosal EGC and mucosal EGC with unfavourable features, a lymphadenectomy is generally performed in these patients. However, there is no consensus on the required extent of the lymphadenectomy. The Japanese Gastric Cancer Association (JGCA) recommends D2 lymphadenectomy for patients with EGC clinically positive node(s) (cN+),[30] but this guideline lacks clear evidence.

For patients without suspicion of positive lymph nodes (cN0), currently no evidence exists that D2 dissection can improve survival rates in EGC. Considering the fact that in EGC the rate of lymph node metastases is relatively low and, when positive, generally confined to the first-tier lymph nodes, D2 resection can probably be omitted in EGC. Therefore, in Europe and the USA D1 resection is advocated for these patients, and also the JGCA recommends a D1 resection for all EGCs that are clinically node negative and do not meet the criteria for EMR or ESD. In Japan and Korea an additional so-called D1+ lymphadenectomy is advocated for submucosal EGC with unfavourable features (poorly differentiated, size >1.5 cm) based on the 5% risk of second-tier lymph nodes.[30] D1+ lymphadenectomy includes a D1 lymphadenectomy plus a selective dissection of second-tier lymph nodes dependent on the location of the tumour (nodes 8a, 9 and 11p in total or proximal gastrectomy; 8a and 9 in distal or pylorus-preserving gastrectomy). However, no randomised controlled studies have been conducted that prove the usefulness of these selective additional lymphadenectomies.

Sentinel node biopsy

In breast cancer and melanoma surgery, sentinel lymph node biopsy (SLNB) has proved to be a valuable tool in lymph node mapping, with a sensitivity of more than 95%. When SLNB is negative in these tumours, lymphadenectomy can safely be omitted.

Obviously, gastric cancer patients with suspicious or proven lymph node metastases are not eligible for SLNB and a routine D2 lymphadenectomy is deployed. Also, in patients with advanced tumours (T3 and more) SLNB seems inappropriate. These patients already have a high probability of having first- or second-tier lymph node metastases. Moreover, in advanced tumours original lymphatic drainage routes might be obstructed or altered, resulting in a lower accuracy of the SLNB.

In EGC the incidence of lymph node metastasis is relatively low, i.e. approximately 3% for mucosal and 20% for submucosal tumours. Consequently, when D1 or D2 lymphadenectomy is performed for these tumours as part of standard surgical treatment, in the majority of patients no lymph node metastases are found. In these patients probably a less extensive resection without lymphadenectomy would probably have resulted in the same excellent disease-free survival rates, but without the inherent surgical morbidity and mortality.

Therefore, SLNB in EGC has been a focus for research in the past 10 years. Many different techniques and protocols have been employed. In most study protocols a double tracer method is preferred using a radioactive colloid, e.g. technetium-99 m, in combination with a dye agent such as isosulfan blue, patent blue violet or indocyanine green. The day before surgery the radioactive colloid is injected endoscopically in four quadrants into the submucosal layer at or in the vicinity of the primary lesion. The dye is injected intraoperatively in the same manner. By this means the sentinel node can be located by both a gamma probe for detection of a radioactive sentinel node and by visualisation of a blue or green coloured sentinel node.[64] Most studies show increased rates of successful identification of sentinel lymph nodes by combining both techniques.[65,66]

Various studies have shown the technical feasibility of SLNB in EGC. However, the accuracy of SLNB in gastric cancer remains to be determined. The difficulty of the SLNB technique in gastric cancer is that, unlike the single-course lymphatic flow in breast cancer, the lymphatic flow of the stomach is multidirectional, which can result in multiple sentinel lymph nodes located in different first-tier lymph node stations (greater and lesser curvature), but also in second-tier stations.[67,68]

✔✔ A meta-analysis[69] of 38 studies with 2128 patients with T1, T2 or T3 gastric cancer showed an identification rate of 93.7%, a sensitivity of 76.9%, a false-negative rate of 23.1% and a negative predictive value of 90.3%. These rates are very disappointing compared to SLNB in breast cancer and melanoma. It seems that identification rate, sensitivity and negative predictive value are decreased with an increase in T stage. For EGC a higher identification rate of 95.6% and an improved sensitivity of 81.6% have been reported.[69]

However, although it has been suggested that SLNB in gastric cancer is a useful tool for individualising the extent of lymphadenectomy in patients,[70] these figures are currently too low to justify the introduction of SLNB as a standard procedure in EGC.

Key points

- EGC is classified by the endoscopic appearance according to the Paris classification.
- This classification helps to predict the depth of infiltration into the submucosal layer and thus the choice between endoscopic or surgical treatment.
- Differentiated EGCs less than 30 mm in size and undifferentiated lesions without ulceration and less than 20 mm in size have a negligible chance of lymph node metastases.
- Endoscopic assessment of depth of infiltration in EGC has similar accuracy compared to endosonography.
- Submucosal dissection allows for an en bloc removal of EGC, full histopathological staging and also minimises the chance of local recurrence.
- Piecemeal resection of EGC is associated with relatively low rates of complete resection as compared to ESD, and local recurrence rates up to 26%.
- The most common complications of ESD/EMR are bleeding, perforations and post-treatment strictures.
- Perforation rates during ESD range from 1–4% in expert hands up to 20% with less expertise.
- Proximal gastrectomy for tumours in the upper third of the stomach is a safe procedure, with survival rates comparable to conventional total gastrectomy.
- Pylorus-preserving gastrectomy is feasible for early tumours in the middle third of the stomach with the distal border at least 3 cm proximal to the pylorus, with survival rates comparable to conventional distal gastrectomy.
- For EGC with unfavourable features (and therefore not eligible for endoscopic resection) local or segmental resection with only limited lymphadenectomy has to be considered investigational.
- Laparoscopic gastric resection for EGC is a technically safe procedure. Although randomised data are lacking, several non-randomised studies have shown that laparoscopic gastric resection may be oncologically justified.
- For EGC without clinical suspicion of positive lymph nodes (cN0), currently no evidence exists that D2 dissection can improve survival rates.
- The role of sentinel node biopsy in gastric cancer still has to be considered investigational.

References

1. The Paris endoscopic classification of superficial neoplastic lesions: esophagus, stomach, and colon: November 30 to December 1, 2002. Gastrointest Endosc 2003;58:S3–43.
2. de Vries AC, van Grieken NC, Looman CW, et al. Gastric cancer risk in patients with premalignant gastric lesions: a nationwide cohort study in the Netherlands. Gastroenterology 2008;134:945–52.
3. Dinis-Ribeiro M, Areia M, de Vries AC, et al. Management of precancerous conditions and lesions in the stomach (MAPS): guideline from the European Society of Gastrointestinal Endoscopy (ESGE), European Helicobacter Study Group (EHSG), European Society of Pathology (ESP), and the Sociedade Portuguesa de Endoscopia Digestiva (SPED). Endoscopy 2012;44:74–94.
4. Capelle LG, de Vries AC, Haringsma J, et al. The staging of gastritis with the OLGA system by using intestinal metaplasia as an accurate alternative for atrophic gastritis. Gastrointest Endosc 2010;71:1150–8.
5. Abe S, Oda I, Shimazu T, et al. Depth-predicting score for differentiated early gastric cancer. Gastric Cancer 2011;14:35–40.
6. Kato H, Haga S, Endo S, et al. Lifting of lesions during endoscopic mucosal resection (EMR) of early colorectal cancer: implications for the assessment of resectability. Endoscopy 2001;33:568–73.
7. Gotoda T, Yanagisawa A, Sasako M, et al. Incidence of lymph node metastasis from early gastric cancer: estimation with a large number of cases at two large centers. Gastric Cancer 2000;3:219–25.
8. Gotoda T, Yamamoto H, Soetikno RM. Endoscopic submucosal dissection of early gastric cancer. J Gastroenterol 2006;41:929–42.
   Based on histopathological assessment of 5265 gastrectomy specimens with formal lymph node dissections, it has been demonstrated that differentiated EGCs less than 30 mm in size and undifferentiated lesions without ulceration and less than 20 mm in size have a negligible risk of lymph node metastases.
9. Puli SR, Batapati Krishna Reddy J, Bechtold ML, et al. How good is endoscopic ultrasound for TNM staging of gastric cancers? A meta-analysis and systematic review. World J Gastroenterol 2008;14:4011–9.
10. Mouri R, Yoshida S, Tanaka S, et al. Usefulness of endoscopic ultrasonography in determining the depth of invasion and indication for endoscopic treatment of early gastric cancer. J Clin Gastroenterol 2009;43:318–22.
11. Okada K, Fujisaki J, Kasuga A, et al. Endoscopic ultrasonography is valuable for identifying early gastric cancers meeting expanded-indication criteria for endoscopic submucosal dissection. Surg Endosc 2011;25:841–8.
12. May A, Gunter E, Roth F, et al. Accuracy of staging in early oesophageal cancer using high resolution endoscopy and high resolution endosonography: a comparative, prospective, and blinded trial. Gut 2004;53:634–40.
13. Dixon MF. Gastrointestinal epithelial neoplasia: Vienna revisited. Gut 2002;51:130–1.
14. Ono H, Kondo H, Gotoda T, et al. Endoscopic mucosal resection for treatment of early gastric cancer. Gut 2001;48:225–9.
15. Hirao M, Masuda K, Asanuma T, et al. Endoscopic resection of early gastric cancer and other tumors with local injection of hypertonic saline–epinephrine. Gastrointest Endosc 1988;34:264–9.
16. Inoue H, Endo M. Endoscopic esophageal mucosal resection using a transparent tube. Surg Endosc 1990;4:198–201.
17. Tada M, Murakami A, Karita M, et al. Endoscopic resection of early gastric cancer. Endoscopy 1993;25:445–50.
18. Alvarez Herrero L, Pouw RE, van Vilsteren FG, et al. Safety and efficacy of multiband mucosectomy in 1060 resections in Barrett's esophagus. Endoscopy 2011;43:177–83.
19. Yahagi N, Neuhaus H, Schumacher B, et al. Comparison of standard endoscopic submucosal dissection (ESD) versus an optimized ESD technique for the colon: an animal study. Endoscopy 2009;41:340–5.
20. Isomoto H, Nishiyama H, Yamaguchi N, et al. Clinicopathological factors associated with clinical outcomes of endoscopic submucosal dissection for colorectal epithelial neoplasms. Endoscopy 2009;41:679–83.
21. Tanaka S, Oka S, Kaneko I, et al. Endoscopic submucosal dissection for colorectal neoplasia: possibility of standardization. Gastrointest Endosc 2007;66:100–7.
22. Nakamoto S, Sakai Y, Kasanuki J, et al. Indications for the use of endoscopic mucosal resection for early gastric cancer in Japan: a comparative study with endoscopic submucosal dissection. Endoscopy 2009;41:746–50.
   Compared to EMR, ESD allows for higher en bloc resection rates (94.3% vs. 53.8%, *P*<0.001) and overall 5-year recurrence-free rates (100% vs. 82.5%, *P*<0.001) for EGCs larger than 10 mm in size.
23. Nasu J, Doi T, Endo H, et al. Characteristics of metachronous multiple early gastric cancers after endoscopic mucosal resection. Endoscopy 2005;37:990–3.
24. Jang JS, Choi SR, Graham DY, et al. Risk factors for immediate and delayed bleeding associated with endoscopic submucosal dissection of gastric neoplastic lesions. Scand J Gastroenterol 2009;44:1370–6.
25. Coda S, Trentino P, Antonellis F, et al. A Western single-center experience with endoscopic submucosal

dissection for early gastrointestinal cancers. Gastric Cancer 2010;13:258–63.

26. Deprez PH, Bergman JJ, Meisner S, et al. Current practice with endoscopic submucosal dissection in Europe: position statement from a panel of experts. Endoscopy 2010;42:853–8.
27. Minami S, Gotoda T, Ono H, et al. Complete endoscopic closure of gastric perforation induced by endoscopic resection of early gastric cancer using endoclips can prevent surgery (with video). Gastrointest Endosc 2006;63:596–601.
28. Jeon SW, Jung MK, Kim SK, et al. Clinical outcomes for perforations during endoscopic submucosal dissection in patients with gastric lesions. Surg Endosc 2010;24:911–6.
29. Manta R, Manno M, Bertani H, et al. Endoscopic treatment of gastrointestinal fistulas using an over-the-scope clip (OTSC) device: case series from a tertiary referral center. Endoscopy 2011;43:545–8.
30. Japanese Gastric Cancer Association. Japanese gastric cancer treatment guidelines 2010 (ver. 3). Gastric Cancer 2011;14:113–23.
31. Kaibara N, Nishimura O, Nishidoi H, et al. Proximal gastrectomy as the surgical procedure of choice for upper gastric carcinoma. J Surg Oncol 1987;36:110–2.
32. Katai H, Sano T, Fukagawa T, et al. Prospective study of proximal gastrectomy for early gastric cancer in the upper third of the stomach. Br J Surg 2003;90:850–3.
33. Shiraishi N, Adachi Y, Kitano S, et al. Clinical outcome of proximal versus total gastrectomy for proximal gastric cancer. World J Surg 2002;26: 1150–4.
34. An JY, Youn HG, Choi MG, et al. The difficult choice between total and proximal gastrectomy in proximal early gastric cancer. Am J Surg 2008;196:587–91.
35. Kondoh Y, Okamoto Y, Morita M, et al. Clinical outcome of proximal gastrectomy in patients with early gastric cancer in the upper third of the stomach. Tokai J Exp Clin Med 2007;32:48–53.
36. Harrison LE, Karpeh MS, Brennan MF. Total gastrectomy is not necessary for proximal gastric cancer. Surgery 1998;123:127–30.
37. Maki T, Shiratori T, Hatafuku T, et al. Pylorus-preserving gastrectomy as an improved operation for gastric ulcer. Surgery 1967;61:838–45.
38. Hiki N, Kaminishi M. Pylorus-preserving gastrectomy in gastric cancer surgery – open and laparoscopic approaches. Langenbeck's Arch Surg 2005;390:442–7.
39. Shibata C, Shiiba KI, Funayama Y, et al. Outcomes after pylorus-preserving gastrectomy for early gastric cancer: a prospective multicenter trial. World J Surg 2004;28:857–61.
40. Nakajima T, Yamaguchi T. Gastric cancer data base in Cancer Institute, Japan, 1946–2004. Tokyo: Kanehara; 2006.
41. Hiki N, Sano T, Fukunaga T, et al. Survival benefit of pylorus-preserving gastrectomy in early gastric cancer. J Am Coll Surg 2009;209:297–301.
42. Seto Y, Nagawa H, Muto Y, et al. Preliminary report on local resection with lymphadenectomy for early gastric cancer. Br J Surg 1999;86:526–8.
43. Seto Y, Yamaguchi H, Shimoyama S, et al. Results of local resection with regional lymphadenectomy for early gastric cancer. Am J Surg 2001;182:498–501.
44. Ohwada S, Nakamura S, Ogawa T, et al. Segmental gastrectomy for early cancer in the mid-stomach. Hepatogastroenterology 1999;46:1229–33.
45. Shinohara T, Ohyama S, Muto T, et al. Clinical outcome of high segmental gastrectomy for early gastric cancer in the upper third of the stomach. Br J Surg 2006;93:975–80.
46. Chen XZ, Hu JK, Yang K, et al. Short-term evaluation of laparoscopy-assisted distal gastrectomy for predictive early gastric cancer: a meta-analysis of randomized controlled trials. Surg Laparosc Endosc Percutan Tech 2009;19:277–84.
47. Kitano S, Shiraishi N, Uyama I, et al., Japanese Laparoscopic Surgery Study Group. A multicenter study on oncologic outcome of laparoscopic gastrectomy for early cancer in Japan. Ann Surg 2007;245:68–72.
48. Lee SW, Nomura E, Bouras G, et al. Long-term oncologic outcomes from laparoscopic gastrectomy for gastric cancer: a single-center experience of 601 consecutive resections. J Am Coll Surg 2010;211:33–40.
    This meta-analysis of six randomised controlled trials and two large retrospective studies showed that laparoscopic gastric resection for EGC is a technically safe procedure.
49. Huscher CG, Mingoli A, Sgarzini G, et al. Laparoscopic versus open subtotal gastrectomy for distal gastric cancer: five-year results of a randomized prospective trial. Ann Surg 2005;241:232–7.
50. Strong VE, Devaud N, Allen PJ, et al. Laparoscopic versus open subtotal gastrectomy for adenocarcinoma: a case–control study. Ann Surg Oncol 2009;16:1507–13.
51. Cho WY, Kim YJ, Cho JY, et al. Hybrid natural orifice transluminal endoscopic surgery: endoscopic full-thickness resection of early gastric cancer and laparoscopic regional lymph node dissection – 14 human cases. Endoscopy 2011;43:134–9.
52. Saka M, Katai H, Fukagawa T, et al. Recurrence in early gastric cancer with lymph node metastasis. Gastric Cancer 2008;11:214–8.
53. Cady B. Lymph node metastases. Indicators, but not governors of survival. Arch Surg 1984;119:1067–72.

54. Bonenkamp JJ, Hermans J, Sasako M, et al. Extended lymph-node dissection for gastric cancer. N Engl J Med 1999;340:908–14.

55. Cuschieri A, Weeden S, Fielding J, et al. Patient survival after D1 and D2 resections for gastric cancer: long-term results of the MRC randomized surgical trial. Surgical Co-operative Group. Br J Cancer 1999;79:1522–30.

56. Hartgrink HH, van de Velde CJ, Putter H, et al. Extended lymph node dissection for gastric cancer: who may benefit? Final results of the randomized Dutch Gastric Cancer Group trial. J Clin Oncol 2004;22:2069–77.

These two large randomised studies compared D1 and D2 resection for gastric cancer. Both studies show no survival benefit or decreased relapse rate, while morbidity and mortality were increased. For EGC currently no evidence exists that D2 resection can improve survival rates.

57. Wu CW, Hsiung CA, Lo SS, et al. Nodal dissection for patients with gastric cancer: a randomised controlled trial. Lancet Oncol 2006;7:309–15.

58. Hirasawa T, Gotoda T, Miyata S, et al. Incidence of lymph node metastasis and the feasibility of endoscopic resection for undifferentiated-type early gastric cancer. Gastric Cancer 2009;12:148–52.

59. An JY, Baik YH, Choi MG, et al. Predictive factors for lymph node metastasis in early gastric cancer with submucosal invasion: analysis of a single institutional experience. Ann Surg 2007;246:749–53.

60. Hayes N, Karat D, Scott DJ, et al. Radical lymphadenectomy in the management of early gastric cancer. Br J Surg 1996;83:1421–3.

61. Popiela T, Kulig J, Kolodziejczyk P, et al., Polish Gastric Cancer Study Group. Long-term results of surgery for early gastric cancer. Br J Surg 2002;89: 1035–42.

62. Nakamura K, Morisaki T, Sugitani A, et al. An early gastric carcinoma treatment strategy based on analysis of lymph node metastasis. Cancer 1999;85:1500–5.

63. Kunisaki C, Shimada H, Nomura M, et al. Appropriate lymph node dissection for early gastric cancer based on lymph node metastases. Surgery 2001;129:153–7.

64. Kitagawa Y, Saikawa Y, Takeuchi H, et al. Sentinel node navigation in early stage gastric cancer – updated data and current status. Scand J Surg 2006;95:256–9.

65. Lee JH, Ryu KW, Kim CG, et al. Sentinel node biopsy using dye and isotope double tracers in early gastric cancer. Ann Surg Oncol 2006;13:1168–74.

66. Park do J, Kim HH, Park YS, et al. Simultaneous indocyanine green and (99m)Tc-antimony sulfur colloid-guided laparoscopic sentinel basin dissection for gastric cancer. Ann Surg Oncol 2011;18:160–5.

67. Kelder W, Nimura H, Takahashi N, et al. Sentinel node mapping with indocyanine green (ICG) and infrared ray detection in early gastric cancer: an accurate method that enables a limited lymphadenectomy. Eur J Surg Oncol 2010;36:552–8.

68. Kitagawa Y, Fujii H, Kumai K, et al. Recent advances in sentinel node navigation for gastric cancer: a paradigm shift of surgical management. J Surg Oncol 2005;90:147–52.

69. Wang Z, Dong ZY, Chen JQ, et al. Diagnostic value of sentinel lymph node biopsy in gastric cancer: a meta-analysis. Ann Surg Oncol 2012;19(5): 1541–50.

A meta-analysis of 38 studies on SLNB for gastric cancer reports a sensitivity of only 76.9% and a false-negative rate of 23.1%. Currently, the reliability of SLNB for gastric cancer is too low for clinical practice.

70. Ichikura T, Chochi K, Sugasawa H, et al. Individualized surgery for early gastric cancer guided by sentinel node biopsy. Surgery 2006;139:501–7.

9

Radiotherapy and chemotherapy in treatment of oesophageal and gastric cancer

Tom Crosby
Adrian Crellin

Introduction

The treatment of oesophagogastric cancer has become more complex, with evidence of the benefits of multimodality therapy. The limitations of surgery alone in producing acceptable long-term survival rates have driven the changing patterns of management of both oesophageal and gastric cancer. Improvements in staging, imaging and pathology have demonstrated that the majority of patients present with either locally advanced or metastatic disease. High local recurrence rates and early failure with metastatic disease are easier to understand in past series of patients who would have been accepted as operable and treated as potentially curable. In addition, the changing pattern of disease, with rapidly increasing rates of adenocarcinoma of the distal oesophagus and oesophagogastric junction but reducing numbers of cancers of the body and antrum of the stomach, challenges the interpretation of historical trials and may necessitate a different approach to treatment.

Oncology is moving steadily towards a more personalised therapeutic approach. The factors that may determine treatment choice can be broadly divided into factors relating to the patient and those to their disease. The former may include age, performance status, comorbidities/physiological fitness and their preference for one treatment modality over another. Disease factors may include macroscopic features such as the location of disease in the oesophagus and stomach and local invasions of mediastinal structures, and microscopic features such as histological type and biological characteristics. Again, more research is required to determine biomarkers that may predict response to specific therapies.

The identification of improved activity when chemotherapy and radiotherapy are given synchronously has already led to chemoradiotherapy (CRT) becoming the primary organ-preserving approach in anal, cervix and certain head and neck cancers, with surgery being reserved for salvage.[1,2] There is now good evidence that primary CRT has a role in oesophageal cancer treatment.

With mounting evidence of the benefit of a multidisciplinary approach to care and assessment, it is important for surgeons and oncologists to understand more of the strengths and weaknesses of their own and each other's treatments. This will necessitate a greater effort to improve and standardise information disclosure regarding different therapeutic approaches. Only then can treatment be truly integrated and improved outcomes achieved with minimal morbidity.

Both oesophageal and gastric cancers have high response rates to chemotherapy, although they are disappointingly short. There is a clearly established role for chemotherapy in palliative treatment of advanced and metastatic disease. It has taken longer to confirm and define the role for its use in the neoadjuvant or adjuvant setting. In the relatively unusual finding of early disease, single modality disease may produce excellent results and certainly does not justify the additional toxicities that accompany multimodality disease. However, in the vast majority of diagnoses suitable for a potentially curative approach, combinations of chemotherapy, radiotherapy and surgery have led to improved outcomes, although the exact role and timing of these modalities is the subject of ongoing research.

The definition of adjuvant treatment and potentially curative therapy is worth stressing. Adjuvant therapy usually means additional treatment given after potentially curative therapy, in an attempt to improve the long-term outcome. Neoadjuvant therapy is the use of a treatment prior to planned definitive therapy such as surgery or radiotherapy. The role of chemotherapy and radiotherapy should be seen in the context of how they combine with surgery to alter patterns of relapse and improve survival or provide a viable alternative to surgery. In this context, surgery can really only be described as potentially curative if the tumour is resected with no residual macroscopic disease and clear histological margins (R0), in the absence of metastatic disease.

The following sections are intended to allow the role of chemotherapy and radiotherapy to be put into context, and the strength of evidence assessed. The sections on potentially curative approaches are more detailed. This is the area in which most treatment will be integrated with surgery in current or future approaches.

Oesophageal cancer

Potentially curative treatment

The following sections will review the numerous possible combinations and trials of combined modality therapy. As well as the use of specific treatment modalities, the timing of such treatment has been extensively studied. Some general principles regarding the timing of adjuvant therapies are outlined.

Theoretical and generic issues of preoperative versus postoperative therapy treatment include:

Advantages

- a more easily defined target volume;
- improved tumour oxygenation at the time of treatment;
- the potential to improve resectability and reduce the impact of tumour cell spillage at surgery;
- improved chance of an R0 resection and thereby the reduction of local recurrence;
- improved chance of treating micrometastatic disease;
- patient likely to be better able to tolerate adjuvant therapy prior to major surgery than following it;
- may improve swallowing and therefore nutrition prior to surgery;
- spare those patients that progress early with metastatic disease major surgery.

Disadvantages

- the overtreatment of some patients that will not benefit from non-targeted therapy as opposed to targeting patients with factors that may determine the likely risk and site of residual disease;
- may make patient less well physiologically prior to major surgery, increasing risk of perioperative morbidity and mortality;
- may allow disease progression prior to definitive treatment.

Preoperative radiotherapy alone

This approach has been shown to be of value in rectal cancer.[3] There have been six randomised trials of preoperative radiotherapy. Three trials were restricted to squamous carcinoma. One of these, by Gignoux et al., reported an improvement in local/regional recurrence (46% vs. 67%).[4] Nygaard et al. report improved survival, but this series is complicated by the inclusion of some patients also receiving chemotherapy.[5] One trial included both squamous and adenocarcinoma,[6] and two do not specify the histology. Overall it is difficult to draw firm conclusions from these trials.

✔✔ A meta-analysis of updated individual patient data from 1147 patients in randomised trials reported a hazard ratio of 0.89 (95% confidence interval (CI) 0.78–1.01) with an absolute survival benefit of 4% at 5 years.[7] This result did not reach conventional statistical significance. The benefit therefore seems likely to be small, if present, and with little evidence of improved resectability.

Postoperative radiotherapy

Postoperative radiotherapy can be challenging in terms of tolerance for the refashioned gastric conduit, avoiding the critical normal tissues such as the spinal cord with a posteriorly placed anastomosis and where the anastomosis is situated some distance proximal to the surgical bed, if both require treatment.

There are four randomised trials in the literature. The numbers are small (totalling 843 adjuvant patients), and three out of the four include only squamous carcinoma. Teniere et al.[8] showed no survival advantage in 221 patients. There was a small improvement in the failure rate but at the cost of significant side-effects. The benefit appears to be limited to node-negative patients. Fok et al.[9] included both adenocarcinoma and squamous carcinoma. Whilst both curative and palliative resections were included, the patients were separately analysed and received different radiotherapy doses. The results show a significant morbidity (37%) and mortality related to bleeding from the transposed intrathoracic stomach. It should be noted that the dose per fraction of the radiotherapy was high (3.5 Gy), which may be significant. There was a lower intrathoracic recurrence rate, particularly relating to tracheobronchial disease.

A larger randomised study from China included 495 well-staged patients with squamous carcinoma randomised to receive either surgery alone (S) or surgery and postoperative radiotherapy (S+R).[10] Whilst there are significant concerns about the ethics (the patients were not aware they were in a trial and so did not give appropriate consent), the study was still published because of its significant results. The surgery appears to be of a high standard and included a radical lymph node dissection. The radiotherapy was wide field and included the bilateral supraclavicular fossae (SCF), mediastinum and anastomosis to an initial dose of 40 Gy. A further 10 Gy was given to the SCF and 20 Gy to the mediastinum by a different technique, allowing a maximum dose to the transposed stomach of 50 Gy. There was a relatively high proportion of earlier stage IIA disease in the study compared with a UK population. The analysis showed a highly significant difference in 1-, 3- and 5-year survival in stage III disease between the S and S+R arms (67.5%, 23.3%, 13.1% vs. 75.5%, 43.2%, 35.1%, respectively). The pattern of relapse was different between the two arms, with significantly fewer recurrences in the neck, SCF and mediastinum. Unlike other studies, toxicity to the transposed stomach was minimal.

The role of postoperative radiotherapy-based treatment in the case of a histological R1 resection is even less clear. There have been no randomised trials addressing this group of patients; indeed, the quality of reporting of circumferential resection margin (CRM) involvement by microscopic disease, which is influenced by postoperative surgical dissection of the operative specimen, is variable. In the absence of randomised evidence, the knowledge that radiotherapy has a proven role in oesophageal cancer probably justifies considering patients with longitudinal resection margin involvement for postoperative radiotherapy on an individual patient basis. When undertaken, there is some evidence that one should attempt to encompass both the anastamosis and the tumour bed but in the case of a high anastomosis for a lower oesophageal cancer, which is difficult to see radiologically, this can be challenging and requires specialised multidisciplinary input. The role for radiotherapy treatment in the case of CRM involvement is unclear, but it would seem sensible to target those patients where the risk of systemic disease relapse is lower, i.e. those with a lower ratio of involved lymph nodes.[11]

✔ There is thus reasonable evidence that postoperative radiotherapy may be offered to pathological stage III squamous carcinoma of the oesophagus. To translate the results into UK practice, where many patients will have had preoperative chemotherapy, would require a step away from a pure evidence base, but is perhaps justifiable given the effect on relapse patterns. For adenocarcinoma the justification is less clear outside the context of a clinical trial. Use for patients with an R1, resection should be given within the context of specialised multidisciplinary team care with adequate expertise in radiology, pathology, surgery and oncology, taking into account risk of local failure, i.e. longitudinal or CRM involved margins, involved lymph node burden and postoperative patient fitness.

Preoperative chemotherapy

Preoperative chemotherapy in both squamous and adenocarcinoma appears to achieve consistently good clinical response rates, ranging from 47% to 61%.[12,13] Early studies, predominantly in squamous carcinoma, used combinations of cisplatin, vindesine and bleomycin. More recently, cisplatin and 5-fluorouracil (5-FU) combinations have been used in important randomised trials. New 5-hydroxytryptamine-3 (5-HT_3) antagonist antiemetic drugs have allowed cisplatin to be used with dramatically reduced toxicity. Protracted venous infusion (PVI) of 5-FU, and more recently capecitabine, an oral 5-FU prodrug, in combination with cisplatin and epirubicin (the ECF regimen) has produced increased response rates in non-randomised studies. These more modern cisplatin–5-FU combinations seem to be active in both squamous[14] and adenocarcinoma,[13] although the benefit of anthracycline therapy, i.e. epirubicin, in squamous cell carcinoma is less certain and is therefore often omitted.

Randomised trials of preoperative chemotherapy

The American Intergroup Trial (INT 0113) produced data on 440 randomised patients with a median follow-up of 46.5 months.[15] Adenocarcinoma (54%) was the predominant histology. The chemotherapy given was three preoperative courses (cisplatin and 5 days of infusional 5-FU) and in stable or responding patients two postoperative courses. Overall, 83% of patients received the intended two preoperative cycles of chemotherapy. However, only 32% of patients received both postoperative chemotherapy cycles. There was no difference in treatment-related mortality between the two arms (6% surgery (S) vs. 7% chemotherapy (C)+surgery (S); P=0.33). On an intent-to-treat basis there was no difference in median survival (16.1 months C+S vs. 14.9 months S), and 1-, 2- and 3-year (23% C+S vs. 26% S) survivals. Disappointingly, there was no difference in the pattern of metastatic disease between the two arms. However, there was a significantly higher rate of R1 resections in the surgery-alone arm.

The Medical Research Council (MRC) OEO2 study is the largest and arguably the most influential trial in this area.[16] A total of 802 patients were randomised to receive two courses of cisplatin and a 4-day infusion of 5-FU followed by surgery (CS) after 3–5 weeks or immediate surgery alone (S) and showed a significant survival advantage for patients receiving preoperative chemotherapy.

The majority of patients (66%) had adenocarcinoma histology. The two arms appear balanced and criticisms of the staging, which was relatively poor by modern standards and could have been as little as a chest radiograph and an abdominal ultrasound, are largely mitigated by the size of the study. The majority of patients in the CS arm received both of the cycles of chemotherapy (90%), with another 6% having just one cycle. The overall operation rate was similar in both arms but there was a significant difference in the microscopic complete resection rate (60% CS vs. 53% S; P<0.0001). There was good evidence for a downstaging effect in terms of size of primary and extent of nodal involvement. The postoperative mortality was equivalent in both arms at 10%.

The overall survival rate was significantly improved with preoperative chemotherapy (P=0.004; hazard ratio 0.79, CI 0.67–0.93), with an estimated reduction in risk of death of 21% and 2-year survival figures of 43% CS vs. 34% S. There was no evidence that the effect of chemotherapy varied with histology. Long-term follow-up with a median follow-up of 6 years has confirmed these results, with 5-year survivals of 23% CS vs. 17% S.[17]

The differing results between the two US and European trials are difficult to explain. Concerns about a low operation rate of 80% in the chemotherapy arm of the Intergroup Trial may reflect the more ambitious and prolonged chemotherapy regimen, leading to more toxicity. In the MRC trial there was no real difference in the rate of death from cancer and one could hypothesise that the important determinant of survival is the achievement of a potentially curative R0 resection, enhanced by the local downstaging effect of chemotherapy (it must remembered this trial was performed in the era prior to improved staging with endoscopic ultrasound (EUS) and computed tomography (CT)/positron emission tomography (PET) scans). Any factor that precludes such a resection, resulting from chemotherapy, such as excess toxicity or delay in surgery in non-responding patients, might counter any gains in the responding patients.

✔✔ An updated Cochrane review of 11 randomised trials involving 2051 patients concludes that there was a 21% increase in survival at 3 years with preoperative chemotherapy, but that statistical significance was not reached until 5 years.[18] Increased toxicity and mortality due to chemotherapy were evident and the pathological complete response (pCR) rate was a disappointing 3%. Preoperative chemotherapy has been adopted as a standard of care in the UK, although chemoradiation is more widely used in the USA.

The recently completed MRC/NCRI trial in the UK (OEO5) compared OEO2 chemotherapy with four cycles of ECX (epirubicin–cisplatin–capecitabine) in adenocarcinoma alone. The high completion rate and positive results of preoperative chemotherapy in the MRC MAGIC (ST02) study[19] for gastric and gastro-oesophageal cancer pointed to the strategy of using a modified ECF regimen, which is accepted in the UK as the best standard of care for advanced gastro-oesophageal cancer, and using it in a neoadjuvant setting to try and improve on the results of OEO2. The results of the REAL2 study,[20] a phase III trial of palliative chemotherapy, showed that the oral fluoropyrimidine (capecitabine) could be substituted for infusional 5-FU with safety and at least equivalent efficacy. The advantage of easier chemotherapy delivery without the use of Hickman lines and their associated morbidity is a step forward. This study is also important in that it places an emphasis on high-quality assurance of staging, surgery, chemotherapy and pathology. There is little doubt that at least one of the reasons for differing results in trials in the whole area of gastro-oesophageal cancer has been a wide variation in the quality of staging modalities and surgery, as well as the heterogeneity in the regimens tested and trial design. The MRC OEO5 trial attempted to set high standards that should translate into improved patient selection and outcomes, even within the control arm.

Postoperative chemotherapy

There are few useful trials that address the question of adjuvant postoperative chemotherapy. The trials reported by Roth et al.[21] and Kelsen et al.[15] both have an adjuvant component, coupled with preoperative treatment. The fact that only 32% completed the postoperative phase in the Intergroup study underlines a problem with this approach.[15] Patients undergoing major resections for oesophageal carcinoma often have a prolonged postoperative phase. The start of chemotherapy may be delayed due to performance status. Patients may also choose not to continue. A strategy that relies solely on postoperative treatment may have significant problems. Improved patient selection and postoperative supportive care may allow this approach to be practical. The MAGIC gastric cancer trial latterly included tumours of the gastro-oesophageal junction and lower oesophagus and intended three postoperative courses of ECF as well as three given preoperatively in the protocol. Again, only 40% completed the postoperative chemotherapy. The trial has shown an improvement in overall survival, as described in the section on gastric cancer,[19] which lends further support for the concept of neoadjuvant chemotherapy for cancers of the oesophagus or gastro-oesophageal junction.

Preoperative chemoradiotherapy

The rationale in using chemotherapy and radiotherapy together is that enhanced tumour cell kill might lead to improved outcomes. Chemotherapy can lead to a decreased ability of tumour cells to repair radiation-induced DNA damage. Many of the commonly used chemotherapy drugs with significant activity in oesophageal and gastric cancer appear to be radiation sensitisers (5-FU, cisplatin, mitomycin C and taxanes). There is good evidence that pCR rates are significantly higher with CRT than with radiotherapy or chemotherapy given alone. There is the significant attraction of achieving enhanced local therapy coupled with a systemic benefit as sought with preoperative chemotherapy alone. When added to surgery, it is not clear that pCR is necessarily the only useful end-point. Preoperative CRT has the added advantage in providing direct evidence to guide the process of developing and optimising combination chemotherapy and radiotherapy schedules for use as definitive treatments.

Both radiotherapy and chemotherapy rely on achieving an acceptable balance between increased response rates in the tumour on one hand and normal tissue morbidity coupled with patient tolerance on the other. Whilst many of the side-effects of chemotherapy are relatively early in presentation, for example hair loss, emesis and myelosuppression, radiotherapy side-effects can present late, from 6 months to years out from treatment. If radical surgery is added in combined modality therapy then the potential for high levels of morbidity becomes significant.

Non-randomised studies of CRT have appeared in the literature since the late 1980s. The review article by Geh et al.[22] summarises 46 trials containing 20 patients or more. Overall, pooled data from these studies show that, of 2704 patients (squamous 68% and adenocarcinoma 32%), 79% were operated on with a pCR rate of 24% of those treated and 32% of those resected. As experience with this modality of treatment has grown, lessons have been learned. Attempts to escalate the dose of radiotherapy can lead to unacceptable rates of morbidity, especially if higher doses per fraction are used.[23,24] Reported CRT-related deaths in the non-randomised series ranged from 0% to 15% (mean 3%). Postoperative deaths ranged from 0% to 29% (mean 9%). Adult respiratory distress syndrome, anastomotic leak and breakdown, pneumonia and sepsis were the commonest causes of death following oesophageal resection. Treatment-related deaths ranged from 3% to 25% (mean 9%) of all patients treated. It seems clear that the risk of chemotherapy-related toxicity, particularly myelosuppression, rises with the number of drugs used and the intensity of the CRT regimen.[25,26] An increased risk of tracheobronchial fistula has been reported.[27] However, most of the reported series did not have the latest sophisticated radiotherapy techniques that allow greater precision and sparing of organs and tissues to within normal tissue tolerance.

Consistent reporting of pathology is important, and a grading of CRT response has been described by Mandard et al.[28] Five grades of response ranging from no identifiable tumour to complete absence of regression allow a more objective approach to be adopted. In this paper the significant predictor of disease-free survival after multivariate analysis was the tumour regression grade. There is evidence that pCR confers a survival advantage over those patients not achieving pCR.[29–34] In **Fig. 9.1**, different comparative outcomes, such as median survival in months, overall or disease-free survival in years, are plotted together in the series, quoting outcomes separately. The importance is in the consistent nature of the difference in outcomes in each series. It becomes clear that prediction of this response prior to treatment either through molecular markers or PET activity after induction chemotherapy alone might allow very different algorithms of treatment modalities (also see Chapter 3).

Table 9.1 summarises nine reported randomised trials of preoperative CRT compared with surgery alone. In four of these the chemotherapy was given sequentially to the radiotherapy and in four synchronously. Two trials using sequential treatment in squamous carcinoma received relatively low doses of radiotherapy and showed no convincing evidence of improved survival with the combined treatment.[6,35] In a larger European Organisation for Research and Treatment of Cancer (EORTC) trial involving 282 patients, the cisplatin chemotherapy was given in close sequence with the radiotherapy.[24] The radiotherapy was given in a split course and at a relatively high dose per fraction (two courses of 18.5 Gy in five daily fractions split 2 weeks apart). The CRT patients were more likely to have a curative resection. The disease-free survival was significantly longer (3-year CRT+S 40% vs. S 28%). There was

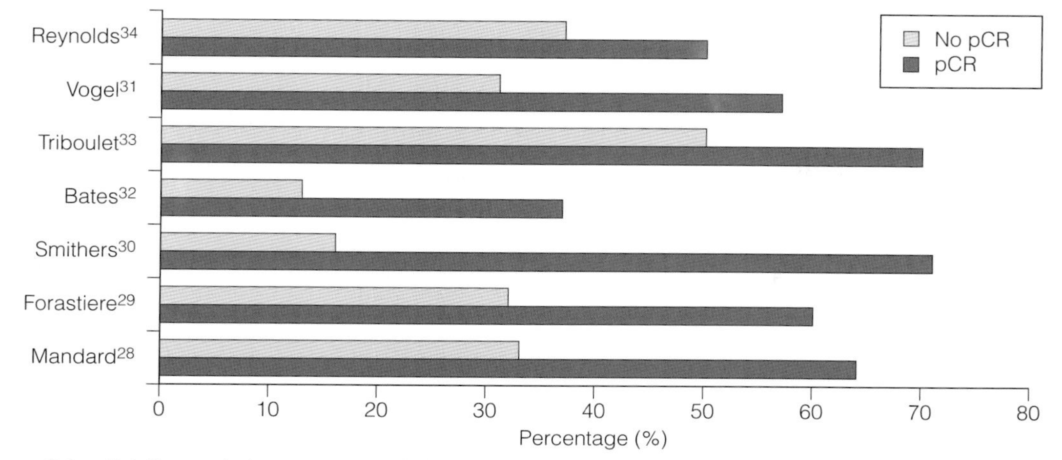

Figure 9.1 • Relative survival outcomes – pathological complete response (pCR) to CRT.

no difference in the overall survival, largely due to a significantly higher postoperative mortality in the CRT arm (12% vs. 4%). Apinop et al.[36] reported a synchronous CRT series of 69 squamous histology patients with no improvement in survival.

There are four larger trials of preoperative synchronous CRT.

✔✔ The Walsh et al. study has been influential in changing practice, particularly in the USA.[37] In 113 patients with adenocarcinoma, cisplatin and 5-FU were given with 40 Gy in 3 weeks of radiotherapy. There was an overall survival benefit in favour of the CRT arm (median 16 months vs. 11 months; 3-year survival 32% vs. 6%). Morbidity in this series was not inconsiderable. The radiotherapy technique and fractionation may explain this. Most open to question, however, is the noticeably poor survival in the surgery alone control arm. The basic standards of staging could potentially have led to an imbalance of true staging in the treatment arms.

The University of Michigan trial[38] randomised 100 patients including both squamous and adenocarcinoma. The surgery was a transhiatal resection. Patients in the CRT arm received 45 Gy in 30 fractions with cisplatin, 5-FU and vinblastine. At first analysis there was no significant difference between the arms but at 3 years a statistically significant benefit to the combined treatment emerged, with overall survival of 32% vs. 15%. A final analysis has shown no survival advantage and demonstrates the danger of early publication of a trial that was essentially underpowered.

The results of the Australasian Gastro-Intestinal Trials Group (AGITG)[39] have been criticised for having a low radiotherapy dose and only one cycle of cisplatin and 5-FU chemotherapy. Although the trial was negative overall there are some clues for the direction of future approaches. There was a significant survival difference in patients with squamous histology (36% of the total) with the addition of CRT and a much higher pathological complete response rate.

The US trial NCCTG-C9781 (CALGB 9781) closed prematurely as a result of poor recruitment due to a reluctance to recruit patients to a trial with a no treatment arm. However, mature results from CALGB 9781 are available and despite small numbers show a significant improvement in overall survival in preoperative CRT compared to surgery alone (5-year survival of 39% vs. 16%).[40] Resection rates were high in the preoperative CRT arm (87%) and there was no increase in operative mortality. The trial included higher quality staging and surgery.

Interpretation of such heterogeneous trials, in the regimen being tested, design and outcomes, is difficult. Nevertheless, a meta-analysis of randomised trials has shown that this approach increases R0 resection rates, reduces locoregional recurrence and improves survival compared with surgery alone.[41] More recently, and not included in the meta-analysis above, a randomised phase III study comparing surgery alone to preoperative CRT has shown a near doubling of overall survival (OS) in favour of the preoperative arm (OS 49 vs. 26 months, hazard ratio (HR) 0.67), a pCR rate of 32% and no increase in surgical mortality (3.8% (S) vs. 3.4% (CRT-S)).[42] In the 'CROSS' trial, 363 patients with operable oesophageal or gastro-oesophageal junction tumours were randomised to surgery alone or to a preoperative CRT regimen of weekly carboplatin (AUC2) and paclitaxel (50 mg/m^2) concurrent

Table 9.1 • Randomised trials of preoperative chemoradiation

Reference	Sequential or concurrent	Squamous or adenocarcinoma	Patients	Chemo*	Radiotherapy dose (Gy)	Resection rate	Mortality in CRT arm	Result†
Nygaard et al.[5]	Seq	Sq	88	Cis–Bleo	35	66%	24%	Negative
Le Prise et al.[35]	Seq	Sq	86	Cis–5-FU	20	85%	8%	Negative
Bosset et al.[24]	Seq	Sq	282	Cis	37	78%	12%	Improved DFS only
Apinop et al.[36]	Con	Sq	69	Cis–5-FU	40	74%	12%	Negative
Walsh et al.[37]	Con	Adeno	113	Cis–5-FU	40	90%	10%	Improved OS
Urba et al.[38]	Con	Adeno/Sq	100	Cis–5-FU–Vbl	45	Not reported	Not reported	Negative
Burmeister et al.[39]	Con	Adeno/Sq	256	Cis–5-FU	35	85%	4.6%	Negative
Tepper et al.[40]	Con	Adeno/Sq	56	Cis–5-FU	50.4	87%	0%	Improved OS
Gaast et al.[42]	Con	Adeno/Sq	363	Carbo–Tax	41.6	90%	3.4%	Improved OS

*Bleo, bleomycin; Carbo, carboplatin; Cis, cisplatin; 5-FU, 5-fluorouracil; Tax, paclitaxel; Vbl, vinblastine.
†DFS, disease-free survival; OS, overall survival.

with radiotherapy (41.4 Gy in 23 fractions). Of the 175 patients assigned to the CRT arm, 163 completed protocol treatment and the study reported a low incidence of grade 3/4 CRT toxicity (haematological, 6.8%; non-haematological, 16%). The R0 resection rates in the surgery and CRT+surgery arms were 67% and 92.3%, respectively (P=0.002). The results of this study, performed in patients with a similar stage and morphological distribution to those in the UK, would suggest that where preoperative CRT is delivered safely, this may lead to a significant improvement in outcome.

Neoadjuvant chemoradiotherapy or chemotherapy?

There are still major questions to be answered, but a surgery-alone arm is not likely to be considered acceptable in the UK or in the USA for stage III disease. The good outcomes from surgery alone in stage I and II disease make neoadjuvant therapy difficult to justify.

Early experience with neoadjuvant CRT in the UK was very variable in terms of its impact on operative risk and toxicity. The results of OEO2 have meant that the UK has continued with a chemotherapy approach in the current OEO5 study.

✔✔ A recent meta-analysis of both chemotherapy and CRT raises some interesting questions.[43] It included 10 randomised neoadjuvant CRT versus surgery-alone trials and eight neoadjuvant chemotherapy versus surgery-alone trials. It concluded that the hazard ratio for CRT was 0.81 (corresponding to a 13% absolute difference in survival at 2 years), with similar results for adenocarcinoma and squamous carcinoma. The hazard ratio for chemotherapy was 0.90 (corresponding to a 7% absolute difference in survival at 2 years), with a marked difference between a benefit demonstrated for adenocarcinoma and no benefit for squamous carcinoma. The results of the most recent Gaast study, not included in the above meta-analysis, performed in patients with a similar stage and morphological distribution to those in the UK would suggest that where preoperative CRT is delivered safely, this may lead to a significant improvement in outcome.

There is rightly a clear separation in future trials for adenocarcinoma and squamous carcinoma. As the trend moves towards squamous cancers being treated with primary CRT, the role of preoperative CRT may be revisited as a means of improving the outcome for patients with adenocarcinoma. The majority of such patients will present with stage III disease (at least T3 with lymph node metastases). Such tumours frequently threaten the circumferential margin of surgical resection (CRM), although a clear plane for surgical excision does not exist as it does for other anatomical sites such as the rectum. Disease present at or within 1 mm of the circumferential margin (R1) occurs in more than 50% of stage III cases[11,44] and is a poor prognostic factor. In the OEO2 study, the 3-year and median survival for patients with R0 and R1 resection were reported as 42.4% vs. 18% and 2.1 years vs. 1.1 years, respectively.[16] Preoperative chemoradiotherapy (CRT) has become a standard management strategy in rectal cancer for patients who have a threatened CRM on preoperative staging.

There has been only one randomised phase III trial comparing preoperative chemotherapy with preoperative CRT. This study by Stahl et al. aimed to recruit 354 patients to detect a 10% improvement in OS in favour of CRT (from 25% to 35%) but closed early as only 126 patients could be recruited in 5 years. Nonetheless, it showed a non-significant trend towards improved 3-year survival in favour of CRT (47.4% vs. 27.7%, P=0.07).[45]

The undoubted extra toxicity may be justified for this selected group and is infinitely preferable to postoperative treatment. New radiotherapy technology allows more accurate treatment delivery and lower morbidity, and when coupled with higher quality surgery and perioperative care should allow the sort of overall results from the Dutch trial[42] to be reproduced. Whatever improvements in locoregional treatments are proposed, the highest risk to be faced and addressed with new trials for stage III adenocarcinoma is ultimate systemic relapse. Trials with new biological agents added to standard chemotherapy or selective CRT are likely to be the next step, with advance knowledge from their use in the advanced and metastatic disease setting.

✔ At present preoperative CRT in the UK should be considered within the context of a clinical trial, or at least within the context of a specialist upper gastrointestinal multidisciplinary team (MDT) that can demonstrate the safe delivery of preoperative CRT. A trial should be designed to directly compare neoadjuvant chemotherapy and neoadjuvant chemoradiotherapy approaches, possibly targeting those patients likely to have an R1 resection.

Definitive radiotherapy and chemoradiotherapy

Surgery as a local treatment modality with neoadjuvant chemotherapy or CRT for stage III disease still remains a gold standard against which new approaches to potentially curative treatment must be compared. However, it is clear that there are long-term survivors in series of definitive non-surgical treatment. With an ageing population it must be remembered that 'inoperable' due to the nature of local disease or comorbidity and performance status does not mean treatment is therefore palliative.

Definitive radiotherapy

✔ With an increasingly elderly population it is not uncommon to be faced with patients who have localised disease on staging, particularly squamous cancers, but who clearly are not candidates for an operation and who, because of comorbidity, may not tolerate the chemotherapy component of a CRT treatment. There still is a role for radical radiotherapy alone.

Classical figures quoted for survival from radical radiotherapy come from the paper from Earlam and Cunha-Melo.[46] Mean survival figures of 8489 patients at 1, 2 and 5 years were 18%, 8% and 6%, respectively. Approximately 50% of patients were treated with curative intent. Older series tend to be of squamous carcinoma treated with radiotherapy alone. Modern radiotherapy in more selected patients can produce impressive survival results. In a series of 101 patients treated at the Christie Hospital in Manchester between 1985 and 1994, 3- and 5-year survival figures of 27% and 21%, respectively, were recorded.[47] There was a slightly better survival for adenocarcinoma, but not reaching statistical significance. The majority of tumours (96/101) were of 5 cm or less in length. Importantly, the only significant prognostic factor was the use of diagnostic CT, introduced during the latter part of the study. This was used to plan the radiotherapy and led to an increase in field sizes. The conclusion of the paper was that radiotherapy provided an effective alternative to surgery and that modern radiotherapy planning techniques may improve results.

There is no reason to compromise on staging or treatment planning standards and with modern technology high doses can be given with low morbidity. A selected series of 51 patients 80 years and over with squamous carcinoma treated with 66 Gy of radiotherapy in Japan produced median survival of 30 months and a 3-year survival rate of 39%.[48]

Definitive chemoradiotherapy

The adoption of CRT stems from high response rates and in particular high pCR rates seen in patients going on to resection. There are four randomised trials comparing radiotherapy alone with CRT. Three of these use low doses or low intensity of chemotherapy. A small series of 59 patients from Brazil did not demonstrate a significant survival advantage.[49] The response rates and 5-year survival rates (6% vs. 16%) were better in the CRT arm but at a cost of increased acute toxicity. An important non-randomised series is reported by Coia et al.[50] Treatment was with infusional 5-FU and mitomycin C with 60 Gy of radiotherapy. Patients with early-stage disease are reported separately. The respective 5-year survival and local failure rates, in clinical stages I and II combined, were 30% and 25%. There was no treatment-related mortality, although there was increased acute toxicity (22% grade III and 6% grade IV).

✔✔ The biggest series with a major impact on treatment patterns has been the RTOG 85-01, Herskovic study.[51] A total of 123 patients were randomised to receive either radiotherapy alone to a dose of 64 Gy or two courses of cisplatin and infusional 5-FU concurrent with 50 Gy of radiotherapy. Two more courses of chemotherapy were scheduled after the completion of the radiotherapy. A summary of the results of the randomised patients is shown in Table 9.2 and demonstrates the significant advantage of combined therapy.

In a confirmatory study, 69 non-randomised patients were treated with the CRT protocol and achieved similar results in terms of median survival and a 3-year survival of 26%. The acute toxicity in the combined treatment arm was significantly higher, with notably haematological and renal pathology and mucositis as the major problems. There was no significant difference in the late complication rates. In all, 80% of patients in the combined modality arm received the protocol treatment. The poor overall survival in the radiotherapy-alone control arm remains a question mark against the study.

Table 9.2 • Summary of results of the RTOG 85-01 study of Al-Sarraf et al. (1997)[51]

	RT	RT+CT	*P* value
Median survival (months)	9.3	14.1	
Overall survival (%):			
• 1-year	34	52	
• 2-year	10	36	
• 5-year	0	30	0.0001
Rate distant metastases (%)	37	21	0.0017
Two-year local recurrence rate (%)	59	45	0.0125
Overall disease free (%)	11	36	<0.001

CT, chemotherapy; RT, radiotherapy.

The high local failure rate of 45% in the Herskovic trial led to the Intergroup study 00123 (Minsky) that compared a regimen similar to the Herskovic regimen (modified with narrower radiotherapy fields, radiotherapy using 1.8 Gy/fraction and an alteration in the chemotherapy schedule to reduce anticipated toxicity), to the same schedule but with a higher dose of radiotherapy (64.8 Gy in 36 fractions).[52] In total, 236 patients, once again predominantly with squamous cell cancer, were randomised within this study. The trial had to be closed prematurely due to an excess of treatment-related deaths in the experimental arm (11 vs. 2), although the majority of these occurred before the higher dose section of the treatment protocol had been received. Although this trial did not show better disease control with higher doses of radiotherapy (56% failure at 2 years compared to 52% in the standard arm) it did demonstrate remarkably consistent outcomes of, approximately 30% survival at 3 years with definitive chemoradiotherapy.

Another approach to improve local control was to use brachytherapy to intensify the radiotherapy dose to the tumour. Study RTOG 92-07 used the 50-Gy external beam and chemotherapy protocol from the Herskovic protocol and added an intraluminal brachytherapy boost with one of two methods of delivery, high dose rate or low dose rate.[53] Six of the 35 patients developed an oesophageal fistula and this toxicity was deemed unacceptable.

Following successful CRT or radiotherapy alone there is a significant rate of benign stricture formation. This ranges from 12%[54] to 25%[50] in more modern studies. However, good swallowing function can be maintained in the majority of patients. Even in those with a benign stricture, a full or soft diet can be maintained by dilations in 71% of cases.[55] The treatment of post-CRT benign stricture with stents has not been successful in the authors' experience and gives rise to mediastinal pain.

The higher pCR rates seen with CRT, the improved local control rates and altered patterns of failure in the literature have all contributed to CRT being largely adopted as a standard of care. The management of patients with CRT is complex and requires good support from specialist nurses and dieticians, and high standards of technical radiotherapy. The risk of morbidity is real but can be overcome. It should be seen as a single integrated modality of therapy rather than two different treatments that happen to be delivered at the same time.

Future directions in definitive chemoradiation

The ability to predict which patients will respond to chemotherapy or CRT would allow greater certainty in a primary non-surgical approach. Molecular markers predicting response to chemotherapy hold some promise.[56–58] Conventional reassessment following treatment, with a negative endoscopic biopsy[35] and CT,[59] appears unreliable. However, the use of a positive surveillance endoscopic biopsy to direct salvage surgery in squamous carcinoma treated with definitive CRT has been reported.[60] Reports of the value of endoscopic ultrasound (EUS) are more variable, with some showing a good correlation with final pathological stage[61] and others suggesting it is not reliable.[62] There are reports advocating that this failure to reliably predict pCR necessitates resection.[34]

✔ There is increasing evidence to show that PET scanning may be extremely useful in predicting which patients are responding to chemotherapy and CRT.[63] Changes in metabolic activity on PET, 14 days after the start of treatment, appear to be significantly correlated with tumour response and patient survival. The ability to predict response in this way might be an attractive tool to determine if definitive CRT should be continued or a change made to a policy of resection. This would avoid surgical delay and increased morbidity in patients who are unlikely to benefit from chemotherapy or CRT. Such a policy would clearly need validation in a trial setting.

Improvements in CRT outcomes are likely to come from refinements in chemotherapy and radiotherapy technique. Results from preoperative phase II studies suggest a steady improvement in pCR rates, with more acceptable toxicity. The rates of pCR range from 24%[31] in 1993 to reports of 56%[64] in 1998. Care must be taken in interpreting the literature as pCR rates can vary depending upon whether rates are quoted as intent to treat or of completed resections, and in the protocols and quality assurance procedures associated with the histological examination. Careful staging can ensure that patients with established metastatic disease are appropriately managed. There has been a trend to accept lower standards of staging in non-surgical series. It is important that all patients who are deemed to have a potentially curative therapy have access to comparable staging, including EUS and PET. In the preoperative setting new protocols can be assessed for toxicity and response rates before use in a phase III randomised setting.[65]

Central to improving treatment strategies is an understanding of patterns of treatment failure. An important series of a detailed analysis of CRT has been published from Australia using combined data from Trans-Tasman Radiation Oncology Group studies.[66] This looks at results from 274 patients treated with definitive CRT and 92 patients treated with preoperative CRT. A summary of survival and

Table 9.3 • Five-year survival and cumulative incidence of relapse in the study of Denham et al. (2003)[66]

Treatment regimen*	Site	Histology	Number	Survival (%)	Local failure (%)	Distant failure (%)
Def CRT	All	All	274	28.8	42.4	33.5
Def CRT	Upper	Squamous	54	49.2	29.9	26.0
Def CRT	Middle	Squamous	81	24.7	41.8	37.3
Def CRT	Lower	Squamous	68	22.0	44.4	29.2
Def CRT	Lower	Adenocarcinoma	54	18.2	50.7	31.9
CRT+surgery	All	All	92	22.5	28.4	43.2
CRT+surgery	Middle	Squamous	31	26.7	30.3	36.4
CRT+surgery	Lower	Squamous	18	23.7	16.7	44.4
CRT+surgery	Lower	Adenocarcinoma	26	3.8	38.5	57.7

*Def CRT, definitive chemoradiation; CRT+surgery, preoperative chemoradiation+surgery.

recurrence patterns is given in Table 9.3. The overall local control rate for definitive CRT is almost 55%, rising to 70% in upper squamous cancers. The striking difference in outcome for these upper cancers includes an apparently lower distant failure rate and improved overall survival. It may be that these tumours are inherently different and respond more like squamous carcinomas of the head and neck. The persisting high distant failure rate in adenocarcinoma treated with CRT and surgery underlines a need for either earlier diagnosis and treatment or improved systemic therapy. There is no doubt that the success of CRT as definitive treatment is determined by similar factors to the outcomes of surgery, namely stage, performance status and the length of the tumour.

There are huge changes in the technology available for radiotherapy treatment. The development of three-dimensional and conformal radiotherapy treatment planning systems directly linked to spiral CT data allows the shape of radiotherapy fields to be individually tailored to an irregular-shaped target volume. In order for this to be successful, however, reliable imaging techniques are essential, including using EUS[67] and PET[68] to help delineate the gross tumour volume, and also localise the tumour on the axial planning CT scans. A reduction in normal tissue damage and so potentially the toxicity of combining therapy will be possible. The ability to define varying dose intensity within a radiotherapy field (intensity-modulated radiotherapy treatment, IMRT) may be helpful in being able to safely increase the dose, especially to tumours in the upper third of the oesophagus. One of the major concerns for tumours in the lower third is the movement of these tumours during treatment as a result of peristalsis, cardiac ejection cycles and especially respiratory motion. This can be up to 2 cm in the superior–inferior direction. There is no doubt that even better distributions of dose can be achieved with proton therapy but availability and cost may preclude this being feasible for some years. Improvements in CRT will also come from a better understanding of the effects on normal tissue near the clinical target volume, such as heart and lung.

The use of new radiosensitising chemotherapy drugs in combination with radiotherapy may allow some small incremental gains in response rates (oxaliplatin/taxanes/capecitabine) and hence local control. Lastly, more attention to the treatment of elective nodal irradiation, perhaps wider fields to a lower dose, may reduce locoregional failure.

The current NCRI study of definitive CRT (SCOPE 1) aims to compare cisplatin and capecitabine with 50 Gy of radiotherapy in the control arm and add the epidermal growth factor receptor (EGFR) monoclonal antibody cetuximab to the investigational arm. There is evidence that one mechanism of radiotherapy resistance is through activation of the EGFR pathways and clinical evidence from a randomised trial in squamous cancer of the head and neck of improved local control and overall survival.[69] This study is important in also defining very high radiotherapy technical standards for the UK, ensuring the accuracy of target volume definition and minimising normal tissue morbidity. It is open to both adenocarcinoma and squamous carcinoma selected by multidisciplinary teams, the entry criteria broadly being patients with disease treatable by chemoradiotherapy who have been deemed unsuitable for surgery due to the extent of local disease, patient comorbidities or patient choice.

Definitive CRT versus surgery

Definitive CRT treatments now report good survival figures[51,59] rivalling those of surgery, stage for stage.[70,71]

✔ In squamous carcinoma there seems to be increasing evidence that a policy of primary CRT with surgery as salvage may be the direction for the future.[72]

Many squamous cancers are in the mid and upper oesophagus and their pattern of lymph node spread is less predictable. These areas can be safely treated with CRT with increasing sophistication. The evidence base for equipoise in efficacy in the treatment of patients with oesophageal adenocarcinoma is less robust. Tumours primarily of the lower oesophagus or limited to the gastro-oesophageal junction might be candidates for CRT but target volumes are more difficult and perhaps CRT should be reserved where a surgical approach is ruled out by age, performance status or comorbidity.

There have been few trials that allow a direct comparison between a primary CRT policy and surgery, and indeed CRT studies may have had a selection bias against them. The results of CRT alone tend to have 5-year survival figures generally comparable to those seen in Tables 9.2 and 9.3, of the order of 30% overall, which are similar to surgical series. Squamous cancers, in particular of the mid and upper thirds, have better outcomes. It does allow CRT to be considered as a viable option to chemotherapy and surgery for adenocarcinoma and as primary treatment for squamous carcinoma.

✔✔ There are two trials that address the additional value of surgery after CRT and would give some support to a selective approach to its use, particularly in squamous carcinoma. The conflicting results of these trials suggest surgery is not routinely necessary following definitive CRT.

In a French study, patients were assessed after induction CRT using 5-FU and cisplatin.[73] If they had achieved an objective response they were randomised (295 of 455 patients) to carry on with CRT or go to surgery. There was no significant difference between the 2-year survival rates for patients who had surgery (33.6%) and those who had CRT alone (39.8%). There were more early deaths in the surgery arm but CRT required more dilatations and stents.

In a German trial, 177 patients with T3 or T4 squamous carcinoma were randomised to receive CRT+surgery or CRT alone.[74] The rate of response to initial CRT was the same for both arms. There was a strong trend towards improved local tumour control in the arm with surgery. In responding patients the 3-year survival (45% and 44%, respectively) was equivalent in both arms, whereas in non-responding patients the rates were 18% and 11%, respectively. The 3-year survival rate improved to 35% in non-responding patients undergoing complete tumour resection, implying that a subgroup of non-responding patients may benefit from surgery as an elective salvage procedure. Longer-term results confirm no clear survival difference between a surgical versus CRT approach. This trial did show that a clinical response to induction chemotherapy may be a valuable surrogate for predicting prognosis.

There is evidence collected from the literature that selected salvage surgery is possible after CRT failure, with acceptable operative mortality of 11.4% and 5-year survival rates of 25–35%.[75] Clearly such a high-risk policy should be after CT-PET restaging and only within the context of a tertiary MDT with audited results for the safe delivery of both chemoradiation and surgery.

Small-cell oesophageal cancer

Small-cell oesophageal cancer (SCOC) is a rare entity, accounting for up to 2.5% of primary oesophageal cancers and associated with a poor prognosis due to a high rate of metastatic disease. It thus requires a distinct approach to management with similarities to primary small-cell lung cancer (SCLC), which has similar histological features.

The literature is made up of small retrospective series from major institutions. It tends to have male preponderance and occurs in the mid and lower oesophagus. Series vary but most, even with staging that would be considered less than optimum today, have a majority of patients with metastases at presentation. The median survival of untreated metastatic patients is less than 3 months.

The treatment of SCOC is dependent on a separation between limited disease and extensive disease. Table 9.4 shows the outcomes in two of the larger

Table 9.4 • Outcomes of small-cell oesophageal cancer series

Date	Series	Patient numbers	Median survival LD	Median survival ED	Overall median survival
2007	Hudson et al.[76]	16	24.4	9.1	13.2
2008	Ku et al.[77]	25	22.5	8.5	19.8

ED, extensive disease; LD, limited disease.

and most recent series in the literature.[76,77] Both have good references and discussion.

✔ The treatment of patients with extensive disease is palliative chemotherapy based on etoposide- and platinum-containing regimens if the performance status allows. Response rates to treatment are high and there is definite improvement in overall survival, but outcomes are universally poor, with median survivals of 8–11 months.

Due to the very high rate of systemic relapse, limited stage disease requires primary treatment with chemotherapy, again based on etoposide- and platinum-containing regimes. There is a role for consolidation treatment to enhance local control and to prevent local symptomatic progression. There are surgical series with good local control rates, but the majority of series concentrate on radiotherapy (doses up to 50 Gy) or chemoradiotherapy as would be considered for SCLC, thus avoiding the mortality risk and morbidity of surgery.

Local control rates with surgery are high but overall prognosis poor, with survival dictated by metastatic disease and median survivals in the range of 15–24 months. There is no literature on prophylactic cranial irradiation, which has been shown to be an advantage in SCLC after successful systemic and local therapy.

Gastric cancer

Potentially curative treatment

Perioperative adjuvant chemotherapy

The goal of systemic therapy for gastric cancer is to reduce the late patterns of failure following successful surgical resection. The pattern of spread includes nodal, transcoelomic and haematogenous. A significant proportion of patients with intra-abdominal, hepatic, peritoneal or omental disease will fail. Extended lymphadenectomy has been advocated to improve the local/regional control rates. Chemotherapy, either systemic or intraperitoneal, has been used to try to reduce the incidence of widespread recurrence. Despite encouraging results for chemotherapy in advanced disease, proof of a benefit for adjuvant postoperative chemotherapy has been elusive. Standard approaches have been with postoperative chemotherapy but more recent studies have looked at a combination of preoperative and postoperative treatment.

There have been a wide range of randomised adjuvant chemotherapy trials. Regimens with significant activity in the advanced disease setting have been tested since the 1980s. There are variations in the surgery used, the timing of the start of chemotherapy and the toxicity, which all make interpretation and comparisons difficult.

✔✔ Three meta-analyses exist.[78–80] In summary, these demonstrate a small survival benefit of borderline significance that was more marked in trials, with greater than two-thirds of patients having node-positive disease.

However, many of the regimens in the older studies have low response rates (10–30%) in advanced disease, compared with the higher expected response of more modern regimens such as ECF.

The MRC STO2 (MAGIC) trial was opened in 1994 and aimed to recruit 500 patients testing the role of three courses of ECF before and after resection in operable gastric cancer. The results suggest a significant downstaging effect of the chemotherapy.[19] As the MRC OEO2 neoadjuvant oesophageal trial was completed, the eligibility criteria were widened in 1999 to include adenocarcinoma of the lower oesophagus. The type of resection was left to the discretion of the participating surgeon and the staging was relatively permissive by modern standards. The arms of the study were well balanced and included 74% stomach, 14% oesophageal and 12% junctional cancers. Toxicity of the chemotherapy was acceptable but only 40% of patients received both cycles of postoperative treatment. In fact, the majority of resections were at least D1, with 40% having a D2. The proportion deemed to have had a potentially curative resection was 10% higher with chemotherapy (79% vs. 69%). There was a significant effect on tumour size, T stage and nodal status. Recent results with a median follow-up of >3 years have demonstrated an improvement in overall survival (hazard ratio of 0.75, P=0.009), with 5-year survival rates of 36% for chemotherapy and surgery vs. 23% for surgery alone. Progression-free survival was also significantly prolonged.

In a similar French multicentre trial, of perioperative fluorouracil plus cisplatin in resectable gastro-oesophageal adenocarcinoma, 224 patients with resectable adenocarcinoma of the lower oesophagus, gastro-oesophageal junction (GEJ) or stomach were randomly assigned to either perioperative chemotherapy and surgery (CS group; n=113) or surgery alone (S group; n=111).[81] Chemotherapy consisted of two or three preoperative cycles of intravenous cisplatin (100 mg/m^2) on day 1, and a continuous intravenous infusion of fluorouracil (800 mg/m^2/day) for 5 consecutive days (days 1–5) every 28 days and three or four postoperative cycles of the same regimen. The CS group had a better overall survival (5-year rate 38% vs. 24%; HR for death: 0.69; 95% CI 0.50–0.95; P=0.02). The postoperative morbidity was similar in the two groups.

✔✔ It is thus reasonable to adopt a standard approach using perioperative chemotherapy for tumours other than early-stage gastric cancer.

The current NCRI study ST03 or 'MAGIC 2' compares three cycles of pre- and postoperative ECX with the addition of bevacizumab and three cycles of maintenance bevacizumab, a humanised monoclonal antibody against vascular endothelial growth factor (VEGF).

Intraperitoneal chemotherapy

The pattern of peritoneal and hepatic recurrence in gastric cancer makes the early use of intraperitoneal chemotherapy attractive. The most positive trial is from Japan,[82] using mitomycin C adsorbed on to activated charcoal, acting as a delayed-release preparation. Fifty patients with serosal involvement were randomised to immediate treatment or observation. A highly significant difference in survival at 2 years was seen (68.6% vs. 26.9%), with the treatment group maintaining its advantage at 3 years. The treatment was reported to be well tolerated. However, when an attempt was made to repeat these results, in an Austrian multicentre study,[83] serious toxicity caused the trial to be suspended. A significantly higher postoperative complication rate (35% vs. 16%) and 60-day mortality rate (11% vs. 2%) were seen in the treatment arm of the study. No benefits were found in overall or recurrence-free survival.

Postoperative chemoradiotherapy

Radiotherapy has not been routinely used in the management of stomach cancer. However, local recurrence can be a significant problem. The stomach and nodal areas are close to many crucial normal tissues with dose-limiting susceptibility to toxicity, such as kidney, spinal cord and small bowel.

In the British Stomach Cancer Group trial,[84] postoperative radiotherapy was one of the arms of the study. The other arms were FAM chemotherapy and a control surgery-only group. There was no difference in survival but the local recurrence rate was significantly better (54% surgery vs. 32% with radiotherapy; $P<0.01$).

✔✔ The American Intergroup INT 0116 (SWOG 9008) study (commonly referred to as the Macdonald study) has produced important results. Postoperative CRT has been reported to show a significant benefit to survival following gastric resection.[85]

The regimen consisted of 5-FU–leucovorin (folinic acid) given in the first and last weeks of radiotherapy (45 Gy) and two 5-day courses of 5-FU–leucovorin given monthly. With a median follow-up of 3.3 years both the disease-free survival (49% vs. 32%) and overall survival (52% vs. 41%) were improved in the CRT arm. There was some significant haematological and gastrointestinal morbidity. However, the treatment-related mortality was only 1%. The need for great care in the technical quality and placement of the radiotherapy was apparent. However, a significant proportion of the patients (54%) had only a D0 resection and the survival in the surgery-alone arm was relatively poor (41% 3-year survival). It is possible that the CRT is making up for less than adequate surgery, and may not translate into routine practice where more extensive surgery is undertaken. It is the most obvious source of criticism of the trial. However, in a subsequent paper,[86] using a different surgical quality assurance measure for the likelihood of undissected disease (the Maruyama Index), the group concluded that surgical undertreatment clearly undermines survival. Major concerns about the toxicity and chemotherapy used and the poor radiotherapy technique are being addressed, which should significantly reduce the potential for long-term morbidity and make the most of sophisticated IMRT and radiotherapy planning techniques. Despite criticisms, postoperative CRT has been patchily adopted throughout the world.

✔✔ Thus there are now two major trials demonstrating improved survival with the addition of perioperative therapy in gastric cancer. One study (MAGIC)[19] involves pre- and postoperative chemotherapy, and the other (INT 0116)[85] the use of postoperative CRT. Whilst one can argue the relative merits of each approach, one certain conclusion is that for all but early-stage tumours surgery alone is no longer a standard of care.

Palliative chemotherapy

Squamous carcinoma of the oesophagus

Cisplatin-containing combination chemotherapy is the standard for the treatment of advanced and recurrent squamous carcinoma. The indications for use are limited by the relative infrequency of the disease, and in particular the age and performance status of patients requiring palliation. Very often the indication is to improve symptoms and quality of life caused by the primary leasion and local therapy with a stent or radiotherapy will be adequate. However, good response rates of the order of 35% can be achieved with cisplatin and 4- or 5-day 5-FU infusion.[87] Response duration is variable and can range from 3 to 6 months. Consideration should be given to consolidation palliative radiotherapy after successful chemotherapy to improve local control where recurrent growth may produce symptoms for patients with a better performance status and expectation of life. There is some evidence that the improved response rates seen with PVI of 5-FU in adenocarcinoma can be achieved in squamous carcinoma.[14] New agents such as paclitaxel are clearly active as single agents but have yet to demonstrate their clear superiority in combination regimens. Some results are promising, with response rates nearer 50%.[88]

Adenocarcinoma of the oesophagus and stomach

Whilst earlier literature tends to report activity in pure gastric cancer, the changing pattern of disease has meant that more recent reports deal with oesophagogastric cancer. The single agents most commonly used in the treatment of advanced oesophagogastric cancer include 5-FU, methotrexate, mitomycin C, the anthracyclines doxorubicin and epirubicin, cisplatin and etoposide. More recently the oral 5-FU prodrugs such as UFT and capecitabine, the taxane drugs, irinotecan and gemcitabine all feature in new phase II studies. Biological agents such as EGFR monoclonal antibodies represent a new potential means of improving outcomes.

✔✔ There are early randomised clinical trials of palliative chemotherapy versus best supportive care that clearly show improved survival (8–12 months chemotherapy vs. 3–5 months best supportive care).[89–91]

The FAM regimen (5-FU, doxorubicin and mitomycin) initially seemed to have a high response rate of 40%.[92] However, in the setting of a randomised trial by the North Central Cancer Treatment Group, it seemed to be no better than 5-FU alone.[93] In an attempt to modulate the activity of 5-FU within the FAM regimen, high-dose methotrexate was given 1 hour before the 5-FU in the FAMTX regimen (fluorouracil, doxorubicin and methotrexate). Klein produced impressive results in a study of 100 patients.[94] The response rate was 58%, with a complete remission rate of 12%. There were only 3% treatment-related deaths and a long-term survival rate of 6%. The response rate seen in subsequent studies was slightly lower but still confirmed acceptable toxicity. This regimen has now been tested against other combinations. A randomised EORTC trial with 208 evaluable patients demonstrated its superiority against FAM.[95] Median survival was better (42 weeks vs. 29 weeks; P=0.004), with 41% and 9% of the FAMTX patients alive at 1 and 2 years, respectively, compared with 22% and 0% for FAM patients. The EAP regimen (etoposide, doxorubicin and cisplatin) was found to have similar survivals, similar overall response rates but lower complete remission rates and was significantly more toxic.[96] The recent EORTC trial has compared three regimens, FAMTX, ELF (etoposide, leucovorin and bolus 5-FU) and FUP (infusional 5-FU and cisplatin), in 399 randomised patients.[97] There was no significant difference in median survivals between the regimens. The response rates were lower than in some previous trials (ELF 9%, FUP 20%, FAMTX 12%) but this trial had tight objective response criteria and required measurable disease. The conclusion is that they all produce modest response with comparable survival and toxicity.

✔✔ The ECF regimen developed at The Royal Marsden Hospital was shown to have high activity against advanced oesophagogastric cancer.[13] It has become widely used in the UK and is well tolerated. Its status as the current gold standard was confirmed in a multicentre randomised trial of ECF against FAMTX.[98] A total of 274 patients with adenocarcinoma or undifferentiated carcinoma of the oesophagus, oesophagogastric junction or stomach were treated.

Patients were predominantly of good performance status with a median age of 60 years. The overall objective response rate was 45% in the ECF arm and 21% in the FAMTX arm (P=0.0002). The response of locally advanced disease to ECF has previously been shown to be higher than in metastatic disease.[13] This was confirmed in both arms of the trial (56% ECF vs. 23% FAMTX). Of the 121 patients receiving ECF, 10 were able to undergo a resection due to improved status, six of whom remain disease free. There were three cases of histological pCR. Only 5% of patients had progression whilst on either chemotherapy regimen.

The 2-year survival figures and median survival were 14% and 8.7 months for ECF and 5% and 6.1 months for FAMTX, respectively (P=0.03).

The ECF results have opened up a grey area in locally advanced gastric and junctional cancer management. Whilst a patient may not be operable, or it may be deemed inadvisable to operate due to the extent of disease at presentation, it may be possible to consider a potentially curative resection in some cases after chemotherapy. The intent of treatment may therefore need to be revisited by close reassessment after chemotherapy. This emphasises the need for teamwork between the surgeon and oncologist within a multidisciplinary setting.

In a study from Leeds of advanced upper gastrointestinal cancer patients, oral UFT and leucovorin were substituted for PVI of 5-FU in ECF in an attempt to create a more practical, acceptable and cheaper alternative (the ECU regimen) without the need for central lines and pumps.[99] In this dose-escalation pilot study 30 patients were treated. Toxicity was acceptable and of 20 assessable patients, nine of the 15 with gastro-oesophageal cancer had an objective response and two of these were complete radiological responses.

The NCRI REAL2 trial was designed to address some practical problems that surrounded delivery of the gold standard ECF regime.[20] Infusional 5-FU has problems associated with Hickman lines, particularly thrombosis and infection. Cisplatin causes renal toxicity and requires prehydration and inpatient admission for higher doses. It tested the toxicity and response rates of oxaliplatin as a substitute for cisplatin, and of capecitabine (an oral fluoropyrimidine) as a substitute for infusional 5-FU in a randomised 2×2 study based on statistics of non-inferiority against ECF.

✔✔ The REAL2 results demonstrated that oxaliplatin can be substituted for cisplatin with less renal toxicity and neutropenia and that capecitabine is a valid substitution for 5-FU.[20] Although a secondary end-point, there was a significant improvement in median survival for the EOX (epirubicin–oxaliplatin–capecitabine) regimen compared to the ECF regimen (11.2 months vs. 9.9 months). There was no significant difference in response rates between regimens and a response rate of 40.7% in the ECF arm.

The EOX regimen has been taken forward as the control arm in the next REAL3 study, with the addition of panitumumab (an EGFR antibody) in the investigational arm. Other attempts to improve treatment outcomes using the addition of docetaxel to cisplatin and 5-FU have uncovered high potential toxicities with neutropenia, treatment withdrawal rates of nearly 50% due to grade 3 and 4 toxicity, and no improvement in response rates or survival, raising a question as to whether a plateau has been nearly reached with conventional approaches to chemotherapy.[100] New biological agents possibly bring new distinctions between different agents even within antibodies to the same receptor and very different response rates of gastric and gastro-oesophageal/oesophageal cancers.[101] This emphasises the need for good tissue collection and analysis in parallel with clinical studies. The recent closure of REAL3 as a result of insufficient benefits seen in the trial arm of EOX plus panitumumab suggests that we have not yet found the right targets or the optimum agents with which to counter these targets.

Trastuzumab (herceptin), a monoclonal antibody against human epidermal growth factor receptor 2 (HER-2; also known as ERBB-2), was investigated in combination with chemotherapy for first-line treatment of HER-2-positive advanced gastric or gastro-oesophageal junction cancer. The ToGA trial was an international phase 3 study undertaken in 594 patients, randomised to capecitabine or fluorouracil plus cisplatin plus or minus trastuzumab.[102] Median overall survival was 13.8 months (95% CI 12–16; 16.0 months in those who would be considered HER-2 positive by today's definition (HER-2 3+ or HER-2 2+ + FISH+)) in those assigned to trastuzumab plus chemotherapy compared with 11.1 months (95% CI 10–13) in those assigned to chemotherapy alone (HR 0.74; P=0·0046). There were no significant differences in toxicities, including cardiac, between the two groups. The proportion of HER-2-positive tumours ranges from approximately 10% to 30% of all gastric cancers, being higher in gastro-oesophageal junctional cancers, Caucasians and intestinal type pathology.

✔✔ Trastuzumab in combination with chemotherapy can be considered as a new standard option for patients with HER-2-positive advanced gastric or gastro-oesophageal junction cancer.[102]

The selection of patients who are likely to benefit from palliative chemotherapy may be helped by the development of prognostic scoring methods. One study has demonstrated that performance status, liver metastases, peritoneal metastases and alkaline phosphatase can be used to separate different risk groups.[103] Problems in the literature with myelosuppression, and in particular toxic deaths, may be avoided by the use of growth factors to reduce the incidence of neutropenic sepsis. Many of the problems of severe emesis have already been improved by the use of 5-HT_3 antiemetic drugs.

Second-line chemotherapy using taxanes and irinotecan has been reported, with some evidence of worthwhile activity. In practice, however, great care will need to be taken in the selection of suitable patients, and such treatment should really only be undertaken within the context of a trial.

The success in palliative chemotherapy has brought about problems and patterns of recurrence that have not been common before. Brain metastases and bone metastases are increasingly seen. Palliative radiotherapy can be helpful in controlling symptoms.

Palliative radiotherapy

External beam radiotherapy

The whole literature surrounding radiotherapy in a palliative setting is poor. Nonetheless, the role of radiotherapy is important. There are many instances where patients have local symptoms from metastatic disease. With a high proportion of patients presenting with T3N1 disease it is not surprising that many will fail despite more complex and aggressive therapy. The pattern of metastases seems already to be changing in that patients are living to get metastases in brain, bone and skin, as well as recurrent nodal masses. These clinical problems are amenable to short fractionated radiotherapy, which provides good symptomatic relief.

The role of external beam radiotherapy to treat dysphagia has changed with the ready availability of oesophageal stents. Radiotherapy can be very effective in relieving dysphagia but it can take weeks to accomplish this, and it can even temporarily worsen symptoms with radiation oesophagitis. The role of radiotherapy following successful stent placement is unproven. A UK trial has been proposed, largely to explore the possibility of improvements in survival and symptom-free survival. The attraction is in achieving a measure of local disease control and in treating the mediastinum. There is also an intermediate group of patients with good performance status and relatively localised disease who are clearly not appropriate for potentially curative treatment. Some short CRT regimes or primary chemotherapy with consolidation radiotherapy have been used, with some suggestion of improved results. This group of patients deserves greater study to optimise palliation.

There is a major difference between the fractionation regimens used in the USA and in the UK. 'Palliative' doses of 40–60 Gy in 4–6 weeks are quoted in the US literature. These are in the radical dose range and are felt to be inappropriate for UK practice, where doses of 20–30 Gy in 1 or 2 weeks are more likely to be used. These can be combined with brachytherapy. Good resolution of tumour and symptom relief in a majority of patients have been reported.[104] Often, however, whichever palliative technique is used first, other modalities have a role for patients with longer survival, to maintain swallowing.

Brachytherapy

Brachytherapy involves the placement of a high-dose-rate radioactive source, usually iridium-192, down the oesophagus in proximity to the tumour. The aim is to get direct tumour cell kill, thereby relieving dysphagia, or in the case of its use as a boost to external beam radiotherapy, to achieve an increased dose to the tumour with minimal dose to surrounding normal tissues. It does not require a general anaesthetic and can be done as a day-case procedure. Occasionally, placement of a nasogastric guide tube is required under endoscopic vision. Pagliero and Rowlands[105] describe a single dose of 15 Gy with a response rate of about 60% measured at 6 weeks from treatment. It can be repeated in cases of symptomatic relapse.

The optimum dose of brachytherapy has been addressed in a randomised trial using three schedules.[106] Three doses and schedules were tested in 172 patients with advanced oesophageal cancer These were 12 Gy/two fractions (A), 16 Gy/two fractions (B) and 18 Gy/three fractions (C).

Patients were assessed for relief of dysphagia and survival. Dose and tumour length were found to be significant for survival on multivariate analysis. Brachytherapy dose had a significant effect on tumour control. Overall survival for the whole group was 19.4% at 1 year.

✓✓ The survival by group, although not statistically significant, suggests a trend towards better outcomes with the higher dose schedules of brachytherapy (at 12 months: A=9.8%, B=22.5%, C=35.3%).[106]

✓✓ There are good published guidelines[107] for the use of brachytherapy, taking into account the potential wide range of applications for this technique.

✓✓ A randomised multicentre trial with 209 patients has shown that single-dose brachytherapy gave better long-term relief of dysphagia than metal stent placement, with equivalent costs.[108] The time to symptom relief was, however, worse for brachytherapy but there were fewer complications.

Future strategies

In order to achieve the best outcomes for patients, assessment, staging and treatment need to be closely coordinated and integrated in a multidisciplinary setting. Poor outcomes from single-modality therapy and increasing evidence of the value of multiple modalities will be powerful drivers towards higher quality and more centralised services. Site specialist clinicians and support services can only meet demands for quality assurance in all possible modalities of treatment with appropriate resources and infrastructure. The essential role of high-quality radiology, including EUS, and expert pathology cannot be underestimated. The routine use of PET, both as a diagnostic tool to pick up early metastatic disease, and also to help target volume localisation in radiotherapy planning and predict response to non-surgical treatment, seems likely to become a key decision-making tool (see Chapter 3). Support services such as specialist nursing and dietetic services are particularly important in this area of disease management.

Radiotherapy is undergoing rapid technological developments through computer technology and improved imaging, both in terms of primary tumour localisation and treatment verification. Intensity-modulated treatment uses computer algorithms to optimise the delivery of radiation and spare normal tissue injury. This more accurate radiotherapy technique may allow safe dose escalation in cancers in the upper third of the oesophagus, where there is close proximity of the target volume to the spinal cord and where radiotherapy doses used are significantly lower than those used to treat hypopharyngeal carcinomas a few centimetres higher. Image-guided radiotherapy used various techniques in target volume localisation and on treatment verification to ensure the target volume is actually being treated every day. This is especially important where the target is prone to movement, for example as a result of respiration. This is particularly important for tumours of the lower third of the oesophagus. The use of evidence-based modern radiotherapy techniques is a prerequisite for dose escalation and for better local disease control if non-surgical therapies are going to be increasingly used with the aim of primary organ preservation.

As with radiotherapy treatments, systemic therapy is moving towards an era of personalised oncology. This is where treatments are selected based on the characteristics of the individual tumour rather than on prognostic risk factors. Many patients will never benefit from current chemotherapy and biological therapies, including monoclonal antibodies, and biomarkers are needed to select those that will benefit the most from what may be relatively toxic and/or expensive treatment. We have seen the first of these in the form of HER-2-positive oesophagogastric cancer, which predicts the benefit of the addition of herceptin to combination chemotherapy.[102] ERCC1 may predict for cisplatin resistance and future studies must define the role of these biomarkers in routine treatment. If the lessons from past trials are to be learned, namely the poor and variable results in control arm treatments, attention will have to be paid to rigorous quality assurance within each area of defined treatment. This will aid the process of new high-quality research trials aiming to develop new treatment strategies.

✔ As chemoradiotherapy emerges as an alternative to radical surgery, particularly in squamous carcinoma, accurately predicting and defining those patients who will achieve good remission prospectively is important, as is the identification of patients who require salvage surgery. New molecular markers may be important tools for the future.

The need for quick assessment by site specialist teams, able to offer a full range of treatments, ranging from complex combined modality therapy all the way through to quick and efficient palliative care, is only likely to be achieved by teamwork and some degree of reorganisation. Reconfiguration of surgical services has probably contributed to improved outcomes from surgery and it is likely that some further specialisation of non-surgical services might reduce variability in therapeutic options being offered to patients and use of new radiotherapy techniques. Ultimately, a greater improved understanding of the epidemiology of these diseases will be necessary to allow the identification of disease at a far earlier stage. The current presentation with predominantly nodal and advanced stage disease is likely to limit the improvements that are possible with existing treatments.

The need for continued randomised trials is important. Major centres with high-quality assurance and good research support can recruit sufficient patients to answer major questions that are important to improve the outcome for these diseases.

Key points

- Chemotherapy and radiotherapy have a major role, integrated with surgery, in the treatment of oesophageal and gastric cancer. Poor outcomes from single-modality therapy and increasing evidence of the value of selective use of multiple modalities are powerful drivers towards higher quality and more centralised services.
- Effective staging is essential as surgery alone is now indicated only for early-stage disease.
- The benefit of preoperative radiotherapy in oesophageal cancer seems to be small.
- Preoperative chemotherapy has been demonstrated to improve survival and is accepted in the UK as a standard of care in oesophageal cancer. Cisplatin–5-FU combinations seem to be active in both squamous carcinoma and adenocarcinoma.
- Postoperative radiotherapy has a possible role in selected cases of oesophageal cancer (e.g. pathological stage III squamous cell carcinoma). The justification is less clear for adenocarcinoma outside the context of a clinical trial.

- An updated Cochrane review of 11 randomised trials concludes that there was a 21% increase in survival at 3 years with neoadjuvant chemotherapy prior to oesophageal resection, but that statistical significance was not reached until 5 years.
- There is good evidence that pCR rates are significantly higher with chemoradiotherapy (CRT) than with radiotherapy or chemotherapy given alone. CRT achieves enhanced local therapy coupled with a systemic benefit.
- The current approach in the UK is to concentrate on preoperative chemotherapy rather than CRT for adenocarcinoma. At present preoperative CRT should only be considered within the context of a clinical trial.
- Surgery remains a gold standard for local treatment against which new approaches to potentially curative treatment must be compared.
- Definitive CRT does provide an alternative to surgery in localised oesophageal cancer.
- In squamous carcinoma there is good evidence that a policy of primary CRT is a sustainable strategy (with or without surgical salvage), with equivalent results to surgery.
- The overall local control rate for definitive CRT is 70% in upper-third squamous cancers, for which it is presently the treatment of choice.
- The ability to predict which patients will respond to chemotherapy or CRT would allow greater certainty in a primary non-surgical approach.
- Better outcomes in gastric cancer can be achieved for all but early-stage tumours with the addition of chemotherapy to surgery (MAGIC).
- The American Intergroup postoperative CRT study has been reported to show a significant benefit to survival following gastric resection. However, it is possible that the CRT is only making up for less than adequate surgery and may not translate into routine practice where appropriate radical surgery is undertaken.
- Chemotherapy and radiotherapy have a major role in the palliative treatment of oesophageal and gastric cancer.
- The UK ECF regimen shows high activity against advanced oesophagogastric cancer but new derivatives such as EOX will be easier and safer to deliver.
- The selection of patients who are likely to benefit from palliative chemotherapy may be helped by the development of prognostic scoring methods.

References

1. Nigro ND, Seydel HG, Considine B, et al. Combined preoperative radiation and chemotherapy for squamous cell carcinoma of the anal canal. Cancer 1983;51:1826–9.
2. Northover JM. Epidermoid cancer of the anus – the surgeon retreats. J R Soc Med 1991;84:389–90.
3. Swedish Rectal Cancer Trial. Improved survival with preoperative radiotherapy in resectable rectal cancer. N Engl J Med 1997;336:980–7.
4. Gignoux M, Roussel A, Paillot B, et al. The value of preoperative radiotherapy in esophageal cancer: results of the EORTC. World J Surg 1987;11:426–32.
5. Nygaard K, Hagen S, Hansen HS, et al. Pre-operative radiotherapy prolongs survival in operable esophageal carcinoma: a randomized, multicentre study of pre-operative radiotherapy and chemotherapy. The Second Scandinavian Trial in esophageal cancer. World J Surg 1992;16:1104–10.
6. Arnott SJ, Duncan W, Kerr GR, et al. Low-dose preoperative radiotherapy for carcinoma of the oesophagus: results of a randomized clinical trial. Radiother Oncol 1992;24:108–13.
7. Arnott SJ, Duncan W, Gignoux M, et al. Preoperative radiotherapy in esophageal carcinoma: a meta-analysis using individual patient data (Oesophageal Cancer Collaborative Group). Int J Radiat Oncol Biol Phys 1998;41:579–83.
8. Teniere P, Hay J, Fingethut A, et al. Postoperative radiation therapy does not increase survival after curative resection for squamous carcinoma of the middle and lower oesophagus as shown by a multi-center controlled trial. Surg Gynaecol Obstet 1991;173:123–30.
9. Fok M, Sham JST, Choy D, et al. Postoperative radiotherapy for carcinoma of the esophagus: a prospective randomized controlled trial. Surgery 1993;113:138–47.
10. Xiao ZF, Yang ZY, Liang J, et al. Value of radiotherapy after radical surgery for esophageal

carcinoma: a report of 495 patients. Ann Thorac Surg 2003;75:331–6.

11. Dexter SP, Sue-Ling H, McMahon MJ, et al. Circumferential resection margin involvement: an independent predictor of survival following surgery for oesophageal cancer. Gut 2001;48(5):667–70.
12. Schlag PM. Randomized trial of preoperative chemotherapy of squamous cell cancer of the esophagus. Arch Surg 1992;127:1446–50.
13. Bamias A, Hill ME, Cunningham D, et al. Epirubicin, cisplatin and protracted venous infusion of 5-fluorouracil for esophagogastric adenocarcinoma. Cancer 1996;77:1978–85.
14. Andreyev HJN, Norman AR, Cunningham D, et al. Squamous oesophageal cancer can be downstaged using protracted venous infusion of 5-fluorouracil with epirubicin and cisplatin (ECF). Eur J Cancer 1995;31A:2209–14.
15. Kelsen DP, Ginsberg R, Pajak TF, et al. Chemotherapy followed by surgery compared with surgery alone for localized esophageal cancer. N Engl J Med 1998;339:1979–84.
16. Medical Research Council Oesophageal Cancer Working Party. Surgical resection with or without preoperative chemotherapy in oesophageal cancer: a randomised controlled trial. Lancet 2002;359:1727–33.
17. Allum WH, Fogaty PJ, Stenning SP, et al. Long term results of the MRC OEO2 randomized trial of surgery with or without preoperative chemotherapy in resectable esophageal cancer. Proc ASCO GI Cancer Symp 2008;abstr. 9.
18. Malthaner R, Fenlon D. Preoperative chemotherapy for resectable thoracic esophageal cancer. Cochrane Database Syst Rev 2003;(4)CD001556.
19. Cunningham D, Allum WH, Stenning SP, et al. Perioperative chemotherapy versus surgery alone for resectable gastroesophageal cancer. N Engl J Med 2006;355:11–20.
20. Cunningham D, Starling N, Rao S, et al. Capecitabine and oxaliplatin for advanced esophagogastric cancer. N Engl J Med 2008;358:36–46.
21. Roth JA, Pass HI, Flanagan MM, et al. Randomized clinical trial of preoperative and postoperative adjuvant chemotherapy with cisplatin, vindesine and bleomycin for carcinoma of the esophagus. J Thorac Cardiovasc Surg 1988;96:242–8.
22. Geh IJ, Crellin AM, Glynne-Jones R. A review of the role of preoperative (neoadjuvant) chemoradiotherapy in oesophageal carcinoma. Br J Surg 2001;88:338–56.
23. Urba SG, Orringer MB, Perez-Tamayo C, et al. Concurrent preoperative chemotherapy and radiation therapy in localized esophageal adenocarcinoma. Cancer 1992;69:285–91.
24. Bosset JF, Gignoux M, Triboulet JP, et al. Chemoradiotherapy followed by surgery compared with surgery alone in squamous-cell cancer of the esophagus. N Engl J Med 1997;337:161–7.
25. MacKean J, Burmeister BH, Lamb DS, et al. Concurrent chemoradiation for oesophageal cancer: factors influencing myelotoxicity. Aust Radio 1996;40:424–9.
26. Minsky BD, Neuberg D, Kelsen DP, et al. Final report of Intergroup trial 0122 (ECOG PE-289, RTOG 90-12): phase II trial of neoadjuvant chemotherapy plus concurrent chemotherapy and high-dose radiation for squamous cell carcinoma of the esophagus. Int J Radiat Oncol Biol Phys 1999;43:517–23.
27. Bartels HE, Stein HJ, Siewert JR. Tracheobronchial lesions following oesophagectomy: prevalence, predisposing factors and outcome. Br J Surg 1998;85:403–6.
28. Mandard AM, Dalibard F, Mandard JC, et al. Pathologic assessment of tumor regression after preoperative chemoradiotherapy of esophageal carcinoma. Cancer 1994;73:2680–6.
29. Forastiere AA, Orringer MB, Perez-Tamayo C, et al. Preoperative chemoradiation followed by transhiatal esophagectomy for carcinoma of the esophagus: final report. J Clin Oncol 1993;11:1118–23.
30. Smithers BM, Devitt P, Jamieson GG, et al. A combined modality approach to the management of oesophageal cancer. Eur J Surg Oncol 1997;23:219–23.
31. Vogel SB, Mendenhall WM, Sombeck MD, et al. Downstaging of esophageal cancer after preoperative radiation and chemotherapy. Ann Surg 1995;221:685–95.
32. Bates BA, Detterbeck FC, Bernard SA, et al. Concurrent radiation therapy and chemotherapy followed by esophagectomy for localized esophageal carcinoma. J Clin Oncol 1996;14:156–63.
33. Triboulet JP, Amrouni H, Guillem P, et al. Long-term results of resected esophageal cancer with complete remission to pre-operative chemoradiation. Ann Chir 1998;52:503–8.
34. Reynolds JV, Muldoon C, Hollywood D, et al. Long-term outcomes following neoadjuvant chemoradiotherapy for oesophageal cancer. Ann Surg 2007;245:707–16.
35. Le Prise E, Etienne PL, Meunier B, et al. A randomized study of chemotherapy, radiation therapy, and surgery versus surgery for localized squamous cell carcinoma of the esophagus. Cancer 1994;73:1779–84.
36. Apinop C, Puttisak P, Preecha N. A prospective study of combined therapy in esophageal cancer. Hepatogastroenterology 1994;41:391–3.
37. Walsh TN, Noonan N, Hollywood D, et al. A comparison of multimodal therapy and surgery for esophageal adenocarcinoma. N Engl J Med 1996;335:462–7.
38. Urba S, Orringer M, Turrisi A, et al. A randomized trial comparing surgery (S) to preoperative concomitant chemoradiation plus surgery in patients (pts) with resectable esophageal cancer (CA): updated analysis. Proc Am Soc Clin Oncol 1997;16:277.

39. Burmeister BH, Smithers BM, Fitzgerald L, et al. A randomised phase III trial of preoperative chemoradiation followed by surgery (CR-S) versus surgery alone (S) for localized resectable cancer of the esophagus. Proc Am Soc Clin Oncol 2002;21:518.
40. Tepper J, Krasna MJ, Niedzwiecki D, et al. Phase III trial of trimodality therapy with cisplatin; fluorouracil, radiotherapy, and surgery compared with surgery alone for esophageal cancer: CALGB 9781. J Clin Oncol 2008;26:1086–92.
41. Urschel JD, Vasan H. A meta-analysis of randomized controlled trials that compared neoadjuvant chemoradiation and surgery to surgery alone for resectable esophageal cancer. Am J Surg 2003;185(6):538–43.
42. van Hagen P, Hulshof MCCM, Lanschot JJB, et al. Preoperative chemoradiotherapy for esophageal or junctional cancer. N Engl J Med 2012;366:2074–84.
43. Gebski V, Burmeister B, Foo K, et al. Survival benefits from neoadjuvant chemoradiotherapy or chemotherapy in oesophageal carcinoma: a meta-analysis. Lancet Oncol 2007;8:226–34.
44. Khan OA, Cruttenden-Wood D, Toh SK. Is an involved circumferential resection margin following oesphagectomy for cancer an important prognostic indicator? Interact Cardiovasc Thorac Surg 2010;11:645–8.
45. Stahl M, Walz MK, Stuschke M, et al. Phase III comparison of preoperative chemotherapy compared with chemoradiotherapy in patients with locally advanced adenocarcinoma of the esophagogastric junction. J Clin Oncol 2009;27:851–6.
46. Earlam R, Cunha-Melo JR. Oesophageal squamous cell carcinoma I. A critical review of radiotherapy. Br J Surg 1980;67:457–61.
47. Sykes AJ, Burt PA, Slevin NJ, et al. Radical radiotherapy for carcinoma of the oesophagus: an effective alternative to surgery. Radiother Oncol 1998;48:15–21.
48. Kawashima M, Kagami Y, Toita T, et al. Prospective trial of radiotherapy for patients 80 years of age or older with squamous cell carcinoma of the esophagus. Int J Radiat Oncol Biol Phys 2006;64:1112–21.
49. Araujo CM, Souhami L, Gil RA, et al. A randomized trial comparing radiation therapy versus concomitant radiation therapy and chemotherapy in carcinoma of the thoracic esophagus. Cancer 1991;67(9):2258–61.
50. Coia LR, Engstrom PF, Paul AR, et al. Long-term results of infusional 5-FU, mitomycin-C, and radiation as primary management of esophageal cancer. Int J Radiat Oncol Biol Phys 1991;20:29–36.
51. Al-Sarraf M, Martz K, Herskovic A, et al. Progress report of combined chemoradiotherapy versus radiotherapy alone in patients with esophageal cancer: an Intergroup study. J Clin Oncol 1997;15:277–84.
52. Minsky BD, Neuberg D, Kelsen DP, et al. Neoadjuvant chemotherapy plus high-dose radiation for squamous cell carcinoma of the esophagus: a preliminary analysis of the phase II Intergroup Trial 0122. J Clin Oncol 1996;14(1):149–55.
53. Gaspar LE, Qian C, Kocha WI, et al. A phase I/II study of external beam radiation, brachytherapy and concurrent chemotherapy in localized cancer of the esophagus (RTOG 92-07): preliminary toxicity report. Int J Radiat Oncol Biol Phys 1997;37(3):593–9.
54. Coia LR, Soffen EM, Schultheiss TE, et al. Swallowing function in patients with esophageal cancer treated with concurrent radiation and chemotherapy. Cancer 1993;71:281–6.
55. O'Rourke IC, Tiver K, Bull C, et al. Swallowing performance after radiation therapy for carcinoma of the esophagus. Cancer 1988;61:2022–6.
56. Ribiero U, Finklestein SD, Safatle-Ribiero A, et al. P53 sequence predicts treatment response and outcome of patients with esophageal carcinoma. Cancer 1998;83:7–18.
57. Yamamoto M, Tsujinaka T, Shiozaki H, et al. Metallothionein expression correlates with the pathological response of patients with esophageal cancer undergoing preoperative chemoradiation therapy. Oncology 1999;56:332–7.
58. Beardsmore DM, Verbeke CS, Davies CL, et al. Apoptotic and proliferative indexes in esophageal cancer: predictors of response to neoadjuvant therapy apoptosis and proliferation in esophageal cancer. J Gastrointest Surg 2003;7:77–87.
59. Jones DR, Parker LA, Detterbeck FC, et al. Inadequacy of computed tomography in assessing patients with esophageal carcinoma after induction chemoradiotherapy. Cancer 1999;85:1026–32.
60. Lim JTW, Truong PT, Berthelet E, et al. Endoscopic response predicts for survival and organ preservation after primary chemoradiotherapy for esophageal cancer. Int J Radiat Oncol Biol Phys 2003;57:1328–35.
61. Giovannini M, Seitz JF, Thomas P, et al. Endoscopic ultrasonography for assessment of the response to combined radiation therapy and chemotherapy in patients with esophageal cancer. Endoscopy 1997;29:4–9.
62. Mallery S, DeCamp M, Bueno R, et al. Pretreatment staging by endoscopic ultrasonography does not predict complete response to neoadjuvant chemoradiation in patients with esophageal carcinoma. Cancer 1999;86:764–9.
63. Wieder HA, Brucher B, Zimmermann F, et al. Time course of tumour metabolic activity during chemoradiotherapy of esophageal squamous cell carcinoma and response to treatment. J Clin Oncol 2004;22:900–8.
64. Raoul JL, Le Prise E, Meunier B, et al. Neoadjuvant chemotherapy and hyperfractionated radiotherapy with concurrent low-dose chemotherapy for squamous cell esophageal carcinoma. Int J Radiat Biol Phys 1998;42:29–34.

65. Crellin AM, Sebag-Montefiore D, Martin I, et al. Preoperative chemotherapy and radiotherapy, plus excision (CARE): a phase II study in esophageal cancer. Proc Am Soc Clin Oncol 2000;19:A1128.
66. Denham JW, Steigler A, Kilmurray J, et al. Relapse patterns after chemo-radiation for carcinoma of the oesophagus. Clin Oncol 2003;15:98–108.
67. Thomas E, Crellin A, Harris K, et al. The role of endoscopic ultrasound (EUS) in planning radiotherapy target volumes for oesophageal cancer. Radiother Oncol 2004;73:149–51.
68. Leong T, Everitt C, Yuen K, et al. A prospective study to evaluate the impact of FDG-PET on CT-based radiotherapy treatment planning for oesophageal cancer. Radiother Oncol 2006;78:254–61.
69. Bonner JA, Harari PM, Giralt JL, et al. Radiotherapy plus cetuximab for squamous-cell carcinoma of the head and neck. N Engl J Med 2006;354:567–78.
70. Chan A, Wong A. Is combined chemotherapy and radiation therapy equally effective as surgical resection in localized esophageal carcinoma? Int J Radiat Oncol Biol Phys 1999;45(2):265–70.
71. Murakami M, Kuroda Y, Nakajima T, et al. Comparison between chemoradiation protocol intended for organ preservation and conventional surgery for clinical T1–T2 esophageal carcinoma. Int J Radiat Oncol Biol Phys 1999;45(2):277–84.
72. Wilson KS, Lim JT. Primary chemotherapy–radiotherapy and selective oesophagectomy for oesophageal cancer: goal of cure with organ preservation. Radiother Oncol 2000;54:129–34.
73. Bedenne L, Michel P, Bouche O, et al. Chemoradiation followed by surgery compared with chemoradiation alone in squamous cancer of the esophagus: FFCD 9102. J Clin Oncol 2007;25:1160–8.
74. Stahl M, Wilke H, Lehmann N, et al. Long-term results of a phase III study investigating chemoradiation with and without surgery in locally advanced squamous cell carcinoma (LA-SCC) of the esophagus. J Clin Oncol 2008;26:(Suppl.):Abstr. 4530.
75. Gardner-Thorpe J, Hardwick R, Dwerryhouse SJ. Salvage oesophagectomy after local failure of definitive chemoradiotherapy. Br J Surg 2007;94:1059–66.
76. Hudson E, Powell J, Mukherjee S, et al. Small cell oesophageal carcinoma: an institutional experience and review of the literature. Br J Cancer 2007;96:708–11.
77. Ku GY, Minsky BD, Rusch VW, et al. Small-cell carcinoma of the esophagus and gastroesophageal junction: review of the Memorial Sloan-Kettering experience. Ann Oncol 2008;19:533–7.
78. Hermans J, Bonenkamp JJ, Ban MC, et al. Adjuvant therapy after curative resection for gastric cancer: a meta-analysis of randomized trials. J Clin Oncol 1993;11:1441–7.
79. Earle CC, Maroun JA. Adjuvant chemotherapy after curative resection for gastric cancer in non-Asian patients: revisiting a meta-analysis of randomised trials. Eur J Cancer 1999;35(7):1059–64.
80. Mari E, Floriani I, Tinazzi A, et al. Efficacy of adjuvant chemotherapy after curative resection for gastric cancer: a meta-analysis of published randomised trials. A study of the GISCAD (Gruppo Italiano per lo Studio dei Carcinomi della Apparato Digerente). Ann Oncol 2000;11(7):837–43.
81. Ychou M, Boige V, Pignon J-P, et al. Perioperative chemotherapy compared with surgery alone for resectable gastroesophageal adenocarcinoma: an FNCLCC and FFCD multicenter phase III trial. Clin Oncol 2011;29(13):1715–21.
82. Hagiwara A, Takahashi T, Kojima O, et al. Prophylaxis with carbon-adsorbed mitomycin against peritoneal recurrence of gastric cancer. Lancet 1992;339(8794):629–31.
83. Rosen HR, Jatzko G, Repse S, et al. Adjuvant intraperitoneal chemotherapy with carbon-adsorbed mitomycin in patients with gastric cancer: results of a randomized multicenter trial of the Austrian Working Group for Surgical Oncology. J Clin Oncol 1998;16(8):2733–8.
84. Hallissey MT, Dunn JA, Ward LC, et al. The second British Stomach Cancer Group trial of adjuvant radiotherapy or chemotherapy in resectable gastric cancer: five-year follow-up. Lancet 1994;343(8909):1309–12.
85. Macdonald JS, Smalley SR, Benedetti J, et al. Chemoradiotherapy after surgery compared with surgery alone for adenocarcinoma of the stomach or gastroesophageal junction. N Engl J Med 2001;345:725–30.
86. Hundahl SA, Macdonald JS, Benedetti J, et al., for the Southwest Oncology Group and the Gastric Intergroup. Surgical treatment variation in a prospective randomized trial of chemoradiotherapy in gastric cancer: the effect of undertreatment. Ann Surg Oncol 2002;9(3):278–86.
87. Bleiberg H, Jacob JH, Bedenne L, et al. A randomized phase II trial of 5-fluorouracil (5FU) and cisplatin (DDP) versus DDP alone in advanced esophageal cancer. Proc Soc Clin Oncol 1991;10:A447.
88. Zhang X, Shen L, Li J, et al. A phase II trial of paclitaxel and cisplatin in patients with advanced squamous-cell carcinoma of the esophagus. Am J Clin Oncol 2008;31:29–33.
89. Murad A, Santiago F, Petroianu A, et al. Modified therapy with 5-fluorouracil, doxorubicin, and methotrexate in advanced gastric cancer. Cancer 1993;72:37–41.
90. Pyrhonen S, Kuitunen T, Nvandoto P, et al. Randomised comparison of fluorouracil, epidoxorubicin and methotrexate (FEMTX) plus supportive care with supportive care alone in patients with non-resectable gastric cancer. Br J Cancer 1995;71:587–91.
91. Glimelius B, Ekstrom K, Hoffman K, et al. Randomized comparison between chemotherapy plus best supportive care with best supportive care in advanced gastric cancer. Ann Oncol 1997;8:163–8.

92. Macdonald J, Schein P, Woolley P, et al. 5-Fluorouracil, doxorubicin and mitomycin (FAM) combination chemotherapy for advanced gastric cancer. Ann Intern Med 1980;93:533–6.

93. Cullinan S, Moertel C, Fleming T, et al. A comparison of three chemotherapeutic regimens in the treatment of advanced pancreatic and gastric cancer. JAMA 1985;253:2061–7.

94. Klein HO. Long term results with FAMTX (5-fluorouracil, adriamycin, methotrexate) in advanced gastric cancer. Cancer Res 1989;9:1025.

95. Wils JA, Klein HO, Wegener DJT, et al. Sequential high-dose methotrexate and fluorouracil combined with doxorubicin: a step ahead in the treatment of advanced gastric cancer. A trial of the European Organisation for Research and Treatment of Cancer Gastrointestinal Tract Cooperative Group. J Clin Oncol 1991;9:827.

96. Kelsen D, Atiq O, Saltz L, et al. FAMTX versus etoposide, doxorubicin and cisplatin: a random assignment in gastric cancer. J Clin Oncol 1992;10:541–8.

97. Vanhoefer U, Rougier P, Wilke H, et al. Final results of a randomized phase III trial of sequential high-dose methotrexate, fluorouracil, and doxorubicin versus etoposide, leucovorin, and fluorouracil versus infusional fluorouracil and cisplatin in advanced gastric cancer: a trial of the European Organization for Research and Treatment of Cancer Gastrointestinal Tract Cooperative Group. J Clin Oncol 2000;18:2648–57.

98. Webb A, Cunningham D, Scarffe JH, et al. Randomized trial comparing epirubicin, cisplatin and fluorouracil versus fluorouracil, doxorubicin, and methotrexate in advanced esophagogastric cancer. J Clin Oncol 1997;15:261–7.

99. Seymour MT, Dent JT, Papamichael D, et al. Epirubicin, cisplatin and oral UFT with leucovorin (ECU): a phase I–II study in patients with advanced upper gastrointestinal tract cancer. Ann Oncol 1999;10(11):1329–33.

100. Van Cutsem E, Moiseyenko V, Tjulandin S, et al. Phase III study of docetaxel and cisplatin plus fluorouracil compared with cisplatin and fluorouracil as first line therapy for advanced gastric cancer: a report of the V325 study group. J Clin Oncol 2006;24:4991–7.

101. Dragovich T, McCoy S, Fenoglio-Preiser C, et al. Phase II trial of erlotinib in gastroesophageal junction and gastric adenocarcinomas: SWOG 0127. J Clin Oncol 2006;24:4922–7.

102. Bang Y-J, Van Cutsem E, Feyereislova A, et al. Trastuzumab in combination with chemotherapy versus chemotherapy alone for treatment of HER2-positive advanced gastric or gastro-oesophageal junction cancer (ToGA): a phase 3, open-label, randomised controlled trial. Lancet 2010;376:687–97.

103. Chau I, Norman A, Cunningham D, et al. Multivariate prognostic factor analysis in locally advanced and metastatic esophago-gastric cancer – pooled analysis from three multicenter, randomized, controlled trials using individual patient data. J Clin Oncol 2004;22:2395–403.

104. Dawes PJDK, Clague MB, Dean EM. Combined external beam and intracavitary radiotherapy for carcinoma of the oesophagus. Brachytherapy 2. In: Proceedings of the 5th International Selectron User's Meeting 1988; Nucleotron International; 1989. p. 442–4.

105. Pagliero KM, Rowlands CG. The place of brachytherapy in the treatment of carcinoma of the oesophagus. Brachytherapy HDR and LDR. In: Proceedings of a brachytherapy meeting: remote afterloading; state of the art; Nucleotron Corporation; 1990. p. 44–51.

106. Sur RK, Donde B, Levin VC, et al. Fractionated high dose rate brachytherapy in palliation of advanced esophageal cancer. Int J Radiat Oncol Biol Phys 1998;40(2):447–53.

107. Gaspar LE, Nag S, Hersokic A, et al. American Brachytherapy Society (ABS) consensus guidelines for brachytherapy of esophageal cancer. Int J Radiat Oncol Biol Phys 1997;38(1):127–32.

108. Homs MY, Steyerberg EW, Eijkenboom WM, et al. Single-dose brachytherapy verus metal stent placement for the palliation of dysphagia from oesophageal cancer: multicentre randomized trial. Lancet 2004;364:1497–504.

Palliative treatments of carcinoma of the oesophagus and stomach

Jane M. Blazeby
Natalie Blencowe

Despite improvements in the detection of oesophageal and gastric cancer the majority of Western patients present with advanced disease that is not amenable to cure. There are also patients with localised disease whose comorbidities or general frailty prohibits radical treatment. In these situations effective palliative therapy is required, with the aim of improving quality of life and maintaining survival with minimum risks until death occurs. This chapter concentrates on treatment modalities used for the palliation of oesophageal and gastric cancer.

Epidemiology and survival

Accurate information about the proportion of patients with oesophageal and gastric cancer who are treated with palliative intent is difficult to obtain. This largely reflects variations in the selection of patients for treatment. National audit data from England and Wales show that about 64% of new patients with oesophageal or gastric cancer undergo primary palliative treatment, although this varies between cancer networks and worldwide.[1–3] Trials continue to examine the role of palliative chemotherapy or radiotherapy in oesophageal cancer, but currently there is no evidence to show a survival benefit when compared to best supportive care.[4] The median survival is less than 8 months and few survive beyond 1 year. It is recommended, therefore, that treatment is tailored to the general status of the patient in order to reduce symptoms with minimal risks and side-effects.[5]

✔✔ There is little evidence to show that any single or combination of palliative treatment modality changes survival for patients not amenable to potentially curative treatment for oesophageal cancer[4]. Future trials comparing palliative treatment modalities should assess survival and health-related quality of life using validated measures.

The resection rate for patients with gastric cancer is greater than that for oesophageal cancer (25%), probably because distal gastrectomy is still widely employed to overcome gastric outlet obstruction even in patients with advanced disease.[1] Gastrojejunostomy (laparoscopic or open) or endoscopic stenting are also commonly performed if the tumour is very advanced or the patient frail. There is a lack of well-designed and conducted trials comparing distal gastrectomy with bypass or duodenal stenting, but systematic reviews comparing gastrojejunostomy with endoscopic stenting suggest that stent placement may be more favourable in patients with a very short life expectancy, although bypass is preferable in patients with a prolonged prognosis.[6,7] The randomised trials examining these issues are often small, however, and well-designed studies are still needed. Palliative chemotherapy, either alone or in combination with biological therapies, may lead to improved survival in gastric cancer. A Cochrane systematic review shows that chemotherapy significantly increases survival in comparison with best supportive care and that combination chemotherapy improves survival compared to single-agent 5-fluorouracil (5-FU).[8] It is also recommended that patients are tested for human epidermal growth factor receptor 2 (HER-2) status and a monoclonal antibody (trastuzumab) be added in patients with HER-2-positive tumours.[8,9] Despite these improvements in the treatment of advanced gastric cancer overall outcomes remain poor, with a median survival of less than 14 months.

Disease stage, age and general performance status influence outcomes and survival, although the effect of age may be largely due to more comorbidity in older patients.[10] Another predictor of mortality is the length of the oesophageal tumour, mainly because this increases the likelihood of nodal involvement with large tumours.[11] All these factors need to be taken into consideration when planning treatment.

Patient selection and multidisciplinary teams

Since the introduction of the National Health Service Cancer Plan in the UK in 2000, treatment decisions for patients with cancer are mandated to be made within the context of a multidisciplinary team.[12] Guidelines for the constitution and processes for upper gastrointestinal multidisciplinary teams have been published and national peer review processes audit team working.[12,13] Teams consist of core members, specialist nurses, gastroenterologists, oncologists, pathologists, radiologists, administrators, palliative medicine experts and surgeons. Additional members may include cytologists, dieticians and researchers from clinical trials units. The aim of the team is to review available evidence for each new patient and make optimal treatment decisions. Evidence includes information about the cell type, disease stage, patient comorbidity and choice, and expert discussion of best available treatments. Although team working has been widely implemented across the UK and is recommended by some continental European centres, in North America a similar role of 'tumour boards' is not mandatory within cancer care.[14] Currently, evidence to support team working is sparse, based upon longitudinal or retrospective case series. It is also uncertain how to best evaluate the quality of multidisciplinary teams because outcomes are dependent upon so many variables. It has been suggested that monitoring implementation of team decisions further evaluates team working. In one centre it has been shown that 15% (95% confidence interval (CI) 10–20%) of team decisions change after the meeting.[15] The most common reason cited for changing team decisions was lack of available information about patient choice and comorbidity. There is also uncertainty whether upper gastrointestinal multidisciplinary teams should routinely discuss patients who develop disease recurrence following radical treatment.[16] If this becomes mandatory in the UK the workload of teams would increase; however, patients with recurrence should be offered the full range of palliative treatments and so this requires further consideration. Team working is an area that is likely to develop over the next decade; professionals may need training in team-working skills and the infrastructure to support these processes is required.[17]

After establishing a diagnosis, new patients require careful assessment to decide whether treatment should be directed towards attempting a cure, or if palliation of symptoms is more appropriate. Careful patient selection has been shown to significantly influence results. Principal factors to consider are the type and stage of the tumour, physical and psychological well-being of the patient, and knowledge of patient preferences. Decisions should be considered in the knowledge of treatment outcomes, including impact on patients' health-related quality of life. **Figs 10.1** and **10.2** illustrate pathways that can be used to select patients for palliative treatment.

✔ Multidisciplinary cancer teams are a mandatory part of cancer care in the UK. The opportunity to elicit multiprofessional expertise in treatment decision-making is likely to benefit patient outcomes, but evidence to support this hypothesis is currently lacking. In the UK, selecting patients for palliative or potentially curative treatment is made within the context of a multidisciplinary team meeting, and full expert review of tumour type and stage, patient comorbidity and their wishes is required to make these decisions.

Fitness for treatment

The place of oesophagectomy in many older patients is often easily settled because of general debilitation or multiple coexistent medical problems. Age in itself does not preclude octogenarians from surgery, but in most series older patients are carefully selected. In general, patients who are not fit enough for oesophagectomy are also unable to tolerate a radical course of radiotherapy or definitive chemoradiation. On the whole, surgery for gastric tumours is better tolerated than oesophageal surgery by the elderly population, but patients still require careful preoperative assessment before undergoing major resection. Anaesthetic assessment for surgery is considered in more detail in Chapter 4.

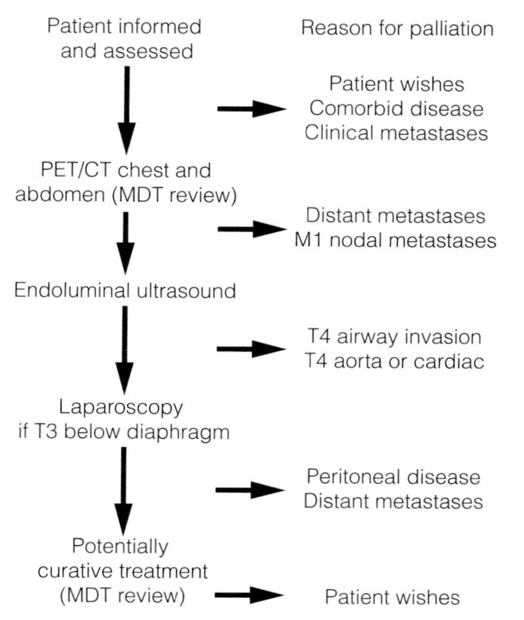

Figure 10.1 • Algorithm for selection for palliative or curative treatment of oesophageal and junctional tumours. CT, computed tomography; MDT, multidisciplinary team; PET, positron emission tomography.

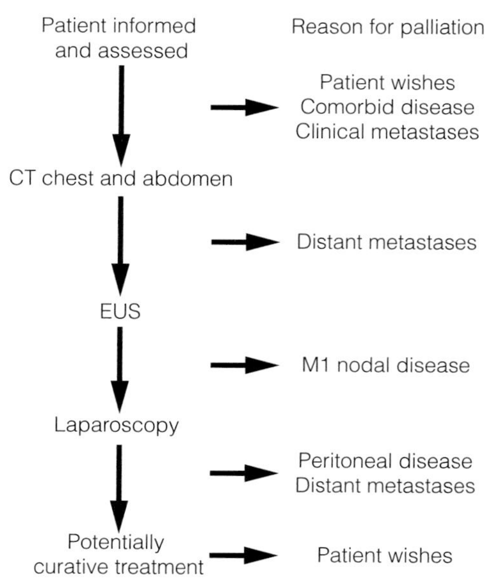

Figure 10.2 • Algorithm for selection for palliative or curative treatment for cancers of the gastric body or antrum. CT, computed tomography; EUS, endoscopic ultrasonography.

Staging investigations

Accurate tumour staging plays a crucial part in any therapeutic protocol, enabling patients to be assigned appropriately to treatments with either curative or palliative intent. Clear evidence of haematogenous tumour spread or irresectability directs patients with oesophageal cancer to palliative treatment. Despite advances in staging procedures, no single investigation is perfect and a small percentage of patients still require exploratory surgery to determine resectability. Palliative resection or bypass surgery to ameliorate bleeding or obstruction may be indicated for some patients with gastric cancer even in the presence of haematogenous tumour spread. The decision to proceed with palliative surgery requires careful consideration, as many patients rapidly deteriorate in this situation.

Patient preferences and information provision

Information about the diagnosis and prognosis of oesophageal and gastric cancer should be offered to all patients and it is essential that a nurse specialist is involved in this process whenever possible. The volume and type of information required will vary between individuals, although evidence from studies of patients' information needs performed in other disease sites generally shows that patients wish to have as much information as possible and prefer the information to be provided by a health professional, as well as in other forms such as a booklet or CD-ROM.[17] It is necessary to inform patients of the potential treatments and alternatives together with treatment-related benefits and risks, both in the short and long term. Surveys of patients' information needs also show that information about impact on health-related quality of life is considered important to patients during treatment decision-making.[18] Ensuring that consultations provide this information in a way that is understood is difficult and requires that professionals are trained. In the UK it is recommended that all specialist cancer teams undergo training in advanced communication skills.[19] All clinicians will be faced with patients who demand every small chance of cure, despite its risks, and others who wish to receive minimal, dignified intervention. Communicating outcomes, providing adequate information and listening to patients' views is necessary so that patients and their families have access to as much information and support as required.

Symptoms and signs of advanced oesophageal and gastric cancer

Tumours of the oesophagus and gastric cardia

Dysphagia is the predominant symptom for most patients with tumours of the oesophagus, oesophagogastric junction or proximal stomach. The progressive nature of malignant dysphagia is usually apparent. Initial difficulties in swallowing solid food may cause bolus obstruction and odynophagia. Solid food intake gradually reduces and patients are finally unable to even swallow saliva. Complete dysphagia may lead to aspiration pneumonia. Less than 5% of patients with oesophageal cancer develop an aero-digestive fistula, but this is generally associated with locally advanced disease and a very poor prognosis. Oesophageal tumours may also present with vomiting, haematemesis or gastro-oesophageal reflux. Many patients present with symptoms of advanced disease including fatigue, anorexia, upper abdominal pain caused by lymphadenopathy, ascites or liver metastases, and constipation. Rapid weight loss frequently occurs because of cancer cachexia exacerbated by poor oral intake. Hoarseness caused by tumour infiltration of the recurrent laryngeal nerves may be the result of advanced local disease or mediastinal recurrence after oesophagectomy.

Tumours of the gastric body and antrum

Gastric cancer commonly has an insidious presentation and some patients have few symptoms. Slow blood loss may eventually result in symptoms of anaemia. Haematemesis is a rare first presentation. Vague upper gastrointestinal problems, such as epigastric discomfort, early satiety and gastro-oesophageal reflux, are common. Tumours of the distal stomach cause outlet obstruction and patients describe epigastric fullness, reflux and nausea, finally leading to effortless vomiting. The presence of an epigastric mass, supraclavicular lymphadenopathy, jaundice, ascites or pleural effusions all reflect advanced disease. Less commonly, bony pain and symptoms of increased intracranial pressure are seen related to metastatic spread. Symptoms of oesophageal and gastric cancer are listed in Box 10.1.

The provision of rapid relief of dysphagia or gastric obstruction for patients with advanced oesophageal and gastric malignancies is the initial priority of palliative treatment for patients who are symptomatic. When patients with disease not amenable to cure have minimal symptoms related to the primary tumour, the main aim of palliative treatment is to extend survival and maintain or improve health-related quality of life. Many patients undergoing palliative treatment will also need dietary advice. Appropriate end-of-life care should be implemented.

Box 10.1 • Symptoms of oesophageal and gastric cancer

Oesophageal cancer
Dysphagia
Odynophagia
Reflux
Chest pain
Haematemesis
Cough
Dyspnoea
Hoarseness

Gastric cancer
Dysphagia
Epigastric fullness/discomfort
Effortless vomiting
Haematemesis
Nausea
Reflux
Symptoms of anaemia

Metastatic disease
Upper abdominal pain
Epigastric fullness/discomfort
Anorexia
Bone pain
Constipation
Dyspnoea
Cough
Weight loss
Fatigue

Palliative treatments for cancer of the oesophagus and gastric cardia

A variety of approaches are available for the palliation of advanced tumours of the oesophagus and gastric cardia. These include rigid plastic tube insertion, self-expanding metal stents (SEMS), brachytherapy, external beam radiotherapy, chemotherapy, chemical and thermal ablation, palliative resection (for gastric cancer) and bypass surgery either as single or combination treatment modalities. These different treatment modalities can treat and palliate the cancers and therefore there is no longer a role for palliative surgery for oesophageal cancer, which has a major detrimental impact on patients' quality of life.[20] Generally, patients undergoing palliative surgery do not have sufficient time to recover from the operation before they experience symptoms of metastatic disease. Historical data also show that palliative resection is associated with high perioperative mortality and morbidity rates. It is possible that the improved surgical techniques and perioperative care may mean that minimal access surgical resection may in certain situations be suitable for the palliation of oesophageal cancer; however, well-designed studies are needed to corroborate this. Evidence for the effectiveness of non-surgical interventions for the palliation of malignant dysphagia in the treatment of primary oesophageal cancer is summarised in a recent Cochrane review that includes 40 studies.[21] Overall, it concluded that SEMS insertion is safe, quick and effective in palliating malignant dysphagia compared to other modalities. High-dose intraluminal brachytherapy may be a suitable alternative and provide additional survival benefit and quality of life. The individual studies examining endoscopic methods of relieving luminal obstruction are considered below, with other sections concentrating on treatments for palliation of other common problems in oesophageal or oesophagogastric junctional cancer:

1. Endoscopic methods of relieving luminal obstruction.
2. Chemotherapy, radiotherapy, chemoradiotherapy and monoclonal antibody treatments.
3. Management of aero-digestive fistulas.
4. Management of recurrent laryngeal nerve palsy.
5. Management of chronic bleeding.

The endoscopic relief of luminal obstruction

Malignant dysphagia may be relieved by stent insertion, brachytherapy, external beam radiotherapy, chemotherapy or tumour ablation with photothermal, photodynamic therapy, or by the injection of cytotoxic substances.[20] Many modalities are complementary and SEMS insertion is safe, effective and quicker in palliating dysphagia compared to other modalities. No one method or combination is greatly superior to the rest in terms of relief of dysphagia, although some evidence is emerging to show better long-term relief of dysphagia with high-dose intraluminal brachytherapy. This might provide a suitable alternative and may provide additional survival with a better quality of life compared to metal stent placement.[22] Historically, dilatation was advocated for the palliation of malignant dysphagia and rigid plastic tubes were inserted following this. Because of the short-lived benefits of dilatation alone and the associated risks of perforation, its use nowadays is reduced to that of a preliminary measure before definitive management of dysphagia. Minimal oesophageal dilatation may be performed to allow insertion of an SEMS or to place a brachytherapy bougie. Guidelines on the use of dilatation in clinical practice recommend careful preparation, polyvinyl wire-guided bougies or hydrostatic balloons.[23] Strictures with severe narrowing and angulation are best negotiated under X-ray screening.

✔✔ A tissue diagnosis is desirable prior to dilatation of a malignant stricture and wherever possible oesophageal dilatation should be undertaken as a planned procedure with informed consent. It should be undertaken by experienced endoscopists with contrast radiology available.

The majority of randomised trials evaluating palliative treatments for dysphagia have been small and single-centred, and may therefore have lacked power to detect differences between treatment arms. Table 10.1 summarises the randomised controlled trials published before the end of 2011, evaluating interventions of the palliation of malignant dysphagia. The table includes only trials that randomised more than a total of 50 patients, excluding smaller studies because they are less likely to influence practice. Even within the included studies, eight (50%) may be at risk of selection bias because methods used to conceal the allocation sequence were unclear (i.e. intervention allocations could have been foreseen before or during enrolment).

Intubation

Intubation is probably the most widely used form of palliation of malignant dysphagia at present and allows rapid relief of dysphagia with associated low morbidity. Prostheses may be placed endoscopically, radiologically or surgically at laparotomy, although there is little place for open insertion of a prosthesis when a tumour is unexpectedly found to be irresectable because endoscopic insertion is safer and has fewer complications. Self-expanding metal stents are now routinely employed for this purpose and plastic rigid tubes are generally no longer in use.[21,24–26]

Table 10.1 • Prospective randomised controlled trials of endoscopic palliation of malignant dysphagia ($n > 50$)

Authors	*n*	Group 1	Group 2	Dysphagia	Clinical outcomes	Health-related quality of life*	Allocation concealment†
Blomberg et al., 2010[62]	72	Antireflux stent (oesophageal Z-stent with antireflux valve)	SEMS: Oesophageal Z-stent, Ultraflex or Wallstent	Worse in Group 2	No difference	In favour of Group 1	B
Verschuur et al., 2008[63‡]	83	SEMS: Ultraflex	SEMS: Polyflex	Worse in Group 1	No difference except more stent migrations in Group 2	Not assessed	B
Verschuur et al., 2008[63‡]	44	SEMS: Ultraflex	SEMS: Niti-S	Worse in Group 1	No difference	Not assessed	B
Conio et al., 2007[27]	101	Self-expandable plastic stent	SEMS: covered Ultraflex	No difference	Morbidity higher with expandable plastic stents	Not assessed	B
Bergquist et al., 2005[40]	65	SEMS	Brachytherapy	Not assessed	Not assessed	In favour of SEMS	B
Shenfine et al., 2009[26]	217	SEMS (then randomised to 18- or 24-mm-diameter stent)	Standard treatment (then randomised to plastic tube or no tube treatment)	Worse quality swallowing with plastic tubes	Survival advantage in standard group randomised to no tube treatment	18-mm stents reported less pain than with 24-mm SEMS	A
Fu et al., 2004[64]	53	SEMS	SEMS and chemotherapy or chemoradiotherapy	No difference	No difference	Not assessed	B
Homs et al., 2004[22,41]	209	SEMS: covered Ultraflex	Brachytherapy	SEMS better short-term relief. Brachytherapy better long-term relief	Morbidity higher with SEMS	In favour of brachytherapy	A
Sabharwal et al., 2003[65]	53	SEMS: covered Wallstent	SEMS: covered Ultraflex	No difference	No difference	Not assessed	A
O'Donnell et al., 2002[66]	50	Cook plastic tube	SEMS: covered Wallstent	No difference	No difference	No difference	A
Canto et al., 2002[67]	56	SEMS	PDT	SEMS better short-term relief, similar long-term relief	Not assessed	In favour of PDT	B

Table 10.1 • (*cont.*) Prospective randomised controlled trials of endoscopic palliation of malignant dysphagia ($n > 50$)

Authors	*n*	Group 1	Group 2	Dysphagia	Clinical outcomes	Health-related quality of life*	Allocation concealment†
Siersema et al., 2001[68]	100	SEMS: covered Wallstent	SEMS: covered Ultraflex or Gianturco Z stent	No difference	No difference	Not assessed	B
Vakil et al., 2001[69]	62	SEMS: covered	SEMS: uncovered	No difference	Fewer reinterventions in covered SEMS group	Not assessed	A
Dallal et al., 2001[29]	65	Nd:YAG laser	SEMS: uncovered Ultraflex	No difference	Morbidity similar, survival better Group 1	Significant HRQOL deterioration in stent group at 1 month	A
Adam et al., 1997[30]	60	SEMS either: covered Wallstent or uncovered Ultraflex	Nd:YAG laser	Worse in Group 2	Stent migration worse in Group 1, covered Wallstent	Not assessed	B
Sargeant et al., 1997[70]	67	Nd:YAG laser	Nd:YAG laser and external beam radiotherapy	Longer treatment intervals in Group 2	No difference	Not assessed	A
Lightdale et al., 1995[33]	218	Nd:YAG laser	Photodynamic therapy + argon pumped dye laser	No difference	Perforations more common in Group 1	Not assessed	A

Note: 30-day mortality rates were similar in all of the above trials.
HRQOL, health-related quality of life; Nd:YAG, neodymium yttrium–aluminium–garnet laser; SEMS, self-expanding metal stent.
*Health-related quality-of-life results in article reported from a valid multidimensional questionnaire.
†The risk of bias in the trial was judged as A = low, B = unclear or C = high, using the Cochrane risk of bias tool assessing allocation concealment.[71] The tool allows an author to judge whether the randomisation process described in the study has clear evidence that the treatment allocation was concealed to the person randomising the patient before the patient is entered into the study.
‡This randomised controlled trial had three treatment arms and subsequently two comparisons.

✔✔ **Self-expanding metal stent insertion is safe, effective and quick in palliating dysphagia compared to other modalities.[21] High-dose intraluminal brachytherapy is a suitable alternative and might provide additional survival benefit with a better quality of life.[22,41,42]**

Self-expanding metal stents (SEMS)

The design of SEMS has evolved since they were first introduced for the palliation of malignant dysphagia in the early 1990s with the introduction of covering and also fixtures to allow endoscopic stent removal. They are made from a flexible metal mesh that expands after deployment for up to 48 hours, leading to rapid relief of dysphagia and creation of an internal luminal diameter of 16–25 mm. Early disadvantages of tumour ingrowth and stent migration have been largely overcome by newer materials and designs, although migration may still occur when stents are placed at the oesophagogastric junction. Although initially stents were expensive (about £500–800), the cost is now reducing. Current design developments are centred upon using expandable plastic rather than metal to reduce the manufacturing costs, and developing removable stents and possibly dissolvable stents to use in temporary settings.[27] Stents nowadays, therefore, may be fully or partially covered (partially covered self-expanding metal stents, PCSEMS). Several studies have investigated the addition of a valve in the distal part of the stent to reduce acid reflux.[28]

Method of insertion

Self-expanding metal stents may be inserted endoscopically or radiologically. There are several designs with very similar delivery devices. The Ultraflex Esophageal Stent (Boston Scientific Inc.) is made of an alloy of titanium and nickel and has a shape 'memory' as well as superelastic behaviour. It is loaded in a small-diameter delivery catheter, constrained in a compressed form by a double plastic membrane. During expansion the stent shrinks by approximately one-third. It is available either uncovered or partially covered. The design incorporates a proximal flare for secure placement and to reduce the possibility of food entrapment. The conical 'Flamingo' Wallstent is designed to reduce problems with migration, and the proximal and distal 1.5 cm of the stent remain uncovered. It may be recovered during deployment and repositioned, provided less than 50% of the endoprosthesis has been released. The Gianturco Z stent also uses stainless steel and it is entirely coated with a polyethylene film. It has long wire hooks at its mid-portion to facilitate anchoring. Unlike the Ultraflex and Wallstents it undergoes very little shortening upon release. A 'windsock' design to reduce the possibility of gastro-oesophageal reflux is available. Other stents are variations on these basic designs. Comparative studies show that reintervention rates for tumour ingrowth are higher with uncovered than covered stents. Other comparative studies of SEMS show conflicting results and although these trials may have design weaknesses, there is currently no good evidence that one design is superior to another in terms of morbidity or relief of dysphagia.

Contraindications to metal stent placement are tumours requiring stent placement within 2 cm of the upper oesophageal sphincter. This is not recommended because of concerns about proximal migration, laryngeal compression, intractable pain and a globus sensation. Relative contraindications to stent placement are more dependent on operator expertise, but these include: total luminal obstruction; non-circumferential tumour growth prohibiting proper anchoring of the prosthesis; almost horizontal orientation of the malignant lumen; prior chemoradiation; and multiangulated lesions, particularly with tumours at the gastro-oesophageal junction. All of these situations render endoscopic intubation hazardous or make the stent less likely to relieve dysphagia.

Preparation

Endoscopic prosthesis insertion is usually possible under intravenous sedation, although some endoscopists continue to use general anaesthesia. Routine monitoring is required with intravenous sedation, as is continual attention to the airway. Saliva and regurgitated fluids should be constantly removed to prevent aspiration during the procedure.

Endoscopic insertion with fluoroscopy

After endoscopic assessment and measurement of the tumour, a guidewire is passed into the stomach (after successful negotiation of the tumour with the endoscope or under fluoroscopic control). Occasionally, dilatation may be required to a minimum of 10 mm before passage of the delivery system over the guidewire. The proximal and distal extents of the tumour may be marked with radio-opaque skin markers or the tumour limitations injected with contrast. The slim delivery device is advanced over the guidewire until the radio-opaque markers of the compressed stent are correctly aligned with the tumour. Once in position the stent is deployed. It is possible to reposition some of the stents after partial deployment. The guidewire and delivery device are then carefully removed under fluoroscopic guidance. After release of the stent, the endoscope may be reinserted to check the final position. Immediate balloon dilatation is recommended to improve expansion and prevent early migration, but may still be performed up to several days after stent insertion.

Radiological insertion

Morphological imaging of the malignant stricture with oral contrast is performed prior to stent insertion. This assesses length and position of the tumour. A fine steerable catheter is then negotiated over a guidewire through the stricture to the stomach and skin markers aligned. The proximal and distal ends of the tumour are marked (similar to endoscopic positioning). Balloon dilatation to 10–15 mm may be performed if the stricture is very narrow. The stent insertion device is then passed safely and positioned radiographically over the guidewire and released according to the type of stent.

Postoperative management

After stent insertion the patient must be instructed to sit upright. Oral fluids are usually allowed the same day unless there is concern about complications or symptoms or signs of perforation. Clinical and radiological examination may be performed to exclude perforation before oral fluids are commenced. Patients should receive written dietary information with advice to chew food carefully and drink regularly during and after meals. A daily intake of 10 mL hydrogen peroxide (20 vol.) is sometimes recommended.

Complications

Even in experienced hands, intubation with SEMS has a procedure-related mortality of about 1–2% and early complication rates of between 0% and 30%. Complications are listed in Box 10.2.

Box 10.2 • Complications of stent insertion

Early complications
Malposition/migration
Incomplete expansion
Oesophageal perforation
Upper gastrointestinal bleeding
Aspiration pneumonia
Pain
Late complications
Migration
Tumour ingrowth or overgrowth
Aspiration pneumonia
Pain
Reflux
Late perforation and fistulation
Disintegration of prosthesis
Stent torsion
Bleeding

Early complications

1. Malposition of the stent may require insertion of a second or even third stent (if the tumour is long). This may overlap the malpositioned stent to adequately cover the tumour.
2. Incomplete stent expansion and early dysphagia may require balloon dilatation if no improvement is seen within 48 hours.
3. Early stent migration. This occurs in about 1% of patients and is more prone in stents placed at the oesophagogastric junction than in stents with both ends anchored within the oesophagus. Endoscopic retrieval may be performed safely, especially with the newer devices. Stents that have migrated into the stomach may also be safely left as they rarely obstruct the pyloric channel or cause intestinal perforation.
4. Oesophageal perforation is the most serious complication and is more likely if the stricture has been dilated before stent insertion, there has been prior use of radiotherapy and/or chemotherapy, if the tumour is sharply angulated or if it extensively encases the oesophagus. Rapid development of subcutaneous emphysema, severe pain, radiological evidence of pneumomediastinum, air under the diaphragm or a pleural effusion should all raise suspicion. The extent of the leak is confirmed by contrast radiography. The most appropriate form of therapy depends on the time of detection and the extent of the leak. If recognised at endoscopy, the insertion of the prosthesis itself may seal off the perforation and prevent mediastinitis. Alternatively, the procedure may be abandoned and conservative treatment undertaken. This involves administration of broad-spectrum antibiotics, cessation of oral intake and feeding either parenterally or by jejunostomy. An intercostal drain may need to be inserted if there is evidence of pleural contamination. Specific management of this serious complication is covered in detail in Chapter 19.
5. Severe upper gastrointestinal haemorrhage occasionally occurs. This is difficult to treat, and only supportive measures may be possible.

Late complications

Long-term problems occur in at least 20% of patients and are most frequently related to eating. Problems often require hospital admission, further endoscopic manoeuvres and occasionally replacement of the prosthesis.

1. Prostheses may block because of tumour overgrowth at either end of the stent or tumour ingrowth through the metallic stent latticework if an uncovered design is used. This leads to recurrent dysphagia and occurs in 5–30% of patients. Tumour ingrowth is best managed with laser, argon-beam coagulation or photodynamic therapy. Overgrowth at either end of the stent may be successfully treated with placement of a second stent.
2. Food bolus obstruction occurs in metallic stents despite their wide diameter. Spontaneous resolution can occur or endoscopy may be required to displace the impacted food bolus into the stomach.
3. Reflux of gastric acid occurs in all patients whenever the tube crosses the gastro-oesophageal junction. It may lead to oesophagitis and occasionally benign stricture formation above the tube. This can be controlled by conservative measures, dilatation and acid suppression therapy. The use of a stent with an antireflux valve may reduce reflux symptoms.
4. Pressure necrosis and late oesophageal perforation leading to mediastinal fistulation has been reported.
5. Stents can fracture or twist, leading to serious morbidity. These are rare problems as most patients do not live long enough. Operative

removal of these tubes is only very occasionally required.
6. Eating difficulties exist due to incomplete relief of dysphagia. Once a prosthesis is in place all food must pass through a tube with a fixed diameter. Patients therefore need appropriate nutritional support and advice.

Manufacturers continue to develop new designs to decrease the risk of migration, increase the ease of insertion and enable stents to be repositioned or extracted. A new self-expanding plastic stent (SEPS) prosthesis has been evaluated but may lead to particular problems of stent migration. However, it is likely that future developments will overcome these issues.[27] Despite the associated morbidity with stent insertion, the immediate relief of dysphagia in one endoscopy session has made intubation an attractively simple palliative treatment, particularly for patients with poor performance status whose life expectancy is short.

Laser treatment

Laser therapy as a treatment for palliation of malignant dysphagia is diminishing because it is time-consuming and requires repeated hospital visits. Where patients are fit enough for multiple hospital treatments they may be offered palliative chemotherapy or brachytherapy. Laser treatment may still be useful for overgrowth or ingrowth of tumour in patients with oesophageal stents and it is valuable for tumours of the cervical oesophagus (where a stent is contraindicated). The principles of tumour ablation with laser treatment are similar to those used in other techniques such as argon-beam coagulation. Successful recanalisation and relief of dysphagia may be achieved after a mean of two treatment sessions, although most patients will continue to manage only semisolid or liquid foods. The mean dysphagia-free interval after laser treatment varies from 4 to 16 weeks. Repeated recanalisations can be performed with a laser or argon beam as many times as necessary.

The most popular type of laser in Britain is the non-contact neodymium yttrium–aluminium–garnet (Nd:YAG) laser. Laser energy is conveyed through a single monofibre, which is enclosed in a Teflon sheath. At an irradiation distance of 5–10 mm, multiple pulses for a duration of about 0.5–1 s are given. It causes tissue necrosis with eventual vaporisation, depending on the power used, the duration of application, the distance between the fibre tip and target, the aim of the application and the colour of the tissue. Coaxial gas (usually CO_2 or NO_2) is administered around the quartz fibre, to cool the probe tip and clear debris. Gas is removed with the suction channel of the endoscope. A nasogastric tube next to the endoscope can be used to vent the oesophagus. The low-power contact Nd:YAG system uses coaxial water to cool the tip, remove debris and reduce adherence of the contact probe. This employs a sapphire tip, which acts like a hot knife. Lower power settings theoretically mean that the chances of perforation by excessive laser energy are reduced. Tissue damage only occurs up to 0.5 mm beyond the treatment site. Each laser treatment session may recanalise the whole or part of the stricture. Some recommend routine endoscopic review at 48–72 hours, when oedema has subsided and accurate assessment of the overall effect can be made. The destroyed tumour may then be evacuated with forceps, polyp graspers, lavage or pushed distally with the endoscope. Others administer treatment as dictated by clinical response.

Endoscopic technique

Laser treatment is usually carried out with intravenous sedation, although some centres use a rigid endoscope requiring general anaesthesia and endotracheal intubation. Those in favour of a rigid scope believe its advantages are that it allows better suction of fluid, smoke and debris, with improved visualisation of the tumour. If a malignant stricture is negotiable, the laser is first applied to the distal end of the tumour. The scope is then withdrawn in a circular fashion into the more proximal tumour. If complete obstruction is encountered, tumours can be vaporised in the antegrade direction or first dilated to allow passage of the endoscope. Antegrade therapy may be more dangerous because information about the luminal axis is lacking and the area first treated rapidly becomes oedematous, thus impairing visualisation and access more distally.

Early complications

The incidence of major complications and mortality (which is in the region of 1–5%) was usually lower for laser destruction than endoscopic intubation with rigid plastic stents. Few studies have compared laser treatment with metal stents (Table 10.1). Early complications after laser treatment are listed in Box 10.3.

1. Chest pain may result from extensive mucosal burning. It is common but not severe.
2. Oesophageal perforation is less common following laser recanalisation than intubation with a rigid endoprosthesis. The risk is about 5% and is said to be related to predilatation rather than a direct complication of the laser treatment.
3. A benign pneumoperitoneum or pneumomediastinum is sometimes detected by chest X-ray after laser treatment. This is thought to be related to

Box 10.3 • Complications of laser treatment

Early complications
Pain
Perforation
Pneumatoperitoneum
Pneumomediastinum
Gastric distension
Bleeding
Aspiration pneumonia
Late complications
Repeated hospital admissions
Tumour recurrence
Benign strictures
Functional swallowing problems

jets of coaxial gas passing through abnormal, often necrotic, tumour tissue. Patients rarely have symptoms. Contrast studies do not show a leak and patients usually make an uneventful recovery.

4. Gastric distension as a result of carbon dioxide infusion can be quite uncomfortable despite adequate decompression. The pain is visceral in nature and may be confused with chest pain from excessive mucosal burning.
5. Haemorrhage after laser treatment is rare, occurring in about 1%.

Late complications

Late complications frequently occur following laser destruction and require repeated endoscopic treatment.

1. The main problem is tumour recurrence. Patients require about monthly treatment sessions. It is perceived by the medical profession that this is burdensome and disruptive, but there have been few studies that have objectively measured patients' views about this matter. Some may feel that continued hospital contact contributes to their sense of well-being.
2. Delayed laser-associated benign strictures can occur in up to 20% of patients. They require repeated dilatation and occasionally stent insertion.
3. Persistent dysphagia for solids. Laser treatment may recanalise 90% of all stenoses, but a wide luminal diameter does not necessarily equate to normal swallowing. Distal tumours may cause 'pseudoachalasia' that impairs swallowing. Residual intramural tumour may cause impaired oesophageal body motility and, together with progressive cachexia, may make it impossible for some patients to take solid foods again.

Combination laser treatment

In view of the varied responses with laser treatment alone, means of improving the efficacy of laser treatment by increasing the period between laser therapy and symptomatic relapse have been explored through combination treatments. Laser therapy can be combined with external- or internal-beam radiotherapy to prolong the interval between treatments, although the patient must attend for radiotherapy, which does increase hospital attendance. Intraluminal radiotherapy is useful for treating mural invasion following laser debulking of the tumour.

Thermal recanalisation or stenting?

Although laser therapy is rapid, safe and effective, and may have superior relief of dysphagia compared to rigid intubation, it also has drawbacks related to the need to attend hospital on a regular basis and the capital cost of the equipment. It may be preferable for non-circumferential, polypoid or exophytic tumours, but it is not suitable for patients with a fistula, an extrinsic lesion causing oesophageal compression, or patients with a diffuse subepithelial tumour. Two randomised controlled trials that included 125 patients comparing SEMS with thermoablative therapy (predominantly laser) showed no evidence to suggest that either modality is different in improving dysphagia, the interval to recurrent dysphagia or procedure-related mortality.[29,30] It is noted, however, that both procedures have certain adverse effects that are more common in each group. Laser may therefore increasingly be viewed as a complementary rather than competing palliative treatment, to deal with tube overgrowth or ingrowth or local recurrence after surgery.

Argon-beam plasma coagulation

High-frequency diathermy electrocoagulation has become widely used for surgical haemostasis and to ablate tumour tissue. The argon-beam coagulator utilises a jet of ionised argon gas to limit conduction of high-frequency electrical energy to the desired point, i.e. tumour and unhealthy tissue. This is readily applied through an endoscope. Once the surface of the tumour has been coagulated and dried, the electrical current passes through to an adjacent area. Unlike laser light, the argon beam will arc to the nearest point of contact. The depth of extension is minimal (2–3 mm) and this reduces the risk of perforation. The gas flow is high, which means that regular aspiration is required to prevent gastric distension. It is not expensive and operator confidence is high, given the low risk of perforation. Because of these pragmatic features it has largely replaced laser treatment as a primary debulking treatment.[31] As with laser treatment, it is time-consuming and there is a need for repeated treatments.

Photodynamic therapy

Photodynamic therapy (PDT) is an investigational treatment that modifies conventional laser treatment. It uses a selective technique that targets tumour tissue and limits damage to adjacent tissue. It essentially has three elements: light, a photosensitising drug (a haematoporphyrin derivative) and oxygen. The drug acting as a photosensitiser is injected intravenously 3–4 days before irradiation of the tumour. Laser light (administered endoscopically) then activates the drug within the tissue. Once stimulated, the photosensitiser interacts with oxygen to create a highly reactive oxygen species that is cytotoxic. Retention of the photosensitiser is longer in dysplastic or frankly neoplastic than normal tissues, at a ratio of about 2:1. Damage to normal tissue heals by regeneration.[32]

Clinical indications

The role of PDT in palliative treatments is yet to be determined and is likely to be small. It may be used to treat patients with small mucosal tumours (uT1, N0) who are unfit or who do not wish to undergo major surgery (see Chapter 6), or it can be used on larger inoperable lesions where other treatments have failed. Two prospective randomised studies have compared PDT with laser therapy.[33,34] There was no evidence to suggest differences between PDT and laser treatment in dysphagia or 30-day mortality and equivocal evidence that PDT decreased the need for repeated endoscopic interventions compared to laser treatment.

Complications

A number of specific complications have been recognised. The activated photosensitiser creates an iatrogenic porphyria, which may persist for up to 6 weeks after injection of the drug and leads to skin photosensitivity. Patients are advised to avoid sunlight. Perforation and fistulas may occur as well as oesophagitis leading to stricture formation. PDT has yet to enter widespread clinical use, partly because of cost. New photosensitisers with shorter durations of action may make the treatment more acceptable. At present, there are no data to support PDT as first-line palliative treatment, but it may be considered for high oesophageal tumours, for salvage treatment if stents have migrated or for stent over/ingrowth.

Bipolar electrocoagulation

Bipolar electrocoagulation (BICAP) is another thermal endoscopic treatment that has been used to relieve dysphagia.[35] Usually 2–4 mm of coagulation occurs at the tumour surface and one or two treatment sessions are required to treat the entire tumour. Although dysphagia may be partially relieved, problems with perforation, fistula formation, strictures and bleeding have occurred, and the technique has never been widely used.

Chemically induced tumour necrosis

The use of intralesional injection of alcohol (usually ethanol) to induce tumour necrosis is a simple and readily available palliative treatment, suitable for exophytic tumours and tumours in the proximal oesophagus.[36,37] It may also be used to control haemorrhage from bleeding tumours.

Endoscopic technique

Patients require intravenous sedation and flexible endoscopy. A sclerotherapy needle is used to inject 0.5- to 1-mL aliquots of alcohol into the protuberant part of the tumour. Endoscopic observation of the tumour blanching and swelling confirms needle position. In patients with long tumours it is best to start injections distally so that induced oedema does not impede the passage of the endoscope. There is no limit to the total volume injected in one session (1–36 mL have been reported). Dilatation is needed if the endoscope is unable to traverse the stricture. Several treatment sessions may be required to improve swallowing, but it usually does so within a week of injection.

Outcome

An improvement in dysphagia score is reported in most patients after treatment with absolute alcohol, although it may be made temporarily worse because of initial tumour oedema and swelling. Retrosternal chest pain and low-grade pyrexia may occur. Perforation and fistula formation have been reported.[38] The pattern of necrosis may be unpredictable and the main disadvantage is the need for repetitive treatments.

✔ Injection of chemicals to relieve malignant dysphagia has all the hallmarks of a good technique, being safe, inexpensive and readily available. The technique is less precise than laser treatment because it is difficult to be sure where the alcohol is going once it enters the tissue. The summaries of the evidence available do not support its use; therefore, it should only be used where other modalities are not available or to temporise a situation before a definitive treatment plan is instituted.

External beam and intracavity radiotherapy

The aim of palliative radiotherapy is to recanalise the oesophagus and inhibit local tumour progression. It may be delivered by an external beam or an intraluminal source (brachytherapy).

External beam radiotherapy

External beam radiotherapy is widely used. It is straightforward to plan and does not require admission to hospital. Regimens are based on 30–60 Gy in 10 or more fractions given over a 5- to 6-week period. Initially, swallowing may deteriorate because of radiation-induced oedema and swelling of the tumour. For patients whose nutrition is at risk prior to treatment, a form of nutritional support may first be required (endoscopic recanalisation or enteral feeding by gastrostomy, jejunostomy or nasogastric tube).

Complications

Side-effects are common and often serious, particularly if initial treatment seems successful: pulmonary fibrosis, fistula and benign stricture formation have all been described. Data from the 1970s show that less than 40% of patients experience acceptable palliation of dysphagia with external beam radiotherapy. Problems with recurrent dysphagia, as a result of cicatricial narrowing of the oesophagus, also occur.[39] As a single modality it has probably been superseded by intracavity irradiation or combination treatment. A new NIHR HTA (National Institute of Health Research, Health Technology Assessment) trial comparing the addition of external beam radiotherapy to SEMS is just starting in the UK. This will provide clarity about whether this leads to improved control of dysphagia in patients with a poor life expectancy.

Brachytherapy (intracavitary irradiation)

The development of the Selectron (Nucleotron, Zeersum, the Netherlands) remote control after-loading machine has generated considerable interest in recent years because it places the radiotherapy source close to the tumour and maximises the tumour radiation dose. It is a simple and safe procedure, and there is no radiation exposure to staff. The brachytherapy applicator, only 8 mm in diameter, is passed over an endoscopically placed guidewire and positioned in the tumour by fluoroscopy. This is immobilised at the mouth or nose. The patient is then transferred to a protected treatment room and connected to the Selectron machine. A microprocessor controls the pneumatic transfer of caesium-137 pellets down a flexible tube inserted into the applicator. The optimal dose is unknown and varies from 15 to 20 Gy to a depth of 1 cm in single or multiple fractions. Treatment may be repeated on alternate days leaving the nasogastric tube in situ or replacing it as necessary, although it is usually given as a single-dose fraction of 10–15 Gy. It is necessary to precisely map the tumour by endoscopy, fluoroscopy or computed tomography, and planning aims to incorporate a few centimetres of normal oesophagus at either end. The great merit of brachytherapy is that the radiation dose is highest to the tumour while adjacent normal tissues are relatively spared. It can be used in combination with other treatments.

Relief of dysphagia and patient-reported outcomes

Two well-designed randomised trials have been reported that compare single-dose brachytherapy (12 Gy) with SEMS (Ultraflex covered stent) in patients not suitable for curative treatment.[22,40,41] The main end-point of these trials was dysphagia. Results showed that SEMS provided better short-term relief of dysphagia but was associated with increased morbidity. Longer-lasting relief of dysphagia was achieved in the brachytherapy group. In the larger trial, survival was similar in both arms (median survival 155 days (95% CI 127–183 days) after brachytherapy and 145 days (95% CI 103–187 days) after stent placement), but morbidity was significantly higher after stent insertion than after brachytherapy. Major complications included perforation, haemorrhage and fistula formation. Major haemorrhage occurred more significantly after metal stent insertion. Other complications include the development of post-irradiation strictures or tracheo-oesophageal fistula. This trial also included a robust assessment of health-related quality of life and costs. Health-related quality-of-life differences between treatments were initially small but increased over time. Indeed, for emotional, cognitive and social function, differences in effect over time were statistically significant and differences were also seen in the dysphagia scale.[41] There were only minor differences in costs between the two treatments. The authors of the trial concluded that brachytherapy should be the primary treatment for palliation of dysphagia from oesophageal cancer.

✔✔ Intracavity irradiation (brachytherapy) with a single high dose appears to be a good palliative treatment of malignant dysphagia. High-quality randomised evidence including patient-reported outcome measures supports this approach.[22,41,42] Changes in the delivery of radiotherapy services may be necessary if this is to be widely adopted in the UK. Selecting patients for this treatment is important and some frail patients will still require immediate relief of dysphagia with a single admission for placement of an SEMS. Otherwise, for patients who require palliation of malignant dysphagia, brachytherapy is recommended if available locally.

Palliative chemotherapy or combination chemoradiotherapy for oesophageal cancer

The role of palliative chemotherapy for oeophageal cancer remains ill defined. The aim of treatment is to control local and distant tumour to improve quality of life and prolong survival. A recent Cochrane systematic review included only two randomised controlled trials, with a total of 42 patients, comparing chemotherapy with best supportive care for metastatic oesophageal cancer.[4] Median survival in the intervention group was 6 months compared to 3.9 in the control group and there was no difference in quality of life (although only one aspect, oral intake, was measured); the small number of included patients means robust conclusions cannot be drawn. In the five randomised trials assessing different chemotherapeutic regimes in 1242 patients, two compared monotherapy with combination treatments and found non-significant improved response rates in the latter group, with similar survival. The remaining three trials compared different combination therapies; no consistent benefit to any specific regimen was observed and it was not possible to perform a formal pooled analysis. Although quality of life was measured, response rates were very poor and validated questionnaires designed specifically for oesophageal cancer patients were not used. There is therefore a need for well-designed trials to assess the effect of palliative chemotherapy on survival and quality of life in patients with advanced oesophageal cancer.

It is possible that combination chemoradiotherapy may improve response rates and survival, although evidence is also limited. Additionally, there is a lack of evidence to support the role of second-line chemotherapy, although a current trial is investigating the use of gefitinib (tyrosine kinase inhibitor) and results are awaited.[43] Patients suitable for palliative chemotherapy often require attention for nutritional needs. If the initial course of chemotherapy can be tolerated and a response achieved, it is possible that relief of dysphagia will occur and last for some months before further progression is experienced.

Epidermal growth factor receptor inhibitors in the palliation of oesophageal cancer

Growth factors such as epidermal growth factor (EGF) and transforming growth factor α (TGFα) that bind and activate the erbB1 receptor, also known as the EGFR, are known to be involved in the mitogenic process in both adenocarcinoma and squamous cell cancer of the oesophagus. EGF over-expression has been found in Barrett's oesophagus and in oesophageal cancers, and a high level of EGFR expression is associated with poor prognosis.[44] Both phase I and II trials have used small-molecule inhibitors to target EGFR and data are encouraging in both oesophageal cancer cell types.[45–48] In the UK, the COG (Cancer Oesophagus Gefitinib) trial has now completed recruitment of over 400 patients and results will be available in 2013.[43]

Aero-digestive fistulas

Aero-digestive fistulas cause paroxysmal coughing fits, aspiration and, if untreated, eventually death from recurrent chest infections. They occur in about 5% of patients with oesophageal cancer, either because of spontaneous necrosis of the tumour and/or local nodes through the oesophageal wall into the bronchial tree, or as a result of treatment. Such fistulas are difficult to treat and life expectancy is usually short. The creation of a cervical oesophagostomy and gastrostomy may relieve symptoms, but is not usually appropriate. Palliative bypass surgery with stomach or colon for interposition is highly invasive and is also not generally recommended because of the poor general health and prognosis of patients in these situations. Endoscopic insertion of a prosthesis is the treatment of choice, although results following the use of rigid prostheses have not been encouraging, despite the availability of modified cuffed prostheses. The use of covered metal stents to seal aero-digestive fistulas seems to be a more promising development, although no randomised trials have been performed.[49] Fistulas close to the cricopharyngeus are particularly difficult to manage. In this situation simultaneous tracheal and oesophageal stenting may be performed. The possibility that an oesophageal prosthesis may cause significant airway compression should always be considered for tumours in the upper half of the oesophagus and particularly when a fistula of the airway is known or suspected. Preliminary bronchoscopy may clarify this and indicate that tracheal stenting may be preferable to oesophageal stenting, or at least should be performed before oesophageal stenting. Tracheal stenting may also be necessary before commencing chemoradiation treatment for T4 tumours close to, but not actually invading, the airway.[50] At present the role of chemotherapy or radiotherapy in this regard needs further evaluation. The endoscopic placement of fibrin tissue glue may be worthwhile where stenting is not achievable.

Recurrent laryngeal nerve palsy

Recurrent laryngeal nerve palsy caused by tumour infiltration results in eating difficulties, a weak voice, poor cough and repeated chest infections because of aspiration pneumonia. Patients are usually hoarse and complain of swallowing difficulties in the oropharyngeal phase. Coughing and a sensation of choking are typical on consuming solids and liquids. The diagnosis is confirmed by laryngoscopy. Endoscopy may be required to exclude other problems contributing to dysphagia. Aspiration can be confirmed during the pharyngeal phase of swallowing on barium studies. The left nerve is more commonly involved because of its intrathoracic course. Teflon injection to re-establish glottic competence should help swallowing, speech and problems with coughing. In a series of 15 patients, all improved except one, who developed stridor and required emergency tracheostomy.[51] Recurrent laryngeal nerve damage at the time of oesophagectomy usually causes a temporary paralysis that resolves within 6 weeks.

Bleeding

Bleeding from inoperable oesophageal and cardia tumours causes problems with refractory anaemia and occasionally acute upper gastrointestinal haemorrhage. It is often difficult to deal with because of the advanced nature of the tumour and it may be a terminal event. Symptoms may be controlled endoscopically using laser energy, adrenaline injection or electrocoagulation. External-beam radiotherapy is also said to reduce bleeding and extend the interval between blood transfusions, although there is no evidence for this practice.

Palliative treatments of tumours of the gastric body and antrum

Patients in whom potentially curative radical surgery for gastric cancer is not appropriate often require palliation of symptoms. Many with advanced disease may be asymptomatic but even for patients with obstructive symptoms or bleeding, palliative chemotherapy is recommended for symptom relief. There are also situations where problems with gastric outlet obstruction or bleeding are severe and palliative surgery or endoscopic therapy is necessary. The role of palliative chemotherapy or radiotherapy, and the management of gastric outflow obstruction and chronic and acute gastric bleeding, will be discussed separately.

Chemotherapy for advanced gastric and oesophagogastric cancer

Systemic chemotherapy is the main treatment option for patients with inoperable gastric tumours. A recent systematic review and meta-analysis of randomised controlled trials on first-line chemotherapy in advanced gastric cancer has summarised current knowledge.[8] Palliative chemotherapy offers survival benefits compared with best supportive care (hazard ratio 0.37, 95% CI 0.24–0.55), which can be interpreted as an improvement in median survival from 4.3 months (best supportive care) to 11 months (chemotherapy). Combination versus single agents also confers survival advantages (hazard ratio 0.82, 95% CI 0.74–0.90). Combinations of 5-FU/cisplatin/anthracycline were found to significantly benefit overall survival compared with 5-FU/cisplatin (hazard ratio 0.77, 95% CI 0.62–0.95) and, similarly, benefits were found when comparing 5-FU/cisplatin/anthracycline with 5-FU/anthracycline (epirubicin). Although the survival benefit of oral 5-FU (capecitabine) compared with intravenous formulations did not reach statistical significance in this review, another meta-analysis confirmed the non-inferiority of capecitabine[52] and a further review found significant survival benefits.[53] This oral preparation is advantageous as it eliminates the need for continuous infusions and associated risks of long-term venous lines, and has been approved by NICE for use in these patients. Evidence also indicates that oxaliplatin is non-inferior to cisplatin in the treatment of advanced gastric cancer.[8,54] Epirubicin, cisplatin/oxaliplatin and capecitabine is therefore recommended to achieve best survival results and minimise rates of toxicity. More recently, the use of monoclonal antibodies has been examined in the context of advanced gastric cancer and in a phase III study median overall survival was 13.8 months (95% CI 12–16 months) in those assigned to trastuzumab (herceptin) plus chemotherapy compared with 11.1 months (95% CI 10–13 months) in those receiving chemotherapy alone (hazard ratio 0.74, 95% CI 0.60–0.91).[9] It is therefore also recommended that patients are routinely tested for HER-2 overexpression and potentially receive trastuzumab in combination with cisplatin and capecitabine. To date, effectiveness of trastuzumab has not been assessed using any other drug combinations.

Irrespective of the positive impact of any of the presently available palliative regimens for gastric cancer, the median survival is only 7–10 months in most large clinical trials. Full, frank and kind discussion with patients considering palliative treatments is therefore recommended. The main drawbacks of chemotherapy are the potential complications. Toxicities include haematological problems, thrombovenous embolism and infective complications. During treatment itself, generic aspects of quality of life deteriorate (physical, role function) but symptoms are relieved (dysphagia, eating restrictions). Patients with a good baseline performance status usually tolerate temporary problems well. Patients require information to help them cope with treatments and to meet information needs, and this will include data about treatment advantages (survival) and disadvantages (morbidity and temporary negative impact on quality of life).

✔✔ Chemotherapy improves survival in advanced gastric cancer in comparison to best supportive care, and combination chemotherapy (most commonly including a platinum and fluoropyrimidine drug) is superior to single-agent treatment[8,54]. Patients should be tested for HER-2 status by immunohistochemistry and those with HER-2 strongly positive tumours should be offered trastuzumab in addition to a standard regimen[9]. Median life expectancy is 9–14 months. Patients require realistic information about expected survival benefits, toxicity and impact on quality of life before undergoing this type of treatment, and further studies comparing novel therapies should include robust assessment of patient experience and detailed assessment of quality of life.

Gastric outlet obstruction

Obstruction associated with cancer of the gastric corpus or antrum can be difficult to manage. Many of these extend proximally to involve extensive segments of the stomach, resulting in interference with both reservoir function and empyting. Resection of the primary tumour may provide symptomatic relief and generally provides a better guarantee of success than bypass surgery. The problem is that many patients with incurable distal gastric cancer with obstruction are nutritionally depleted and frail. Surgery may therefore be best avoided, as patients never sufficiently recover from surgery to benefit from it during their remaining life (median survival 6 months). There are also differing opinions about the type of palliative gastrectomy that should be performed in this situation (subtotal or total). In the Western world, where morbidity associated with total gastrectomy is high, it is not generally recommended for palliative purposes. The role of gastric resection in linitis plastica remains controversial. It probably has little to offer for those patients who additionally have peritoneal or liver metastasis or contiguous organ involvement, where life expectancy is very poor at around only 4 months. Patients with linitis plastica who have disease limited to the stomach or regional lymph nodes may, however, survive beyond 12 months and thus be appropriately palliated by total gastrectomy. In the authors' unit palliative total gastrectomy is rarely performed for linitis plastica. Wherever possible, endoscopic palliative treatment of obstructive symptoms or palliative chemotherapy is offered to these patients, in combination with support from palliative care services.

Patients with non-resectable distal lesions may undergo gastrojejunostomy. The loop of jejunum is anastomosed close to the greater curve of the stomach. There is little consensus regarding anterior or posterior loops. The latter may theoretically be more prone to recurrent obstruction due to proximity to the tumour. The Devine exclusion bypass operation for inoperable antral tumours was thought to increase survival by preventing recurrent tumour obstructing the gastrojejunostomy.[55] There is some evidence that laparoscopic gastrojejunostomy for palliation of incurable gastric outlet obstruction causes less morbidity than standard open surgery. Systematic reviews of the role of stents versus gastrojejunostomy for the palliation of gastric outlet obstruction suggest that stent placement may be associated with more favourable results in patients with a relatively short life expectancy and that gastrojejunostomy was the recommended palliative treatment in patients with a better prognosis.[6,7]

Metal stents can be more successfully placed across recurrent tumours at oesophagojejunal anastomoses and in recurrent peritoneal disease causing high small-bowel obstruction following total gastrectomy. Recanalisation of the gastric outlet with laser coagulation has not been used successfully. The insertion of nasogastric tubes, percutaneous endoscopically placed feeding tubes and jejunostomies enables nutrition to be delivered to

✔ Duodenal stents may be used as first-line treatment in patients with a poor prognosis requiring palliation of gastric outlet obstruction. Fitter patients with longer life expectancy may benefit more from surgical gastrojejunostomy. High-quality evidence with large clinical trials is still required to compare these treatment modalities.

patients with inoperable tumours. These manoeuvres alone, however, fail to palliate most of the patient's symptoms. Many believe that such palliation merely perpetuates suffering except in situations where they are used as an adjunct to recanalisation. They may be indicated to provide preliminary nutritional support in patients selected for palliative chemotherapy.

Chronic bleeding

Surgery remains a useful therapeutic manoeuvre to palliate the symptoms and problems of chronic blood loss from gastric tumours. Laser therapy can successfully achieve haemostasis in bleeding gastric malignancies and there are increasing reports of argon-beam coagulation to limit bleeding from gastric tumours.[56] Both methods require repeated hospital admissions. Radiotherapy may also be used to control chronic bleeding from gastric tumours, although there are no published data to support this practice.

Summary

The number of therapeutic options available for the palliation of patients with oesophageal and gastric cancer has increased significantly over the past decade. No single treatment completely relieves all symptoms without side-effects and median life expectancy for patients with either tumour type is only between 6 and 12 months. Common clinical situations such as the management of fistulas, high oesophageal tumours and bleeding inoperable gastric lesions continue to present formidable management problems. The introduction of self-expanding metal stents, argon-beam coagulation, brachytherapy, chemotherapy and combination treatments offers new hope, although evidence of significant survival benefits or improvements in quality of life with new treatments has yet to be realised. The increasing centralisation of cancer services in order to provide high-technology specialised care may improve outcomes and increase recruitment into national randomised trials that focus on palliative treatments. There are still many patients who present with advanced disease who are severely debilitated and have a limited life expectancy. Such patients need to be identified early to prevent travelling long distances to a centre with specialised endoscopic facilities only to find that treatment has to be performed more than once. Genuine efforts should be made to see if patients with very short survival times (less than 4 weeks) can be identified and perhaps spared unnecessarily aggressive attempts at palliation.

There remains a need to define outcomes for patients with inoperable malignancies of the upper gastrointestinal tract. Although it would be useful to standardise dysphagia scores and improve audit, in the palliative setting the most important outcome should be patients' assessment of benefits of treatment. The use of self-report quality-of-life questionnaires in clinical practice will provide such data, although at present these are mainly research tools.[57–59] The role of the specialist upper gastrointestinal nurse to support patients undergoing palliative treatment and to provide nutritional support is increasing, and links between palliative care and upper gastrointestinal cancer teams need to be well established and used.[60,61]

The selection of palliation for patients with advanced disease is difficult. Every patient is unique with regard to tumour histology, stricture location, clinical stage, premorbid state and emotional requirements. Choosing one technique over another must be justifiable on the grounds of treatment efficacy, ease of application, overall adaptability to other therapeutic areas and patient acceptance, while minimising both complications and cost. Skilled multidisciplinary teams with a thorough understanding of all the available palliative treatments are needed and close liaison with palliative care services is essential to minimise suffering.

Key points

- Patients with oesophageal cancer selected for palliative treatment have a median survival of less than 8 months and few survive beyond 1 year. There is little evidence to show that any single or combination of palliative treatment modalities changes survival for patients with incurable oesophageal cancer.
- The median survival for patients with gastric cancer undergoing palliative treatment is poor; 50% of patients die within 8 months of diagnosis and the remainder within 2 years. Combination chemotherapy increases survival compared with best supportive care, and it is recommended for patients with sufficient performance status and desire to undergo this intervention. Recent evidence shows that patients fit for palliative chemotherapy should be tested for HER-2 status and monoclonal antibodies (trastuzumab) be added in patients with HER-2-positive tumours.

- Palliative treatment decisions should be taken in the context of a multidisciplinary team meeting and recommendations subsequently shared with the patient. Patients require information that is imparted kindly but truthfully and it should include data about likely survival benefits and impact of treatment of symptom relief and quality of life.
- Accurate tumour staging and assessment of patient comorbidity and choice play a critical part in any therapeutic protocol, enabling patients to be assigned appropriately to treatments with either curative or palliative intent.
- Surgery has a limited role to play in palliative treatments of cancer of the oesophagus and stomach. Subtotal gastrectomy may be useful to palliate outlet obstruction in patients with a reasonable prognosis and it will allow them to undergo palliative chemotherapy. The role of palliative total gastrectomy is very limited to patients with advanced disease causing intractable dysphagia or bleeding. It is possible that death will occur from disease recurrence before the benefits of surgery are realised.
- Self-expanding metal stent insertion provides quick, effective relief of malignant dysphagia. Single high-dose brachytherapy provides better long-term relief of dysphagia than self-expanding metal stents, and survival benefit. There is no longer a role for intubation with rigid plastic prostheses.
- Laser treatment may be preferable for non-circumferential, polypoid or exophytic tumours, while intubation is preferable in sclerotic stenosing tumours.
- Injection of chemicals to relieve malignant dysphagia has all the hallmarks of a good technique, being safe, inexpensive and readily available. There is little evidence to support this technique, however, and it is only recommended for use if alternatives are not available or to temporise a situtation.
- Palliative chemotherapy has an increasingly important role to play in advanced oesophageal cancer and tumours of the oesophagogastric junction, but currently evidence to routinely support its role is lacking.
- The main drawbacks of palliative chemotherapy for gastric cancer are the potential complications and reduction in quality of life. Patients with a good baseline performance status, however, usually tolerate temporary problems well.
- The selection of palliation for patients with advanced disease is difficult and requires skilled motivated input from multidisciplinary teams with a thorough understanding of all the available palliative treatments and awareness of the patient's individual needs.

References

1. National Oesophago-Gastric Cancer Audit. Third annual report. London: The NHS Information Centre; 2010.
2. Ajani JA, Barthel JS, Bentrem DJ, et al. Esophageal and esophagogastric junction cancers. J Natl Compr Canc Netw 2011;9(8):830–87.
3. Yada I, Wada H, Shinoda M, et al. Thoracic and cardiovascular surgery in Japan during 2001: annual report by the Japanese Association for Thoracic Surgery. Jpn J Thorac Cardiovasc Surg 2003;51(12): 699–716.
4. Homs MY, Gaast A, Siersema PD, et al. Chemotherapy for metastatic carcinoma of the esophagus and gastro-esophageal junction. Cochrane Database Syst Rev 2009;(4)CD004063.
5. Allum WH, Blazeby JM, Griffin SM, et al. Guidelines for the management of oesophageal and gastric cancer. Gut 2011;60(11):1449–72.
6. Jeurnink SM, van Eijck CH, Steyerberg EW, et al. Stent versus gastrojejunostomy for the palliation of gastric outlet obstruction: a systematic review. BMC Gastroenterol 2007;7:18.
7. Ly J, O'Grady G, Mittal A, et al. A systematic review of methods to palliate malignant gastric outlet obstruction. Surg Endosc 2010;24(2):290–7.
8. Wagner AD, Unverzagt S, Grothe W, et al. Chemotherapy for advanced gastric cancer. Cochrane Database Syst Rev 2010;(3):CD004064.
9. Bang YJ, Van Cutsem E, Feyereislova A, et al. Trastuzumab in combination with chemotherapy versus chemotherapy alone for treatment of HER2-positive advanced gastric or gastro-oesophageal junction cancer (ToGA): a phase 3, open-label, randomised controlled trial. Lancet 2010;376(9742):687–97.
10. Bartels H, Stein HJ, Siewert JR. Preoperative risk analysis and postoperative mortality of oesophagectomy for resectable oesophageal cancer. Br J Surg 1998;85(6):840–4.

11. Eloubeidi MA, Desmond R, Arguedas MR, et al. Prognostic factors for the survival of patients with esophageal carcinoma in the U.S.: the importance of tumor length and lymph node status. Cancer 2002;95(7):1434–43.
12. The NHS cancer plan. London: Department of Health; 2000.
13. Executive NHS. Improving outcomes in upper-gastrointestinal cancers. The Manual. 2001.
14. Fleissig A, Jenkins V, Catt S, et al. Multidisciplinary teams in cancer care: are they effective in the UK? Lancet Oncol 2006;7(11):935–43.
15. Blazeby JM, Wilson L, Metcalfe C, et al. Analysis of clinical decision-making in multi-disciplinary cancer teams. Ann Oncol 2006;17(3):457–60.
16. Strong S, Blencowe NS, Fox T, et al. The role of multi-disciplinary teams in decision making for patients with recurrent malignant disease. Palliat Med 2012;26(7):954–8.
17. Rutten LJ, Arora NK, Bakos AD, et al. Information needs and sources of information among cancer patients: a systematic review of research (1980–2003). Patient Educ Couns 2005;57(3):250–61.
18. Thrumurthy SG, Morris JJ, Mughal MM, et al. Discrete-choice preference comparison between patients and doctors for the surgical management of oesophagogastric cancer. Br J Surg 2011;98(8):1124–31.
19. Cancer reform strategy. Department of Health; 2007.
20. Blazeby JM, Farndon JR, Donovan J, et al. A prospective longitudinal study examining the quality of life of patients with esophageal carcinoma. Cancer 2000;88(8):1781–7.
21. Sreedharan A, Harris K, Crellin A, et al. Interventions for dysphagia in oesophageal cancer. Cochrane Database Syst Rev 2009;(4): CD005048.
22. Homs MY, Steyerberg EW, Eijkenboom WM, et al. Single-dose brachytherapy versus metal stent placement for the palliation of dysphagia from oesophageal cancer: multicentre randomised trial. Lancet 2004;364(9444):1497–504.
23. Riley SA, Attwood SE. Guidelines on the use of oesophageal dilatation in clinical practice. Gut 2004;53(Suppl. 1):i1–6.
24. Knyrim K, Wagner HJ, Bethge N, et al. A controlled trial of an expansile metal stent for palliation of esophageal obstruction due to inoperable cancer. N Engl J Med 1993;329(18):1302–7.
25. Siersema PD, Hop WC, Dees J, et al. Coated self-expanding metal stents versus latex prostheses for esophagogastric cancer with special reference to prior radiation and chemotherapy: a controlled, prospective study. Gastrointest Endosc 1998;47(2):113–20.
26. Shenfine J, McNamee P, Steen N, Bond J, Griffin SM. A randomized controlled clinical trial of palliative therapies for patients with inoperable esophageal cancer. Am J Gastroenterol. 2009;104(7):1674–85.
27. Conio M, Repici A, Battaglia G, et al. A randomized prospective comparison of self-expandable plastic stents and partially covered self-expandable metal stents in the palliation of malignant esophageal dysphagia. Am J Gastroenterol 2007;102(12):2667–77.
28. Power C, Byrne PJ, Lim K, et al. Superiority of anti-reflux stent compared with conventional stents in the palliative management of patients with cancer of the lower esophagus and esophago-gastric junction: results of a randomized clinical trial. Dis Esophagus 2007;20(6):466–70.
29. Dallal HJ, Smith GD, Grieve DC, et al. A randomized trial of thermal ablative therapy versus expandable metal stents in the palliative treatment of patients with esophageal carcinoma. Gastrointest Endosc 2001;54(5):549–57.
30. Adam A, Ellul J, Watkinson AF, et al. Palliation of inoperable esophageal carcinoma: a prospective randomized trial of laser therapy and stent placement. Radiology 1997;202(2):344–8.
31. Manner H, May A, Rabenstein T, et al. Prospective evaluation of a new high-power argon plasma coagulation system (hp-APC) in therapeutic gastrointestinal endoscopy. Scand J Gastroenterol 2007;42(3):397–405.
32. Barr H, Dix AJ, Kendall C, et al. Review article: the potential role for photodynamic therapy in the management of upper gastrointestinal disease. Aliment Pharmacol Ther 2001;15(3):311–21.
33. Lightdale CJ, Heier SK, Marcon NE, et al. Photodynamic therapy with porfimer sodium versus thermal ablation therapy with Nd:YAG laser for palliation of esophageal cancer: a multicenter randomized trial. Gastrointest Endosc 1995;42(6):507–12.
34. Heier SK, Rothman KA, Heier LM, et al. Photodynamic therapy for obstructing esophageal cancer: light dosimetry and randomized comparison with Nd:YAG laser therapy. Gastroenterology 1995;109(1):63–72.
35. Jensen DM, Machicado G, Randall G, et al. Comparison of low-power YAG laser and BICAP tumor probe for palliation of esophageal cancer strictures. Gastroenterology 1988;94(6):1263–70.
36. Nwokolo CU, Payne-James JJ, Silk DB, et al. Palliation of malignant dysphagia by ethanol induced tumour necrosis. Gut 1994;35(3):299–303.
37. Payne-James JJ, Spiller RC, Misiewicz JJ, et al. Use of ethanol-induced tumor necrosis to palliate dysphagia in patients with esophagogastric cancer. Gastrointest Endosc 1990;36(1):43–6.
38. Chung SC, Leong HT, Choi CY, et al. Palliation of malignant oesophageal obstruction by endoscopic alcohol injection. Endoscopy 1994;26(3):275–7.
39. Earlam R, Cunha-Melo JR. Oesophageal squamous cell carcinoma: I. A critical review of surgery. Br J Surg 1980;67(6):381–90.

40. Bergquist H, Wenger U, Johnsson E, et al. Stent insertion or endoluminal brachytherapy as palliation of patients with advanced cancer of the esophagus and gastroesophageal junction. Results of a randomized, controlled clinical trial. Dis Esophagus 2005;18(3):131–9.

41. Homs MY, Essink-Bot ML, Borsboom GJ, et al. Quality of life after palliative treatment for oesophageal carcinoma – a prospective comparison between stent placement and single dose brachytherapy. Eur J Cancer 2004;40(12):1862–71.

42. Polinder S, Homs MY, Siersema PD, et al. Cost study of metal stent placement vs single-dose brachytherapy in the palliative treatment of oesophageal cancer. Br J Cancer 2004;90(11):2067–72.

43. Ferry D. Phase III randomised, double-blind, placebo-controlled trial of gefitinib versus placebo in oesophageal cancer progressing after chemotherapy, http://public.ukcrn.org.uk/search/StudyDetail.aspx?StudyID=1754; [accessed 5.03.12].

44. Yacoub L, Goldman H, Odze RD. Transforming growth factor-alpha, epidermal growth factor receptor, and MiB-1 expression in Barrett's-associated neoplasia: correlation with prognosis. Mod Pathol 1997;10(2):105–12.

45. Ferry D. Phase II, trial of gefitinib (ZD1839) in advanced adenocarcinoma of the oesophagus incorporating biopsy before and after gefitinib. J Clin Oncol 2004;22(Suppl. 14):4021.

46. Assersohn L, Brown G, Cunningham D, et al. Phase II study of irinotecan and 5-fluorouracil/leucovorin in patients with primary refractory or relapsed advanced oesophageal and gastric carcinoma. Ann Oncol 2004;15(1):64–9.

47. Lordick F, von Schilling C, Bernhard H, et al. Phase II trial of irinotecan plus docetaxel in cisplatin-pretreated relapsed or refractory oesophageal cancer. Br J Cancer 2003;89(4):630–3.

48. Ferry DR, Anderson M, Beddard K, et al. A phase II study of gefitinib monotherapy in advanced esophageal adenocarcinoma: evidence of gene expression, cellular, and clinical response. Clin Cancer Res 2007;13(19):5869–75.

49. Cook TA, Dehn TC. Use of covered expandable metal stents in the treatment of oesophageal carcinoma and tracheo-oesophageal fistula. Br J Surg 1996;83(10):1417–8.

50. Ellul JP, Morgan R, Gold D, et al. Parallel self-expanding covered metal stents in the trachea and oesophagus for the palliation of complex high tracheo-oesophageal fistula. Br J Surg 1996;83(12):1767–8.

51. Griffin SM, Chung SC, van Hasselt CA, et al. Late swallowing and aspiration problems after esophagectomy for cancer: malignant infiltration of the recurrent laryngeal nerves and its management. Surgery 1992;112(3):533–5.

52. Norman G, Soares M, Peura P, et al. Capecitabine for the treatment of advanced gastric cancer. Health Technol Assess 2010;14(Suppl. 2):11–7.

53. Okines A, Chau I, Cunningham D. Capecitabine in gastric cancer. Drugs Today (Barc) 2008;44(8):629–40.

54. Chong G, Cunningham D. Can cisplatin and infused 5-fluorouracil be replaced by oxaliplatin and capecitabine in the treatment of advanced oesophagogastric cancer? The REAL 2 trial. Clin Oncol (R Coll Radiol) 2005;17(2):79–80.

55. Kwok SP, Chung SC, Griffin SM, et al. Devine exclusion for unresectable carcinoma of the stomach. Br J Surg 1991;78(6):684–5.

56. Heindorff H, Wojdemann M, Bisgaard T, et al. Endoscopic palliation of inoperable cancer of the oesophagus or cardia by argon electrocoagulation. Scand J Gastroenterol 1998;33(1):21–3.

57. Blazeby JM, Conroy T, Bottomley A, et al. Clinical and psychometric validation of a questionnaire module, the EORTC QLQ-STO 22, to assess quality of life in patients with gastric cancer. Eur J Cancer 2004;40(15):2260–8.

58. Lagergren P, Fayers P, Conroy T, et al. Clinical and psychometric validation of a questionnaire module, the EORTC QLQ-OG25, to assess health-related quality of life in patients with cancer of the oesophagus, the oesophago-gastric junction and the stomach. Eur J Cancer 2007;43(14):2066–73.

59. Blazeby JM, Conroy T, Hammerlid E, et al. Clinical and psychometric validation of an EORTC questionnaire module, the EORTC QLQ-OES18, to assess quality of life in patients with oesophageal cancer. Eur J Cancer 2003;39(10):1384–94.

60. Nicklin J, Blazeby JM. Anorexia in patients dying from oesophageal and gastric cancers. Gastrointest Nurs 2003;1:35–9.

61. Irving M. Oesophageal cancer and the role of the nurse specialist. Nurs Times 2002;98:38–40.

62. Blomberg J, Wenger U, Lagergren J, et al. Antireflux stent versus conventional stent in the palliation of distal esophageal cancer. A randomized, multicenter clinical trial. Scand J Gastroenterol 2010;45(2):208–16.

63. Verschuur EM, Repici A, Kuipers EJ, et al. New design esophageal stents for the palliation of dysphagia from esophageal or gastric cardia cancer: a randomized trial. Am J Gastroenterol 2008;103(2):304–12.

64. Fu JH, Rong TH, Li XD, et al. Treatment of unresectable esophageal carcinoma by stenting with or without radiochemotherapy. Zhonghua Zhong Liu Za Zhi 2004;26(2):109–11.

65. Sabharwal T, Hamady MS, Chui S, et al. A randomised prospective comparison of the Flamingo Wallstent and Ultraflex stent for palliation of dysphagia associated with lower third oesophageal carcinoma. Gut 2003;52(7):922–6.

66. O'Donnell CA, Fullarton GM, Watt E, et al. Randomized clinical trial comparing self-expanding metallic stents with plastic endoprostheses in the palliation of oesophageal cancer. Br J Surg 2002;89(8):985–92.
67. Canto MI, Smith C, McClelland L, et al. Randomized trial of PDT vs. stent for palliation of malignant dysphagia: cost-effectiveness and quality of life. Gastrointest Endosc 2002;55(5):Ab100.
68. Siersema PD, Hop WC, van Blankenstein M, et al. A comparison of 3 types of covered metal stents for the palliation of patients with dysphagia caused by esophagogastric carcinoma: a prospective, randomized study. Gastrointest Endosc 2001;54(2):145–53.
69. Vakil N, Morris AI, Marcon N. A prospective, randomized, controlled trial of covered expandable metal stents in the palliation of malignant esophageal obstruction at the gastroesophageal junction. Am J Gastroenterol 2001;96:1791–6.
70. Sargeant IR, Tobias JS, Blackman G, et al. Radiotherapy enhances laser palliation of malignant dysphagia: a randomised study. Gut 1997;40(3):362–9.
71. Higgins JP, Altman DG, Gotzsche PC, et al. The Cochrane Collaboration's tool for assessing risk of bias in randomised trials. Br Med J 2011;343:d5928.

11

Other oesophageal and gastric neoplasms

Richard H. Hardwick

Introduction

This chapter will cover a less common group of upper gastrointestinal tumours whose treatment has changed greatly in the past decade; some can be cured by surgery alone while others are managed almost exclusively by chemotherapy. By far the largest group are the gastrointestinal stromal tumours (GISTs). A large part of this chapter will therefore cover the presentation, diagnosis and management of upper gastrointestinal GISTs. Better understanding of the pathophysiology of these interesting tumours has occurred simultaneously with the introduction of effective medical treatment in the form of imatinib (Glivec®, Novartis Pharma AG, Basel, Switzerland). The importance of accurate histological diagnosis of gastric tumours cannot be overemphasised; the treatment and prognosis of gastric lymphoma is very different from adenocarcinoma and this will be covered in its own section, as will gastric carcinoid. In the final section on 'rarities' we will look briefly at leiomyomas, leiomyosarcomas and small cell tumours of the oesophagus.

Gastrointestinal stromal tumours (GISTs)

Pathophysiology

GISTs are soft-tissue sarcomas of mesenchymal origin that arise in the gastrointestinal tract; they are rare, representing 0.1–3% of all gut tumours and 5% of all soft-tissue sarcomas.[1] Historically, these tumours were considered to be of smooth muscle origin and were generally regarded as leiomyomas (benign) or leiomyosarcomas (malignant). Electron microscopy and immunohistochemical studies indicated, however, that only a minority of stromal tumours have the typical features of smooth muscle, with some having a more neural appearance and others appearing undifferentiated.[2] 'Gastrointestinal stromal tumour' was subsequently introduced as being a more appropriate term for these neoplasms, with the variable histological features (smooth muscle, neural or undifferentiated) considered to be of little clinical relevance. Gastrointestinal autonomic nerve tumour (GANT) was also introduced to describe sarcomas with ultrastructural evidence of autonomic nervous system differentiation,[3] but these tumours are now recognised as a variant of GIST.[4] The discovery of CD34 expression in many GISTs suggested that they were a specific entity,[5] distinct from smooth muscle tumours. It was also observed that GISTs and the interstitial cells of Cajal (ICCs) express the receptor tyrosine kinase KIT (CD117).[6] This has led to the now widely accepted classification of mesenchymal tumours of the gastrointestinal (GI) tract into GISTs, true smooth muscle tumours and, far less frequently, true Schwann cell tumours.[7] GISTs are microscopically classified into three histological subtypes: spindle cell (70%), epithelioid (20%) and mixed (10%). Immunohistochemically, more than 90% of GISTs stain positive for CD117. A new antibody, DOG-1, is also highly sensitive and specific for GISTs.[8] The commonest sites of mutations in the c-*kit* gene are in exon 11 (60–70%), followed by exon 9 (18%), and exons 13 and 17 (3%). It is important that an experienced pathologist examines the immunohistochemical profile of any mesenchymal tumour as CD117-positive staining can be seen in other tumours such as seminomas, small-cell lung cancer, thyroid cancer and melanomas.

Incidence and malignant potential

Studies using diagnostic markers including CD117 immunoreactivity have shown that GISTs are under-diagnosed.[6] The morphological spectrum of GISTs was also wider than previously recognised. The estimated annual incidence of GISTs is around 15 per million,[9] which equates to approximately 900 new cases per year in the UK. A true measure of the incidence, prevalence and ratio of 'benign' to 'malignant' GISTs may not be possible as these tumours appear to possess varying degrees of malignant potential. The size of the tumour, the symptoms at diagnosis, the organ of origin (small-bowel GISTs have the worst prognosis) and mitotic count seem to be the most important factors when assessing prognosis.[10]

> A scheme for defining the risk of aggressive behaviour in GIST based on tumour size and mitotic count has been proposed[11] (**Fig. 11.1**). Most GISTs <2 cm have negligible mitotic activity (usually <5 per 50 high-power fields), and are considered very low or low risk in all sites when completely removed. Large tumours have a much poorer prognosis, even after apparently complete resection (**Fig. 11.2**).[12]

Disease-specific survival after complete resection of primary GIST is based on tumour size. Eighty patients underwent gross resection of primary GISTs. Patients with tumours >10 cm (n=27) had significantly worse survival than those with tumours between 6 and 10 cm (n=30) or ≤5 cm (n=23).

Patient demographics and anatomical distribution

No marked sex difference is apparent for GISTs. Two larger series of malignant GI sarcomas did, however, demonstrate a slight male predominance.[12,13] The age distribution appears to be unimodal, with a median age at presentation of 58 years (range 16–94). The peak incidence in men occurs in the fifth decade, slightly before that in women, where it peaks in the sixth decade. The median age at presentation appears constant in several series, ranging from 58 to 61 years.[14] Only 1–2% of GISTs present in patients before 30 years of age.[12]

Most GISTs arise in the stomach or small intestine, and infrequently in the oesophagus, mesentery, omentum, colon or rectum[13,15] (Table 11.1). Approximately 10–30% of GISTs are overtly malignant at presentation;[16] the principal sites of metastasis are the liver and the peritoneal cavity, and spread to lymph nodes is very rare.[12]

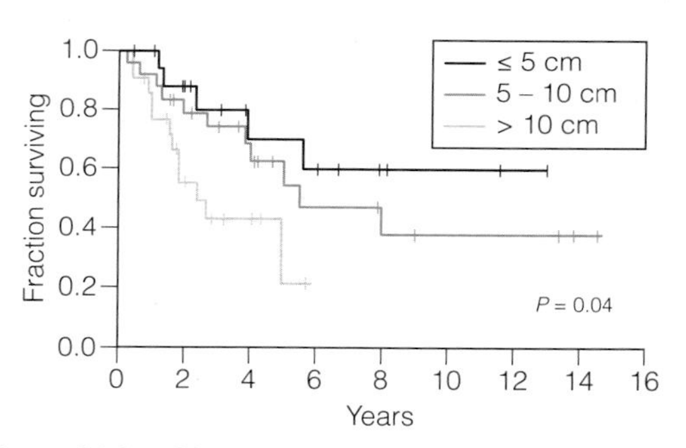

Figure 11.2 • Disease-specific survival after resection of primary GIST.[12] Eighty patients underwent gross resection of primary GISTs. Patients with tumours >10 cm (n=27) had significantly worse survival than those with tumours between 6 and 10 cm (n=30) or ≤5 cm (n=23).

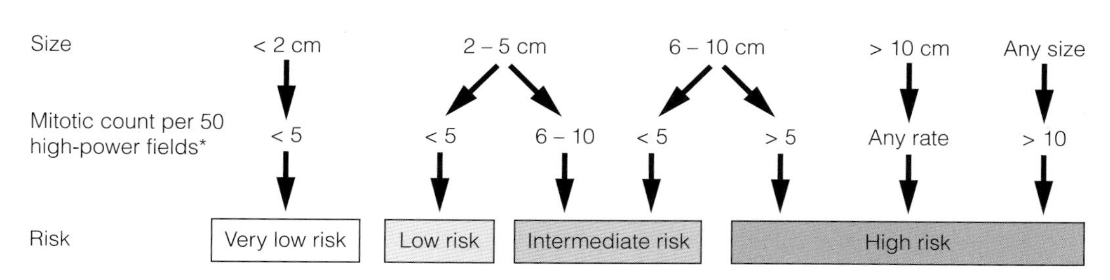

Figure 11.1 • Algorithm based on the consensus approach for assessing the risk of malignancy of GIST reached at National Institutes of Health workshop.[11]

Presentation

The symptoms of GISTs are non-specific and depend on the size and location of the lesion. Small GISTs (2 cm or less) are usually asymptomatic and are detected during investigations or surgical procedures for unrelated disease. The vast majority of these are of low risk for malignancy.[17] In many cases the mucosa is normal so that endoscopic biopsies are unremarkable. Incidental discovery accounts for approximately one-third of cases.[18]

The most common symptom is GI bleeding, which is present in approximately 50% of patients[19] (Table 11.2). In addition, systemic symptoms such as fever, night sweats and weight loss are common in GIST and rare in other sarcomas. Patients with larger tumours may experience abdominal discomfort or develop a palpable mass.[20]

Table 11.1 • Anatomical site of GISTs

Site	Percentage
Stomach	60–70%
Small intestine	20–30%
Oesophagus, mesentery, omentum, colon or rectum	10%

Table 11.2 • Symptoms of GIST at diagnosis[19]

Symptoms	Incidence
Abdominal pain	20–50%
Gastrointestinal bleeding	50%
Gastrointestinal obstruction	10–30%
Asymptomatic	20%

GISTs are often clinically silent until they reach a large size, bleed or rupture. Symptomatic oesophageal GISTs, although rare, typically present with dysphagia, while gastric and small-intestinal GISTs often present with vague symptoms leading to their eventual detection by gastroscopy or radiology. Most duodenal GISTs occur in the second part of the duodenum, where they push or infiltrate into the pancreas.[21]

Investigation

Approximately 60% of GISTs are submucosal and grow towards the lumen where, if in the proximal GI tract, they may be visualised endoscopically as smooth submucosal projections. If a small submucosal mass is seen as an incidental finding at the time of endoscopy, endoscopic ultrasound (EUS) should be the first investigation, as a significant proportion will be due to extrinsic impression from normal adjacent structures, e.g. gall bladder in the antrum, and spleen in the proximal stomach. If this is the case, no further investigation is required. For larger palpable masses, or where the patients present with haemorrhage, abdominal pain or obstruction, computed tomography (CT) is usually the first investigation after endoscopy to both assess the primary and look for metastases.[22]

Endoscopic ultrasound (EUS)

The classical features are of a hypoechoic mass contiguous with the fourth (muscularis propria) or second (muscularis mucosae) layers of the normal gut wall, both of which are hypoechoic (**Fig. 11.3a,b**). The EUS features most predictive of 'benign' tumours are regular margins, tumour size ≤30 mm and a homogeneous echo pattern. Larger tumours with irregular extraluminal margins and cystic spaces are more likely to behave aggressively.[23,24]

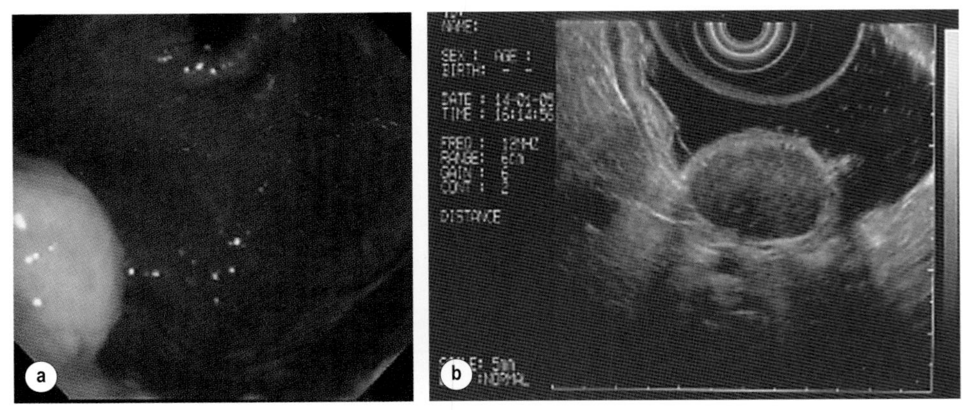

Figure 11.3 • **(a)** Endoscopic view of a small incidental gastric GIST. **(b)** A 12-MHz EUS image of the incidental gastric GIST seen in (a), showing the lesion arising from the muscularis propria.

To further aid diagnostic accuracy it is possible to use a linear EUS scope through which needle aspirates and core biopsies can be taken without breaching surgical resection planes. EUS with fine-needle aspiration (EUS-FNA) in experienced hands has a diagnostic accuracy of up to 97% for GIST lesions,[25] is becoming more widely available and should be considered in the diagnostic work-up of a possible GIST lesion if the result could change clinical management.

CT scanning

GIST imaging by CT typically shows an extraluminal mass, often with central necrosis, arising from the digestive tract wall.[18] Small tumours typically appear as sharply margined, smooth-walled, homogeneous, soft-tissue masses with moderate contrast enhancement.[26] Large tumours tend to have mucosal ulceration, central necrosis and cavitation, and heterogeneous enhancement following i.v. contrast.[26] As well as defining the presence and nature of a mass, if possible, the likely organ of origin should be defined. Multiplanar reconstruction can assist this, particularly with large masses. Negative oral contrast (e.g. water) and intravenous contrast for the assessment of gastric GISTs is recommended. CT of chest, abdomen and pelvis is recommended for staging of GIST, with the exception of small incidental tumours or when a patient presents as an emergency requiring urgent surgery. With regards to assessing treatment response, traditional CT criteria (RECIST criteria) have been shown to be inaccurate for measuring GIST response to imatinib and the Choi criteria are recommended (10% reduction in size and 15% reduction in density).[27]

Magnetic resonance imaging (MRI)

In general, MRI offers no additional information regarding the intralesional tissue characterisation of primary GISTs. However, MRI provides excellent soft-tissue contrast resolution and direct multiplanar imaging, which can help delineate the relationships of the tumour and adjacent organs, and is useful in anorectal disease.[26]

Positron emission tomography (PET)

PET scanning using a standard fluorodeoxyglucose (FDG)-PET technique has proven extremely useful in the prediction of tumour response to the tyrosine kinase inhibitor imatinib (Glivec, Norvartis Pharma AG) now used in the treatment of unresectable and metastatic malignant GISTs.[28] Glucose uptake of the tumours decreases within a few hours to days of the start of treatment, which can be verified with FDG-PET.[17] The PET scan can be utilised to distinguish between tumour progression and increase in volume due to intratumoral bleeding. PET scan responses have also been demonstrated to predict subsequent tumour volume reductions found on CT or MRI.[29]

GIST syndromes

Families have been reported with single-base 'gain of function' mutation in the kinase domain of *KIT*. The resultant effect is the development of multiple GISTs in the small bowel. Diffuse hyperplasia of spindle-shaped cells within the myenteric plexus at sites unaffected by GIST formation was also noted.[30,31] The association of three uncommon neoplasms – gastric GIST, functioning extra-adrenal paraganglionoma and pulmonary chondroma – was first reported in 1977 and has since been recognised as 'Carney's triad' (**Fig. 11.4**).[32] A subsequent review of 79 cases demonstrated that, unlike isolated sporadic GIST, where no significant sex difference was noted, 85% were female.[33] Twenty-two per cent of the patients had all three tumours; the remainder had two of the three, usually the gastric and pulmonary lesions. Adrenocortical adenoma has since been identified as a new constituent of the disorder. The presence of two of the three main tumours is considered sufficient for the syndrome.

Treatment and prognosis (Box 11.1)

A chest, abdominal and pelvic CT should be included in the preoperative assessment for all patients. If the tumour is located in the right or left upper quadrant then the patient should have an endocrine assessment to exclude a large functioning adrenal tumour. Male patients (under the age of 40 years) presenting with large centrally placed retroperitoneal tumours should have α-fetoprotein and β-human chorionic gonadotrophin levels measured to exclude non-seminomatous germ-cell tumour.

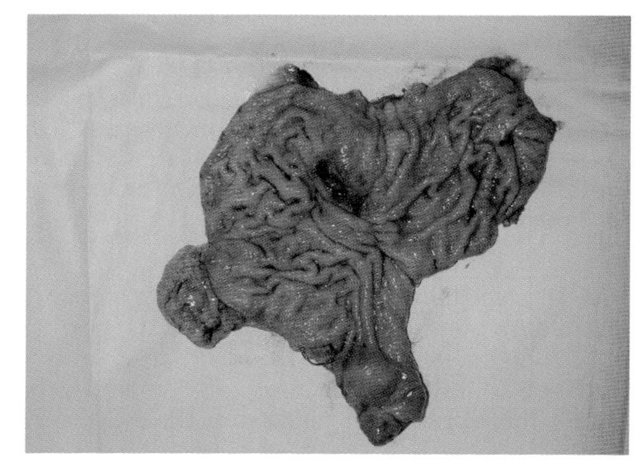

Figure 11.4 • Specimen from completion gastrectomy for bleeding GIST (ulcer clearly visible) in a 34-year-old woman with Carney's triad.

Box 11.1 • Principles of GIST treatment

Locoregional disease

Principles of surgery

- A wide local resection with macroscopic and microscopic removal of the entire tumour is recommended (R0)
- The surgeon should aim to preserve function, but not at the expense of an R0 resection
- Extended lymphadenectomy is normally not required
- Some small tumours may be resected laparoscopically
- Where adjacent organs are involved, en bloc resection is recommended whenever possible – input from other specialist surgeons should be considered prior to embarking on a resection
- Endoscopic resection is not recommended

Unresectable and/or metastatic disease

- Conventional cytotoxic chemotherapy and radiotherapy are not recommended
- Imatinib should be used as treatment for unresectable and/or metastatic GISTs
- The recommended starting dose of imatinib is 400 mg/day

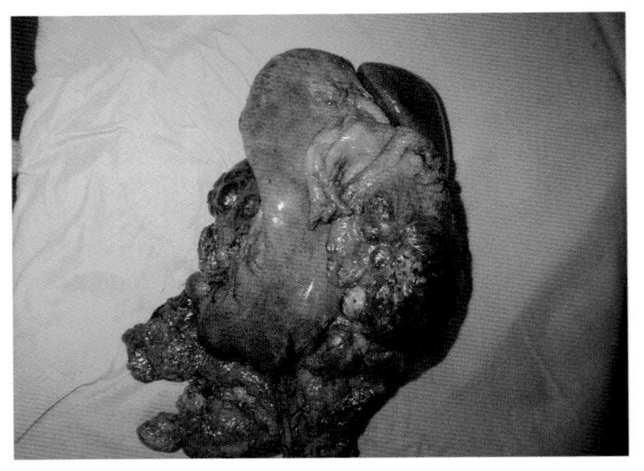

Figure 11.5 • Operative specimen following en bloc total gastrectomy, splenectomy and distal pancreatectomy for locally advanced GIST.

Percutaneous (ultrasound or CT) or laparoscopically guided biopsies should not be used in resectable disease due to the risk of tumour rupture or seeding, unless it may result in a change of treatment.[17] Laparoscopy may be considered in the staging of large lesions to exclude peritoneal metastases but an exploratory laparotomy is usually required to decide whether a large primary tumour is technically resectable or not.

✔ The main goal of GIST management is complete macroscopic and microscopic removal of the tumour, i.e. R0 resection.[34] Complete excision offers a good chance of cure and must be attempted whenever possible; the presence of a positive resection margin or tumour rupture leads to a significant reduction in survival.[35] In one study, only 11% of patients died of recurrent disease after R0 resection compared with 75% of those in whom the resection was R1 or R2, with a median follow-up of 2.2 years.[14]

At all sites the extent of resection is therefore dictated by the size of the tumour and its location in relation to, or invasion of, adjacent structures (**Fig. 11.5**). Oesophagectomy is the standard procedure for oesophageal GISTs but these are very rare and submucosal lesions in the oesophagus are much more likely to be leiomyomas. EUS-FNA core biopsy from these lesions is recommended to make a preoperative diagnosis so that surgical planning is appropriate.[25] Oesophageal GISTs and leiomyosarcomas require an oesophagectomy whereas leiomyomas can safely be enucleated without removing the oesophagus.

In the stomach, R0 resection may involve a partial, subtotal or total gastrectomy, although 'wedge' excision and 'sleeve' resections are also frequently performed to preserve as much stomach as possible. Small gastric lesions lend themselves well to laparoscopic resection (**Fig. 11.6a–c**). Resection of GIST tumours arising at the gastro-oesophageal junction creates particular problems as a poor quality of life may result from simple excision with anastomosis of stomach to oesophagus. Alternatively, reconstruction using a short jejunal interposition should be considered for these patients, the 'Merendino procedure' (**Fig. 11.7**),[36] as it results in a better quality of life compared to an oesophagogastric anastomosis.[37] The most important factors, as stated, are that the tumour is not ruptured and that negative resection margins are obtained. Simple enucleation of the tumour is inadequate as these lesions do not possess a true capsule. Direct invasion of adjacent structures occurs in 10–15% of GISTs and surgery in such cases should include en bloc resection of involved adjacent organs.[12,14] Nodal metastases are extremely rare and routine extended lymph node dissection is therefore unjustified.[38]

As very few studies address the issue of GISTs found incidentally, there are no clear data to support one definitive management plan over another. In their study of 39 GISTs, which included 16 identified incidentally, Ludwig and Traverso concluded that as a consequence of the frequency of serious complications in symptomatic patients, complete excision should also be recommended for asymptomatic patients.[39] However, the UK guidelines for the management of GISTs recommend that small asymptomatic incidental lesions can be treated

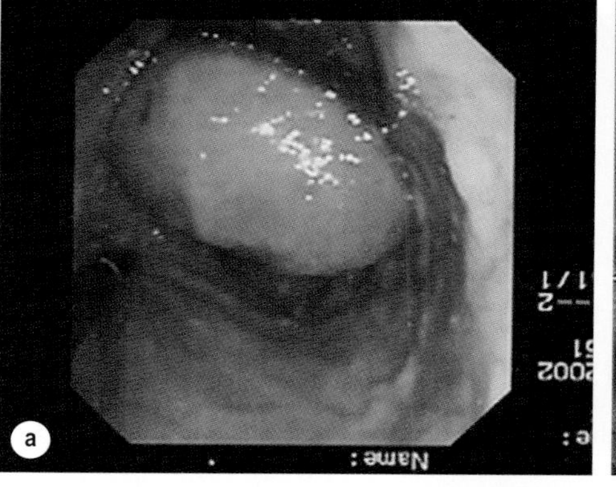

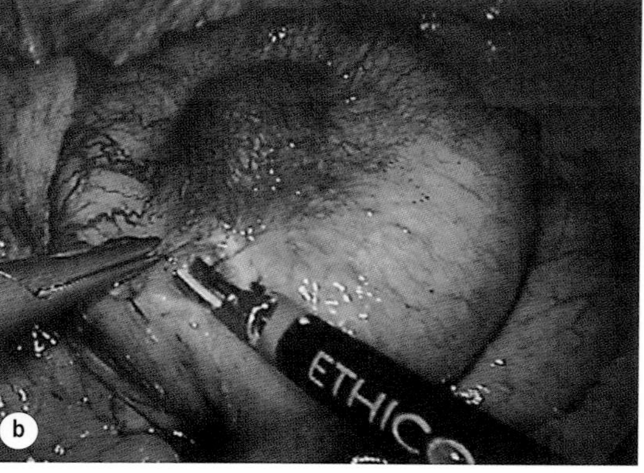

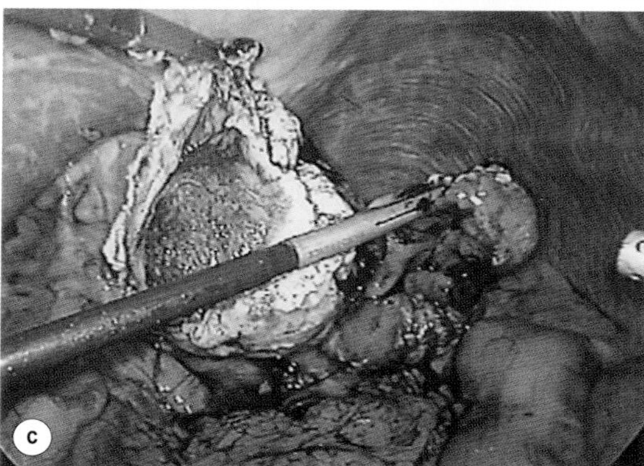

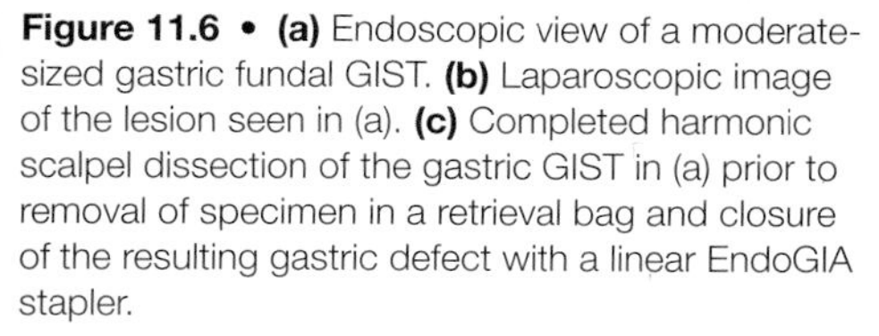

Figure 11.6 • (a) Endoscopic view of a moderate-sized gastric fundal GIST. **(b)** Laparoscopic image of the lesion seen in (a). **(c)** Completed harmonic scalpel dissection of the gastric GIST in (a) prior to removal of specimen in a retrieval bag and closure of the resulting gastric defect with a linear EndoGIA stapler.

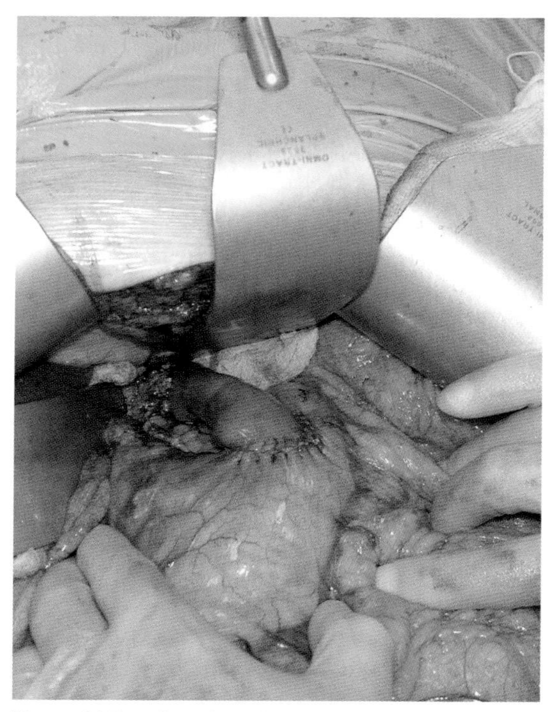

Figure 11.7 • Completed Merendino procedure showing distal anastomosis between the jejunal interposition and the stomach.

conservatively, particularly if serial examination shows no change in size over 1–2 years.[40] However, there are no long-term studies of the natural history of these lesions, and surgeons should explain these uncertainties to their patients and discuss the pros and cons of resection before proceeding to surgery. In patients with borderline fitness for resection, or those who decline surgery at initial presentation, monitoring the lesion with EUS and/or CT for evidence of enlargement is acceptable so long as the results of surveillance influence the final management.

Imatinib

Imatinib mesylate is a receptor tyrosine kinase inhibitor that inhibits the constitutively activated tyrosine kinases of ABL (including the stable transfection product fusion kinase BCR-ABL seen in chronic myeloid leukaemia), platelet-derived growth factor receptor (PDGFR) and KIT. The drug is administered orally, and its use, dosage and side-effect profile are well established following use in the treatment of chronic myeloid leukaemia. It has very little effect on normal cells, where the kinase is not constitutively active. Experiments on human tumour cell lines dependent upon the KIT pathway demonstrate that imatinib blocks the kinase activity of KIT, arrests proliferation and causes apoptotic cell death.[41] Imatinib is generally well tolerated, although most patients experience some mild or moderate adverse events. Serious adverse events occur in around 20% of patients, the most serious of which is life-threatening tumour haemorrhage in approximately 5%.

Unresectable or metastatic disease

Prior to the introduction of imatinib mesylate, patients with advanced GISTs faced severe morbidity and short life expectancy. Untreated, the median overall survival for unresectable or metastatic disease is around 12 months (ranging from 2 to 20 months).[42] Conventional chemotherapy and radiotherapy is ineffective in patients with metastatic GISTs.[43]

Early phase 1 studies of imatinib (then coded ST1571) took the oncology world by storm.[44] Never before had response rates of 80–90% been seen in metastatic sarcomas and a new era of 'smart' compounds was born. Over 50% of patients with metastatic or unresectable GISTs will survive more than 5 years if treated with imatinib.

✓✓ In a randomised controlled trial of 147 patients with metastatic or unresectable GISTs the median survival was 54 months regardless whether the 400- or 600-mg dose regimen of imatinib was used.[45] A larger phase III trial recruited 746 patients and compared 400 mg with 800 mg imatinib and again found no difference in survival between the two doses, but 33% of patients on the lower dose who progressed appeared to stabilise when transferred to the higher dose.[46] Similar results were obtained from an even larger randomised trial involving 946 patients, although a longer progression-free survival was seen for patients on the higher dose of imatinib.[47]

Although 80% of GISTs respond to imatinib, 20% demonstrate initial resistance to the drug and, of those that respond initially, some will develop late resistance.[48]

Adjuvant therapy post-resection

✓✓ The role of imatinib in the adjuvant setting has now been investigated in randomised controlled trials in the USA, Europe and Australasia. The ACOGSOG Z9001 study examined the role of adjuvant therapy for 12 months post-curative resection for GISTs greater than 3 cm in diameter and found improvement in progression-free survival but not overall survival for those patients given imatinib versus placebo.[49]

✓✓ The SSG XVIII study randomised patients with high-risk resected GISTs to 12 months versus 36 months of adjuvant imatinib and found significant improvement in both progression-free and overall survival for the patients having the longer course of treatment.[50] Imatinib is now licensed in the USA and Europe for resected GIST patients deemed at high risk of recurrence.

Surgery has a limited role in metastatic disease except when patients present with low-volume liver metastases; about a third of such patients may be cured by hepatic resection.[51] In selected patients with large incurable tumours, surgery may play a limited role in palliation of symptoms, but whether to operate is best decided by a multidisciplinary team who have expertise in GIST management.[52] Downsizing of unresectable primary tumours and hepatic metastasis following treatment with imatinib can render lesions resectable, but long-term survival is uncommon, particularly if imatinib resistance has developed.[53] Randomised studies in the USA and Europe are under way to assess the value of neoadjuvant imatinib for unresectable GISTs that might be rendered resectable (and potentially curable).

Gastric lymphoma

Primary gastric lymphoma is rare, accounting for about 5% of gastric tumours but one of the commonest sites for 'extranodal' lymphoma.[54] It is twice as common in men as in women and median age of diagnosis is 60–65 years,[55,56] except in human immunodeficiency virus (HIV)-infected patients, who develop the disease earlier.[57] It often presents with the same non-specific signs of dyspepsia and vague epigastric discomfort seen in both benign peptic ulceration and gastric adenocarcinoma. However, it may take longer than epithelial cancer to grow and cause persistent pain and weight loss. Diagnosis is by endoscopy and biopsy. It is essential that patients who fulfil the National Institute for Clinical Excellence (NICE) criteria for urgent upper GI endoscopy are referred and that the endoscopist performs a thorough investigation and takes adequate diagnostic biopsies.[58] If the biopsies are non-diagnostic they should be repeated immediately; accurate histological diagnosis is essential as the treatment and prognosis of gastric lymphoma is very different from adenocarcinoma.

Staging

Once a diagnosis of gastric lymphoma is made the paient should undergo a CT scan of chest, abdomen and pelvis, an endoluminal ultrasound (EUS), as this is the most accurate way of assessing depth

Table 11.3 • Modified Blackledge system for staging gastrointestinal lymphoma[61]

Stage I	Tumour confined to GI tract without serosal penetration: Single primary or multiple non-contiguous lesions
Stage II	Tumour extends into abdomen nodes from the primary: II_1 Local nodes (regional gastric) II_2 Distant nodes (para-aortic or intercaval)
Stage II_E	Perforation of the serosa with involvement of adjacent structures: e.g. stage II_E (pancreas) or stage II_E (colon) Also patients who present with perforated tumours and peritonitis
Stage IV	Disseminated extranodal disease (lung, bone marrow, etc.) or supradiaphragmatic nodal involvement

of invasion and regional node involvement,[59,60] and a bone marrow aspirate to look for distant spread of the disease. Many staging systems have been employed over the years but the most clinically useful is the modified Blackledge system[61] (Table 11.3).

Classification

Low-grade MALT lymphomas arise from the mucosa-associated lymphoid tissue, hence MALT, and behave in an indolent fashion. The WHO classifies MALT as extranodal marginal zone B-cell lymphomas and they are a form of non-Hodgkin's lymphoma.[58,62,63] Men and women are equally affected and they account for about 4% of all gastric tumours and 50% of gastric lymphomas.[64,65]

✔ Low-grade gastric MALT lymphomas are associated with *Helicobacter pylori* (HP) infection and early tumours will often regress with HP eradication therapy.[58,66] More advanced lesions that involve the full thickness of the stomach wall and have spread to local lymph nodes are much less likely to regress with HP eradication.[67]

Histopathologically they can be difficult to differentiate from chronic gastritis and experienced pathologists will look for lymphoepithelial lesions that are diagnostic.[68] Treatment of stage I disease is with HP eradication and 6-monthly endoscopic biopsy for 2 years. More advanced tumours, those that persist after HP eradication or those that recur are treated with chlorambucil and rituximab, and those with large-cell transformation require CHOP chemotherapy (cyclophosphamide, doxorubicin, vincristine and prednisolone) and rituximab.[69,70] Surgery is very rarely indicated for low-grade MALT lymphomas.

High-grade MALT lymphomas and diffuse B-cell lymphomas do not regress with HP eradication. Histologically they consist of sheets of destructive blast cells, do not contain lymphoepithelial lesions, and have frequent mitoses and apoptotic bodies.[71] They may resemble diffuse carcinomas, sarcomas, T-cell lymphomas and even metastatic melanoma.

✔✔ A randomised controlled trial of treatment with CHOP alone versus CHOP and rituximab showed improved 5-year survival from 63% to 76%.[72] A large randomised trial involving 589 patients with diffuse B-cell gastric lymphoma compared four treatment arms: surgery alone, surgery with radiotherapy, surgery with CHOP, and CHOP alone. Aviles et al. found that CHOP alone gave the best 10-year survival rates and had the lowest morbidity.[73]

Surgery, therefore, has a limited role in the modern management of gastric lymphoma.[74] It is used for resection of locoregional disease if medical treatment fails or in the emergency setting for bleeding or perforation.

Neuroendocrine gastroenteropancreatic tumours (GEP-NETs)

GEP-NETs are classified into intestinal neuroendocrine tumours (carcinoids), accounting for about two-thirds, and pancreatic endocrine tumours (PETs), accounting for the remaining one-third. Gastric carcinoid tumours make up just under 2% of all gastric neoplasms and there is some evidence that the incidence has been rising over the past two to three decades.[75] The appendix is the commonest site for carcinoid tumours (48%), followed by the rectum (17%) and the ileum (12%); the stomach only accounts for 9%.[76,77] Carcinoid tumours have characteristic histological and ultrastructural features and contain chromogranin A (CgA).[77] They were first described by Oberndorfer in 1907, who named them 'karzinoide', meaning 'carcinoma-like' in recognition of their more benign behaviour compared to adenocarcinomas.[78] Gastric carcinoids arise from histamine-containing enterochromaffin-like (ECL) cells, which are found in the fundus and body of the stomach. Gastric acid is produced by parietal cells when they are stimulated by gastrin directly (secreted by the G cells in the gastric antrum) or by histamine released locally by ECL cells when these are stimulated by gastrin. Negative feedback is provided by D cells that release somatostatin (SST) when stimulated by rising luminal H^+ concentrations; SST binds to G cells and ECL cells and inhibits the production of gastrin and histamine, respectively, hence reducing stimulation to parietal cells to produce acid. In patients with chronic atrophic gastritis the lack of acid production by parietal cells results in decreased SST levels, with excess production of gastrin and an over-stimulation of ECL cells. As gastrin is trophic to ECL cells, this can lead to ECL hyperplasia, dysplasia and eventually carcinoid tumour.

Presentation, classification and treatment

Gastric carcinoids are often discovered incidentally during upper GI endoscopy. Alternatively, they may present with bleeding (iron deficiency anaemia or frank GI blood loss), abdominal pain or dyspepsia. Rarely, they present late with metastatic disease and symptoms from the release of bioactive substances. Atypical carcinoid syndrome is due to histamine release and presents with a patchy cutaneous flush, oedema, watering eyes, bronchoconstriction and headaches, whereas classical carcinoid syndrome presents with cutaneous flushing, bronchospasm and diarrhoea, and is probably due to circulating serotonin and tachykinins.[79] Diagnosis is made by histology of endoscopic biopsies and the argyrophil reaction with the presence of CgA mRNA or protein.[80] Raised plasma CgA is a very sensitive and specific test for diagnosing metastatic carcinoid in patients with suspected carcinoid syndrome.[77] Initial staging is by EUS and CT. Gastric carcinoid tumours express somatostatin-2 receptors and these will bind the synthetic octapeptide, octreotide; radiolabelled octreotide is used in the OctreoScan™.

✔✔ In a prospective study, Gibril et al.[81] found this test to have positive and negative predictive values of 63% and 97%, respectively, for the detection of gastric carcinoid and its use should be considered in all patients with carcinoid tumours.

There are a number of different classification systems for GEP-NETs. The WHO classification separates tumours on the basis of differentiation; the European Neuroendocrine Tumour Society (ENETS) classification has three groups (G1-3) based upon mitotic count and Ki67 index; and the TNM classification separates tumours according to the extent of the local tumour, regional lymph nodes and distant metastases (Tis-4, N0–1, M0–1).[82] Gastric carcinoids are usefully classified according to their behaviour and are rare under the age of 50 years.[83] Type I tumours are the commonest (75%), arise in patients with chronic atrophic gastritis (often those with pernicious anaemia) and are more common in women than men (3:1). They are usually small, well-differentiated polypoid lesions that behave in a benign fashion but, when larger (1–2 cm), can occasionally metastasise to regional lymph nodes. Small lesions (<1 cm) can be removed by endoscopic mucosal resection (EMR), although long-term follow-up for this treatment is lacking.

✔ The gold standard treatment for a lesion under 2 cm diameter is local surgical resection and antrectomy, as this reduces gastrin levels.[84] Background ECL hyperplasia will often regress after antrectomy. Surgery may be open or laparoscopic depending upon local preference and experience. Patients should have endoscopic surveillence after surgery and the prognosis is excellent, with >90% 5-year survival.

Type II gastric carcinoids are rare (8%) and occur in patients with a gastrinoma as part of the autosomal dominant disorder multiple endocrine neoplasia syndrome type 1 (MEN-1). They have an intermediate behaviour between type I and type III carcinoids, with a 10–30% risk of metastasising. For early lesions the treatment is the same as for type I tumours, although great care should be taken to find and remove the gastrinoma whenever possible. Prognosis is again good, with about 70% 5-year survival, but the MEN-1 syndrome dictates outcome more than the carcinoid tumour.[85]

✔ Type III lesions constitute 21% of gastric carcinoids and are much more aggressive.[86] They usually present as a large ulcerating solitary mass, sometimes with liver metastases, and are not associated with atrophic gastritis, MEN-1 or hypergastrinaemia. Treatment for non-metastatic type III tumours is by gastrectomy, usually total, with clearance of the local lymph nodes (D2 resection).[87] Local resection is not recommened for these tumours. Survival is around 50% at 5 years.[88]

For patients with symptomatic metastatic carcinoid the initial treatment of choice is with somatastatin analogues such as octreotide or lanreotide, which is longer acting.[85] Phase II trials of the monoclonal antibody bevacizumab[89] have shown promise and phase III studies are now awaited. Surgery can play an important role in the management of metastatic GEP-NETs by reducing tumour mass (debulking) and can occasionally be curative when an R0 resection is possible, particularly for liver metastases.[90] Radiofrequency ablation and embolisation/chemoembolisation can similarly be used with success to treat isolated hepatic lesions.

Rarities

Leiomyomas are benign smooth muscle tumours of the upper GI tract, are usually located in the oesophagus and may be very large at presentation.[91] They may present as an incidental submucosal swelling found at endoscopy or with dysphagia or, rarely, with GI bleeding. Similar lesions found in the stomach are nearly always GISTs. Incidental leiomyomas of the oesophagus can be treated conservatively, although an EUS to confirm the diagnosis is recommended and a follow-up EUS examination 1–2 years later will provide reassurance that the lesion is not growing. Symptomatic leiomyomas can be excised by dividing the muscularis propria and enucleating the lesion without disrupting the mucosa. This is usually done now using minimally invasive techniques (thoracoscopically).[92] Leiomyosarcomas look exactly like their benign counterparts but behave differently. A large submucosal lesion in the oesophagus (>2 cm) or one that is enlarging rapidly should be treated as potentially malignant. EUS-guided fine-needle or core biopsy of such a lesion is now possible and should be attempted if leiomyosarcoma is suspected.[93] If confirmed, or doubt continues after biopsy, a formal oesophagectomy is recommended, as long-term survival is dependent upon achieving an R0 resection.[94]

Small-cell carcinoma of the oesophagus is thankfully rare. It has an even worse prognosis than squamous or adenocarcinoma. As with most oesophageal tumours it presents late and has already spread to locoregional nodes when diagnosed.[95] Even radical surgery with three-field lymph node resection results in 5-year survival of less than 10%. Treatment should therefore be by chemoradiation as this will occasionally result in a cure and, if it does not, provides moderately good palliation with less morbidity than radical surgery. There are no randomised studies of treatment but much has been extrapolated from experience with small-cell tumours of the lung.

Key points

- Complete surgical resection (R0) of gastric GISTs is often curative and is the treatment of choice whenever possible.
- Patients who have had resection of a high-risk GIST benefit from adjuvant imatinib.
- Metastatic and unresectable GISTs should be treated with 400 mg imatinib daily in the first instance and their overall care managed by a multidisciplinary team.
- Gastric carcinoid tumours are now classified as a subgroup of gastroenteropancreatic neuroendocrine tumours (GEP-NETs).
- Type I gastric carcinoids can safely be treated with minimal surgery (including endoscopic resection) and have a good prognosis, whereas type III carcinoid tumours require a gastrectomy and nodal resection and have a poorer prognosis.
- Low-grade B-cell gastric MALT lymphoma is caused by *Helicobacter pylori* (HP) and will often regress after HP eradication therapy.
- Surgery has a limited role in the treatment of gastric lymphoma and primary treatment is usually with chemotherapy.
- Submucosal lesions in the oesophagus are usually leiomyomas and, if symptomatic, can be enucleated thoracoscopically.

References

1. Rossi CR, Mocellin S, Mencarelli R, et al. Gastrointestinal stromal tumors: from a surgical to a molecular approach. Int J Cancer 2003;107(2):171–6.
2. Mazur MT, Clark HB. Gastric stromal tumors. Reappraisal of histogenesis. Am J Surg Pathol 1983;7(6):507–19.
3. Walker P, Dvorak AM. Gastrointestinal autonomic nerve (GAN) tumor. Ultrastructural evidence for a newly recognized entity. Arch Pathol Lab Med 1986;110(4):309–16.
4. Lee JR, Joshi V, Griffin Jr. JW, et al. Gastrointestinal autonomic nerve tumor: immunohistochemical and molecular identity with gastrointestinal stromal tumor. Am J Surg Pathol 2001;25(8):979–87.

5. Romert P, Mikkelsen HB. c-kit immunoreactive interstitial cells of Cajal in the human small and large intestine. Histochem Cell Biol 1998;109(3):195–202.
6. Kindblom LG, Remotti HE, Aldenborg F, et al. Gastrointestinal pacemaker cell tumor (GIPACT): gastrointestinal stromal tumors show phenotypic characteristics of the interstitial cells of Cajal. Am J Pathol 1998;152(5):1259–69.
7. Joensuu H, Kindblom LG. Gastrointestinal stromal tumors – a review. Acta Orthop Scand 2004; 75(311):62–71.
8. Kim KH, Nelson SD, Kim DH, et al. Diagnostic relevance of overexpressions of PKC-theta and DOG-1 and KIT/PDGFRA gene mutations in extragastrointestinal stromal tumors: a Korean six-centers study of 28 cases. Anticancer Res 2012;32(3):923–37.
9. Nilsson B, Bumming P, Meis-Kindblom JM, et al. Gastrointestinal stromal tumors: the incidence, prevalence, clinical course, and prognostication in the preimatinib mesylate era – a population-based study in western Sweden. Cancer 2005;103(4):821–9.
10. Hassan I, You YN, Shyyan R, et al. Surgically managed gastrointestinal stromal tumors: a comparative and prognostic analysis. Ann Surg Oncol 2008;15(1):52–9.
11. Fletcher CD, Berman JJ, Corless C, et al. Diagnosis of gastrointestinal stromal tumors: a consensus approach. Hum Pathol 2002;33(5):459–65.
12. DeMatteo RP, Lewis JJ, Leung D, et al. Two hundred gastrointestinal stromal tumors: recurrence patterns and prognostic factors for survival. Ann Surg 2000;231(1):51–8.
13. Emory TS, Sobin LH, Lukes L, et al. Prognosis of gastrointestinal smooth-muscle (stromal) tumors: dependence on anatomic site. Am J Surg Pathol 1999;23(1):82–7.
14. Langer C, Gunawan B, Schuler P, et al. Prognostic factors influencing surgical management and outcome of gastrointestinal stromal tumours. Br J Surg 2003;90(3):332–9.
15. Lee YT. Leiomyosarcoma of the gastro-intestinal tract: general pattern of metastasis and recurrence. Cancer Treat Rev 1983;10(2):91–101.
16. Miettinen M, El-Rifai W, Sobin LH., et al. Evaluation of malignancy and prognosis of gastrointestinal stromal tumors: a review. Hum Pathol 2002;33(5):478–83.
17. Connolly EM, Gaffney E, Reynolds JV. Gastrointestinal stromal tumours. Br J Surg 2003;90(10): 1178–86.
18. Bucher P, Villiger P, Egger JF, et al. Management of gastrointestinal stromal tumors: from diagnosis to treatment. Swiss Med Wkly 2004;134(11–12): 145–53.
19. Lehnert T. Gastrointestinal sarcoma (GIST) – a review of surgical management. Ann Chir Gynaecol 1998;87(4):297–305.
20. DeMatteo RP. The GIST of targeted cancer therapy: a tumor (gastrointestinal stromal tumor), a mutated gene (c-kit), and a molecular inhibitor (STI571). Ann Surg Oncol 2002;9(9):831–9.
21. Berman J, O'Leary TJ. Gastrointestinal stromal tumor workshop. Hum Pathol 2001;32(6):578–82.
22. Joensuu H, Fletcher C, Dimitrijevic S, et al. Management of malignant gastrointestinal stromal tumours. Lancet Oncol 2002;3(11):655–64.
23. Palazzo L, Landi B, Cellier C, et al. Endosonographic features predictive of benign and malignant gastrointestinal stromal cell tumours. Gut 2000;46(1):88–92.
24. Chak A, Canto MI, Rosch T, et al. Endosonographic differentiation of benign and malignant stromal cell tumors. Gastrointest Endosc 1997;45(6):468–73.
25. Akahoshi K, Sumida Y, Matsui N, et al. Preoperative diagnosis of gastrointestinal stromal tumor by endoscopic ultrasound-guided fine needle aspiration. World J Gastroenterol 2007;13(14):2077–82.
26. Lau S, Tam KF, Kam CK, et al. Imaging of gastrointestinal stromal tumour (GIST). Clin Radiol 2004;59(6):487–98.
27. Benjamin RS, Choi H, Macapinlac HA, et al. We should desist using RECIST, at least in GIST. J Clin Oncol 2007;25(13):1760–4.
28. Antoch G, Kanja J, Bauer S, et al. Comparison of PET, CT, and dual-modality PET/CT imaging for monitoring of imatinib (STI571) therapy in patients with gastrointestinal stromal tumors. J Nucl Med 2004;45(3):357–65.
29. Stroobants S, Goeminne J, Seegers M, et al. 18FDG-Positron emission tomography for the early prediction of response in advanced soft tissue sarcoma treated with imatinib mesylate (Glivec). Eur J Cancer 2003;39(14):2012–20.
30. Isozaki K, Terris B, Belghiti J, et al. Germline-activating mutation in the kinase domain of KIT gene in familial gastrointestinal stromal tumors. Am J Pathol 2000;157(5):1581–5.
31. O'Brien P, Kapusta L, Dardick I, et al. Multiple familial gastrointestinal autonomic nerve tumors and small intestinal neuronal dysplasia. Am J Surg Pathol 1999;23(2):198–204.
32. Carney JA, Sheps SG, Go VL, et al. The triad of gastric leiomyosarcoma, functioning extra-adrenal paraganglioma and pulmonary chondroma. N Engl J Med 1977;296(26):1517–8.
33. Carney JA. Gastric stromal sarcoma, pulmonary chondroma, and extra-adrenal paraganglioma (Carney Triad): natural history, adrenocortical component, and possible familial occurrence. Mayo Clin Proc 1999;74(6):543–52.
34. Demetri GD, Benjamin RS, Blanke CD, et al. NCCN Task Force report: management of patients with gastrointestinal stromal tumor (GIST) – update of the NCCN clinical practice guidelines. J Natl Compr Canc Netw 2007;5(Suppl. 2):S1–30.

35. Ng EH, Pollock RE, Romsdahl MM. Prognostic implications of patterns of failure for gastrointestinal leiomyosarcomas. Cancer 1992;69(6):1334–41.

36. Merendino KA, Thomas GI. The jejunal interposition operation for substitution of the esophagogastric sphincter; present status. Surgery 1958;44(6): 1112–5.

37. Stein HJ, Feith M, Mueller J, et al. Limited resection for early adenocarcinoma in Barrett's esophagus. Ann Surg 2000;232(6):733–42.

38. Dematteo RP, Heinrich MC, El-Rifai WM, et al. Clinical management of gastrointestinal stromal tumors: before and after STI-571. Hum Pathol 2002;33(5):466–77.

39. Ludwig DJ, Traverso LW. Gut stromal tumors and their clinical behavior. Am J Surg 1997;173(5): 390–4.

40. UK GIST Consensus Group. Guidelines for the management of gastrointestinal stromal tumours (GISTs). 2005.Available from http://www.augis.org; [accessed 03.11.12].

41. Tuveson DA, Willis NA, Jacks T, et al. STI571 inactivation of the gastrointestinal stromal tumor c-KIT oncoprotein: biological and clinical implications. Oncogene 2001;20(36):5054–8.

42. Katz SC, DeMatteo RP. Gastrointestinal stromal tumors and leiomyosarcomas. J Surg Oncol 2008;97(4):350–9.

43. Van Glabbeke M, van Oosterom AT, Oosterhuis JW, et al. Prognostic factors for the outcome of chemotherapy in advanced soft tissue sarcoma: an analysis of 2,185 patients treated with anthracycline-containing first-line regimens – a European Organization for Research and Treatment of Cancer Soft Tissue and Bone Sarcoma Group Study. J Clin Oncol 1999;17(1):150–7.

44. van Oosterom AT, Judson I, Verweij J, et al. Safety and efficacy of imatinib (STI571) in metastatic gastrointestinal stromal tumours: a phase I study. Lancet 2001;358(9291):1421–3.

45. Blanke CD, Demetri GD, von Mehren M, et al. Long-term results from a randomized phase II trial of standard- versus higher-dose imatinib mesylate for patients with unresectable or metastatic gastrointestinal stromal tumors expressing KIT. J Clin Oncol 2008;26(4):620–5.

46. Blanke CD, Rankin C, Demetri GD, et al. Phase III randomized, intergroup trial assessing imatinib mesylate at two dose levels in patients with unresectable or metastatic gastrointestinal stromal tumors expressing the kit receptor tyrosine kinase: S0033. J Clin Oncol 2008;26(4):626–632.
A randomised study of 400 mg vs 800 mg imatinib in unresectable or metastatic GIST. No difference was found in median survival between the two groups.

47. Verweij J, Casali PG, Zalcberg J, et al. Progression-free survival in gastrointestinal stromal tumours with high-dose imatinib: randomised trial. Lancet 2004;364(9440):1127–34.
Another randomised study (946 patients) comparing 800 mg with 400 mg imatinib found some small improvement in progression-free survival for the higher dose.

48. Van Glabbeke M, Verweij J, Casali PG, et al. Initial and late resistance to imatinib in advanced gastrointestinal stromal tumors are predicted by different prognostic factors: a European Organisation for Research and Treatment of Cancer–Italian Sarcoma Group–Australasian Gastrointestinal Trials Group study. J Clin Oncol 2005;23(24):5795–804.

49. DeMatteo RP, Ballman KV, Antonescu CR, et al. Adjuvant imatinib mesylate after resection of localised, primary gastrointestinal stromal tumour: a randomised, double-blind, placebo-controlled trial. Lancet 2009;373(9669):1097–104.

50. Joensuu H, Eriksson M, Sundby Hall K, et al. One vs three years of adjuvant imatinib for operable gastrointestinal stromal tumor: a randomized trial. JAMA 2012;307(12):1265–72.

51. DeMatteo RP, Shah A, Fong Y, et al. Results of hepatic resection for sarcoma metastatic to liver. Ann Surg 2001;234(4):540–8.

52. Barnes G, Bulusu VR, Hardwick RH, et al. A review of the surgical management of metastatic gastrointestinal stromal tumours (GISTs) on imatinib mesylate (Glivec). Int J Surg 2005;3(3):206–12.

53. Sym SJ, Ryu MH, Lee JL, et al. Surgical intervention following imatinib treatment in patients with advanced gastrointestinal stromal tumors (GISTs). J Surg Oncol 2008;98(1):27–33.

54. Sandler RS. Has primary gastric lymphoma become more common? J Clin Gastroenterol 1984;6(2): 101–7.

55. Cogliatti SB, Schmid U, Schumacher U, et al. Primary B-cell gastric lymphoma: a clinicopathological study of 145 patients. Gastroenterology 1991;101(5):1159–70.

56. Weingrad DN, Decosse JJ, Sherlock P, et al. Primary gastrointestinal lymphoma: a 30-year review. Cancer 1982;49(6):1258–65.

57. Imrie KR, Sawka CA, Kutas G, et al. HIV-associated lymphoma of the gastrointestinal tract: the University of Toronto AIDS-Lymphoma Study Group experience. Leuk Lymphoma 1995;16(3–4):343–9.

58. Stolte M. *Helicobacter pylori* gastritis and gastric MALT-lymphoma. Lancet 1992;339(8795): 745–6.

59. Caletti G, Fusaroli P, Togliani T, et al. Endosonography in gastric lymphoma and large gastric folds. Eur J Ultrasound 2000;11(1):31–40.

60. Yucel C, Ozdemir H, Isik S. Role of endosonography in the evaluation of gastric malignancies. J Ultrasound Med 1999;18(4):283–8.

61. Rohatiner A, d'Amore F, Coiffier B, et al. Report on a workshop convened to discuss the pathological

and staging classifications of gastrointestinal tract lymphoma. Ann Oncol 1994;5(5):397–400.

62. Isaacson P, Wright DH. Extranodal malignant lymphoma arising from mucosa-associated lymphoid tissue. Cancer 1984;53(11):2515–24.
63. Parsonnet J, Hansen S, Rodriguez L, et al. *Helicobacter pylori* infection and gastric lymphoma. N Engl J Med 1994;330(18):1267–71.
64. Shimm DS, Dosoretz DE, Anderson T, et al. Primary gastric lymphoma. An analysis with emphasis on prognostic factors and radiation therapy. Cancer 1983;52(11):2044–8.
65. Sutherland AG, Kennedy M, Anderson DN, et al. Gastric lymphoma in Grampian Region: presentation, treatment and outcome. J R Coll Surg Edinb 1996;41(3):143–7.
66. Pinotti G, Zucca E, Roggero E, et al. Clinical features, treatment and outcome in a series of 93 patients with low-grade gastric MALT lymphoma. Leuk Lymphoma 1997;26(5–6):527–37.
67. Montalban C, Manzanal A, Boixeda D, et al. Treatment of low-grade gastric MALT lymphoma with *Helicobacter pylori* eradication. Lancet 1995;345(8952):798–9.
68. Chan JK. Gastrointestinal lymphomas: an overview with emphasis on new findings and diagnostic problems. Semin Diagn Pathol 1996;13(4):260–96.
69. Raderer M, Chott A, Drach J, et al. Chemotherapy for management of localised high-grade gastric B-cell lymphoma: how much is necessary? Ann Oncol 2002;13(7):1094–8.
70. Wohrer S, Puspok A, Drach J, et al. Rituximab, cyclophosphamide, doxorubicin, vincristine and prednisone (R-CHOP) for treatment of early-stage gastric diffuse large B-cell lymphoma. Ann Oncol 2004;15(7):1086–90.
71. Hiyama T, Haruma K, Kitadai Y, et al. Clinicopathological features of gastric mucosa-associated lymphoid tissue lymphoma: a comparison with diffuse large B-cell lymphoma without a mucosa-associated lymphoid tissue lymphoma component. J Gastroenterol Hepatol 2001;16(7):734–9.
72. Coiffier B, Lepage E, Briere J, et al. CHOP chemotherapy plus rituximab compared with CHOP alone in elderly patients with diffuse large-B-cell lymphoma. N Engl J Med 2002;346(4):235–42.
    A randomised study investigating the value of rituximab when added to standard chemotherapy for treating gastric lymphoma.
73. Aviles A, Nambo MJ, Neri N, et al. The role of surgery in primary gastric lymphoma: results of a controlled clinical trial. Ann Surg 2004;240(1):44–50.
    A large and important study randomising 589 patients to four treatment arms. Surgery did not improve survival and CHOP chemotherapy came out on top.
74. Popescu RA, Wotherspoon AC, Cunningham D, et al. Surgery plus chemotherapy or chemotherapy alone for primary intermediate- and high-grade gastric non-Hodgkin's lymphoma: the Royal Marsden Hospital experience. Eur J Cancer 1999;35(6):928–34.
75. Hodgson N, Koniaris LG, Livingstone AS, et al. Gastric carcinoids: a temporal increase with proton pump introduction. Surg Endosc 2005;19(12):1610–2.
76. Berge T, Linell F. Carcinoid tumours. Frequency in a defined population during a 12-year period. Acta Pathol Microbiol Scand 1976;84(4):322–30.
77. Kidd M, Modlin IM, Mane SM, et al. RT–PCR detection of chromogranin A: a new standard in the identification of neuroendocrine tumor disease. Ann Surg 2006;243(2):273–80.
78. Oberndorfer S. Karzinoid tumoren des dunndarms. Frankf Z Pathol 1907;1:237–40.
79. Conlon JM, Deacon CF, Richter G, et al. Circulating tachykinins (substance P, neurokinin A, neuropeptide K) and the carcinoid flush. Scand J Gastroenterol 1987;22(1):97–105.
80. Nobels FR, Kwekkeboom DJ, Coopmans W, et al. Chromogranin A as serum marker for neuroendocrine neoplasia: comparison with neuron-specific enolase and the alpha-subunit of glycoprotein hormones. J Clin Endocrinol Metab 1997;82(8):2622–8.
81. Gibril F, Reynolds JC, Lubensky IA, et al. Ability of somatostatin receptor scintigraphy to identify patients with gastric carcinoids: a prospective study. J Nucl Med 2000;41(10):1646–56.
    A blinded prospective study of 162 patients with Zollinger–Ellison syndrome comparing the results of radionuclear studies with gastric biopsies looking for gastric carcinoid tumours.
82. Oberg K, Akerstrom G, Rindi G, et al. Neuroendocrine gastroenteropancreatic tumours: ESMO Clinical Practice Guidelines for diagnosis, treatment and follow-up. Ann Oncol 2010;21(Suppl. 5):v223–7.
83. Modlin IM, Kidd M, Latich I, et al. Current status of gastrointestinal carcinoids. Gastroenterology 2005;128(6):1717–51.
84. Dakin GF, Warner RR, Pomp A, et al. Presentation, treatment, and outcome of type 1 gastric carcinoid tumors. J Surg Oncol 2006;93(5):368–72.
85. Modlin IM, Latich I, Kidd M, et al. Therapeutic options for gastrointestinal carcinoids. Clin Gastroenterol Hepatol 2006;4(5):526–47.
86. Rindi G. Clinicopathologic aspects of gastric neuroendocrine tumors. Am J Surg Pathol 1995;19(Suppl. 1):S20–9.
87. Modlin IM, Kidd M, Lye KD. Biology and management of gastric carcinoid tumours: a review. Eur J Surg 2002;168(12):669–83.
88. Modlin IM, Lye KD, Kidd M. A 50-year analysis of 562 gastric carcinoids: small tumor or larger problem? Am J Gastroenterol 2004;99(1):23–32.

89. Yao JC, Phan A, Hoff PM, et al. Targeting vascular endothelial growth factor in advanced carcinoid tumor: a random assignment phase II study of depot octreotide with bevacizumab and pegylated interferon alpha-2b. J Clin Oncol 2008;26(8):1316–23.
90. Akerstrom G, Hellman P. Surgery on neuroendocrine tumours. Best Pract Res Clin Endocrinol Metab 2007;21(1):87–109.
91. Pompeo E, Francioni F, Pappalardo G, et al. Giant leiomyoma of the oesophagus and cardia. Diagnostic and therapeutic considerations: case report and literature review. Scand Cardiovasc J 1997;31(6):361–4.
92. Roviaro GC, Maciocco M, Varoli F, et al. Videothoracoscopic treatment of oesophageal leiomyoma. Thorax 1998;53(3):190–2.
93. Stelow EB, Jones DR, Shami VM. Esophageal leiomyosarcoma diagnosed by endoscopic ultrasound-guided fine-needle aspiration. Diagn Cytopathol 2007;35(3):167–70.
94. Rocco G, Trastek VF, Deschamps C, et al. Leiomyosarcoma of the esophagus: results of surgical treatment. Ann Thorac Surg 1998;66(3):894–7.
95. Yun JP, Zhang MF, Hou JH, et al. Primary small cell carcinoma of the esophagus: clinicopathological and immunohistochemical features of 21 cases. BMC Cancer 2007;7:38.

12

Pathophysiology and investigation of gastro-oesophageal reflux disease

John M. Findlay
Nicholas D. Maynard

Introduction

Gastro-oesophageal reflux disease (GORD) describes symptoms or mucosal damage caused by reflux of gastric contents into the oesophagus.[1] Symptoms are variable and along with damage are associated with many permutations of motility, endoscopic and physiological abnormalities. GORD is the major factor leading to the increasing incidence of oesophageal adenocarcinoma,[2] and is one of the commonest health problems in the developed world.

Epidemiology

Gastro-oesophageal reflux is universal, and as such can be viewed as a normal physiological process. Such physiological episodes are asymptomatic and rapidly cleared. They occur mainly after meals, in the upright position and when awake.[3,4] By contrast, pathological reflux results in chronic symptoms or mucosal damage. However, the subjectivity of symptoms is such that the boundary between the two is blurred, with many people viewing occasional reflux symptoms as normal, without seeking medical attention. For example, the reflux of air (belching) due to gastric distension is a universal experience, yet depending upon frequency and patient perception may be either normal or or a symptom of GORD. Unsurprisingly, the epidemiology of GORD is difficult to determine. A 2011 population-based cohort study of 45 000 people from Norway[5] found the prevalence of any symptoms to be 41%, weekly symptoms to be 17% and severe symptoms to be 6.7% The figures had increased by 30%, 24% and 47%, respectively, over the previous decade. Incidence of any symptoms was 3%, with that of severe symptoms 0.2%, with spontaneous resolution of these symptoms occurring in 2% and 1%, respectively. A systematic review of 15 studies estimated a similar prevalence of weekly symptoms in 10–20% in the Western world (5% in Asia).[6]

✔ One large population-based study and one systematic review estimated the Western prevalence of symptomatic GORD (at least weekly heartburn/acid regurgitation) to be 10–20%.[5,6]

These findings were similar to a smaller Finnish study of 1562 consecutive patients referred for endoscopy. With the caveat of this selection bias, the overall incidence was estimated as 3%, of which 2% had endoscopic mucosal damage.[7] Two additional studies have reached similar conclusions, with 32–38% of those with symptoms having normal endoscopies.[8,9] Importantly, the converse may be true, with up to 20% of those with oesophagitis or Barrett's being asymptomatic.[10]

✔ Two studies of patients with reflux symptoms found a normal oesophagus on endoscopy in 32% and 38% of subjects.[8,9] Up to 20% of those with oesophagitis or Barrett's oesophagus are asymptomatic.[10]

Traditionally, GORD has been viewed as a spectrum of a single disease, with endoscopy-negative

Box 12.1 • Distinct subgroups of GORD

- Symptomatic endoscopy-negative (non-erosive) GORD
- Oesophagitis and erosive reflux
- Barrett's oesophagus

symptoms at the mild end, increasing grades of oesophagitis representing progressively severe disease, culminating in Barrett's metaplasia.[1] However, this approach is undermined by a number of clinical, endoscopic and physiological findings, suggesting that the three may in fact be distinct groups and disease processes in themselves (Box 12.1).[11,12] Most importantly, endoscopic progression from one end of the spectrum to the other is rare.[12]

Symptoms

Symptoms tend to occur in combination rather than isolation, and are classed as typical and atypical. Typical symptoms comprise heartburn, acid brash and regurgitation ('volume reflux'). Heartburn is defined as discomfort or burning behind the sternum; regurgitation as the perception of flow of gastric contents into the oro/hypopharynx. Intermittent dysphagia may also occur. Atypical symptoms include non-heartburn chest pain, epigastric pain and bloating, and can blur with other functional symptoms of the gastrointestinal tract so that even if excessive reflux is demonstrated physiologically, attributing causality may be difficult. Extra-oesophageal manifestations occur in the upper aerodigestive tract and lungs. GORD may be associated with a changing/hoarse voice, pharyngitis, tonsillitis and sinusitis, 'globus' symptoms (resulting from cricopharyngeal dysfunction) as well as throat clearing, chronic cough, dental decay and poor oral hygiene. GORD has also been implicated in exacerbations of asthma, possibly due to micro-aspiration.

Symptoms typically vary between the three GORD groups discussed above. Those with symptomatic endoscopy-negative disease (or non-erosive reflux) tend to have severe, often atypical symptoms with variable response to acid suppression (presumably representing oesophageal hypersensitivity to acid and non-acid reflux).[12] By contrast, those with erosive reflux and oesophagitis tend towards more typical symptoms responding well to acid suppression.[12] Finally, those with Barrett's often have minimal symptoms, possibly due to the relative insensitivity of metaplastic epithelium to acid.[13]

These discrepancies emphasise the challenging multifactorial nature of GORD; central to its understanding is normal oesophageal anatomy and physiology.

Normal oesophageal anatomy

The oesophagus is a muscular tube, approximately 25 cm in length. It extends from the pharynx to the stomach, and is subdivided into three (arbitrary) anatomical segments: cervical, thoracic and abdominal. The cervical oesophagus (approximately 5 cm long) is a direct continuation of the hypopharynx, between cricopharyngeus and the thoracic inlet (T1). The thoracic segment (approximately 18 cm) ends at T10 at the oeophageal hiatus. The abdominal oesophagus (approximately 1–2 cm) ends at the gastro-oesophageal junction.

The muscle configuration of the body of the oesophagus is unique, with both smooth and striated muscle comprising a single functional unit. The muscularis propria consists of outer longitudinal and inner circular layers (the former spiralling slightly). These are exclusively striated muscle at the proximal end (including cricopharyngeus), mixing progressively with smooth muscle over the proximal and middle thirds. The lower third is entirely composed of smooth muscle. The epithelial lining is non-keratinising stratified squamous, abruptly becoming glandular columnar (evident endoscopically as the z-line) at the level of, or at a variable distance above, the gastro-oesophageal junction.

Between the mucosa and muscularis mucosa, and the circular muscle layer, lies the submucosa, which contains neurovascular and support tissue. Blood supply is predominantly from the inferior thyroid arteries, direct aortic branches and left gastric artery for the cervical, thoracic and abdominal segments, respectively. Parasympathetic innervation is predominantly from the vagus nerves, with some indirect contribution proximally from the recurrent laryngeal nerves. Sympathetic innervation is from the middle cervical ganglion proximally, and upper four thoracic ganglia distally. The oesophagus has two sphincters: upper and lower. The former comprises the inferior constrictor muscle, cricopharyngeus and proximal oesophageal muscle. The latter is less discrete and is discussed in greater depth later.

Normal oesophageal physiology

On swallowing the upper and lower oesophageal sphincters relax, and the food or liquid bolus is propelled distally by peristalsis to the stomach. The responsible mechanisms involve complicated coordination between central and local neuromuscular mechanisms. Peristalsis is the sequential contraction of the oesophageal body. Animal models demonstrate progression aborally in both longitudinal and circular layers, without torque.[14] Primary peristalsis is instigated centrally in the swallowing centre by swallowing, with the wave arising in the pharynx. A persistent bolus distends the oesophagus, triggering local neural mechanisms and a secondary peristaltic wave.[15] Tertiary contractions are aberrant, synchronous contractions of oesophageal segments, which play no role in peristalsis. During peristalsis, the oesophageal body contracts segmentally, with the greatest pressure at the mid-point of the contracted segment, a few centimetres behind the bolus[16] (**Fig. 12.1**).

Whether the longitudinal and circular layers contract synchronously or not is disputed. A number of studies have suggested that the circular layer initially hyperpolarises, to contract two seconds after the longitudinal layer.[17–19] However, this has been disputed, and it has been suggested that any delay is a function of the manometric techniques used.[20] In any case, the involvement of both layers confers mechanical advantages, with longitudinal contractions shortening the circular layer, allowing greater contractile force. In addition, contraction of both reduces wall tension at the site of contraction.[21]

Primary peristalsis is initiated centrally (via the vagus) and modified peripherally (via local myogenic and neuronal mechanisms). Vagal efferents from the nucleus ambiguous initiate skeletal muscle contraction, and those from the dorsomotor nucleus innervate smooth muscle. These do so via intrinsic neurons of the myenteric plexus (between the muscle layers). Modification within the oesophageal body occurs in response to volume, temperature and acid receptors, with central feedback via vagal afferents. Warm boluses initiate an exaggerated peristaltic wave, whereas cold boluses (e.g. ice cream) may not provoke distal peristalsis.[22] This is true for wet and dry swallows, respectively. In addition, oesophageal acid receptors are believed to allow protective clearance of refluxate. Crucial to successful peristalsis is the oesophageal latency period. Following initial stimulation of the circular muscle layers, a variable period of membrane hyperpolarisation occurs, primarily mediated by intrinsic nitric oxide inhibition.[23] This period increases progressively, moving distally along the oesophageal body, with greater inhibitory inhibition.[24] Initial (or deglutitive) inhibition describes a refractory period of the oesophageal body due to myogenic and inhibitory properties. Swallowing for a second time within seconds causes the first peristaltic wave to be aborted.[25] This allows rapid sequences of swallows (used primarily for drinking).

Antireflux mechanisms

A positive pressure gradient of approximately 10 mmHg exists between the stomach and oesophagus. The stomach and abdominal oesophagus lie within 5 mmHg of positive intra-abdominal pressure, with the thoracic oesophagus exposed to 5 mmHg of negative pressure. That gastro-oesophageal reflux is the exception rather than the rule is due to several factors: the lower oesophageal sphincter (LOS), the

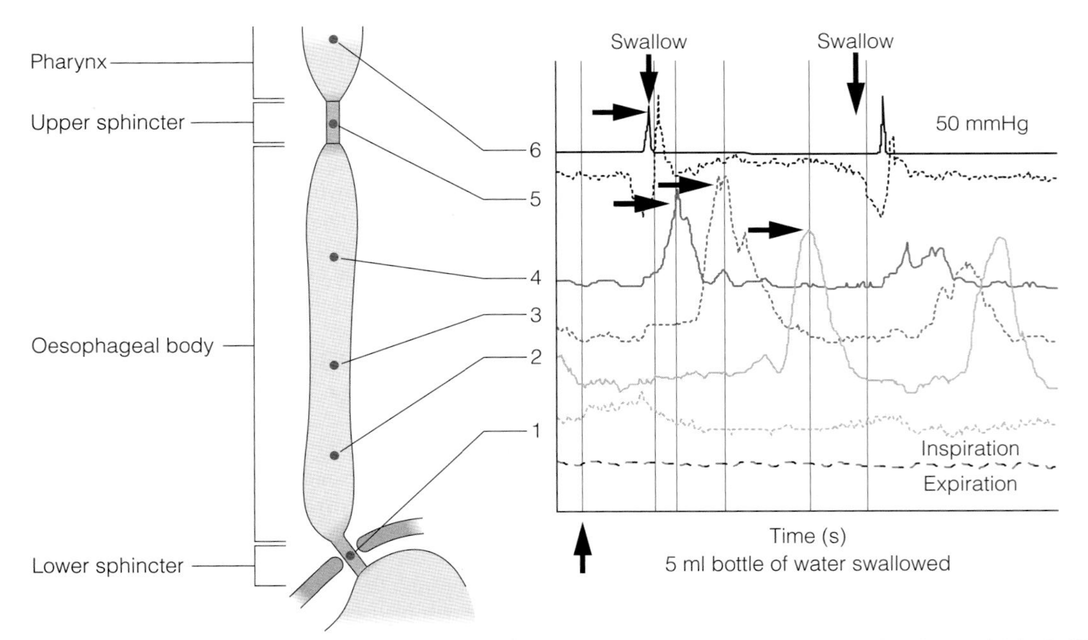

Figure 12.1 • A standard six-sensor manometry trace of normal oesophageal peristalsis. Adapted from Anggiansah A, Marshal R. Use of the oesophageal laboratory, 1st edn. Oxford: Isis Medical Media, 2000. With permission from Isis Medical Media.

Box 12.2 • Antireflux mechanisms

Intrinsic oesophageal mechanism

- Lower oesophageal sphincter
- Basal tone
- Adaptive pressure changes

Extrinsic mechanisms

- Diaphragmatic sphincter
- Distal oesophageal compression
- Angle of His
- Mucosal rosette
- Phreno-oesophageal ligament

diaphragmatic sphincter or 'pinch-cock', distal oesophageal compression, and other mechanical barriers such as the cardio-oesophageal angle (of His) and the mucosal rosette (Box 12.2).

Lower oesophageal sphincter

The LOS is the primary antireflux mechanism. Although not an anatomically discrete sphincter, it is a resting high-pressure zone in the distal oesophagus, which relaxes appropriately to allow swallowing, belching and vomiting.[26] It is composed of specialised smooth muscle, arranged in either clasp or sling formation, running in the distal 1–4 cm of the oesophagus and blending with the cardia.[27] The basal tone of the LOS is both intrinisic (inherent muscular properties) and extrinsic (excitatory cholinergic vagal input). Clasp and sling fibres vary in resting tone and responsiveness to stimulation; sling fibres have lower tone but greater responsiveness, probably due to differing proportions of contractile proteins. These fibres are also asymmetrically arranged, potentially accounting for the longitudinal and radial asymmetry of basal pressure (being greatest posteriorly and on the right).[28] LOS muscle cells are tonic, and as such distinct from the phasic cells of the oesophageal body (which have no intrinsic tone).

Neurological control of the LOS is complicated. Central control is mediated by vagal efferents originating in the dorsal motor nucleus (with excitatory cell bodies cephalad and inhibitory cells caudally).[29] Sensory feedback from the LOS is relayed via the tractus solitarius. Central neurotransmitters include glutamate, adrenaline, dopamine, acetylcholine and nitric oxide. Peripherally, vagal fibres synapse in the myenteric plexus via acetylcholine.[30] Both atropine and vagotomy reduce resting LOS pressure significantly.[31] Nitric oxide is the primary inhibitory neurotransmitter of the LOS: in murine models nitric oxide knockout increases resting LOS pressure and prevents the transient LOS relaxations (TLOSRs) required for swallowing[32] (**Fig. 12.2**). This inhibition may be further modified by the interstitial cells of Cajal.[33]

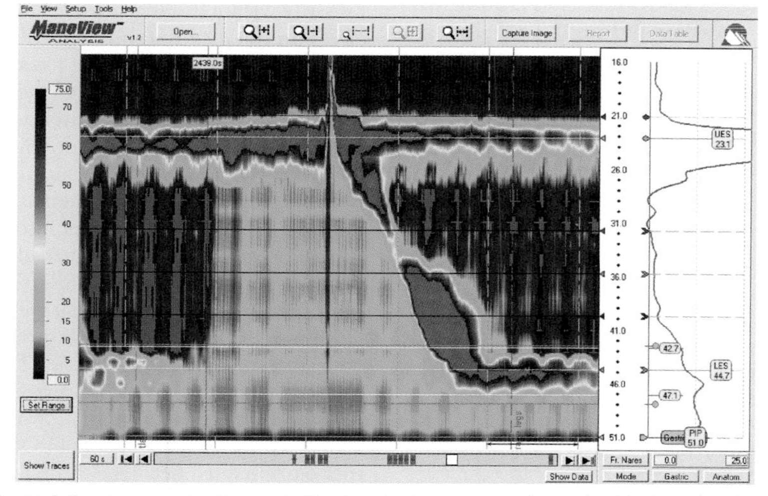

Figure 12.2 • High-resolution manometry demonstrating transient lower oesophageal sphincter relaxation (TLOSR). The upper oesophageal sphincter is demonstrated by the upper red and yellow zone, and the LOS by the lower red and yellow zone. On relaxation of the lower oesophageal sphincter a common cavity is created between the stomach and oesophagus – demonstrated by the light blue zone on the spatiotemporal plot (centre). These events are also observed on the axial pressure plot (right). The event is terminated and oesophagus cleared by primary peristalsis with intra-oesophageal pressure returning to baseline levels. Images acquired by 36-channel SSI Manoscan 360. Reproduced from Fox MR, Bredenoord AJ. Oesophageal high-resolution manometry: moving from research into clinical practice. Gut 2008; 57(3):405–23. With permission from BMJ Publishing Group Ltd.

LOS resting pressure varies physiologically, in particular reducing with meals.[34] It also reduces in response to pharyngeal tactile stimulation (in the absence of swallowing or peristalsis).[35] In control subjects, transient increases in intra-abdominal pressure (e.g. induced by straight leg raising, coughing and straining) are met with reflex increase in LOS pressure that is both greater and faster than the increase in gastric pressure.[36] This response is due in part to neuromuscular reflexes (vagally mediated) and transmitted pressure from the crus of the diaphragm. Similarly, protective increases in pressure occur in response to drops in intrathoracic pressure.[37]

TLOSRs are appropriate short-lived (usually less than 10 seconds) relaxations instigated by primary or secondary peristalsis, gastric distension and vomiting.[38,39] In asymptomatic controls, TLOSRs account for 94% of reflux episodes,[40] primarily occurring after meals and when upright rather than supine[34,41] (correlating with the distribution of asymptomatic physiological reflux episodes discussed above). Fifty per cent of TLOSRs result in reflux episodes.[40,42] Their genesis is incompletely understood, but seems to be a vagally mediated response to proximal gastric distension sensed by mechanoreceptors.[41,43] Fundoplication reduces the frequency of TLOSRs, potentially via reducing cardiac distensibility.[44,45] Manometrically, TLOSRs are similar to the belch reflex, and many reflux episodes follow belching,[46,47] suggesting that the former are aberrations of the latter. Pathological and physiological (swallow-induced) TLOSRs appear to be distinct, with pathological lasting longer (up to 45 seconds).[48]

In a small controlled study of patients with oesophagitis, pathological reflux was found to be due to three primary mechanisms: TLOSRs (65%), spontaneous reflux due to low resting LOS pressure (18%) and transient increased intra-abdominal pressure (17%).[40] However, the commonest mechanisms vary between individuals.

✔ Overall, pathological reflux is due to three primary mechanisms: TLOSRs (65%), a hypotensive LOS (18%) and transient increases in intra-abdominal pressure (17%).[40] However, these proportions vary widely within individuals.

Diaphragmatic sphincter

The slings of the right crus constitute a ‘pinchcock’ mechanism. In the absence of a hiatus hernia, it is difficult to separate the relative contributions of the diaphragmatic sphincter and LOS. In those with a surgically resected LOS, however, a basal high-pressure zone is detectable (oscillating in line with ventilation), suggesting that the diaphragmatic sphincter has a tonic component.[50] Such increases in high-pressure zone pressure with inspiration are abolished with curare in feline models, so as with the LOS the diaphragmatic sphincter seems to have both basal and reactive tonicity.[51] These increases in pressure are related to depth of inspiration[49] and are maximal during sleep (when the gastro-oesophageal pressure gradient is greatest).[52] Functionally, in the absence of a hiatus hernia, both LOS and diaphragmatic sphincter contribute to the high-pressure zone.[53] However, the mechanism of diaphragmatic sphincter relaxation differs neurochemically and functionally. Oesophageal distension (due to swallowing) triggers incomplete diaphragmatic sphincter relaxation, whereas TLOSRs cause complete relaxation.[54] As with the LOS, this relaxation is both central and local. Central control is mediated via vagal afferents modifying control of the diaphragm,[55] although this may be distal to the medulla in site.[56] Local control may be due to stretching of diaphragmatic sphincter fibres by contraction of longitudinal oesophageal fibres.[57] Variation in the distensibility of the diaphragmatic sphincter affects reflux; greater distensibility predisposes to more reflux episodes.[58]

Distal oesophageal compression

The abdominal oesophagus is exposed to positive pressure within the abdomen. This has a compressive effect on the distal oesophagus/LOS, with a shorter length correlating with more frequent reflux.[59] This is particularly important with increasing age and a recumbent position. The phreno-oesophageal ligament is a prolongation of abdominal fascia originating from the abdominal surface of the diaphragm, which anchors the oesophagus. As it approaches the oesophagus, it decussates into upper and lower leaves. The former inserts just above the squamocolumnar junction, with the latter inserting a few centimetres below, but is less well defined and often absent. The upper leaf inserts into the submucosa and intramuscular septae. This fibromuscular anchor is not absolute, allowing the oesophagus to slide 2 cm cranially when swallowing and, crucially, up to 4 cm during TLOSRs.[60,61] Whether the oesophagus herniates into the thorax under physiological conditions is unlikely, however, as the diaphragmatic hiatus moves almost as far cranially. This arrangement serves to keep the distal oesophagus within this positive pressure environment, ensuring that any increases in intra-abdominal pressure are transmitted to the LOS.[62] Anatomical variations in strength and height of insertion of the phreno-oesophageal ligament presumably influence the length of oesophagus to which this applies. Disruption of the ligament predisposes to sliding hiatus hernias, although the hernia sac will still envelop the LOS within the physiological (but not anatomical) abdomen.

Other mechanical barriers

The acute angle of the gastro-oesophageal junction may represent a partial barrier to reflux, functioning as a 'flap valve' (the cardio-oesophageal angle of His). This angle disappears after death, suggesting that the angle is maintained by tonic contraction of the oblique sling fibres of the cardia.[63] This 'valve' lies below the physiological high-pressure zone determined with radiological contrast, and so its contribution is therefore limited. The mucosal rosette of the gastro-oesophageal junction is also reported to act as a partial barrier.

Oesophageal mucosal acid defence mechanisms

The main defence mechanisms comprise oesophageal clearance and tissue resistance. Reflex peristalsis is induced by oesophageal acid receptors and aided by gravity, both of which are impaired, particularly during sleep.[64]

The oesophagus has a number of further protective mechanisms, both intrinsic and extrinsic, termed tissue resistance. These are such that continuous in vivo exposure of oesophageal epithelium to hydrochloric acid and pepsin does not cause damage for 1 hour.[65] Mechanisms are classed as pre-epithelial, epithelial and post-epithelial. Pre-epithelial resistance is conferred by the oesophageal buffer layer, augmented by saliva. In contrast to the gastroduodenal buffer layer, the (non-Barrett's) oesophageal epithelium lacks a mucous gel barrier and the ability to secrete bicarbonate. However, the buffer needs only to raise pH above 3 to prevent pepsin-induced damage.[66]

This buffer is augmented by the neutralising properties of saliva. Swallowing saliva contributes to approximately 5% of acid clearance by neutralising acid remaining after peristaltic clearance.[67] It has a pH of 7.02,[68] but the solubility of its mucins means that it cannot contribute permanently to the oesophageal buffer.[69] Consequently, when salivary production and primary oesophageal peristalsis cease at night, the oesophagus is particularly vulnerable.[70]

The epithelium itself possesses a combination of properties: a protective transmural electrochemical gradient, tight cell junctions, pH-dependent cation channels and intracellular buffers. Post-epithelial characteristics include adaptive perfusion and epithelial repair. For refluxed acid to cause epithelial cell death, hydrogen ions must enter the epithelial cytosol in sufficient quantities and for long enough to disrupt cytosol homeostasis and induce apoptosis/necrosis. One mechanism is transit of acid into the intercellular space, disrupting cell junctions and increasing permeability into the space, resulting in greater levels of acid. However, acid levels below that required to cause cellular damage may still be symptomatic. Nociceptors underlying heartburn can be found within the intercellular space within three cell layers of the oesophageal lumen,[71] thus helping to explain the existence of heartburn without frank oesophagitis. Quite why pain and oesophagitis may be independent is not clear. Potentially this represents visceral hypersensitivity,[72] or a reduction in acid sensitivity due to chronic reflux acid.[73]

Risk factors for reflux

The complexity of the body's control of swallowing and reflux means that there are numerous opportunities for disruption (and therefore pharmacological and surgical intervention). Pathological reflux is caused by excessive frequency of TLOSRs, inadequate high-pressure zone resting pressure, and inability of the LOS and diaphragmatic sphincter to compensate for increases in abdominal pressure. A number of factors have been implicated in these mechanisms (Table 12.1).

Inherited factors

A small number of studies have demonstrated the role of a positive family history. A parental history

Table 12.1 • Risk factors for GORD

Inherited	Demographic	Lifestyle	Medical	Structural
Family history	Increasing age (weak)	Smoking Alcohol Obesity	Comorbidities (gastrointestinal, cardiac, psychological) Gastric dysfunction Anticholisterases Negative *H. pylori* status	Hiatus hernia Oesophageal dysmotility

of GORD conferred an odds ratio (OR) of 1.5 in one study,[74] with an OR of 2.6 when symptoms are extended to that of an immediate relative.[75] In the latter study, no association was found with GORD prevalence between spouses, implying genetic effects to be greater than shared environmental effects (although this has been disputed).[76] Greater concordance has also been demonstrated between monozygotic than dizygotic twins.[74]

Demographic factors

No association between sex and GORD has been demonstrated. Findings assessing age have been equivocal; both European and US studies assessing symptomatology have found contradictory results. Overall, a marginally increased risk with increasing age seems likely (OR 1.1)[77] up to the age of 55, and possibly beyond.[78]

Lifestyle factors

Longitudinal studies show that smoking increases the risk of GORD (OR 1.1–2.6)[77,78] due to a chronic reduction in LOS pressure, combined with acute provocation of reflux (via coughing/deep inspiration). Particular foods and drinks are often felt to predispose to reflux episodes, although a Swedish case–control study of over 1000 subjects found no association between an extensive range of foodstuffs (including chocolate, coffee, onions and acidic fruits) and chronic symptoms of reflux (although the authors admit this may be due to avoidance in sufferers).[79] The study also found no correlation between portion size and eating late in the evening (albeit with the same caveat). Coffee is consistently cited as a factor, although one not demonstrated by additional studies.[74] Any underlying mechanism is believed to be due to caffeine-mediated inhibition of phosphodiesterase, inducing LOS relaxation.[80] Alcohol is generally agreed to lead to reflux – the US study above[78] found an OR of 1.8 between alcohol consumption and GORD. Again, this is thought to be via a reduction in LOS pressure, combined with direct irritation.[80]

Obesity has been repeatedy shown to correlate with GORD, with ORs between 1.3[78] and 2.8.[77] A meta-analysis of nine studies found an OR of 1.4 for a body mass index (BMI) of 25–30, and 1.9 for a BMI greater than 30.[81] Multiple mechanisms have been proposed: impaired LOS pressure, increased intra-abdominal pressure and delayed gastric emptying.[81] A combination of GORD and obesity is a potent risk factor for oesophageal adenocarcinoma.[82] The effect of weight loss on symptoms varies between studies, having been shown to improve symptoms[83] or have no effect.[84] Pregnancy induces progesterone-mediated LOS relaxation, in addition to increasing abdominal pressure.

Medical factors

GORD has been associated with a number of gastrointestinal and extragastrointestinal conditions, including irritable bowel syndrome, peptic ulceration, angina,[78] psychosomatic symptoms, anxiety and depression.[75,85] Anticholinergic medications increase risk (OR 1.5),[74] but non-steroidal anti-inflammatory drugs do not.

Gastric function can influence GORD via a number of mechanisms. Overall, *Helicobacter pylori* seems to protect against GORD and its complications, via atrophic gastritis.[86] A Japanese study found *H. pylori* to be present in 71% of controls, 30% of those with oesophagitis and almost 0% of those with Barrett's.[87] However, this relationship is not simple, and is dependent upon site of infection, extent and strain type. Indeed, antral infection induces acid hypersecretion and therefore may increase GORD. *Helicobacter pylori* eradication might therefore worsen GORD rates – however, associations with gastric carcinoma and ulceration are strong, and in practice eradication does not hamper treatment of oesophagitis with proton-pump inhibitors.[88] The hypersecretion of acid seen in Zollinger–Ellison syndrome is unsurprisingly associated with higher rates of GORD and oesophagitis;[89] however, supraphysiological levels of acid secretion in those with 'normal' GORD has not been demonstrated.[90] Delayed gastric emptying seems a plausible factor in GORD, and a recent study reported a prevalence of 26% in those with GORD.[91] The consequent distension hypothetically may induce more TLOSRs and acid secretion, although this is unproven.

Hiatus hernia

For the reasons outlined above, sliding hiatus hernia is a strong risk factor for GORD. A multicentric study found the endoscopic prevalence of hiatus hernia overall to be 5.8%, rising to 32% in those with oesophagitis. One radiological study of those with oesophagitis found a much higher rate of 90%.[92] Two-thirds of those with a hiatus hernia have GORD, and oesophagitis is more common.[93] The underlying mechanisms involve both an increase in duration and frequency of reflux episodes[94] (**Fig. 12.3**).

> ✔ Hiatus hernia is a strong risk factor for GORD, present in 32% of those with oesophagitis;[92] two-thirds of those with a hernia have GORD.[93]

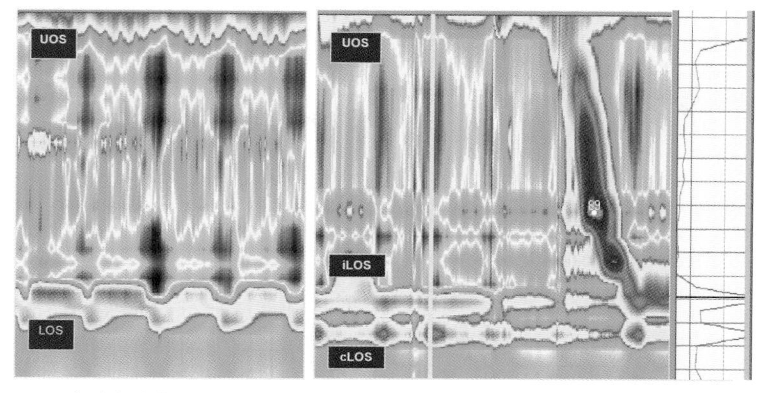

Figure 12.3 • High-resolution manometry showing a single high-pressure zone in the lower oesophagus crossing the diaphragm on the left (LOS). In this spatiotemporal plot higher pressures are presented in the yellow–red spectrum and lower pressures in the green–blue spectrum. On the right there is separation of the lower oesophageal high-pressure zone (iLOS) and the high-pressure zone created by the diaphragmatic crura (cLOS) suggestive of a transient hiatus hernia. The longitudinal red and yellow zone on the right demonstrates the propagation of a peristaltic wave down the oesophagus. LOS, lower oesophageal sphincter; cLOS, crural LOS; iLOS, intrinsic LOS; UOS, upper oesophageal sphincter. Reproduced from Fox MR, Bredenoord AJ. Oesophageal high-resolution manometry: moving from research into clinical practice. Gut 2008; 57(3):405–23. With permission from BMJ Publishing Group Ltd.

Oesophageal dysmotility and GORD: cause or effect?

Oesophageal dysmotility (as distinct from inappropriate TLOSR and low resting LOS) is a common finding in GORD. This exists in many guises, but predominantly that of hypomotility and ineffective peristalsis. It remains unclear whether dysmotility predisposes to GORD, whether GORD predisposes to dysmotility, or indeed to what extent dysmotility is responsible for symptoms.

As discussed above, peristaltic acid clearance is an integral component of the body's antireflux mechanism. Surrogate radiological and manometric simulation using barium fluoroscopy in one study demonstrated complete clearance with a single effective peristaltic wave greater than 20 mmHg.[94] In 1968, Booth et al.[95] described their standard acid clearance test, having demonstrated that those with GORD required more swallows to clear acid than controls. However, whilst subsequent studies have confirmed this, the utility of this test is very limited by both poor sensitivity and specificity[96] for assessing GORD. The potential role of reduced or delayed acid clearance in GORD as a function of dysmotility is plausible and supported by a number of studies. Pathological reflux episodes last longer than physiological episodes, and this has been suggested to be due to impaired acid clearance. Corroborating evidence by DeMeester et al.[97] expanded upon the different patterns of reflux seen between cases and controls. The former experienced longer nocturnal supine episodes, compared with the more physiological transient upright episodes in the latter. These nocturnal episodes are due to reduced peristaltic acid clearance,[97] both in terms of reduced frequency and probably quality of peristaltic waves,[98,99] compounded by a lack of gravitational clearance.[100] Elevating the head of the bed compensates partially, and improves both acid clearance and microscopic oesophagitis.[101]

> ✔ **Pathological reflux differs from physiological reflux. In the former, episodes are primarily supine or nocturnal and last longer. This is probably due in part to impaired acid clearance (both quality and quantity of protective peristalsis).[98–100]**

In one of the first such studies, Olsen and Schlegel[102] assessed motility in 50 subjects with oesophagitis, finding normal activity in 28%, incoordinated peristalsis in 32%, hypotensive peristalsis in 37% and complete motor failure in 8%. Progressively worse motility was seen with worsening degrees of oesophagitis. In a separate study, 48% of those with severe oesophagitis displayed peristaltic dysfunction.[103] A later study supported this, finding nonspecific dysmotility or aperistalsis in 64% of those with benign peptic stricutres, compared to 32% of those with non-stricturing GORD.[104]

It is highly relevant, of course, that oesophageal sensitivity to acid is often reduced,[1] and this combination of motor and sensory dysfunction may lead to particularly severe acid exposure, with resultant significant mucosal damage.[105] Abnormal motility has been found in 46% of those with Barrett's oesophagus, with a longer segment correlating with worse motility.[106] These findings have recently been corroborated in a 1000-patient (with proven GORD) study by Diener et al.[107] Peristalsis was normal in 56%, ineffective (hypotensive or incoordinated) in 21% and non-specifically abnormal in 23%. Those with ineffective peristalsis had worse symptoms, slower acid clearance and greater mucosal injury.

Whether this dysmotility with consequent delayed acid clearance is a primary phenomenon or occurs secondary to reflux-induced damage is unclear. Eriksen et al.,[108] using the solid bolus oesophageal egg transit test, compared the transit times of those with GORD and controls. Whilst delayed transit times correlated with the frequency of prolonged reflux episodes, no correlation was demonstrated between symptoms and oesophagitis and motility. The study authors argued that this dysmotility may be a primary phenomenon. Contradictory evidence exists in the form of improvements in oesophageal motility seen after antireflux surgery.[109] Other studies have found no such improvements, despite objective improvements in reflux, suggesting that either reflux-induced dysmotility may be permanent or it is a primary phenomenon.[110,111] Perhaps both may be true, with reflux-induced dysmotility perpetuating a vicious cycle of impaired peristalsis and LOS function.

Certainly, molecular mechanisms exist for this. Inflammation has been shown to impair both oesophageal motility and LOS function. Proinflammatory cytokines such as interleukin (IL)-1B, IL-6 and IL-8 have been shown to inhibit in vitro motility.[112] IL-1B induces prostaglandin E2 (PGE2)-mediated relaxation of the LOS,[113] and IL-6 induces PGE2- and platelet activating factor-mediated relaxation of the LOS.[114] Inflammation also increases nitric oxide and consequent inhibition of motility.[115]

✔ Dysmotility is common in GORD, present in 44%. Those with ineffective peristalsis have worse symptoms, acid clearance and mucosal damage.[107] As motility worsens, so does severity of oesophagitis and Barrett's.[103,105] What is not clear is whether dysmotility causes, results from or is synergistic with GORD.

Role of duodenogastric reflux

Whilst gastric acid (potentiated by pepsin) is the predominant source of inflammation and symptoms, the role of non-acidic duodenogastric reflux is not as clear cut. Observationally, oesophagitis is more common in those with both acid and duodenal reflux, compared with acid alone,[116] and duodenal reflux is more frequently seen in those with peptic strictures and Barrett's.[117] Bile acids contribute to the sequence of oesophagitis, metaplasia and dysplasia, and with progressively severe disease (from endoscopy-negative reflux, to simple oesophagitis, to peptic stricturing, and on to Barrett's metaplasia and finally dysplasia) so the relative proportion of bile acids in the refluxate increases.[118] Despite this, abolition of acid seems adequate to prevent progression.[119] Bile acids cause pain independently of acid,[120] but the two are probably synergistic, with biliary reflux the lesser culprit.[121,122] Duodenogastric reflux is difficult to assess, but can be detected using bilirubin as a surrogate (via spectrophotometry).[123] This topic is being further assessed by the use of impedance techniques.

✔ Duodenogastric reflux is synergistic with acid reflux, with increasing levels of bilious reflux correlating with worsening oesophagitis.[118] However, abolition of acid alone is usually adequate. With advances in impedance techniques, the role of duodenogastric reflux should be better delineated.

Investigation and diagnosis

The oesophagus is readily accessible, and so a large array of investigations have been developed. Flexible endoscopy and simple contrast radiology are widely available, with more specialist investigations such as physiology and manometry confined largely to tertiary centres, and yet more specialist techniques (such as aspiration studies) restricted to research.

Symptomatic diagnosis

Symptoms alone have limited utility. Whilst heartburn and regurgitation are typical symptoms and highly suggestive of GORD, their utility is limited by subjectivity and lack of evidence comparing them with investigations. One systematic review concluded that reflux symptoms had limited sensitivity (30–76%) and specificity (62–96%) in diagnosing oesophagitis.[119] One meta-analysis reported response of chest pain to proton-pump inhibitors to be suggestive of GORD, but significantly less specific (74%) and sensitive (80%) than 24-hour pH studies.[120] A number of standardised symptom questionnaires have been developed to aid diagnosis, but these are limited in terms of their diagnostic validity.[121] They may have a greater role to play in assessing and standardising functional end-points of treatment (particularly in clinical trials), such as the Reflux Questionnaire (ReQuest).[122]

Symptoms have limited diagnostic utility, with or without oesophagitis.[119] Symptomatic response to proton-pump inhibitors is more useful, but still significantly less specific (74%) and sensitive (80%) than 24-hour pH studies.[120]

Endoscopy

Flexible endoscopy is typically first line for investigation of oesophageal symptoms. The current UK National Institute for Health and Clinical Excellence (NICE) guidelines endorsed by the British Society of Gastroenterology suggest urgent endoscopy for patients of *any* age with dyspeptic symptoms plus any of: chronic gastrointestinal bleeding, progressive unintentional weight loss, progressive dysphagia, persistent vomiting, iron deficiency anaemia, epigastric mass or suspicious contrast swallow radiology. In those aged 55 years or more, unexplained and persistent dyspepsia alone mandates endoscopy.[121] In reality, endoscopy is used much more liberally. It allows diagnosis via inspection of the mucosa, and biopsy for histology, as well as various therapeutic interventions. Clues towards underlying dysmotility may be apparent, such as a dilated oesophagus, the presence of food residue and diverticula. Oesophagitis and Barrett's mucosa indicate reflux, but a subset of those with GORD will have normal endoscopies. Consequently, whilst the sensitivity and specificity of diagnosing mucosal lesions is high (and assessment of oesophagitis is reliable between observers),[122] those for diagnosing GORD are low relative to 24-hour pH monitoring. The roles of newer techniques (such as high-resolution, narrow-band and chromendoscopy) have yet to be determined.

Contrast radiology

Contrast radiology, whilst lacking the ability to biopsy and perform therapeutic procedures, has an important complementary role to endoscopy. A double-contrast barium swallow is highly sensitive at diagnosing significant complications of GORD (mucosal abnormalities such as strictures or malignancy).[123] It will also demonstrate associated anatomical abnormalities such as hiatus hernias and diverticula, and may give useful information as to motility via the presence and quality of peristalsis. In particular it may demonstrate the classical appearances of achalasia or diffuse oesophageal spasm ('corkscrew oesophagus'). However, the diagnostic ability of contrast radiology for GORD is limited; radiological features of finely nodular or granular mucosa may be visualised, or frank reflux may occur during the study. One review found radiological evidence of reflux in just 35% of symptomatic patients.[124] One study (*n* = 112) compared barium swallow to 24-hour pH monitoring, concluding that just 30% of those with pH monitoring-diagnosed GORD had radiological abnormalities.[125] This poor sensitivity may be somewhat improved by provocative manoeuvres (such as the water siphon test).

Contrast radiology has a limited role in diagnosing GORD, with abnormal studies in just 35% of those with symptoms[124] and 30% of those with pH.[125] However, it is much more sensitive for structural complications of GORD and may demonstrate alternate diagnoses such as achalasia.[123]

pH studies

Since the original description in 1969 by Spencer, advances in nasogastric pH catheters, portable digital recorders and computer software have allowed 24-hour ambulatory pH studies to become widely available. Of great importance is the ability of the patient to mark symptoms by pressing a button, allowing correlation of symptoms with reflux episodes (**Fig. 12.4**). Computer analysis of the resultant data generates multiple variables, which are then compared to those of controls (Table 12.1). Indications for 24-hour pH monitoring include refractory typical symptoms, assessment of atypical symptoms and suspected motility disorders (as pH studies are usually combined with manometry), and as such are a prerequesite when considering anti-reflux surgery.[124]

Positioning of the pH probe 5 cm above the top of the LOS is crucial. Too low and the probe will dip into the stomach on swallowing, too high and reflux will be underestimated. As distance from nose to LOS is variable, manometry is required to determine location. When the probe registers a pH less than 4, it records a reflux episode lasting usually until the pH rises above 5 (or 4 in some laboratories). One limitation is that a prolonged reflux episode may be a single episode (implying poor clearance) or multiple overlapping transient episodes. In the case of doubt (e.g. whether the probe is too low and generating a falsely positive reading), a second probe can be positioned cranially to the first. Multiple probes may also be placed higher to assess more proximal symptoms (such as chronic cough).

Twenty-four-hour studies are considered the gold standard, although there is some evidence that shorter studies may be representative and better tolerated.[126] Antireflux medications are usually stopped to increase

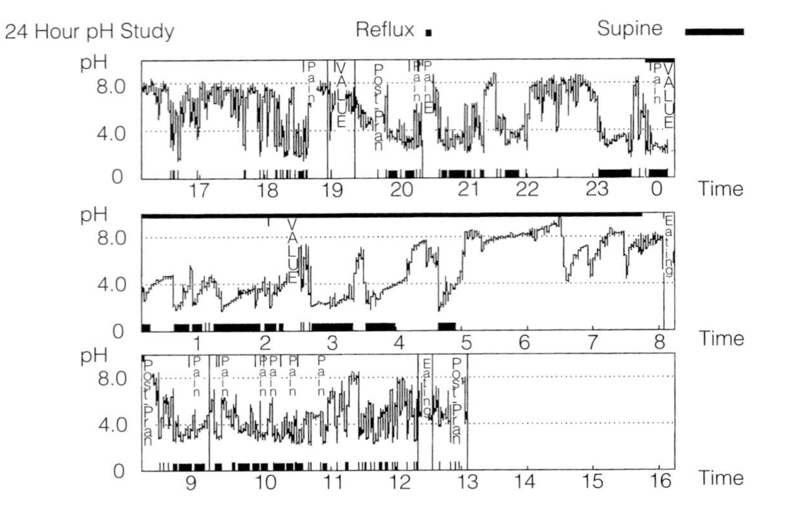

Figure 12.4 • A 24-hour pH study showing excessive acid reflux in a patient with Barrett's oesophagus. Note the correlation of the patient's pain with acid in the oesophagus.

Table 12.2 • Findings of pH study conducted on patient illustrated in Fig. 12.4

	Total	Upright	Supine	Eating	Postprandial	Fasting
Duration (h)	20:48	12:50	7:58	0:55	2:30	0:00
No. of reflux episodes	123	106	17	1	19	–
Time below pH 4.0 (min)	426:34	228:19	198:15	0:03	53:17	–
Time below pH 4.0 (%)	34.1	29.6	41.4	0.1	35.5	–
No. of episodes >5 min	24	15	9	0	4	–
Longest reflux (min)	42:27	27:15	42:27	0:03	12:16	–

Table 12.3 • Scores according to Johnson and DeMeester for pH <4 for findings in Table 12.1 (study of patient illustrated in Fig. 12.4)

Component	Patient value	Normal values	Score
Total time (%)	34.1	4.45	24.96
Upright time (%)	29.6	8.42	12.64
Supine time (%)	41.4	3.45	41.77
No. of episodes	123	46.90	9.08
No. >5 min	24	3.45	20.62
Longest episode	42:27	19.80	5.54
Composite score			**114.61**
A normal composite score is <14.72			

diagnostic yield,[127] although performing the test whilst on treatment may be useful in assessing refractory symptoms. Patients should take a normal diet, but complete a food and drink diary to allow elimination of acidic foodstuffs from the analysis.

Parameters generated include the number of reflux episodes, those that are prolonged beyond 5 minutes and the total reflux time (expressed as a percentage of the study time). This should be less than 5% of a 24-hour period.[128] These parameters can be subdivided into periods, such as when supine or upright. These may then be used to generate composite scores with reference to controls. The most commonly used is the DeMeester score. This combines the parameters in Tables 12.2 and 12.3 (number of episodes, number over 5 minutes and longest episode, with total reflux, upright and supine times (weighted towards supine)).[129] A normal value is <14.72.

However, the presence of increased reflux and symptoms does not prove causality as the mere presence of acid in the oesophagus often correlates poorly with symptoms and inflammation. Correlation of episodes with symptoms is therefore central to diagnosis. A patient with both an abnormal study and symptoms does not necessarily have GORD if these symptoms occur in the absence of a reflux episode. In contrast, the patient with a normal study but typical symptoms coinciding with proven reflux episodes may well have GORD. This is further complicated by the controversy regarding performing studies on or off medical treatment. An abnormal pH study off treatment implies reflux, yet if treatment does not improve symptoms, the relevance of this reflux is questionable. To this end, three symptom-reflux values are usually generated (with a reflux episode generally considered to cause symptoms if occurring in the preceding 2 minutes).

Symptom Index (SI) is the proportion of symptoms relating to reflux:

$$\text{SI} = (\text{Number of reflux - related symptom episodes / Total symptom episodes}) \times 100$$

An SI of 50% or more is usually considered to be positive, although with the caveats that it does not take account of the frequency or severity of symptoms. Consequently, in those with frequent reflux episodes or infrequent symptoms these may coincide with symptoms purely by chance.[130] Despite this, a positive SI has been demonstrated to correlate with greatest improvement with proton-pump inhibitor acid suppression.[131]

The **Symptom Sensitivity Index (SSI)** takes into account the number of reflux episodes:

$$\text{SSI} = (\text{Number of reflux - related symptom episodes / Number of reflux episodes}) \times 100$$

An SSI ≥10% is considered positive, and strengthening evidence of GORD.

The **Symptom Association Probability (SAP)** was introduced by Weuston and colleagues, and represents a more complex probability calculation. This aims to calculate the probability that the association of reflux and symptoms is not due to chance. This is performed by generating a 2 × 2 contingency table analysing each 2-minute segment of the study period. An SAP >95% represents a P value <0.05 and so is considered positive. Whilst the caveat of probability should not be forgotten, it has been shown to have (limited) success in predicting successful response to both proton-pump inhibitors[132] and antireflux surgery.[133]

The **Ghillebert Probability Estimate (GPE)** was similarly developed to assess the probability of symptoms occurring by chance. It uses a binomial formula, inputting the number of symptom episodes, the number occurring within 2 minutes of demonstrated reflux, and the individual probability of an episode of pain coinciding with reflux.[134]

The concordance of SI, SAP and GPE was assessed in a recent study of 772 subjects. SAP and GPE were extremely concordant, with major discordance in 2.8%. GPE underestimated symptom association, whereas SAP overestimated. This discordance increased with greater frequency of symptoms and total reflux time. Similarly, SI became discordant with SAP when symptoms were less frequent than two or greater than 18. The authors concluded that SAP and GPE were interchangable.[130] Taghavi et al.,[132] using 50% reduction in heartburn with proton-pump inhibitor treatment as an end-point, calculated positive predictive vaules of SI (73%), SSI (81%) and SAP (79%). The imperfect diagnostic and predictive characteristics of these indices reinforce the need to interpret pH studies within the context of symptoms, endoscopic and radiological findings, manometry and any response to acid suppression. This is especially so when considering surgical intervention.

✔ Twenty-four-hour pH studies are the traditional gold standard of diagnosis,[135] although their sensitivity and specificity are imperfect, as are derivative symptom-reflux values. Consequently, it remains crucial to interpret them within their clinical, endoscopic and manometric contexts; this is particularly so when considering antireflux surgery.

Wireless pH monitoring

A major drawback to catheter-based pH studies is the catheter; this may preclude testing in the 5–10% who are intolerant,[73] or inhibit the ability to eat or function normally in the remainder (due to discomfort or social embarrassment), possibly causing a false-negative test. Wireless capsule-based systems have been designed to avoid this. The second major drawback is reproducibility; significant day-to-day variation occurs (up to the order of 3.2),[136] with overall reproducibility of 70–80%.[137]

The Bravo® pH system (Medtronic, Minneapolis, MN, USA) is a wireless capsule system that may avoid both disadvantages (**Fig. 12.5**). It consists of a 26 mm × 6 mm capsule with an antimony electrode and radiofrequency transmitter, which is placed endoscopically 6 cm above the z-line (the high pressure zone being 1–1.5 cm above the squamocolumnar junction). Data are transmitted to a recorder attached to the patient's belt. It is better tolerated than

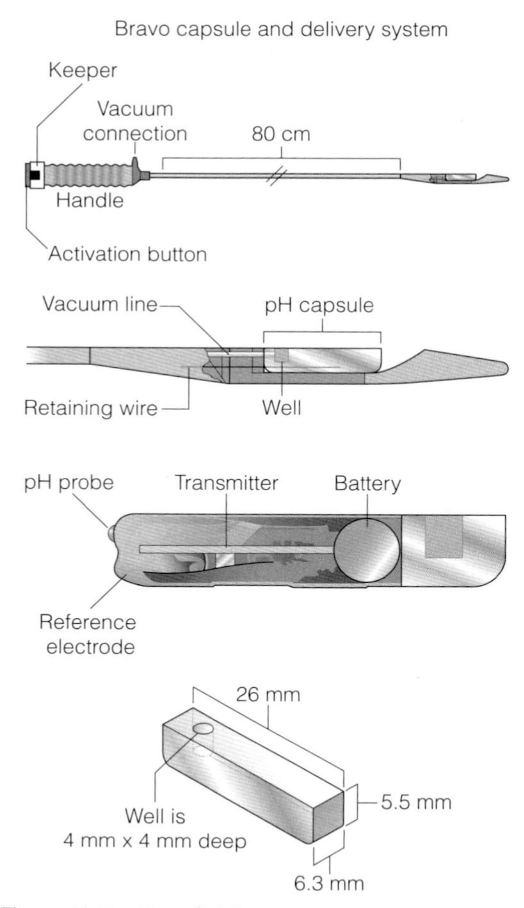

Figure 12.5 • Bravo® delivery system and capsule. The delivery system is inserted in the same way as a nasogastric tube, although it is usually delivered orally. Markings on the side depict the distance from the incisors. The capsule is deployed 6 cm above the anatomical z-line (or 5 cm above the proximal LOS high-pressure zone). The delivery system is then retracted and the receiver is synchronised. It remains attached to the patient (via belt clip or shoulder pouch) for 48 hours at least. Capsules all fall off inevitably within 10 days (usually 5–7). Complications requiring early removal are almost unheard of. Reprinted by permission from Macmillan Publishers Ltd: Pandolfino JE, Richter JE, Ours T et al. Ambulatory oesophageal pH monitoring using a wireless system. Am J Gastroenterol 2003; 98 (4):740–9, copyright 2003.

conventional catheter-based studies[138] and allows prolonged measurement (up to 96 hours), which may be particularly useful in those with intermittent symptoms.[139] One study found the Bravo® system to under-record acid exposure, although it concluded that this did not affect sensitivity provided it was allowed for.[140] It has a particularly useful role in those intolerant of a catheter (and as such is recommended by NICE for this subgroup;[141] the largest study to date successfully used the Bravo® system in 129 of 134 (96%) patients who failed a catheter system.[142] The authors also reported less oropharyngeal discomfort, dysphagia and chest pain.

There are a number of disadvantages, however. Foremost is that of cost. A very small minority develop pain on implantation of the capsule, requiring removal. Furthermore, one small study reported that 25% of patients experienced significant hypercontractillity on placement of the capsule, leading to chest pain in six of 40.[143]

Oesophageal impedance monitoring

Multichannel intraluminal impedance (MII) was described by Silny in 1991[144] and represents a novel direction in monitoring of refluxate. Impedance is the opposite of current flow, measured by detecting resistance to alternating current. This allows detection and differentiation of gas and liquid reflux (irrespective of pH). Paired electrodes are placed in the oesophageal lumen, separated by a non-conducting catheter (**Fig. 12.6**). The circuit is completed by ions within the oesophageal mucosa and lumen, the availability of which varies with luminal content.

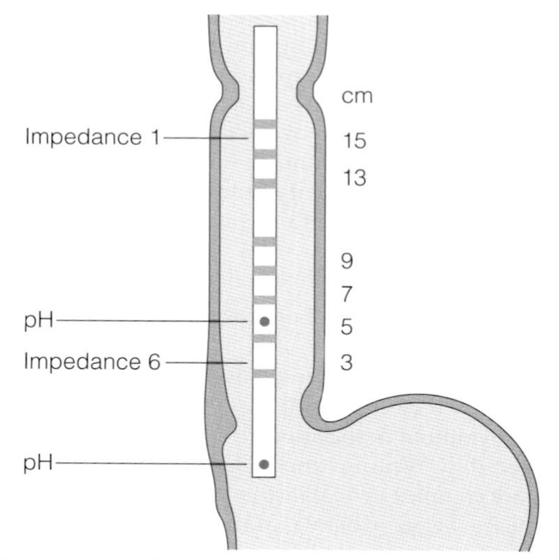

Figure 12.6 • Example of impedance catheter. This one has six impedance sensors and two pH sensors. Reprinted by permission from Macmillan Publishers Ltd: Sifrim D, Blondeau K. Technology insight: the role of impedance testing for esophageal disorders. Nat Clin Pract Gastroenterol Hepatol 2006; 3(4):210–9, copyright 2006.

When empty, ionic conduction is relatively stable. The presence of liquid (either swallowed or refluxing), with its greater ionic concentration, improves conduction and therefore impedance drops. Conversely, the presence of air reduces conduction and increases impedance. Impedance for both returns to baseline when the refluxate has been cleared. Multiple electrodes along the catheter determine the direction of flow. Sensitivity is high, and boluses of just 1 mL can be detected.[145]

MII can therefore determine the following:

- whether the bolus is swallowed or refluxed;
- how long it takes to be swallowed or cleared;
- the velocity of transit;
- whether the bolus is liquid or gas;
- how proximally reflux extends;
- whether superimposed episodes of reflux occur (re-reflux).

Importantly, MII cannot determine the volume of refluxate.

The combination of MII and pH monitoring is easily achieved with a nasogastric catheter. MII–pH can be used to characterise the following for reflux episodes:

- nature (i.e. gas, liquid or mixed);
- acidity (acidic, weakly acidic or weakly alkaline);
- height (of reflux episode);
- the presence of a bolus;
- acid clearance;
- superimposed reflux.

This more comprehensive assessment allows a more sensitive approach to reflux, correlating symptoms beyond the somewhat arbitrary threshold of a pH of 4 for reflux.[146] This is important for both gastroduodenal reflux and postprandial reflux (which may be non-acidic yet still symptomatic). It also allows consideration of the role of disturbances of bolus transport in oesophageal symptoms. It is reproducible[147] and, consequently, MII–pH represents the most sensitive investigation for GORD, potentially increasing the detection of pathological reflux by a factor of four[148,149] and improving symptom correlation by 10–20%.[150] It has a particularly useful role in investigating the troublesome subgroup increasingly referred to surgeons: those with symptoms despite acid suppression. This group are often considered not to have GORD as determined by conventional pH studies, yet may be shown to have symptoms correlating with non-acidic or weakly acidic reflux.[151] Consequently, a negative MII–pH study is a more discriminatory tool in the selection of patients who will benefit from antireflux surgery.[148]

✔ The combination of multichannel intraluminal impedance and pH monitoring is the most powerful diagnostic test for GORD, although it is not readily available. It is up to 400% more sensitive than pH studies alone,[148,149] with 10–20% greater symptom correlation.[150]

Manometry

Oesophageal manometry is the gold standard of assessment tools for motor function. Whilst there are no diagnostic criteria for GORD, manometry has a number of important functions. The role of dysmotility in GORD has been discussed, but it is important to exclude those with reflux-type symptoms due to a formal dysmotility disorder (in whom treatment will be entirely different). The typical example is achalasia; oesophageal stasis, with bacterial fermentation and production of lactic acid, may cause heartburn, odynophagia and volume reflux indistinguishable from GORD. However, fundoplication will be disastrous. Manometry allows the position of the high-pressure zone to be determined, and therefore accurate placement of pH catheters. It also allows detection of those with GORD and major defects in peristalsis, which may impair surgical outcomes.

Standard static manometry

This measures a number of parameters. Multiple pressure sensors can be used to map and characterise peristalsis, and determine the resting and functional pressures of the oesophageal sphincters. Consequently, circumferential contraction, peristaltic wave duration and velocity can be determined. Normal peristaltic sequences (as previously discussed) consist of upper and lower oesophageal sphincter relaxation, followed by segmental contraction of adjacent oesophageal body segments, coordinated to give a smooth peristaltic wave. Contractions typically last for up to 6 seconds (in individual segments) and can reach pressures of 180 mmHg distally, with an overall velocity of 5 cm/s.[151]

There are two major options available: intraluminal solid-state transducers versus water-perfused assemblies connected to external transducers. Ultimately both are roughly equivalent, with the exceptions of pharyngeal pressures (best assessed with solid-state transducers), the ability to use larger numbers of recording points (perfused systems) and better assessment of the LOS (sleeve-perfused systems). Perhaps most significantly, perfused systems are cheaper.

Measurements are taken using a manometry catheter, with multiple measurement ports. This is passed nasogastrically, then withdrawn from the stomach via the LOS, with the multiple ports used to estimate resting sphincter pressure and length. The ports are then positioned within the oesophageal body (with at least three placed 5 cm apart, although typically five to eight are used). Motility is then assessed using the standard 10 wet swallow test, with amplitudes, coordination and velocity compared to control values. Abnormal contractions (either simultaneous or non-peristaltic) can also be characterised. Water-perfused systems can be combined with a sleeve device that straddles the LOS, to allow for axial movement of the sphincter.

Clearly, this limited assessment has a number of caveats. Firstly, measuring just 10 of the approximately 1000–2000 peristaltic swallows occurring per day means that intermittent or subtle dysmotility may be missed. Secondly, the experimental conditions are different to those of normal swallows; small-volume water swallows may not trigger symptoms occurring during normal activity. This is particularly true of GORD (with often postprandial symptoms triggered by physical activity or position). Thirdly, anatomical resolution is limited: focal anatomical or physiological abnormalities may lie between measurement ports and be missed. In addition, the presence of a hiatus hernia may distort the position of the LOS and affect its measurement. However, the availability and cost-effectiveness of standard manometry is such that it is the commonest investigation used in assessing motility.[152] Although diagnosis may be limited to characteristic disorders such as achalasia and diffuse oesophageal spasm (with the rest characterised as inneffective or non-specific dysmotility), this may be adequate for the purposes of GORD assessment.

High-resolution manometry (HRM)

To circumvent some of these limitations, Clouse and Staiano developed HRM.[153,154] A larger number of more closely spaced ports has become possible with the development of both micromanometric solid-state and perfused transducers. Up to 36 pressure sensors can be used to generate a three-dimensional representation, combining time, position and amplitude with greatly increased spatial resolution. This can be represented as a two-dimensional plot, with pressure represented with a colour spectrum (**Fig. 12.7** and **12.8**), and allows better characterisation of peristalsis.[152] This has three specific advantages within the assessment of GORD: firstly, associated or causative dysmotility can be better defined; secondly, acid clearance can be better predicted; and thirdly the LOS can be better assessed (in both function and

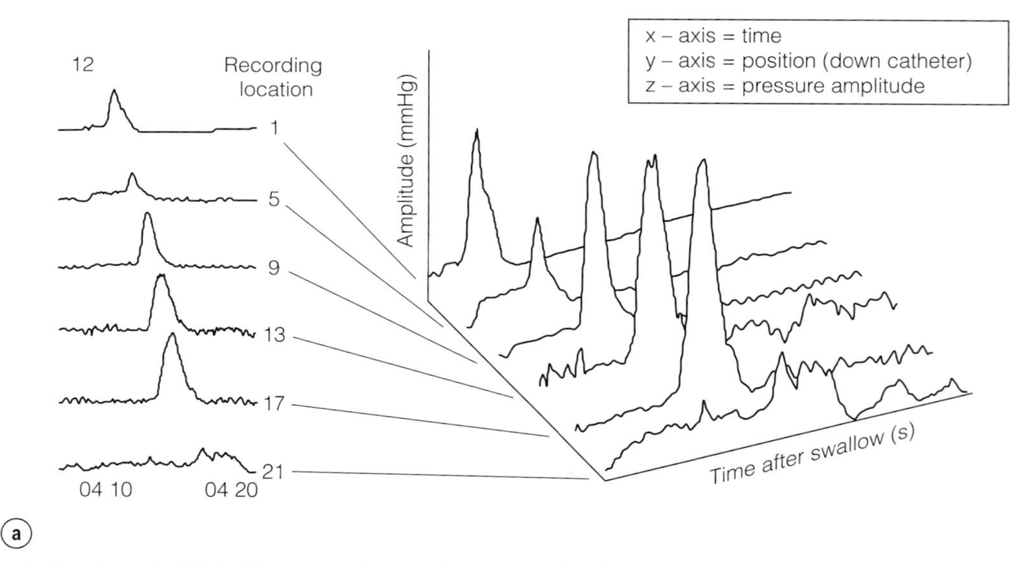

Figure 12.7 • (a) Early 1990s (Clouse and Staiano), foundations of HRM laid: time, catheter position and average pressure were reconstructed into pseudo-3-D 'topographic plots' that demonstrated the functional anatomy of the oesophagus. **(b)** Topographic display of normal oesophageal pressure data. The pseudo-3-D surface plot displays the characteristic peaks and troughs of the peristaltic pressure wave proceeding from the proximal oesophagus (background), until it merges with the LOS after contraction (foreground). The contour plot of the same swallow superimposed at the top of the figure demonstrates how 3-D data are represented using concentric rings at 10-mmHg intervals to indicate increasing amplitudes. Reproduced from Clouse RE, Staiano A, Bickston SJ et al. Characteristics of the propagating pressure wave in the oesophagus. Dig Dis Sci 1996; 41(12):2369–76. Used with permission from the American Physiological Society.

(Continued)

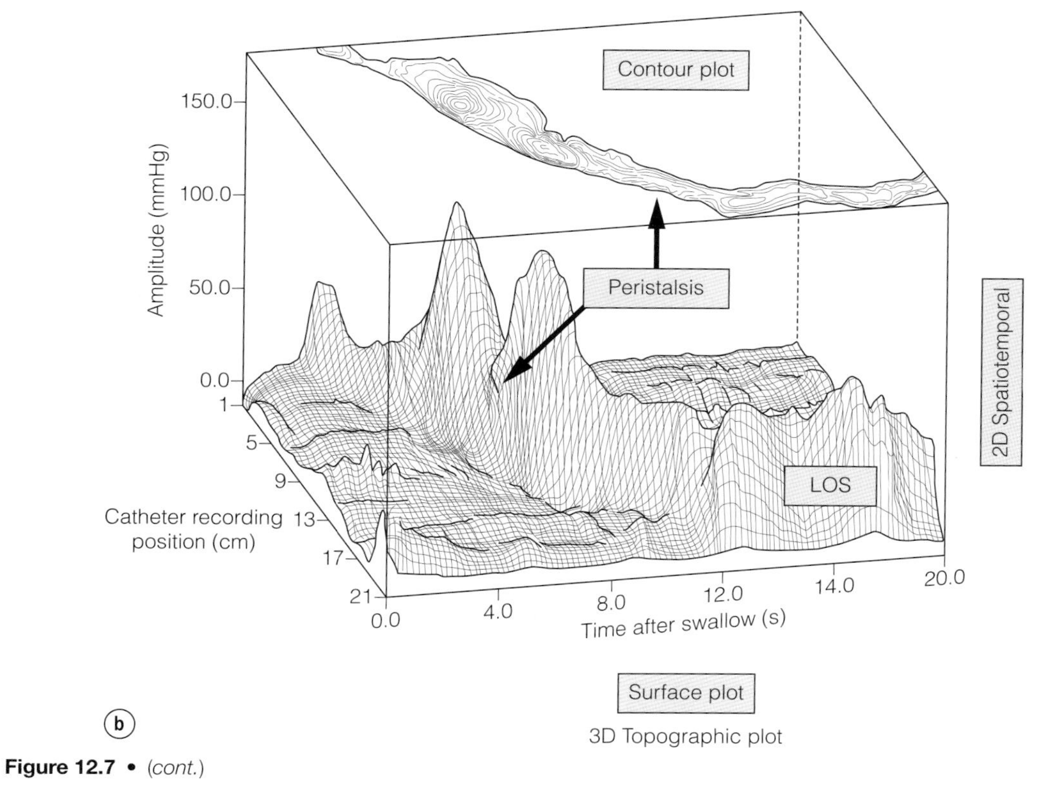

(b)

Figure 12.7 • *(cont.)*

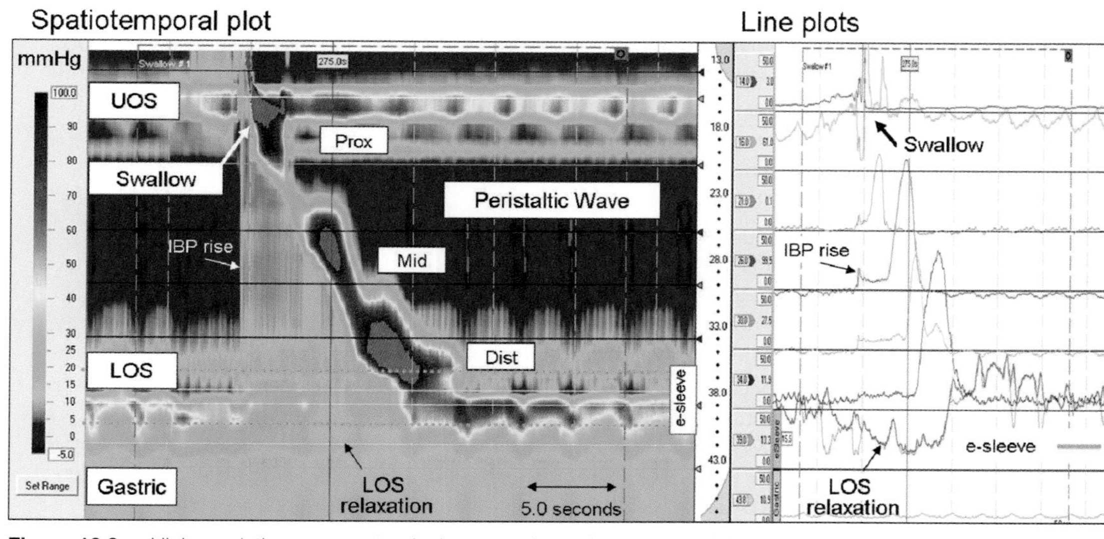

Figure 12.8 • High-resolution manometry depicts oesophageal pressure activity from the pharynx to the stomach via pressure sensors spaced at <2 cm intervals apart. Recordings can be analysed and presented either as line plots (similar to conventional manometry) or spatiotemporal plots. The spatiotemporal plot presents the same information as the line plots. Time is on the *x*-axis, distance from the nares is on the *y*-axis and pressure amplitude on the *z*-axis (each pressure is assigned a colour (legend left)). The segmental functional anatomy of the oesophagus is clearly demonstrated. The synchronous relaxation of the upper oesophageal sphincter (UOS) and LOS (deglutitive inhibition) is obvious, as is the increasing pressure and duration of the peristaltic wave as it passes distally. The virtual 'e-sleeve' application provides a summary measurement of LOS pressure and relaxation (bold brown line plot). Similar to a conventional sleeve sensor, the maximum pressure over a 6-cm distance is displayed. Images acquired by 36-channel SSI Manoscan 360. Reproduced from Fox MR, Bredenoord AJ. Oesophageal high-resolution manometry: moving from research into clinical practice. Gut 2008; 57(3):405–23. With permission from BMJ Publishing Group Ltd.

anatomy; Table 12.4).[152] A sophisticated development is that of the 'e-sleeve'. This is a software emulation of the sleeve device of standard pull-through manometry. This allows better characterisation of the LOS and also more rapid positioning of the catheter array. Furthermore, HRM can be used more easily to assess the dynamics of more frequent liquid swallows, and also solids, which may improve the sensitivity of GORD assessment (by being more physiologically representative and challenging).[153–155] Manometry can be combined with MII to provide a valuable functional perspective.[156]

Table 12.4 • Comparison between standard and high-resolution manometry

	Conventional pull-through manometry	Conventional sleeve manometry	High-resolution manometry
Costs	Inexpensive	Inexpensive	Expensive
Execution	Relatively elaborate and time consuming	Relatively elaborate and time consuming	Relatively simple and fast
Interpretation	Requires experience	Requires experience	Relatively easy
Measuring LOS function and relaxation	Limited	Yes	Yes
Measuring UOS function and relaxation	No	Limited	Yes

LOS, lower oesophageal sphincter; UOS, upper oesophageal sphincter.
Reproduced from Fox MR, Bredenoord AJ. Oesophageal high-resolution manometry: moving from research into clinical practice. Gut 2008; 57(3):405–23. With permission from BMJ Publishing Group Ltd.

Key points

- The oesophagus is a sophisticated peristaltic tube, protected by a sphincter at either end.
- The high-pressure zone of the lower oesophagus is formed from the LOS and diaphragmatic sphincter, and regulated by a complicated interplay of local and central, and myo- and neurogenic factors.
- Reflux occurs due to permutations of aberrant transient LOS relaxation (TLOSR), low resting LOS pressure and increases in gastric pressure.
- Oesophageal acid clearance is important in limiting both the symptoms and damage of reflux, and is a function of dysmotility.
- The role of dysmotility (as cause, effect or innocent bystander) in GORD remains controversial.
- The combination of motor and sensory dysfunction may lead to particularly severe acid exposure and significant mucosal damage.
- Endoscopy has an important role in excluding cancer, detecting Barrett's metaplasia, and assessing oesophagitis and hiatus hernia.
- Contrast swallows are less sensitive, although they provide greater clues as to function and motility.
- Twenty-four-hour ambulatory pH studies are currently the gold standard test for diagnosis of GORD, although may be superseded by combination impedance studies. Wireless pH monitoring is in the early stages of use, but seems to increase diagnostic reproducibility and sensitivity, although it is expensive and requires endoscopy.
- The total acid reflux time is the most reproducible and useful single measurement. pH measured 5 cm above the LOS should be less than 4 for less than 5% of the time measured.
- The DeMeester score is the most commonly used validated score for assessing GORD. It takes into account the number and duration of reflux episodes in both supine and upright positions. A normal score is ≤14.72.
- Symptom–reflux association is crucial to both making a diagnosis and considering surgery; the most commonly used indices are:
  - Symptom Index (SI);
  - Symptom Sensitivity Index (SSI);
  - Symptom Association Probability (SAP).

- Standard manometry is a static test of oesophageal motility (peristaltic coordination, amplitude and velocity) and LOS function, routinely combined with 24-hour pH studies. It is useful in assessing associated dysmotility and excluding major dysmotility disorders masquerading clinically as GORD.
- High-resolution manometry uses multiple pressure sensors to map oesophageal and LOS functional anatomy in much greater detail, and to generate three-dimensional representations of motility. It allows much more detailed assessment of motility (including within the context of GORD).
- Multichannel intraluminal impedance (MII) uses electrical impedance (via a nasogastric catheter) to detect non or weakly acidic reflux. It is particularly useful in those with symptoms despite maximal medical therapy, in assessing acid clearance in those with dysmotility, and in assessing duodenogastric reflux. It can be combined with 24-hour pH studies and manometry, and as such represents the most sensitive test available for GORD.

References

1. Fox M, Forgacs I. Gastro-oesophageal reflux disease. Br Med J 2006;332(7533):88–93.
2. Lagergren J, Bergstrom R, Lindgren A, et al. Symptomatic gastroesophageal reflux as a risk factor for oesophageal adenocarcinoma. N Engl J Med 1999;340(11):825–31.
3. Johnson LF, DeMeester TR. Twenty-four-hour pH monitoring of the distal oesophagus. A quantitative measure of gastroesophageal reflux. Am J Gastroenterol 1974;62(4):325–32.
4. Dent J, Dodds WJ, Friedman RH, et al. Mechanism of gastroesophageal reflux in recumbent asymptomatic human subjects. J Clin Invest 1980;65(2):256–67.
5. Ness-Jensen E, Lindam A, Lagergren J, et al. Changes in prevalence, incidence and spontaneous loss of gastro-oesophageal reflux symptoms: a prospective population-based cohort study, the HUNT study. Gut 2012;61(10):1390–7.
6. Dent J, El-Serag HB, Wallander MA, et al. Epidemiology of gastro-oesophageal reflux disease: a systematic review. Gut 2005;54(5):710–7.
7. Voutilainen M, Sipponen P, Mecklin JP, et al. Gastroesophageal reflux disease: prevalence, clinical, endoscopic and histopathological findings in 1,128 consecutive patients referred for endoscopy due to dyspeptic and reflux symptoms. Digestion 2000;61(1):6–13.
8. Johansson KE, Ask P, Boeryd B, et al. Oesophagitis, signs of reflux, and gastric acid secretion in patients with symptoms of gastro-oesophageal reflux disease. Scand J Gastroenterol 1986;21(7):837–47.
9. Fuchs KH, DeMeester TR, Albertucci M. Specificity and sensitivity of objective diagnosis of gastroesophageal reflux disease. Surgery 1987;102(4):575–80.
10. Sloan S, Rademaker AW, Kahrilas PJ. Determinants of gastroesophageal junction incompetence: hiatal hernia, lower oesophageal sphincter, or both. Ann Intern Med 1992;117(12):977–82.
11. Fitzgerald RC, Onwuegbusi BA, Bajaj-Elliott M, et al. Diversity in the oesophageal phenotypic response to gastro-oesophageal relux: immunological determinants. Gut 2002;50(4):451–9.
12. Vela MF, Camacho-Lobato L, Srinivasan R, et al. Simultaneous intraesophageal impedance and pH measurement of acid and nonacid gastroesophageal reflux: effect of omeprazole. Gastroenterology 2001;120(7):1599–606.
13. Rex DK, Cummings OW, Shaw M, et al. Screening for Barrett's esophagus in colonoscopy patients with and without heartburn. Gastroenterology 2003;125(6):1670–7.
14. Dodds WJ, Stewart ET, Hodges D, et al. Movement of the feline esophagus associated with respiration and peristalsis. An evaluation using tantalum markers. J Clin Invest 1973;52(1):1–13.
15. Castell D. Anatomy and physiology of the oesophagus and its sphincters. In: Castell DO, Richter JE, Dalton CB, editors. Esophageal motility testing. New York: Elsevier Science; 1987. p. 13–27.
16. Clouse RE, Staiano A, Bickston SJ, et al. Characteristics of the propagating pressure wave in the esophagus. Dig Dis Sci 1996;41(12):2369–76.
17. Sugarbaker DJ, Rattan S, Goyal RK. Mechanical and electrical activity of oesophageal smooth muscle during peristalsis. Am J Physiol 1984;246(2, Pt 1):G145–50.
18. Sugarbaker DJ, Rattan S, Goyal RK. Swallowing induces sequential activation of esophageal longitudinal smooth muscle. Am J Physiol 1984;247(5, Pt 1):G515–9.
19. Pouderoux P, Lin S, Kahrilas PJ. Timing, propogation, coordination, and effect of esophageal shortening during peristalsis. Gastroenterology 1997;112(4):1147–54.
20. Bhall V, Liu J, Puckett JL, et al. Symptom hypersensitivity to acid infusion is associated with hypersensitivity of esophageal contracility. Am J Physiol Gastrointest Liver Physiol 2004;287(1):G65–71.

21. Pal A, Brasseur JG. The mechanical advantage of local longitudinal shortening on peristaltic transport. J Biomech Eng 2002;124(1):94–100.
22. Winship DH, Viegas de Andrade SR, Zboralske FF. Influence of bolus temperature on human oesophageal motor function. J Clin Invest 1970;49(2):243–50.
23. Gidda JS, Goyal RK. Regional gradient of local inhibition and refractoriness in esophageal smooth muscle. Gastroenterology 1985;89(4):843–51.
24. Crist J, Gidda JS, Goyal RK. Intramural mechanism of esophageal peristalsis: roles of cholinergic and noncholinergic nerves. Proc Natl Acad Sci U S A 1984;81(11):3595–9.
25. Meyer GW, Gerhardt DC, Castell DO. Human esophageal response to rapid swallowing: muscle refractory period or neural inhibition? Am J Physiol 1981;241:G129–36.
26. Higgs B, Shorter RG, Ellis H. A study of the anatomy of the human esophagus with special reference to the gatroesophageal sphincter. J Surg Res 1965;5(11):503–7.
27. Liebermann-Meffert D. What anatomic structures are undoubtedly responsible for gastroesophageal competence. Gastroenterology 1979;76:31–9.
28. Bemelman W, Van Der Hulst V, Dijkhuis T, et al. The lower oesophageal sphincter shown by a computerized representation. Scand J Gastroenterol 1990;25:601–8.
29. Rossiter CD, Norman WP, Jain M, et al. Control of the lower esophageal sphincter pressure by two sites in dorsal motor nucleus of the vagus. Am J Physiol 1990;259(6, Pt 1):G899–906.
30. Gonella J, Niel JP, Roman C. Vagal control of lower oesophageal sphincter motility in the cat. J Physiol 1977;273(3):647–64.
31. Rattan S, Goyal RK. Neural control of the lower oesophageal sphincter: influence of the vagus nerves. J Clin Invest 1974;54(4):899–906.
32. Mashimo H, He XD, Huang PL, et al. Neuronal constructive nitric oxide synthetase is involved in murine enteric inhibitory neurotransmission. J Clin Invest 1996;98(1):3–13.
33. Ward SM, Morris G, Reese L, et al. Interstitial cells of Cajal mediate enteric inhibitory neurotransmission in the lower esophageal and pyloric sphincters. Gastroenterology 1998;115(2):314–29.
34. Dent J, Dodds WJ, Friedman RH, et al. Mechanism of gastroesophageal reflux in recumbent asymptomatic human subjects. J Clin Invest 1980;65(2):256–67.
35. Dodds WJ, Dent J, Hogan WJ, et al. Effect of atropine on esophageal motor function in humans. Am J Physiol 1981;240(4):G290–6.
36. Mittal RK, Fisher M, McCallum RW, et al. Human lower esophageal sphincter pressure response to increased intra-abdominal pressure. Am J Physiol 1990;258(4, Pt 1):G624–30.
37. Mittal RK, Rochester DF, McCallum RW. Electrical and mechanical activity in the human lower esophageal sphincter during diaphragmatic contraction. J Clin Invest 1988;81(4):1182–9.
38. Dent J. A new technique for continuous sphincter pressure measurement. Gastroenterology 1976;71(2):263–7.
39. Mittal RK, McCallum RW. Characteristics of transient lower oesophageal sphincter relaxation in humans. Am J Physiol 1987;252(5, Pt 1):G636–41.
40. Dodds WJ, Dent J, Hogan WJ, et al. Mechanisms of gastroesophageal reflux in patients with reflux esophagitis. N Engl J Med 1982;307(25):1547–52.
41. Wyman JB, Dent J, Heddle R, et al. Control of belching by the lower oesophageal sphincter. Gut 1990;31(6):639–46.
42. Dent J, Holloway RH, Toouli J, et al. Mechanisms of lower oesophageal sphincter incompetence in patients with symptomatic gastrooesophageal reflux. Gut 1988;29(8):1020–8.
43. Penagini R, Carmagnola S, Cantu P, et al. Mechanoreceptors of the proximal stomach: role in triggering transient lower oesophageal sphincter relaxation. Gastroenterology 2004;126(1):49–56.
44. Ireland AC, Holloway RH, Toouli J, et al. Mechanisms underlying the antireflux action of fundoplication. Gut 1993;34(3):303–8.
45. Scheffer RC, Akkermans LM, Bais JE, et al. Elicitation of transient lower oesophageal sphincter relaxations in response to gastric distension and meal ingestion. Neurogastroenterol Motil 2002;14(6):647–55.
46. Barham CP, Gotley DC, Mills A, et al. Precipitating causes of acid reflux episodes in ambulant patients with gastro-oesophageal reflux disease. Gut 1995;36(4):505–10.
47. Barham CP, Gotley DC, Miller R, et al. Pressure events surrounding oesophageal acid reflux episodes and acid clearance in ambulant healthy volunteers. Gut 1993;34(4):444–9.
48. Holloway RH, Penagini R, Ireland AC. Criteria for objective definition of transient lower esophageal sphincter relaxation. Am J Physiol 1995;268(1, Pt 1):G128–33.
49. Welch RW, Gray JE. Influence of respiration on recordings of lower oesophageal sphincter pressure in humans. Gastroenterology 1982;83(3):590–594.
50. Klein WA, Parkman HP, Dempsey DT, et al. Sphincterlike thoracoabdominal high pressure zone after esophagogastrectomy. Gastroenterology 1993;105(5):1362–9.
51. Boyle JT, Altschuler SM, Nixon TE, et al. Role of the diaphragm in the genesis of lower esophageal sphincter pressure in the cat. Gastroenterology 1985;88(3):723–30.
52. Mittal RK, Rochester DF, McCallum RW. Effect of the diaphragmatic contraction on lower oesophageal sphincter pressure in man. Gut 1987;28(12):1564–8.

53. Kaye M, Showater J. Manometric configuration of the lower oesophageal sphincter in normal human subjects. Gastroenterology 1971;61:213–23.
54. Mittal RK, Holloway RH, Penagini R, et al. Transient lower esophageal sphincter relaxation. Gastroenterology 1995;109(2):601–10.
55. Altschuler SM, Boyle JT, Nixon TE, et al. Simultaneous reflex inhibition of lower esophageal sphincter and crural diaphragm in cats. Am J Physiol 1985;249(5, Pt 1):G586–91.
56. Oyer LM, Knuth SL, Ward DK, et al. Patterns of neural and muscular electrical activity in the costal and crural portions of the diaphragm. J Appl Physiol 1989;66:2092–100.
57. Liu J, Puckett JL, Takeda T, et al. Crural diaphragm inhibition during esophageal distension correlates with contraction of the esophageal longitudinal muscle in cats. Am J Physiol 2005;288:G927–32.
58. Pandolfino JE, Shi G, Trueworthy B, et al. Esophagogastric junction opening during relaxation distinguishes nonhernia reflux patients, hernia patients, and normal subjects. Gastroenterology 2003;125(4):1018–24.
59. Joelsson BE, DeMeester TR, Skinner DB, et al. The role of the oesophageal body in the antireflux mechanism. Surgery 1982;92(2):417–24.
60. Edmundowicz SA, Clouse RE. Shortening of the esophagus in response to swallowing. Am J Physiol 1991;260(3, Pt 1):G512–6.
61. Shi G, Pandolfino JE, Joehl RJ, et al. Distinct patterns of oesophageal shortening during primary peristalsis, secondary peristalsis and transient lower oesophageal sphincter relaxation. Neurogastroenterol Motil 2002;14(5):505–12.
62. De Caestecker J, Heading R. The pathophysiology of reflux. In: Hennessy TPJ, Cuschieri A, Bennett JR, editors. Reflux oesophagitis. London: Butterworth; 1989. p. 1–36.
63. Atkinson M, Summerling M. The competence of the cardia after cardiomyotomy. Gastroenterologia 1954;92:123–34.
64. Madsen T, Wallin L, Boesby S, et al. Oesophageal peristalsis in normal subjects. Influence of pH and volume during imitated gastro-oesophageal reflux. Scand J Gastroenterol 1983;18(4):513–8.
65. Salo JA, Lehto VP, Kivilaakso E. Morphological alterations in experimental esophagitis. Light microscopic and scanning and transmission electron microscopic study. Dig Dis Sci 1983;28(5):440–8.
66. Tobey NA, Hosseini SS, Caymaz-Bor C, et al. The role of pepsin in acid injury to esophageal epithelium. Am J Gastroenterol 2001;96(11):3062–70.
67. Helm JF, Dodds WJ, Pelc LR, et al. Effect of oesophageal emptying and saliva on clearance of acid from the oesophagus. N Engl J Med 1984;310(5):284–8.
68. Helm JF, Dodds WJ, Hogan WJ, et al. Acid neutralizing capacity of human saliva. Gastroenterology 1982;83(1, Pt 1):69–74.
69. Arul GS, Moorghen M, Myerscough N, et al. Mucin gene expression in Barrett's oesophagus: an in situ hybridisation and immunohistochemical study. Gut 2000;47(6):753–61.
70. Lichter I, Muir RC. The pattern of swallowing during sleep. Electroenceph Clin Neurophysiol 1975;38(4):427–32.
71. Rodrigo J, Hernández CJ, Vidal MA, et al. Vegetative innervation of the esophagus. III. Intraepithelial endings. Acta Anat (Basel) 1975;92(2):242–58.
72. Mehta AJ, De Caestecker JS, Camm AJ, et al. Sensitization to painful distention and abnormal sensory perception in the esophagus. Gastroenterology 1995;108(2):311–9.
73. Lee J, Anggiansah A, Anggiansah R, et al. Effects of age on the gastroesophageal junction, oesophageal motility, and reflux disease. Clin Gastroenterol Hepatol 2007;5(12):1392–8.
74. Mohammed I, Cherkas LF, Riley SA, et al. Genetic influences in gastro-oesophageal reflux disease: a twin study. Gut 2003;52(8):1085–9.
75. Locke 3rd GR, Talley NJ, Fett SL, et al. Risk factors associated with symptoms of gastroesophageal reflux. Am J Med 1999;106(6):642–9.
76. Diaz-Rubio M, Moreno-Elola-Olaso C, Rey E, et al. Symptoms of gastro-oesophageal reflux: prevalence, severity, duration and associated factors in a Spanish population. Aliment Pharmacol Ther 2004;19(1):95–105.
77. Kotzan J, Wade W, Yu HH, et al. Assessing NSAID prescription use as a predisposing factor for gastroesophageal reflux disease in a Medicaid population. Pharm Res 2001;18(9):1367–72.
78. Ruigómez A, García Rodríguez LA, Wallander MA, et al. Natural history of gastro-oesophageal reflux disease diagnosed in general practice. Aliment Pharmacol Ther 2004;20(7):751–60.
79. Kahrilas PJ, Gupta RR. Mechanisms of acid reflux associated with cigarette smoking. Gut 1990;31(1):4–10.
80. Castell DO. Diet and the lower esophageal sphincter. Am J Clin Nutr 1975;28:1296–8.
81. Hampel H, Abraham NS, El-Serag HB. Meta-analysis: Obesity and the risk for gastroesophageal reflux disease and its complications. Ann Intern Med 2005;143(3):199–211.
82. Whiteman DC, Sadeghi S, Pandeya N, et al. Combined effects of obesity, acid reflux and smoking on the risk of adenocarcinomas of the oesophagus. Gut 2008;57(2):173–80.
83. Fraser-Moodie CA, Norton B, Gornall C, et al. Weight loss has an independent beneficial effect on symptoms of gastro-oesophageal reflux in

patients who are overweight. Scand J Gastroenterol 1999;34(4):337–40.

84. Kjellin A, Ramel S, Rossner S, et al. Gastroesophageal reflux in obese patients is not reduced by weight reduction. Scand J Gastroenterol 1996;31:1047–51.

85. Hu WH, Wong WM, Lam CL, et al. Anxiety but not depression determines health care-seeking behaviour in Chinese patients with dyspepsia and irritable bowel syndrome: a population-based study. Aliment Pharmacol Ther 2002;16(12):2081–8.

86. Vicari JJ, Peek RM, Falk GW, et al. The seroprevalence of cagA-positive *Helicobacter pylori* strains in the spectrum of gastroesophageal reflux disease. Gastroenterology 1998;115(1):50–7.

87. Abe Y, Ohara S, Koike T, et al. The prevalence of *Helicobacter pylori* infection and the status of gastric acid secretion in patients with Barrett's esophagus in Japan. Am J Gastroenterol 2004;99(7):1213–21.

88. Muramatsu A, Azuma T, Okajima T, et al. Evaluation of treatment for gastro-oesophageal reflux disease with a proton pump inhibitor, and relationship between gastro-oesophageal reflux disease and *Helicobacter pylori* infection in Japan. Aliment Pharmacol Ther 2004;20(Suppl. 1):102–6.

89. Miller LS, Vinayek R, Frucht H, et al. Reflux esophagitis in patients with Zollinger–Ellison syndrome. Gastroenterology 1990;98(2):341–6.

90. Hirschowitz BI. A critical analysis, with appropriate controls, of gastric acid and pepsin secretion in clinical esophagitis. Gastroenterology 1991;101(5):1149–58.

91. Buckles DC, Sarosiek I, McMillin C, et al. Delayed gastric emptying in gastroesophageal reflux disease: reassessment with new methods and symptomatic correlations. Am J Med Sci 2004;327:1–4.

92. Baldi F, Ferrarini F, Labate A, et al. Prevalence of esophagitis in patients undergoing routine upper endoscopy: a multicenter survey in Italy. In: DeMeester TR, Skinner DB, editors. Esophageal disorders: pathophysiology and therapy. New York: Raven Press; 1985. p. 213–9.

93. Savas N, Dagli U, Sahin B. The effect of hiatal hernia on gastroesophageal reflux disease and influence on proximal and distal esophageal reflux. Dig Dis Sci 2008;53(9):2380–6.

94. Kahrilas PJ, Dodds WJ, Hogan WJ. Effect of peristaltic dysfunction on oesophageal volume clearance. Gastroenterology 1988;94(1):73–80.

95. Booth DJ, Kemmerer WT, Skinner DB. Acid clearing from the distal oesophagus. Arch Surg 1968;96(5):731–4.

96. Barham CP, Gotley DC, Mills A, et al. Oesophageal acid clearance in patients with severe reflux oesophagitis. Br J Surg 1995;82(3):333–7.

97. DeMeester TR, Johnson LF, Joseph GJ, et al. Patterns of gastroesophageal reflux in health and disease. Ann Surg 1976;184(4):459–70.

98. Lichter I, Muir RC. The pattern of swallowing during sleep. Electroenceph Clin Neurophysiol 1975;38(4):427–32.

99. Orr WC, Robinson MG, Johnson LF. Acid clearance during sleep in the pathogenesis of reflux esophagitis. Dig Dis Sci 1981;26(5):423–7.

100. Kjellen G, Tibbling L. Influence of body position, dry and water swallows, smoking, and alcohol on oesophageal acid clearing. Scand J Gastroenterol 1978;13(3):283–8.

101. Johnson LF, DeMeester TR. Evaluation of elevation of the head of the bed, bethanechol, and antacid form tablets on gastroesophageal reflux. Dig Dis Sci 1981;26(8):673–80.

102. Olsen AM, Schlegel JF. Motility disturbances caused by esophagitis. J Thorac Cardiovasc Surg 1965;50(5):607–12.

103. Kahrilas PJ, Dodds WJ, Hogan WJ, et al. Esophageal peristaltic dysfunction in peptic esophagitis. Gastroenterology 1986;91(4):897–904.

104. Ahtaridis G, Snape Jr WJ, Cohen S. Clinical and manometric findings in benign peptic strictures of the oesophagus. Dig Dis Sci 1979;24(11):858–61.

105. Jones MP, Sloan SS, Jovanovic B, et al. Impaired egress rather than increased access: an important independent predictor of erosive oesophagitis. Neurogastroenterol Motil 2002;14(6):625–31.

106. Shah AK, Wolfsen HC, Hemminger LL, et al. Changes in oesophageal motility after porfimer sodium photodynamic therapy for Barrett's dysplasia and mucosal carcinoma. Dis Esophagus 2006;19(5):335–9.

107. Diener U, Patti MG, Molena D, et al. Esophageal dysmotility and gastroesophageal reflux disease. J Gastrointest Surg 2001;5(3):260–5.

108. Eriksen CA, Sadek SA, Cranford C, et al. Reflux oesophagitis and oesophageal transit: evidence for a primary oesophageal motor disorder. Gut 1988;29(4):448–52.

109. Escandell AO, De Haro LFM, Paricio PP, et al. Surgery improves defective oesophageal peristalsis in patients with gastro-oesophageal reflux. Br J Surg 1991;78:1095–7.

110. Eckardt VF. Does healing of esophagitis improve oesophageal motor function. Dig Dis Sci 1988;33(2):161–5.

111. Baldi F, Ferrarini F, Longanesi A, et al. Oesophageal function before, during, and after healing of erosive oesophagitis. Gut 1988;29(2):157–60.

112. Reider F, Cheng L, Harnett KM, et al. Gastroesophageal reflux disease-associated esophagitis induces endogenous cytokine production leading to motor abnormalities. Gastroenterology 2007;132:154–65.

113. Cheng L, Cao W, Behar J, et al. Inflammation induced changes in arachidonic acid metabolism in cat LES circular muscle. Am J Physiol Gastrointest Liver Physiol 2005;288:G787–97.
114. Eastwood GL, Beck BD, Castell DO, et al. Beneficial effect of indomethacin on acid-induced esophagitis in cats. Dig Dis Sci 1981;26(7):601–8.
115. Tomita R, Tanjoh K, Fujisaki S, et al. Physiological studies on nitric oxide in the lower esophageal sphincter of patients with reflux esophagitis. Hepatogastroenterology 2003;50(49):110–4.
116. Vaezi MF, Richter JE. Contribution of acid and duodenogastro-oesophageal reflux to oesophageal mucosal injury and symptoms in partial gastrectomy patients. Gut 1997;41(3):297–302.
117. Stein HJ, Barlow AP, DeMeester TR, et al. Complications of gastroesophageal reflux disease: role of the lower esophageal sphincter, esophageal acid/alkaline exposure and duodenogastric reflux. Ann Surg 1992;216:35–43.
118. Nehra D, Howell P, Williams CP, et al. Toxic bile acids in gastro-oesophageal reflux disease: influence of gastric acidity. Gut 1999;44(5):598–602.
119. Moayyedi P, Talley NJ, Fennerty MB, et al. Can the clinical history distinguish between organic and functional dyspepsia? JAMA 2006;295(13):1566–76.
120. Cremonini F, Wise J, Moayyedi P, et al. Diagnostic and therapeutic use of proton pump inhibitors in non-cardiac chest pain: a metaanalysis. Am J Gastroenterol 2005;100(6):1226–32.
121. NICE. Dyspepsia: Management of dyspepsia in adults in primary care. London, UK: National Institute for Health and Clinical Excellence; 2004.
122. Lundell LR, Dent J, Bennett JR, et al. Endoscopic assessment of oesophagitis: clinical and functional correlates and further validation of the Los Angeles classification. Gut 1999;45(2):172–80.
123. Levine MS, Chu P, Furth EE, et al. Carcinoma of the esophagus and esophagogastric junction: sensitivity of radiographic diagnosis. Am J Roentgenol 1997;168(6):1423–6.
124. Ott DJ. Gastroesophageal reflux: what is the role of barium studies? Am J Roentgenol 1994;162(3):627–9.
125. Chen MY, Ott DJ, Sinclair JW, et al. Gastroesophageal reflux disease: correlation of esophageal pH testing and radiographic findings. Radiology 1992;185(2):483–6.
126. Dobhan R, Castell DO. Prolonged intraesophageal pH monitoring with 16-hr overnight recording. Comparison with "24-hr" analysis. Dig Dis Sci 1992;37(6):857–64.
127. Kushnir VM, Sayuk GS, Gyawali CP. The effect of antisecretory therapy and study duration on ambulatory esophageal pH monitoring. Dig Dis Sci 2011;56(5):1412–9.
128. Bodger K, Trudgill N. Guidelines for oesophageal manometry and pH monitoring. BSG Guidelines in Gastroenterology; 2006. p. 1–11.
129. Johnson LF, DeMeester TR. Twenty-four-hour pH monitoring of the distal oesophagus. A quantitative measure of gastroesophageal reflux. Am J Gastroenterol 1974;62(4):325–32.
130. Kushnir VM, Sathyamurthy A, Drapekin J, et al. Assessment of concordance of symptom reflux association tests in ambulatory pH monitoring. Aliment Pharmacol Ther 2012;Mar 20. Epub ahead of print.
131. Watson RG, Tham TC, Johnston BT, et al. Double blind cross-over placebo controlled study of omeprazole in the treatment of patients with reflux symptoms and physiological levels of acid reflux – the "sensitive oesophagus". Gut 1997;40(5):587–90.
132. Taghavi SA, Ghasedi M, Saberi-Firoozi M, et al. Symptom association probability and symptom sensitivity index: preferable but still suboptimal predictors of response to high dose omeprazole. Gut 2005;54(8):1067–71.
133. Diaz S, Aymerich R, Clouse R, et al. The symptom association probability (SAP) is superior to the symptom index (SI) for attributing symptoms to gastroesophageal reflux: validation using outcome from laparoscopic antireflux surgery (LARS). Gastroenterology 2002;122:A75.
134. Ghillebert G, Janssens J, Vantrappen G, et al. Ambulatory 24 hour intraoesophageal pH and pressure recordings v provocation tests in the diagnosis of chest pain of oesophageal origin. Gut 1990;31(7):738–44.
135. Gotley D, Cooper M. The investigation of gastrooesophageal reflux. Surg Res Commun 1987;2:1–17.
136. Wiener GJ, Morgan TM, Copper JB, et al. Ambulatory 24-hour oesophageal pH monitoring. Reproducibility and variability of pH parameters. Dig Dis Sci 1988;33(9):1127–33.
137. Bredenoord AJ, Weusten BL, Smout AJ. Symptom association analysis in ambulatory gastrooesophageal reflux monitoring. Gut 2005;54(12):1810–7.
138. Pandolfino JE, Richter JE, Ours T, et al. Ambulatory oesophageal pH monitoring using a wireless system. Am J Gastroenterol 2003;98(4):740–9.
139. Scarpulla G, Camilleri S, Galante P, et al. The impact of prolonged pH measurements on the diagnosis of gastroesophageal reflux disease: 4-day wireless pH studies. Am J Gastroenterol 2007;102(12):2642–7.
140. des Varannes SB, Mion F, Ducrotté P, et al. Simultaneous recordings of oesophageal acid exposure with conventional pH monitoring and a wireless system (Bravo). Gut 2005;54(12):1682–6.
141. NICE. Catheterless Oesophageal pH Monitoring. National Institute for Health and Clinical Excellence; July 2006.

142. Sweis R, Fox M, Anggiansah R, et al. Patient acceptance and clinical impact of Bravo monitoring in patients with previous failed catheter-based studies. Aliment Pharmacol Ther 2009;29(6):669–76.

143. Tharavej C, Hagen JA, Portale G, et al. Bravo capsule induction of esophageal hypercontractility and chest pain. Surg Endosc 2006;20(5):783–6.

144. Silny J. Intraluminal multiple electric impedance procedure for measurement of gastrointestinal motility. J Gastrointest Motil 1991;3:151–62.

145. Srinivasan R, Vela MF, Katz PO, et al. Esophageal function testing using multichannel intraluminal impedance. Am J Physiol Gastrointest Liver Physiol 2001;280(3):G457–62.

146. Sifrim D, Castell D, Dent J, et al. Gastro-oesophageal reflux monitoring: review and consensus report on detection and definitions of acid, non-acid, and gas reflux. Gut 2004;53(7):1024–31.

147. Bredenoord AJ. Impedance–pH monitoring: new standard for measuring gastro-oesophageal reflux. Neurogastroenterol Motil 2008;20(5):434–9.

148. Mainie I, Tutuian R, Agrawal A, et al. Combined multichannel intraluminal impedance–pH monitoring to select patients with persistent gastro-oesophageal reflux for laparoscopic Nissen fundoplication. Br J Surg 2006;93(12):1483–7.

149. Shay S, Richter J. Direct comparison of impedance, manometry, and pH probe in detecting reflux before and after a meal. Dig Dis Sci 2005;50(9):1584–90.

150. Bredenoord AJ, Weusten BL, Curvers WL, et al. Determinants of perception of heartburn and regurgitation. Gut 2006;55(3):313–8.

151. Anggiansah A, Marshal R. Use of the oesophageal laboratory. 1st ed. Oxford: Isis Medical Media; 2000.

152. Fox M, Hebbard G, Janiak P, et al. High-resolution manometry predicts the success of oesophageal bolus transport and identifies clinically important abnormalities not detected by conventional manometry. Neurogastroenterol Motil 2004;16(5):533–42.

153. Fox MR, Bredenoord AJ. Oesophageal high-resolution manometry: moving from research into clinical practice. Gut 2008;57(3):405–23.

154. Fox M. Multiple rapid swallowing in idiopathic achalasia: from conventional to high resolution manometry. Neurogastroenterol Motil 2007;19(9):780–1;author reply 782.

155. Fox M, Young A, Anggiansah R, et al. A 22 year old man with persistent regurgitation and vomiting: case outcome. Br Med J 2006;333(7559):133–7.

156. Tutuian R, Vela MF, Balaji NS, et al. Esophageal function testing with combined multichannel intraluminal impedance and manometry: multicenter study in healthy volunteers. Clin Gastroenterol Hepatol 2003;1(3):174–82.

13

Treatment of gastro-oesophageal reflux disease

David I. Watson

Introduction

Gastro-oesophageal reflux disease (GORD) is common, affecting between 10% and 40% of the population of most Western countries.[1,2] It is difficult to establish if the incidence of GORD is increasing but it is certainly the case that more and more patients are being treated for reflux. This is reflected in a dramatic rise in the overall cost of medical therapy for GORD in many countries over recent decades. In addition, the incidence of distal oesophageal adenocarcinoma is increasing,[3] which provides circumstantial evidence that complications of gastro-oesophageal reflux, such as the development of Barrett's oesophagus, are also increasing.

GORD is caused by excessive reflux of gastric contents, which contain acid and sometimes bile and pancreatic secretions, into the oesophageal lumen. Pathological reflux leads to heartburn, upper abdominal pain and the regurgitation of gastric contents into the oropharynx. A multifactorial aetiology is most likely. Hiatus herniation is associated with reflux in approximately half of the patients who undergo surgical treatment.[4,5] This results in widening of the angle of His, effacement of the lower oesophageal sphincter and loss of the assistance of positive intra-abdominal pressure acting on the lower oesophagus. Reduced lower oesophageal sphincter pressure is also often found. In patients with normal resting lower oesophageal sphincter pressure, reflux may result from an excessive number of transient lower oesophageal sphincter relaxation events.[6] Other factors that might contribute to reflux are abnormal oesophageal peristalsis (which causes poor clearance of refluxed fluid) and delayed gastric emptying.

The treatment of reflux is incremental, commencing with medical measures, surgery being reserved for patients with more severe disease who either fail to respond adequately to medical treatment or who do not wish to take lifelong medication. In basic terms, medical therapy treats the effects of reflux, as the underlying reflux problem is not corrected, and treatment is usually continued indefinitely.[7] In contrast, surgery aims to be curative, preventing reflux by reconstructing an antireflux valve at the gastro-oesophageal junction.[6,8] In the past, surgery was reserved for patients with complicated reflux disease or those with very severe symptoms. However, since the introduction of laparoscopic surgical approaches some surgeons advocate utilising surgery at earlier stages in the course of reflux disease. Endoscopic (transoral) antireflux procedures have also been developed, although the outcomes following these treatments have been disappointing.

Medical treatment

Simple measures

Simple measures can be helpful for the management of patients who experience mild symptoms. These include antacids, avoiding precipitating factors, e.g. spicy foods and alcohol, weight loss (when appropriate), avoiding cigarette smoking, modification of the timing and quantity of meals (e.g. not going to bed with a full stomach), and raising the bed head.

Unfortunately, these measures are rarely effective for patients with moderate to severe disease, and most patients who present for surgery cannot be adequately treated with these measures.

H_2-receptor antagonists

When first used in the 1970s, histamine type 2 (H_2)-receptor antagonists, which reduce the production of gastric acid, revolutionised the medical approach to duodenal ulcer disease. However, they were less effective for reflux disease and although they sometimes relieve mild to moderate reflux symptoms, few patients achieve complete relief of symptoms.[9] With the current widespread availability of proton-pump inhibitors, H_2-receptor antagonists are now rarely used as first-line medical therapy.

Proton-pump inhibitors

Proton-pump inhibitors (omeprazole, lanzoprazole, pantoprazole, rabeprazole and esomeprazole) were introduced into clinical practice in the late 1980s.[7] Proton-pump inhibitors are much more effective at symptom relief and achieve better healing of oesophagitis than H_2-receptor antagonists. However, in patients with severe oesophagitis (Savary Miller grade 2/3) there is a high treatment failure rate,[10] and many patients who initially achieve good symptom control develop 'breakthrough' symptoms at a later date, requiring an increased dose of medication to maintain symptom control. Failure may be due to inadequate acid suppression, although in some cases bile or duodenal refluxate may play a role. In patients who respond well to proton-pump inhibitors, symptoms usually recur rapidly (sometimes in less than 24 hours) following cessation of medication, and for this reason lifelong medical treatment is likely to be required.[7] The long-term use of proton-pump inhibitors appears generally safe. One study has shown, however, that long-term use can be associated with the development of atrophic gastritis with intestinal metaplasia in patients with concurrent *Helicobacter pylori* infection.[11] Long-term use can also be associated with parietal cell hyperplasia.[12] This latter phenomenon may be the reason why symptoms recur rapidly in some patients on cessation of therapy, and may be another reason why some patients require escalating dosages of proton-pump inhibitors to control their symptoms.

Prokinetic agents

Cisapride is the only prokinetic agent that has been shown to be better than placebo for the treatment of reflux.[13] It acts by improving acid clearance from the distal oesophagus by accelerating gastric emptying. Its therapeutic benefit is similar to that of the H_2-receptor antagonists. Hence, its clinical role has been limited since proton-pump inhibitors became widely available. An incidence of cardiac arrhythmias in the 1990s led to its withdrawal in most parts of the world.

Surgical treatment

The principle of surgery for gastro-oesophageal reflux disease is to create a mechanical antireflux barrier between the oesophagus and stomach. This therefore works independently of the composition of the refluxate, so whilst medical therapy is effective in relieving symptoms for many patients with acid reflux, only surgery achieves effective control of duodeno-gastro-oesophageal reflux.

Selection criteria for surgery

As a general rule, all patients who undergo antireflux surgery should have objective evidence of reflux. This may be the demonstration of erosive oesophagitis on endoscopy or an abnormal amount of acid reflux demonstrated by 24-hour pH monitoring. Neither of these tests is sufficiently reliable to base all preoperative decisions on their outcome,[14] as a number of patients with troublesome reflux will have either a normal 24-hour pH study or no evidence of oesophagitis at endoscopy (and, very occasionally, both). For this reason the tests have to be interpreted in the light of the patient's clinical presentation, and a final recommendation for surgery must be based on all available clinical and objective information.[14] More recently, impedance monitoring (in combination with pH monitoring) has been used to measure 'volume' reflux, although the additional information obtained from this investigation appears unlikely to influence surgical decision-making.[15]

Patients selected for surgery fall into two groups: (1) patients who have failed to respond (or have responded only partially) to medical therapy; (2) patients whose symptoms are fully controlled by medications, but who do not wish to continue with medication throughout their lives. The first group represents the large majority of patients. The latter group are more likely to be younger patients who face decades of acid suppression to alleviate their symptoms. In the first group, the response to surgery is usually more certain if the patient has had a good response to acid suppression in the past, or at least has had some symptom relief from medication. In patients who have had no response to proton-pump inhibitors, particularly those presenting with atypical symptoms, their symptoms are often due to something other than reflux, despite concurrent objective evidence of reflux (which may be incidental and/or asymptomatic). Such patients will usually not benefit from antireflux surgery.

Failure of medical treatment can be defined as continuing symptoms of reflux while on an adequate dose of acid suppression. In most countries this means at least a standard dose of a proton-pump inhibitor for a minimum period of 3 months. Proton-pump inhibitors are more effective for the control of the symptom of heartburn than volume regurgitation, and it is the latter symptom that is often the dominant problem in patients who have failed on medical therapy.

Patients can be further subdivided into: (i) those with complicated reflux disease; and (ii) those who have straightforward disease without complications.

Patients with complicated reflux disease

Reflux with stricture formation

In the past, surgery was the only effective treatment for strictures, and when the stricture was densely fibrotic this even meant resection of the oesophagus. Fortunately, it is now unusual to see patients with such advanced strictures since proton-pump inhibitors became available, so that the role of surgery seems to have lessened.[16] Strictures in young and fit patients are usually best treated by antireflux surgery and dilatation. However, many patients who develop strictures are elderly or infirm and the use of proton-pump inhibitors with dilatation is usually effective in this group.

Reflux with respiratory complications

When gastro-oesophageal regurgitation spills over into the respiratory tree, this can cause chronic respiratory illness, such as recurrent pneumonia, asthma or bronchiectasis. This is a firm indication for antireflux surgery, as the predominant action of proton-pump inhibitors is to block acid secretion and the volume of reflux is not greatly altered.

Reflux with throat symptoms

Halitosis, chronic cough, chronic laryngitis, chronic pharyngitis, chronic sinusitis and loss of enamel on teeth are sometimes attributed to gastro-oesophageal reflux. Whilst there is little doubt that on occasions such problems do arise in refluxing patients, these problems in isolation are not reliable indications for surgery. Whether or not these symptoms will be relieved following surgery is unpredictable. If symptoms are associated with typical reflux symptoms such as heartburn and/or regurgitation, then response rates of approximately 80% are reported, whereas throat symptoms in the absence of typical reflux symptoms respond poorly to surgery, with success rates of less than 50% reported.[17]

Columnar-lined (Barrett's) oesophagus

Patients with Barrett's oesophagus who have reflux symptoms should be selected for surgery on the basis of their symptoms and their response to medications, not simply because they have a columnar-lined oesophagus.[18] There is some experimental evidence to suggest that continuing reflux may be deleterious in regard to malignant change in oesophageal mucosa,[19] and one prospective randomised trial has suggested that antireflux surgery gives superior results to drug therapy in this patient group.[19] However, proton-pump inhibitors were only introduced into the medical arm of that trial in its later years.

There is also evidence that abolition of symptoms with proton-pump inhibition does not equate to 'normalising' the pH profile in a patient's oesophagus.[20] Since antireflux surgery does abolish acid reflux, this may become a further reason to recommend surgery in patients with Barrett's oesophagus. However, there is only limited evidence that either surgical or medical treatment of reflux in patients with Barrett's oesophagus consistently leads to regression of the columnar lining.[21] A report by Gurski et al.[22] suggested that although fundoplication is not followed by a reduction in the length of Barrett's oesophagus, it can be followed by 'histological' regression. In 68% of patients in this study with low-grade dysplasia, there was regression to non-dysplastic Barrett's mucosa. Equally, studies have shown that combining medical or surgical therapy with argon-beam plasma coagulation, photodynamic therapy or radiofrequency ablation of the columnar lining achieves complete or near complete reversion to squamous mucosa.[23–25] There is no evidence to support that antireflux surgery reduces the risk of dysplastic or neoplastic progression of Barrett's oesophagus.

✔ Longer-term follow-up from a randomised trial of ablation versus surveillance in patients with Barrett's oesophagus who had a undergone a fundoplication showed a reduction in the length of Barrett's oesophagus in both study groups, although to a greater extent following ablative therapy.[26]

Patients with uncomplicated reflux disease

Medical therapy, in the form of proton-pump inhibitors, is so effective that only a minority of patients do not get substantial or complete relief of their symptoms using these agents. Despite this, patients continue to present for antireflux surgery in large numbers for reasons already discussed. An additional factor that has emerged is the rising incidence of adenocarcinoma of the cardia associated with gastro-oesophageal reflux disease.[3] Whether antireflux surgery is more effective than long-term proton-pump inhibition at preventing the development of columnar-lined oesophagus and subsequently carcinoma of the lower oesophagus is controversial. If duodenal fluid has a role in the pathogenesis of adenocarcinoma of the oesophagus, then antireflux surgery would be preferable to acid suppression alone in patients with Barrett's oesophagus, and of course it may also prevent the development of Barrett's oesophagus in the first place. However, this hypothesis is not adequately tested and at present there is insufficient evidence to support a position that antireflux surgery should be performed to prevent subsequent malignant transformation.

Medical versus surgical therapy

The issue of the most appropriate treatment for gastro-oesophageal reflux disease has long been a subject of disagreement between surgeons and gastroenterologists. However, most would agree that a single management strategy is unlikely to be appropriate for all patients. Equally, there is a need for better comparative data for medical versus surgical therapy. Eight randomised trials[19,27–39] have been reported that have investigated this issue, but five of these were completed or commenced before the availability of both laparoscopic antireflux surgery and proton-pump inhibitor medication. All of these trials recruited patients who had reflux symptoms that were well controlled by medical therapy. In the latter trials this entailed complete symptom control with a proton-pump inhibitor at trial commencement, thereby excluding patients with uncontrolled symptoms. Hence, the majority of patients who are currently selected for surgery were excluded from the surgical arms of these trials, i.e. patients with a poor response to a proton-pump inhibitor.

In 1992, Spechler[28] reported a trial of 247 patients (predominantly men) randomised to either continuous medical therapy with an H_2 blocker, medical therapy for symptoms only or an open Nissen fundoplication. Overall patient satisfaction was highest following surgery at 1 and 2 years follow-up. However, neither the surgical nor medical treatment investigated is now considered optimal. The longer-term outcomes from this study were published in 2001, with median follow-up of approximately 7 years and with proton-pump inhibitors now used for the medically treated patients.[40] Follow-up was not complete and only 37 (45%) surgical patients were available for late follow-up, with 23% of the original surgical group lost to follow-up, and 32% died during follow-up. The later results did, however, show reasonable outcomes in both the medically and surgically treated groups. However, 62% of the surgical patients consumed antireflux medications at late follow-up, although when these medications were ceased in both study groups the surgical group had significantly fewer reflux symptoms than the medical group, suggesting that most of the surgical patients did not actually need the medications!

In 2003, Parrilla et al.[29] reported a randomised trial that randomised 101 patients with Barrett's oesophagus. Medical therapy was initially an H_2 blocker and later a proton-pump inhibitor. A satisfactory clinical outcome was achieved at 5 years follow-up in 91% of each group, although medical treatment was associated with a poorer endoscopic outcome. Progression to dysplasia was similar in both groups.

In 2000, Lundell et al.[30,31,39] reported a trial of proton-pump inhibitor medication versus open antireflux surgery. Three hundred and ten patients were randomised, and antireflux surgery achieved a better outcome at up to 3 years follow-up. Later reports of 7 years follow-up in 228 patients, and 12 years follow-up in 124, confirmed that surgery still achieved better reflux control than medication, although dysphagia and various wind-related side-effects were more common after fundoplication.[39,41]

Rhodes et al. reported the first randomised trial to compare proton-pump inhibitor medication with laparoscopic Nissen fundoplication; 217 patients were enrolled. Surgery was followed by less oesophageal acid exposure 3 months after treatment and better symptom control at 12 months.[32,33,42] A similar study by Anvari et al. enrolled 104 patients into a trial of proton-pump inhibitor therapy versus laparoscopic Nissen fundoplication.[34–36] Follow-up at 12 months and 3 years demonstrated better control of reflux and better quality of life in the patients who underwent surgery.

In 2009, Lundell et al.[37] reported the outcomes for a further multicentre randomised trial of laparoscopic Nissen fundoplication versus esomeprazole proton-pump inhibitor therapy (20–40 mg per day). This trial, which was funded by the pharmaceutical company that provided the medical therapy, enrolled 554 patients and outcomes at up to 3 years have been reported. Similar success rates of approximately 90% were reported for each treatment.

✔✔ It could be contended from the results of all of these trials that the majority of patients who have gastro-oesophageal reflux sufficient to require treatment with a proton-pump inhibitor should at least be offered the opportunity to undergo surgical correction of their reflux irrespective of whether their symptoms are well controlled by medication or not. The clinical trials all support an ongoing and important role for surgery in the treatment of reflux, and potentially a wider role in the management of reflux if offered to proton-pump inhibitor-dependent patients with symptoms that are well controlled by medication.

Pros and cons of antireflux surgery

Advantages

The advantages of surgery are clear. An operation is the only treatment that actually treats the cause rather than the effect, i.e. stops reflux of gastric contents into the oesophagus. Hence patients treated by surgery can usually eat whatever foods they choose, they can lie flat and bend over and do not need to take any tablets.

Disadvantages

The main disadvantage is operative morbidity (see discussion of complications). Laparoscopic surgery has greatly reduced the pain associated with open surgery; however, most patients experience some difficulty in swallowing in the immediate postoperative period, albeit temporary for the majority.[43] The time taken to improve is variable, often several months.[5] Furthermore, most patients experience early satiety leading to postoperative weight loss.[5] In the patients who are overweight at the time of surgery (the majority!) this may be seen as an advantage. This restriction on meal size also usually disappears over a few months.

Fundoplication produces a one-way valve; thus, patients have to be forewarned that they may not be able to belch effectively after the operation, especially in the first 6–12 months after surgery, and hence they should be cautious about drinking gassy drinks.[44] This applies particularly to patients who undergo a Nissen (total) fundoplication. For similar reasons, patients will be unable to vomit after an effective procedure, and should be informed of this. Failure to belch swallowed gas leads to increased passage of flatus after the procedure.[45] Patients who undergo a partial fundoplication (particularly anterior) have a lower incidence of these problems.[4] Despite these negative sequelae, the overwhelming majority of patients claim that the disadvantages are far outweighed by the advantages of the operation.[4,43,46] To date it has not been possible to predict preoperatively those patients who will develop problems following surgery.

Preoperative investigations

Apart from the assessment of each patient's general suitability for surgery by determining comorbidities, some specific investigations should be performed before undertaking antireflux surgery.

Endoscopy

Endoscopy is essential. It enables oesophagitis to be documented (confirming reflux disease), strictures to be dilated, and other gastro-oesophageal pathology to be excluded, documented and treated. The position of the squamocolumnar junction and the presence and size of any hiatus hernia is also assessed. The presence of a large hiatus hernia is not a contraindication to a laparoscopic approach, although the surgery is technically more difficult.[47]

Manometry

✔ Manometry is used to exclude primary motility disorders such as achalasia. It is also able to document the adequacy of oesophageal peristalsis.[14] The presence of weak or poorly propagated peristalsis is not a contraindication to antireflux surgery. Although many surgeons recommend a tailored approach to patient selection by choosing a partial fundoplication in patients with poor peristalsis,[48,49] there is no strong evidence to support this.[50,51] Evidence from randomised trials[52–55] has shown good results following the Nissen procedure in patients with poor peristalsis, suggesting that tailoring with a posterior partial fundoplication is not necessary. Nevertheless, common sense suggests that a partial fundoplication procedure is probably safer in patients with a true adynamic oesophagus and especially in patients with systemic scleroderma, in whom our preference would be to use an anterior partial fundoplication.[56]

Oesophageal pH monitoring

While many surgeons advocate the routine assessment of patients with 24-hour ambulatory pH monitoring before antireflux surgery, we use a selective approach. This test is not sufficiently accurate to be regarded as the 'gold standard' for the investigation of reflux, and if an abnormal pH profile is used to select patients for surgery, up to 20% of patients who have oesophagitis and typical reflux symptoms will be excluded unnecessarily from antireflux surgery. Hence, we apply this investigation in patients with endoscopy-negative reflux disease and in patients with atypical symptoms.[14] This test's ability to clarify whether symptoms are associated with reflux events is useful.

Other investigations

The role of bile reflux monitoring remains undefined in gastro-oesophageal reflux disease, although it has been suggested that it may be helpful in patients who fail to respond to acid suppression. This is measured using either 'Bilitec' or multichannel intraluminal impedance (MII) monitoring. 'Bilitec' measures intra-oesophageal bilirubin as an indirect marker of duodeno-oesophageal reflux, but has largely been superseded by MII, which measures 'volume' reflux. However, at this time, MII has only a limited role in the selection of patients for surgery.[15]

Antireflux surgery

To the non-surgeon, it might seem that there is a bewildering array of operations available for the treatment of reflux. In fact, the fundoplication introduced by Rudolf Nissen in 1956, or some variant of it, remains overwhelmingly the most popular antireflux operation in the world today. The principles of fundoplication are to mobilise the lower oesophagus, wrap the fundus of the stomach, either partially or totally, around the oesophagus, and then stabilise this new anatomy long term. When the oesophageal hiatus is enlarged, it is narrowed by sutures to prevent paraoesophageal herniation postoperatively and also to prevent the wrap being pulled up into the chest. Complications of reflux such as fibrotic stricturing with shortened oesophagus are seen rarely compared to the past. In the circumstance of true oesophageal shortening, an oesophageal lengthening (Collis) procedure can be undertaken to provide a long enough oesophagus to reach the abdomen. The upper lesser curvature of the stomach is used to produce the new oesophagus and the stomach is then wrapped around this. However, in our experience the Collis procedure is now not indicated or required during primary antireflux surgery.

Mechanisms of action of antireflux surgery

Total fundoplications, such as the Nissen, or partial fundoplications, whether anterior or posterior, probably all work in a similar fashion.[8,57] The mechanisms of action of an antireflux operation are not completely clear; they may work as much in a mechanical as physiological fashion, as these procedures are effective not only when placed in the chest in vivo,[58] but also on the benchtop, i.e. ex vivo.[8] Some of the proposed mechanisms include:

1. The creation of a floppy valve by maintaining close apposition between the abdominal oesophagus and the gastric fundus. As intragastric pressure rises the intra-abdominal oesophagus is compressed by the adjacent fundus.
2. Exaggeration of the flap valve at the angle of His.
3. Increase in the basal pressure generated by the lower oesophageal sphincter.
4. Reduction in the triggering of transient lower oesophageal sphincter relaxations.
5. Reduction in the capacity of the gastric fundus, thereby speeding proximal and total gastric emptying.
6. Prevention of effacement of the lower oesophagus (which effectively weakens the lower sphincter).

Since the procedures seem to work, even ex vivo,[8] it seems likely that the first two mechanisms account for the efficacy of the majority of antireflux procedures. Equally, the increase in lower oesophageal sphincter pressure following surgery is not important, and in some partial fundoplication procedures there is very little increase in pressure, yet reflux is well controlled.[4,59] The trend towards increasingly looser and shorter total fundoplications or greater use of partial fundoplication procedures suggests that there is no such thing as a fundoplication that is 'too loose'.

Techniques of antireflux surgery

As ever, when there are a variety of different operations performed for the same underlying condition, this denotes that no single procedure yields perfect results, i.e. 100% reflux control with minimal side-effects. All techniques have their advocates. Published reports can be found that support every known procedure, and it is probably better to consider results from randomised trials when assessing the merits of these procedural variants (see below) rather than relying on uncontrolled outcomes reported by advocates of a single procedure. Equally, the experience of the operating surgeon is of great importance for achieving a good postoperative outcome.[60] Variability can be reduced, but not eliminated, by detailed technical descriptions and effective surgical training. Over the last 20 years, a minimally invasive laparoscopic approach has become standard for primary antireflux surgery, making surgery more acceptable to patients and their physicians.

Nissen fundoplication (**Figs 13.1** and **13.2**)

Nissen originally described a procedure that entailed mobilisation of the oesophagus from the diaphragmatic hiatus, reduction of any hiatus hernia into the abdominal cavity, preservation of the vagus nerves and mobilisation of the posterior gastric fundus around behind the oesophagus, without dividing the short gastric vessels, and suturing of the posterior fundus to the anterior wall of the fundus using non-absorbable sutures, thereby achieving a complete wrap of stomach around the intra-abdominal oesophagus.[61] The original fundoplication was 5 cm in length and an oesophageal bougie was not used to calibrate the wrap. This is now the commonest antireflux operation performed worldwide.

✓ Because this procedure was associated with an incidence of persistent postoperative dysphagia, gas bloat syndrome and an inability to belch, the procedure has been progressively modified in an attempt to improve the long-term outcome. Most surgeons now agree that calibration of the wrap with a large (52 Fr) intra-oesophageal bougie, and shortening the fundoplication to 1–2 cm in length, achieves a better outcome.[62] Furthermore, whilst the need for routine hiatal repair was uncertain in the era of open surgery, most surgeons routinely include this step during laparoscopic antireflux surgery. Omission of this step is associated with a higher incidence of postoperative hiatal herniation.[63] The hepatic branch of the vagus nerve is usually preserved during this procedure.

Controversy still exists about the need to divide the short gastric vessels to achieve full fundal mobilisation. The so-called floppy Nissen procedure described by Donahue and Bombeck[64] relies on extensive fundal mobilisation. On the other hand, the modification of the Nissen fundoplication using the anterior fundal wall alone, also first described by Nissen and Rossetti,[61,65] does not require short gastric vessel division to construct the fundoplication. This simplifies the dissection, although more judgment and experience may be required to select the correct piece of stomach to use for the construction of a sufficiently loose fundoplication. Both procedures have their advocates, and good results (90% good or excellent long-term outcome) have been reported for both variants.[62,65] Nevertheless, strong opinions are held about whether the short gastric vessels should be divided or not, and this controversy has been heightened by the introduction of laparoscopic fundoplication.

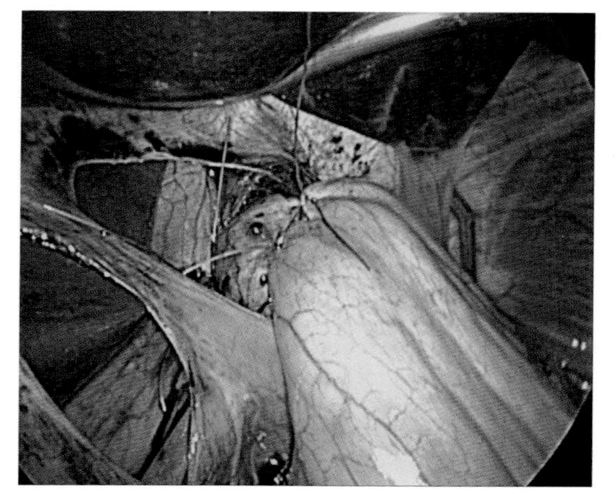

Figure 13.2 • Laparoscopic view of completed Nissen fundoplication.

Posterior partial fundoplication (**Fig. 13.3**)

A variety of fundoplication operations have been described in which the fundus is wrapped partially round the back of the oesophagus, with the aim of reduction of the possible side-effects of total fundoplication due to overcompetence of the cardia, i.e. dysphagia and gas-related problems. Toupet described a posterior partial fundoplication in which the fundus is passed behind the oesophagus and sutured to the left lateral and right lateral walls of the oesophagus, as well as to the right diaphragmatic pillar, creating a 270° posterior fundoplication.[66] A very similar procedure was described by Lind et al.[67] This entails a 300° posterior fundoplication, which is constructed by suturing the fundus to the oesophagus at the left and right lateral positions,

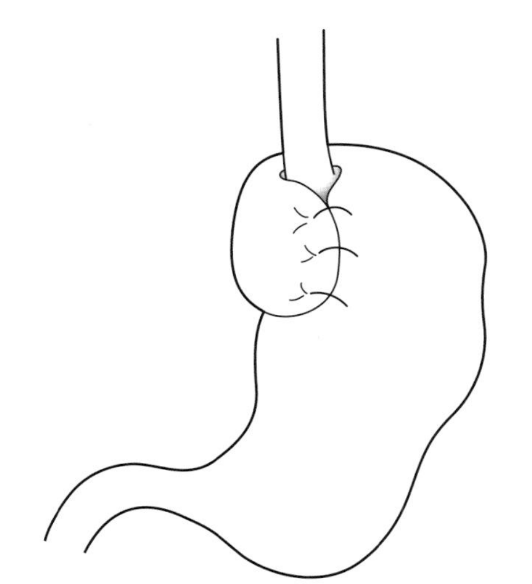

Figure 13.1 • Nissen fundoplication.

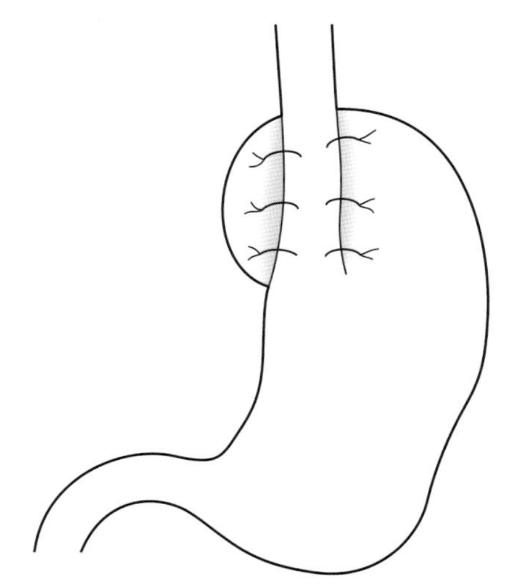

Figure 13.3 • Posterior partial fundoplication.

and additionally anteriorly on the left, leaving a 60° arc of oesophageal wall uncovered. The hiatus is repaired if necessary.

Anterior partial fundoplication

Several anterior partial fundoplication procedures have been described, and all purport to reduce the incidence of dysphagia and other side-effects. The Belsey Mark IV procedure, popular in thoracic practice up the early 1990s, entails a 240° anterior partial fundoplication that is usually performed through a left thoracotomy approach.[68] The distal oesophagus is mobilised, sutured to the gastric fundus and sutured to the diaphragm. Any hiatus hernia is repaired, and the anterior two-thirds of the abdominal oesophagus is covered by the fundoplication. The open thoracic access required is associated with significant morbidity, and for this reason it has fallen from favour since the arrival of laparoscopic antireflux surgery. A minimally invasive thoracoscopic approach was described 15 years ago,[69] although clinical outcomes have never been reported, and this procedure is rarely performed.

The Dor procedure is an anterior hemifundoplication that involves suturing of the fundus to the left and right sides of the oesophagus.[70] The Dor procedure is commonly used in combination with an abdominal cardiomyotomy for achalasia as it is unlikely to cause dysphagia, and it may reduce the risk of gastro-oesophageal reflux following cardiomyotomy.

A 120° anterior fundoplication has also been described.[59] This entails reduction of any hiatus hernia, posterior hiatal repair, suture of the posterior oesophagus to the hiatal pillars posteriorly, suture of the fundus to the diaphragm to accentuate the angle of His, and creation of an anterior partial fundoplication by suturing the fundus to the oesophagus on the right anterolateral aspect. Satisfactory medium-term reflux control following open surgery has been reported for this procedure, and a low incidence of gas-related problems. However, published laparoscopic experience is more limited.

We have reported the results from prospective randomised trials of laparoscopic anterior 180° partial fundoplication and laparoscopic anterior 90° partial fundoplication versus a Nissen procedure[4,71–75] (see below). The anterior 180° fundoplication procedure entails hiatal repair, suture of the distal oesophagus to the hiatus posteriorly, and construction of an anterior fundoplication that is sutured to the oesophagus and the hiatal rim on the right and anteriorly (**Figs 13.4** and **13.5**). The anterior 90° partial fundoplication procedure entails hiatal repair, posterior oesophagopexy, narrowing of the angle of His and construction of a limited anterior fundoplication that covers the left anterolateral aspect of the oesophagus (**Fig. 13.6**). These variants of anterior fundoplication show promise.

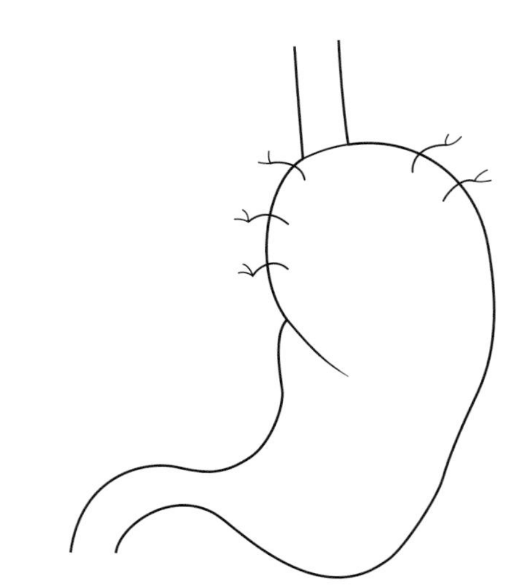

Figure 13.4 • One-hundred-and-eighty-degree anterior partial fundoplication performed by the transabdominal route.

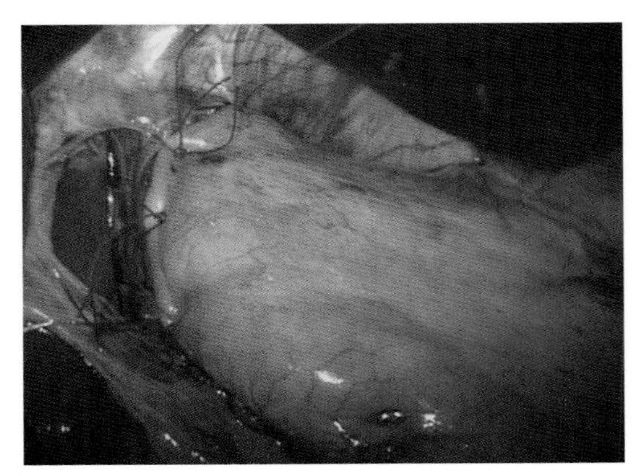

Figure 13.5 • Laparoscopic view of completed 180° anterior partial fundoplication.

Other antireflux procedures

Hill procedure

Hill described a procedure that is often regarded as a gastropexy rather than a fundoplication.[76] However, it also plicates the cardia and when examined endoscopically the intragastric appearances are similar to a fundoplication. The procedure entails suturing the anterior and posterior phreno-oesophageal bundles to the pre-aortic fascia and the median arcuate ligament. Whilst excellent results have been reported by Hill and colleagues,[77] it has not

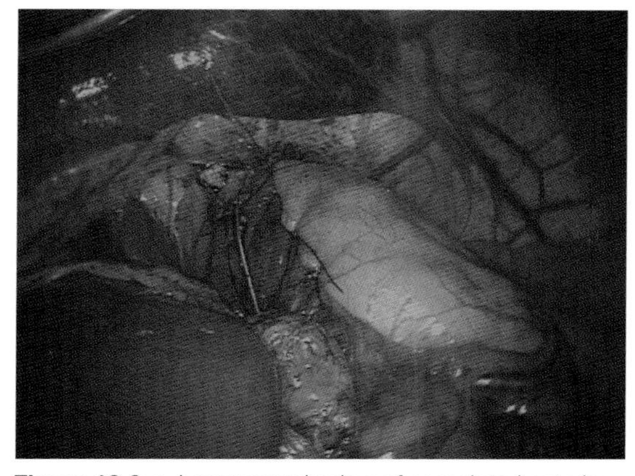

Figure 13.6 • Laparoscopic view of completed anterior partial fundoplication. This particular fundoplication was fashioned as a 90° wrap, leaving an area of exposed oesophagus on the right side.

been applied widely because most surgeons have difficulty understanding the anatomical principles and, in particular, the phreno-oesophageal bundles are not clear structures. Hill also emphasises the need for intraoperative manometry. This is not widely available, limiting the dissemination of his technique.

Collis procedure (**Fig. 13.7**)

The Collis procedure is useful for patients whose oesophagogastric junction cannot be reduced below the diaphragm.[78] However, this situation is very rare in current practice. The Collis procedure entails the construction of a tube of gastric lesser curve to recreate an abdominal length of oesophagus, around which a fundoplication can then be constructed to help with oesophageal shortening. It is often constructed by using a circular end-to-end stapler to create a transgastric window; a linear cutting stapler is used from this hole up to the angle of His to construct the neo-oesophagus. Laparoscopic and thoracoscopic techniques for this procedure have been described, although longer-term outcomes are not available.[79,80] A disadvantage of this procedure is that the gastric tube does not have peristaltic activity and furthermore it can secrete acid. This leads to a poorer overall success rate for this procedure, although some of this could be due to the end-stage nature of the reflux disease that led to the choice of this procedure in the first place.

Augmentation of the lower oesophageal sphincter

LINX®

In 2010, Bonavina et al.[81] described a new approach to surgery for gastro-oesophageal reflux that entailed augmentation of the lower oesophageal sphincter with an implantable string of interlinked titanium beads with magnetic cores. This device (LINX Reflux Management System, Torax Medical, Shoreview, MN) is placed laparoscopically around the gastro-oesophageal junction, and aims to control reflux, but still allow normal swallowing and belching. Experience is limited to a case series of 44 patients followed for up to 2 years.[81] A success rate of approximately 90%, as measured by both clinical scores and pH monitoring, has been reported, and this appears similar to the success rate following fundoplication. It is easy to place, so the potential benefits in comparison to standard Nissen are a standard approach and the relative lack of hiatal

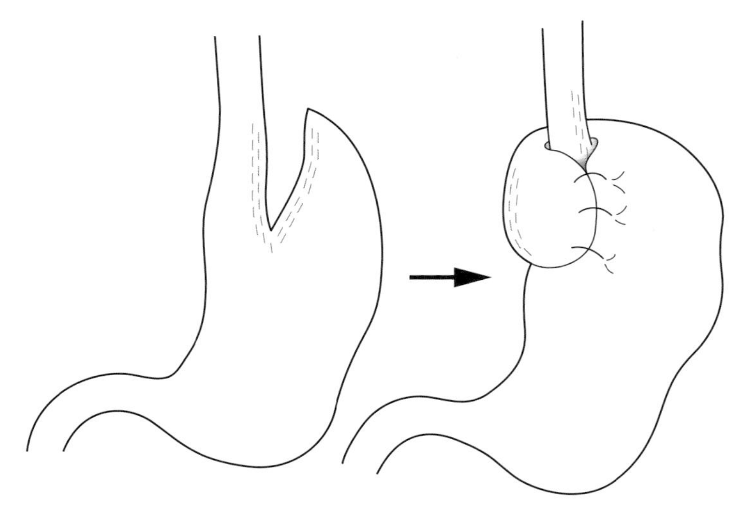

Figure 13.7 • Collis gastroplasty, with subsequent Nissen fundoplication.

dissection. Clinicians familiar with the Angelchik prosthesis will be wary of placing a foreign body around the distal oesophagus, although placement appears to be safe. The outcomes of larger series and longer-term randomised comparative trials are required to prove clinical and cost-effectiveness before this procedures enters wide clinical practice.[82]

EndoStim®

Based on the premise of a dysfunctional sphincter, an innovative new approach to the management of GORD uses an implantable system to deliver electrical stimulation to the lower oesophageal sphincter in order to normalise its function and prevent acid reflux. The EndoStim® device is commercially available in the UK (CE-mark approved). A laparoscopic technique is used to implant the system's electrodes into the distal oesophageal muscle layers using minimal hiatal dissection. A wirelessly programmable pacemaker is then placed subcutaneously. It is thought that the avoidance of a 'wrap' will reduce the negative sequelae associated with various fundoplications. Also, the electrical stimulation is 'tailored' to the individual patient's GORD profile in terms of the number and timing of impulses. Initial data are promising when placed in patients at least partially responsive to proton-pump inhibition, with hiatal hernia ≤3 cm and only mild to moderate oesophagitis. Most importantly, implantation and electrical stimulation were safe. However, a well-designed, randomised, sham-control trial is needed to validate this approach.[83]

Controversies and comparisons

Complete or partial fundoplication?

Because fundoplication is associated with an incidence of postoperative dysphagia, gas bloat and other gas-related symptoms such as increased flatulence, the relative merits of the Nissen fundoplication procedure versus various partial fundoplication variants have been debated for many years. The introduction of laparoscopic approaches only served to heighten this controversy. On the one hand, the Nissen procedure produces an overcompetent gastro-oesophageal junction, which is the cause of some of the problems with dysphagia and gas bloat. On the other hand, it has been suggested that partial fundoplications reduce the risk of over-competence, but perhaps at the expense of a less durable antireflux repair.

Many prospective randomised trials of Nissen versus a partial fundoplication have been performed. DeMeester et al.[84] had the distinction of reporting the first randomised study in the field of surgery for reflux disease in 1974. Their trial randomised 45 patients to undergo either a Nissen, Hill or Belsey procedure, and they followed up their patients for 6 months after surgery. The dysphagia and recurrent reflux rates were similar for all three procedures. However, the number of patients was too small to allow a meaningful comparison to be made.

Nissen versus posterior fundoplication

Eleven randomised trials have compared a Nissen with a posterior partial fundoplication. Some of the trials contribute little to the pool of evidence as they are either small and underpowered, or only reported very-short-term outcomes.[53,85–88]

Lundell et al.[89] reported the outcomes of the first large trial of Nissen versus a posterior (Toupet) partial fundoplication; 137 patients were enrolled. The early outcomes at 6 months follow-up were similar. At 5 years follow-up[90] reflux control and dysphagia rates were also similar, although flatulence was commoner after Nissen fundoplication at 2 and 3 years but not at 4 or 5 years follow-up. Re-operation was more common following Nissen fundoplication, with one patient in the posterior fundoplication group undergoing further surgery for severe gas bloat symptoms and five of the Nissen group undergoing re-operation for postoperative paraoesophageal herniation. A reanalysis of the data from this trial[45] sought to answer the question of whether a tailored approach to antireflux surgery should be applied. There were no demonstrable disadvantages for the Nissen procedure in those patients who had manometrically abnormal peristalsis before surgery. In 2011, minimum follow-up of 18 years was reported.[91] The outcomes at this very late follow-up were equivalent, with success rates of more than 80% reported for both procedures, and no significant differences in the incidence of side-effects at late follow-up, suggesting that the mechanical side-effects following Nissen fundoplication improve progressively with very-long-term follow-up.

Zornig et al.[92] reported a trial that enrolled 200 patients to either total fundoplication with division of the short gastric vessels or posterior fundoplication. One hundred patients had normal preoperative oesophageal motility and 100 had 'abnormal' motility. At 4 months follow-up an overall good outcome was obtained in about 90% of patients in each group, and reflux control was equivalent. Short-term dysphagia was less common following posterior partial fundoplication, and no correlation was seen between preoperative oesophageal motility and outcome, providing no support for the selective application of a partial fundoplication in patients with abnormal preoperative motility. The 2-year follow-up outcomes were similar.[55] Eighty-five per cent of each group were satisfied with their clinical outcome, and dysphagia remained significantly more common after Nissen fundoplication (19 vs. 8 patients).

A study by Guérin et al.[93] enrolled 140 patients. At 3 years follow-up 118 patients were evaluated and no outcome differences could be identified. Similarly, Booth et al.[54] enrolled 127 patients in a trial of Nissen versus Toupet fundoplication, Khan et al.[94] enrolled 121 patients in another trial, and Shaw et al.[95] enrolled 100. Each of these trials showed no differences in reflux control 1 year after surgery. Although dysphagia was more common following Nissen fundoplication in Booth et al.'s trial, there were no differences in the prevalence of side-effects in the other trials. Subgroup analysis in Booth et al.'s and Shaw et al.'s trials did not reveal any differences between patients with or without poor preoperative oesophageal motility.

✔✔ If one combines all the data of the Nissen versus posterior fundoplication trials together, the available evidence supports the view that side-effects are less common following a posterior partial fundoplication, particularly for wind-related problems. The hypothesis that dysphagia is less of a problem following a posterior partial fundoplication has only been substantiated by two of the 11 trials.

Nissen versus anterior fundoplication

Six trials have evaluated Nissen versus anterior partial fundoplication. In 1999 we reported the first prospective randomised trial to compare a Nissen fundoplication with an anterior partial fundoplication technique.[4] Both procedures were performed laparoscopically. This study enrolled 107 patients to undergo either a Nissen or anterior partial fundoplication. The partial fundoplication variant entailed a 180° fundoplication that was anchored to the right hiatal pillar and the oesophageal wall (Figs 13.4 and 13.5). Whilst no overall outcome differences between the two procedures were demonstrated at 1 and 3 months follow-up, at 6 months patients who underwent an anterior fundoplication were less likely to experience dysphagia for solid food, were less likely to be troubled by excessive passage of flatus, were more likely to be able to belch normally, and the overall outcome was better. The outcomes at 5 years confirmed the results of the initial report.[71] Reflux control was slightly better after Nissen fundoplication, but this was offset by significantly less dysphagia, less abdominal bloating and better preservation of belching, resulting in a greater proportion of patients reporting a good or excellent overall outcome 5 years after anterior fundoplication (94% vs. 86%). At 10 years follow-up, however, there were no significant outcome differences for the two procedures, with equivalent control of reflux, and no differences for side-effects,[74] a similar outcome to the very late follow-up for the Lundell and colleagues, trial of Nissen versus posterior partial fundoplication.[91]

Baigrie et al.[96] reported 2-year follow-up from a similar study in which 161 patients underwent either a Nissen or anterior 180° partial fundoplication. This trial demonstrated equivalent control of reflux symptoms and less dysphagia following anterior 180° partial fundoplication, although the incidence of re-operation for recurrent reflux was higher after anterior fundoplication. Cao et al.[97] reported 5-year outcomes for a similar trial that enrolled 100 patients. Reflux control was similar for the two procedures, and flatulence was less common after anterior 180° partial fundoplication. Raue et al.[98] reported equivalent outcomes at 18 months mean follow-up in a smaller trial that enrolled 64 patients.

Two further trials have compared a laparoscopic anterior 90° partial fundoplication with a Nissen fundoplication. In the first of these, 112 patients were enrolled in a multicentre randomised trial conducted in six cities in Australia and New Zealand.[72,75] Side-effects were significantly less common following anterior 90° fundoplication, although this was offset by a slightly higher incidence of recurrent reflux at 6 months follow-up.[72] At 5 years the outcomes were similar for side-effects, although reflux was worse after the partial fundoplication.[75] Satisfaction with the overall outcome was similar for both fundoplication types. Similar outcomes were reported from a parallel single-centre randomised trial that enrolled 79 patients – fewer side-effects offset by more reflux.[73]

Anterior versus posterior partial fundoplication

Two randomised trials have directly compared anterior versus posterior partial fundoplication. Hagedorn et al.[99–101] randomised 95 patients to undergo either a laparoscopic posterior (Toupet) or anterior 120° partial fundoplication. Their results showed better reflux control, but more side-effects following posterior partial fundoplication. Unfortunately, the clinical and objective outcomes following anterior 120° fundoplication in this trial were much worse than the outcomes from other randomised and non-randomised studies. The average exposure time to acid (pH <4) was 5.6% following anterior fundoplication in their study, whereas in other studies this figure is reported to be between 2.5% and 2.7%,[4,72] suggesting that the procedure performed in the study of Hagedorn et al. was less effective and therefore different to the procedures performed in other studies. More recently, Khan et al.[102] reported 6 months follow-up from a trial that enrolled 103 patients to undergo anterior 180° versus posterior partial fundoplication. Reflux control was also better after posterior partial fundoplication, but offset by more side-effects.

✔✔ Currently, the overall results from the eight trials that included an anterior fundoplication suggest that anterior fundoplication variants achieve satisfactory control of reflux, a reduced incidence of post-fundoplication dysphagia and other side-effects, and a good overall clinical outcome. However, the reduced incidence of troublesome side-effects is, to some extent, offset by a higher risk of recurrent reflux. Nevertheless, excellent long-term outcomes and good reflux control have been reported in a series of 548 patients who underwent anterior 180° partial fundoplication, with approximately 90% of patients highly satisfied with the clinical outcome at up to 10 years follow-up.[103]

Division/no division of short gastric vessels

Until the 1990s the issue of division versus non-division of the short gastric vessels was rarely discussed. However, following anecdotal reports of increased problems with postoperative dysphagia following laparoscopic Nissen fundoplication without division of the short gastric vessels,[104,105] this aspect of surgical technique became a much debated topic. Routine division of the short gastric vessels during fundoplication, to achieve full fundal mobilisation and thereby ensure a loose fundoplication, is thought by some to be an essential step during laparoscopic (and open) Nissen fundoplication.[62] This opinion was popularised by the publication of studies that compared experience with division of the short gastric vessels with historical experience with a Nissen fundoplication performed without dividing these vessels.[62,64,104,105] However, other uncontrolled studies of Nissen fundoplication either with or without division of the short gastric vessels confuse the issue further, as good results have been reported whether these vessels were divided or not.[62,65]

Six randomised trials have been reported that investigate this aspect of technique. Luostarinen et al.[106,107] reported the outcome of a small trial of division versus no division of the short gastric vessels during open total fundoplication. Fifty patients were entered into this trial and a later report[107] described outcomes following median 3-year follow-up. Both procedures effectively corrected endoscopic oesophagitis. However, there was a trend towards a higher incidence of disruption of the fundoplication (5 vs. 2) and reflux symptoms (6 vs. 1) in patients whose short gastric vessels were divided, and 9 of 26 patients who underwent vessel division developed a postoperative sliding hiatus hernia, compared to only 1 of 24 patients whose vessels were kept intact. The likelihood of long-term dysphagia or gas-related symptoms was not influenced by mobilising the gastric fundus in this trial.

In 1997 we reported a randomised trial that enrolled 102 patients undergoing a laparoscopic Nissen fundoplication to have a procedure either with or without division of the short gastric vessels.[5] No difference in overall outcome was demonstrated at initial follow-up of 6 months and the trial failed to show that dividing the short gastric vessels during laparoscopic Nissen fundoplication reduced the incidence or severity of early postoperative dysphagia, or the outcome of any objective investigations. At 5 and 10 years follow-up,[108,109] both procedures were equally durable in terms of reflux control and the incidence of postoperative dysphagia. At 5 years follow-up division of the short gastric vessels was associated, with more flatulence and bloating, and greater difficulties with belching.

Blomqvist et al.[110,111] reported the outcome of a similar trial that enrolled 99 patients. At 12 months and 10 years follow-up, this study also showed that dividing the short gastric vessels did not improve the outcome. A recent meta-analysis of larger data with 12 years follow-up, generated by combining the raw Adelaide and Swedish data, confirmed equivalent reflux control, but more bloating after division of the short gastric vessels.[112]

Farah et al.,[113] Kösek et al.[114] and Chrysos et al.[115] all reported trials that showed equivalent reflux control and postoperative dysphagia irrespective of whether the short gastric vessels were divided or not. However, as with the Adelaide and Swedish data, they also demonstrated an increased incidence of bloating symptoms after division of the short gastric vessels.

✔✔ The belief that dividing the short gastric vessels will improve the outcome following laparoscopic total fundoplication is not supported by the results of any published trials. Furthermore, dividing the vessels increases the complexity of the procedure and actually produced a poorer outcome in three of the six trials due to an increase in the incidence of bloating symptoms.

Laparoscopic antireflux surgery

Laparoscopic Nissen fundoplication was first reported in 1991[116,117] and rapidly established itself as the procedure of choice for reflux disease, with the vast majority of antireflux procedures now performed this way. The results of several large series with long-term clinical follow-up have now been published.[118,119] These confirm that laparoscopic Nissen fundoplication is effective, and that 10 years after surgery it achieves an excellent clinical outcome in more than 85–90% of patients. Furthermore, with even longer follow-up, it is likely that this procedure will be as durable as open fundoplication, where a 70–80% success rate can be expected at up to 25 years follow-up.[120]

However, several complications unique to the laparoscopic approach have been described (see below). Dysphagia could be more common following laparoscopic fundoplication, although this may be due to the more intense nature of the prospective follow-up applied in many centres. Furthermore, in our experience dysphagia has been less of a problem after fundoplication than it was before surgery, with a reduction in the incidence from approximately 30% before surgery to less than 10% at 12 months following surgery,[4,5] and for the majority of these patients dysphagia has not been troublesome in the long term.

Up to 10% of patients are dissatisfied. Some of this dissatisfaction is because of a complication of the original surgery. In our experience this has usually been either the development of a paraoesophageal hernia or because of continuing troublesome dysphagia (with either the wrap or the hiatus being too tight). Some patients are dissatisfied, however, even though their reflux has been cured and they have not had any complications.[121] This is usually because they do not like the flatulence that can follow the procedure. It is also important to recognise that there is a learning curve associated with this form of surgery, and we have demonstrated that the first 20 patients in an individual surgeon's experience are associated with a higher complication rate, and as experience increases the re-operation rates fall to below 5%.[60] There are no specific contraindications to the laparoscopic approach, and the repair of giant hiatal hernias and re-operative antireflux surgery are both feasible (although technically more demanding).

There are some differences between the management of patients during and after laparoscopic and open fundoplication procedures. Laparoscopic surgery may increase the risk of thromboembolic complications (see below) and therefore prophylaxis for deep vein thrombosis is mandatory. Other differences are primarily due to the accelerated recovery following laparoscopic surgery. Our practice is to avoid the use of a nasogastric tube, commence oral intake within 6 hours of surgery, and to arrange a barium meal X-ray the day after surgery to check the postoperative anatomy at a time when problems are easily corrected. Since implementing this approach, a similar strategy has been applied to patients undergoing open surgery (usually revision procedures), and this has facilitated a quicker recovery in some of these patients too.

Laparoscopic versus open antireflux surgery

Non-randomised comparisons between open and laparoscopic fundoplication generally showed that laparoscopic surgery required more operating time than the equivalent open surgical procedure,[122,123] that the incidence of postoperative complications was reduced, the length of postoperative hospital stay was shortened by 3–7 days, patients returned to full physical function 6–27 days quicker, and overall hospital costs were reduced. The efficacy of reflux control appeared to be similar between the two approaches. Ten randomised controlled trials have been reported that compare a laparoscopic fundoplication with its open surgical equivalent.[124–138] Nine of these investigated a Nissen fundoplication and one study compared laparoscopic versus open posterior partial fundoplication.[132] The early reports that described follow-up extending up to 12 months confirmed advantages for the laparoscopic approach, albeit less dramatic than the advantages expected from the results of non-randomised studies. More recently, longer-term outcomes from some studies have been reported.[133,135,137,139,140]

Early reports from smaller trials[125–127] that each enrolled 20–42 patients demonstrated equivalent short-term clinical outcomes, shortening of the postoperative stay by about 1 day (3 vs. 4 median), longer operating times (extended by approximately 30 minutes), and an overall reduction in the incidence of postoperative complications following laparoscopic Nissen fundoplication. The reduction in the length of the postoperative hospital stay by only 1 day was unexpected. This was achieved entirely by a shorter hospital stay following open fundoplication, suggesting that at least some of the apparent benefits of the laparoscopic approach have been due to a general change in management policy to encourage earlier oral intake, avoiding nasogastric tubes and encouraging earlier discharge from hospital.

Chrysos et al.[128] reported 12 months follow-up for a trial that enrolled 106 patients. Both approaches achieved effective reflux control, post-fundoplication dysphagia was similar, and the laparoscopic approach was followed by fewer complications, a quicker recovery and fewer symptoms of epigastric bloating and distension. Similar 12-month postoperative outcomes were demonstrated by Ackroyd et al.[138] in a trial that enrolled 99 patients.

Håkanson et al.[132] enrolled 192 patients into a trial of laparoscopic versus open posterior partial fundoplication. Their results were similar to the trials of laparoscopic versus open Nissen fundoplication. Early complications were more common after open surgery, the length of the hospital stay was longer (5 vs. 3 days) and return to work was slower (42 vs. 28 days). However, this was offset by a higher incidence of early side-effects and recurrent reflux in the laparoscopic group. At 3 years follow-up, however, there were no outcome differences, satisfaction with the surgery was similar for the two groups, and the need for re-operative surgery of any sort was not influenced by the choice of technique.

Laine et al.[124] reported 110 patients randomised to undergo laparoscopic or open Nissen fundoplication. As with the other trials, hospital stay was shorter, being halved from 6.4 to 3.2 days and patients returned to work quicker (37 vs. 15 days), but operating time was also prolonged by 31 minutes. Subsequent reports from this group[137,140] described 11- and then 15-year follow-up in 86 patients. Whilst symptom control and side-effects were similar at late follow-up and 82% of the laparoscopic surgery group were satisfied with the late outcome, the incidence of wrap disruption at endoscopic assessment was significantly higher following open surgery (40% vs. 13%) and there were 10 incisional hernias, all following the open technique. Similar outcomes were reported by Nilsson et al.[136] in a smaller trial that followed patients for 5 years.

The study that created the most controversy in this area was published by Bais et al. in 2000.[129] This multicentre study initially enrolled 103 patients. The early (3 months) results of this trial showed a disadvantage for the laparoscopic approach and the trial was stopped early because of an excess of adverse end-points. The investigators were criticised for terminating the trial prematurely,[141,142] as it can be argued that the conclusions were misleading. The decision to stop the trial was based primarily on postoperative dysphagia within the first 3 months. Other studies have reported that most patients who undergo a Nissen fundoplication still have some dysphagia 3 months after surgery,[5,130] but that this dysphagia usually subsides as time passes. Hence, a follow-up period of 3 months is too short for the end-point of dysphagia to be adequately assessed. Subsequent reports of 5- and 10-year follow-up from this trial[133,139] confirmed the validity of this critique. With further enrolment boosting the number of patients to 177, no differences in symptoms or subjective outcome could be demonstrated at late follow-up. In addition, 24-hour pH monitoring confirmed equivalent reflux control. At 10-year follow-up, there was a higher rate of surgical reintervention following open surgery, mainly due to an excess of incisional hernias. Hence, the late results of this trial actually support the application of laparoscopic antireflux surgery.

✔✔ If the overall results of these trials are synthesised, it is clear that laparoscopic antireflux surgery has short- and long-term advantages over the open approach in terms of reduced overall morbidity, quicker recovery and fewer incisional hernias. In addition, control of reflux and risk of side-effects at late follow-up (up to 15 years) is not influenced by the choice of a laparoscopic approach. For these reasons the laparoscopic approach offers advantages, and it has effectively superseded the open approach for most clinical situations.

Complications of laparoscopic antireflux surgery

As experience with laparoscopic approaches for antireflux surgery became standard practice, complications unique to the laparoscopic approach emerged (Box 13.1). These include postoperative

Box 13.1 • Unique or common complications following laparoscopic antireflux surgery

- Pneumothorax[143]
- Pneumomediastinum[144]
- Pulmonary embolism[145,146]
- Injury to major vessels[147]
- Paraoesophageal hiatus hernia[63,148]
- Hiatal stenosis[149]
- Mesenteric thrombosis[150,151]
- Bilobed stomach[145]
- Oesophageal perforation[145,146,152–154]
- Gastric perforation[145,146,152]
- Duodenal perforation[155]
- Bowel perforation[154]
- Cardiac laceration and tamponade[156]
- Pleuropericarditis[157]
- Necrotising fasciitis[158]

paraoesophageal hiatus hernia, re-operation for dysphagia, and gastrointestinal perforation. Nevertheless, the risk of complications should be balanced against the advantages of the laparoscopic approach, as the overall complication rate is reduced following laparoscopic surgery.[139] The likelihood of complications can be influenced by a number of factors, including surgeon experience and expertise, operative technique and perioperative care. Furthermore, the final outcome of some complications can be moderated significantly by applying appropriate early management strategies.

Complications that are more common following laparoscopic antireflux surgery

Paraoesophageal hiatus hernia

Paraoesophageal hiatus herniation was thought to be an uncommon finding following open fundoplication, presenting usually in the late follow-up period, although its frequency was probably underestimated in the past. Most large series of laparoscopic procedures report the occurrence of paraoesophageal herniation following surgery (**Fig. 13.8**), particularly in the immediate postoperative period.[63,148,158] The incidence of this complication ranges up to 7% in published reports,[63] and it seems that this is exacerbated by some factors inherent in the laparoscopic approach. These include a tendency to extend laparoscopic oesophageal dissection further into the thorax than during open surgery, an increased risk of breaching the left pleural membrane[143] and the effect of reduced postoperative pain. Loss of the left pleural barrier can allow the stomach to slide more easily into the left hemithorax, and less pain permits more abdominal force to be transmitted to the hiatal area during coughing, vomiting or other forms of exertion in the initial postoperative period, pushing the stomach into the thorax, as the normal anatomical barriers have been disrupted by surgical dissection. Early resumption of heavy physical work has also been associated with acute herniation. Strategies are available that can reduce the likelihood of herniation. Routine hiatal repair has been shown to reduce the incidence by approximately 80%.[63] In addition, excessive strain on the hiatal repair during the early postoperative period should be avoided by the routine use of antiemetics, and advising patients to avoid excessive lifting or straining for about 1 month following surgery.

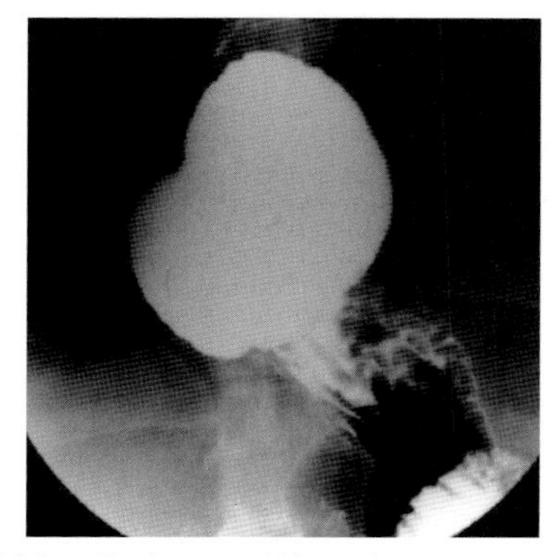

Figure 13.8 • Barium meal X-ray demonstrating a large paraoesophageal hiatus hernia 3 months after laparoscopic fundoplication.

Dysphagia

The debate in the laparoscopic era is whether dysphagia is more likely to occur following laparoscopic antireflux surgery. Nearly all patients, including those who undergo a partial fundoplication, experience dysphagia requiring dietary modification in the first weeks to months following laparoscopic surgery. However, it is dysphagia that is severe enough to need further surgery that is of most concern. Early severe dysphagia requiring surgical revision has been reported in a number of series.[149,159,160] Conversion of a Nissen fundoplication to a partial fundoplication has been performed for troublesome dysphagia following both open and laparoscopic techniques, usually with success.[160,161]

More common with the laparoscopic approach, however, is the problem of a tight oesophageal diaphragmatic hiatus causing dysphagia[149,161] (**Figs 13.9** and **13.10**). Two factors may cause this problem: over-tightening of the hiatus during hiatal repair and excessive perihiatal scar tissue formation. Many surgeons use an intra-oesophageal bougie to distend the oesophagus, to assist with calibration of the hiatal closure. However, this will not always prevent over-tightening from occurring. If a problem does arise in the immediate postoperative period, it can usually be corrected by early laparoscopic reintervention with release of one or more hiatal sutures. Later narrowing of the oesophageal hiatus due to postoperative scar tissue formation in the second and third postoperative weeks, even in patients not undergoing initial hiatal repair, has also been described. In our experience, endoscopic dilatation with standard bougies usually only provides temporary relief of symptoms rather than a long-term solution. Correction of this problem often requires widening of the diaphragmatic hiatus. This can be achieved by a laparoscopic approach, with anterolateral division of the hiatal ring and adjacent diaphragm until the hiatus is sufficiently loose.

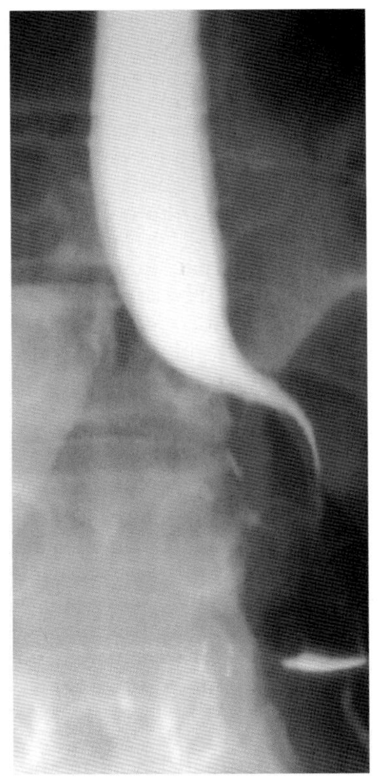

Figure 13.9 • Barium meal X-ray demonstrating usual appearance following laparoscopic Nissen fundoplication.

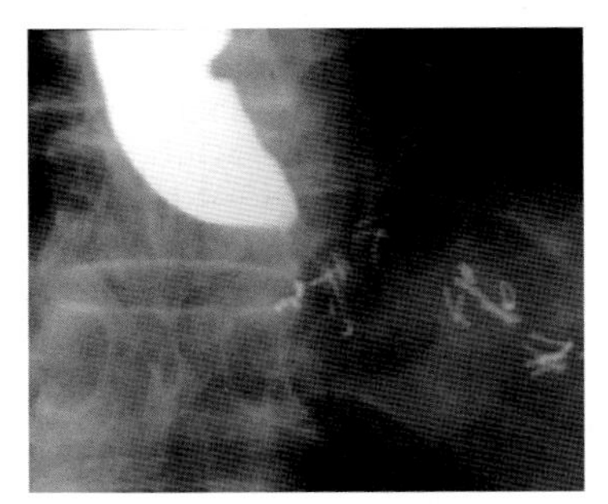

Figure 13.10 • Day 2 postoperative barium meal in a patient with total dysphagia following Nissen fundoplication due to a tight oesophageal hiatus. The problem was corrected by widening the hiatus and removing the hiatal repair sutures.

An alternative strategy, which is sometimes successful, is pneumatic balloon dilatation (using a 30-mm-diameter balloon).

Pulmonary embolism

Pulmonary embolism was more common in some of the early reports of laparoscopic Nissen fundoplication[145] and in particular following conversion of cases to open surgery, suggesting that prolonged operating times might be an important aetiological factor. In addition, several mechanical factors inherent in the laparoscopic antireflux surgery environment create a scenario in which venous thrombosis is more likely. The combination of head-up tilt of the operating table, intra-abdominal insufflation of gas under pressure and elevation of the legs in stirrups greatly reduces venous flow in the leg veins, potentially predisposing patients to deep venous thrombosis. This problem can be minimised by the routine use of vigorous antithromboembolism prophylaxis, including low-dose heparin, antiembolism stockings and mechanical compression of the calves.

Complications unique to laparoscopic antireflux surgery

Bilobed stomach

A technical error described during early experiences with laparoscopic Nissen fundoplication is the 'bilobed stomach'.[145] This occurs when too distal a piece of stomach is used to form the Nissen fundoplication wrap, usually the gastric body rather than the fundus, resulting in a bilobular-shaped stomach (**Fig. 13.11**). Most patients are asymptomatic; in extreme cases it is possible for the upper part of the stomach to become obstructed at the point of constriction in the gastric body, resulting in postprandial abdominal pain, which requires surgical revision (**Fig. 13.12**). Checking carefully to ensure that the correct piece of stomach (the fundus) is used for construction of the fundoplication prevents this problem from arising.

Pneumothorax

Intraoperative pneumothorax occurs in up to 2% of patients due to injury to the left pleural membrane

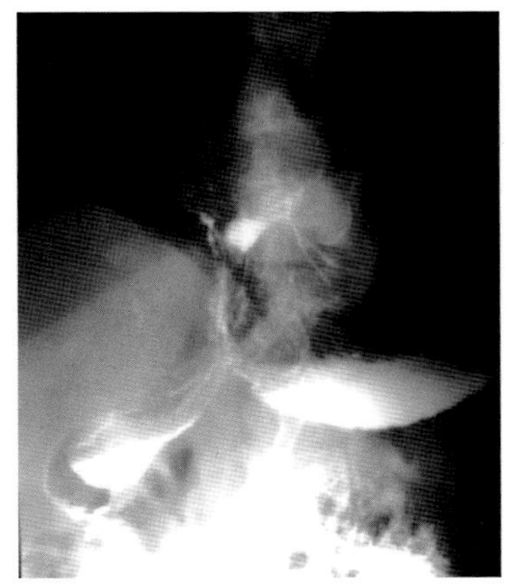

Figure 13.11 • Barium meal image of a 'bilobed' stomach. This patient continues to have an excellent clinical result at 7 years follow-up.

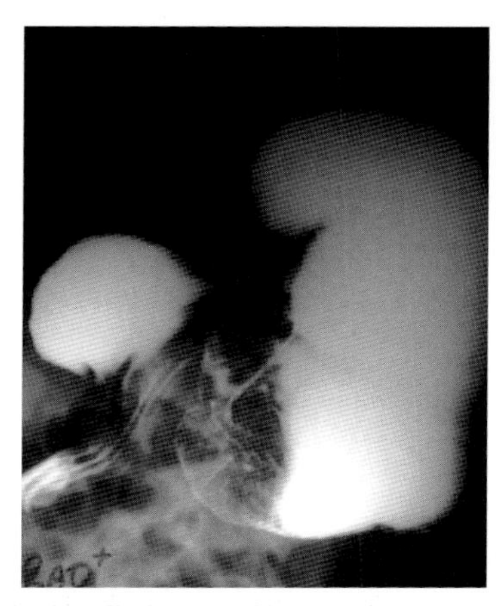

Figure 13.12 • Barium meal image of a more severe 'bilobed' stomach. This patient developed gastric obstruction and required surgical revision.

during retro-oesophageal dissection, particularly if dissection is directed too high within the mediastinum.[143] This is more likely to occur during dissection of a large hiatus hernia. Careful dissection behind the oesophagus, ensuring that the tips of instruments passed from right to left behind the oesophagus do not pass above the level of the diaphragm, and experience with laparoscopic dissection at the hiatus reduce its likelihood. The occurrence of a pneumothorax does not usually require the placement of a chest drain, as CO_2 gas in the pleural cavity is rapidly reabsorbed at the completion of the procedure, allowing the lung to re-expand rapidly.

Vascular injury

Vascular injury to the inferior vena cava, the left hepatic vein and the abdominal aorta have all been reported.[147,162] This problem may be associated with aberrant anatomy, inexperience, the excessive use of monopolar diathermy cautery dissection, the incorrect application of ultrasonic shears, or a combination of these. Intraoperative bleeding more commonly follows inadvertent laceration of the left lobe of the liver by the liver retractor or other instrument and haemorrhage from poorly secured short gastric vessels during fundal mobilisation. A rare complication is cardiac tamponade, which has been reported twice,[156,163] once due to laceration of the right ventricle by a liver retractor and once due to an injury of the cardiac wall from a suture needle. The proximity of the heart, inferior vena cava and aorta to the distal oesophagus renders potentially life-threatening injuries a possibility if surgeons are unfamiliar with the laparoscopic view of hiatal anatomy. Nevertheless, the risk of perioperative haemorrhage during and after antireflux surgery is probably reduced by a laparoscopic approach, as is the likelihood of splenectomy.

Perforation of the upper gastrointestinal tract

Oesophageal and gastric perforation are specific risks, with an incidence of approximately 1%.[45,155] Gastric perforation of the cardia can result from excessive traction by the surgical assistant. Perforation of the back wall of the oesophagus usually occurs during dissection of the posterior oesophagus. The anterior oesophageal wall is probably at greatest risk when a bougie is passed to calibrate the fundoplication or the oesophageal hiatus. All these injuries can be repaired by suturing either laparoscopically or by an open technique. Awareness that injury can occur enables surgeons to institute strategies that reduce the likelihood of their occurrence. Furthermore, injury is less likely with greater experience.

Mortality

Deaths have been reported following laparoscopic antireflux procedures. Causes include peritonitis secondary to duodenal perforation,[155] thrombosis of the superior mesenteric artery and the coeliac axis,[150] and infarction of the liver.[164] However, the overall mortality of laparoscopic antireflux surgery is probably less than 0.1%.

Avoiding complications following laparoscopic antireflux surgery and minimising their impact

To avoid or minimise complications following a laparoscopic antireflux procedure, a range of strategies should be considered and applied whenever possible. Most agree that the oesophageal hiatus should be narrowed or reinforced with sutures, irrespective of whether a hiatus hernia is present or not.[63] A barium swallow examination on the first or second postoperative day should be used to confirm that the fundoplication is in the correct position and that the stomach is entirely intra-abdominal. If there is any uncertainty endoscopic examination may clarify the situation. If the appearances are not acceptable, or if other problems such as severe dysphagia or excessive pain occur, then re-exploration should be performed, as early laparoscopic reintervention is associated with minimal morbidity and usually delays the patient's recovery by only a few days. Most complications requiring reintervention can be readily dealt with laparoscopically within a week of the original procedure.[43] Beyond this time, however, laparoscopic re-operation becomes difficult, and for this reason we have a relatively low threshold for laparoscopic re-exploration in the first postoperative week if early problems arise.

If complications become apparent at a later stage, laparoscopic re-operation may still be feasible if an experienced surgeon is available.[161] However, the likelihood of success is reduced in the intermediate period following the original procedure, and in this case waiting until scar tissue has matured (i.e. at least 3–6 months) simplifies subsequent dissection and increases the likelihood of completing the procedure laparoscopically.

Synthesis of the results from prospective randomised trials

The results of randomised trials can be assessed together to facilitate the development of guidelines for antireflux surgery (Box 13.2). Some of these will meet with wide acceptance as they support the current body of thought of the international surgical community. However, others are controversial, as they do not support the opinions of the majority of experts in the field.

Most surgeons performing surgery for reflux agree that the laparoscopic approach has been a major advance in surgical technique for antireflux surgery and that this has led to surgery becoming a more attractive management option. Controversy, however, will be raised by conclusions drawn about division of the short gastric blood vessels, and the place of partial fundoplications in the surgeon's armamentarium.

Box 13.2 • Evidence from prospective randomised trials for antireflux surgery

- Laparoscopic Nissen fundoplication is associated with fewer complications overall and a shorter convalescence than open Nissen fundoplication*
- The longer-term outcome following laparoscopic Nissen fundoplication is at least as good as the equivalent open surgical procedure*
- Division of the short gastric blood vessels does not improve the outcome following Nissen fundoplication*
- The incidence of recurrent reflux is similar following posterior partial fundoplication and Nissen fundoplication*
- The incidence of dysphagia is probably less following posterior partial fundoplication compared to Nissen fundoplication*
- The incidence of dysphagia and 'gas-related' complications is reduced following anterior partial fundoplication*
- Partial fundoplications are associated with fewer wind-related problems than total fundoplication*

*All statements are supported by evidence from more than one randomised trial.

✓✓ The longer-term outcomes from published trials that have investigated division of the short gastric vessels clearly support the position that this manoeuvre is not necessary for the creation of a satisfactory Nissen fundoplication and that it actually increases the likelihood of bloating side-effects.

Evidence has now emerged from the larger trials of posterior versus Nissen fundoplication that demonstrate advantages for the posterior partial fundoplication technique. Whilst the combined data from the reported trials can be confusing, with most of the smaller trials showing no advantages for posterior partial fundoplication, the larger trials do support the proposition that this technique reduces the risk of gas-related side-effects and might reduce the risk of post-fundoplication dysphagia. However, the magnitude of these differences is probably less than for anterior partial versus Nissen fundoplication. Six of eight randomised trials support the anterior partial fundoplication approach, although poor results were reported in one study.[99] However, longer-term results for the anterior partial fundoplication techniques do confirm its efficacy as an antireflux procedure.[71,103]

The large caseload of many surgical units performing laparoscopic surgery for gastro-oesophageal reflux continues to provide impetus for further trials of antireflux surgery techniques, and these are contributing to the rapidly expanding evidence base from which future conclusions will be drawn.

Endoscopic therapies for reflux

Over the last decade, endoscopic procedures for the treatment of reflux have emerged as they offer the potential for reflux control without abdominal wall incisions These approaches appeal to patients and physicians and can be broadly categorised into four types (Box 13.3). Three of these approaches aim to narrow the gastro-oesophageal junction by using radiofrequency energy,[165] injection of an inert substance[166] or endoscopic suturing.[167] Since the early 2000s these procedures have been applied with enthusiasm, particularly in the USA. However, none of these treatments apply the established principles that underpin the efficacy of antireflux surgery (see 'Mechanism of action of antireflux operations' section above) and the clinical outcomes were all predictably disappointing.[168] More recently, however, a fourth technique has been described that constructs an anterior partial fundoplication using a totally endoscopic (transoral) technique.[169] Because the latter approaches aim to fix the fundus of the stomach to a length of intra-abdominal oesophagus,

Box 13.3 • Endoscopic antireflux procedures

Procedures that narrow the gastro-oesophageal junction

Radiofrequency

- Stretta procedure

Polymer injection

- Enteryx
- Gatekeeper
- PMMA (Plexiglas microspheres)

'Suturing'

- EndoCinch
- NDO Plicator

Procedure that aims to create a partial fundoplication

- EsophyX endoluminal fundoplication procedure

first principles suggest that these approaches should be more successful, although the clinical reality has also been disappointing.

Radiofrequency

The Stretta procedure[165] used a purpose-built device to apply radiofrequency energy to the muscular layer of the oesophageal wall at the gastro-oeosophageal junction. The device comprised a 30-mm-diameter balloon, four 5.5-mm-long retractable stylet electrodes and a mucosal irrigation system. It was passed over an endoscopically placed guidewire and positioned at the gastro-oesophageal junction. The electrodes were deployed to puncture the oesophageal wall, and radiofrequency energy was applied to cauterise the oesophageal muscle. The Stretta procedure generated fibrosis in the muscle layer with the aim of tightening the gastro-oesophageal junction. In general, patients were only selected for this treatment if they had mild grades of reflux. Whilst short-term follow-up of case series suggested reduced reflux symptoms and reduced oesophageal acid exposure, the magnitude of the reduction in acid exposure was disappointing, and most patients continued to have abnormal reflux after treatment.[170] A randomised trial that compared the Stretta procedure with a sham endoscopy showed no differences at 6 months follow-up.[171] The trial demonstrated a large placebo effect in the sham controls, and this should be remembered when considering the outcomes of any antireflux therapy. The company that made the device closed in 2006.

Polymer injection

Polymer injection (and similar procedures) aimed to add bulk to the gastro-oesophageal junction, thereby narrowing it, to reduce reflux. The most popular of these procedures was Enteryx.[166] The procedure entailed endoscopic injection of 5–8 mL of a bioinert polymer into the plane between the circular and longitudinal muscle of the distal oesophagus, to create a ring of polymer just above the gastro-oesophageal junction. Initial reports suggested success rates of 70–80% at 12 months follow-up.[166] However, the results from a randomised sham-controlled trial were also unimpressive, with no difference in acid exposure (11.2% vs. 12.7%) at 3 months follow-up. This trial also demonstrated a significant placebo effect, with 41% of the sham-treated patients able to cease proton-pump inhibitor medication, compared to 68% of the treated group.[172] Unfortunately, there were also some catastrophic complications, including four deaths,[173,174] and the manufacturer withdrew the procedure. A similar product, the Gatekeeper reflux repair system, was also withdrawn from clinical use.[175]

Endoscopic suturing

EndoCinch

The EndoCinch (Bard Endoscopic Technologies, Murray Hill, NJ) procedure entailed the endoscopic placement of two 3-mm-deep sutures into adjoining gastric mucosal folds immediately below the gastro-oesophageal junction, to create pleats to narrow this region. The sutures were not deep enough to include the underlying muscle. Case series demonstrated improvements in symptoms and distal oesophageal acid exposure (15.4% to 8.7%).[176] However, as with the other endoscopic procedures, reflux was only cured in a minority, and 90% of sutures disappeared within 12 months.[177] In a randomised sham-controlled trial, oesophageal acid exposure was similar in the treated and sham groups, and the results of this trial did not compare well with the outcomes for laparoscopic antireflux surgery.[177]

NDO Plicator

The NDO Plicator (NDO Surgical, Mansfield, MA) represented the first attempt to perform a more 'surgical' procedure via a transoral approach. It used a flexible overtube that could be retroflexed in the stomach. A screw device penetrated and retracted the gastro-oesophageal junction, and a full-thickness plication of the cardia was fashioned to narrow the gastro-oesophageal junction. This was secured with a pre-tied pledgeted suture. For the first time, a sham-controlled trial[178] actually showed a significant reduction in oesophageal acid exposure (measured by ambulatory pH monitoring) from 10% to 7% at 3 months following treatment. However, acid exposure was not restored to normal in most patients, and the degree of improvement was certainly inferior to the 0–2.5% expected following laparoscopic fundoplication.[4,89] At 3 months follow-up, 50% of patients were able to cease proton-pump inhibitor medication compared to 25% of the sham-treated patients. Again, these results are inferior to those of laparoscopic antireflux surgery and it is likely that this procedure does not create a true fundoplication. The company making this device closed in 2008.

Endoscopic fundoplication

Unlike the previous procedures, the EsophyX (Endogastric Solutions, Washington) procedure aims to construct an actual fundoplication.[179] This procedure requires general anaesthesia and two operators. A standard endoscope is passed through the device (**Figs 13.13** and **13.14**) and both are passed transorally into the stomach. The endoscope is retroflexed for vision and a screw device anchors tissue at the gastro-oesophageal junction to retract it caudally. A plastic arm (tissue mould) then compresses the fundus against the side of the oesophagus, and polypropylene fasteners are passed between the oesophagus and the gastric fundus to anchor these structures. Multiple fasteners are applied to fashion a 200–300° anterior partial fundoplication.

Some cases series report promising short-term outcomes, with claimed success rates of 55–80% at up to 2 years follow-up,[179,180] but lower success rates for normalisation of oesophageal acid exposure.[179] In general, however, this procedure has been restricted to patients with milder degrees of reflux, i.e. no circumferential ulcerative oesophagitis, Barrett's oesophagus, hiatus hernia ≥3 cm or a body mass index >30. Whilst most patients recover uneventfully, significant complications have also been reported, including bleeding, pneumoperitoneum and oesophageal perforation. Cadière et al.[179] reported a series of 86 patients, followed for 12 months. Eighty-one per cent of patients were not using proton-pump inhibitor medication and 56% claimed cure of their reflux. Postoperative pH monitoring, however, revealed that only 37% of patients had a normal pH study following the EsophyX procedure. The results from this experience suggest that in some patients a fundoplication can be constructed, but perhaps not reliably. Other experience is also less than satisfactory. We recently reported a three-centre experience of 19 EsophyX procedures.[181] Only five patients were able to stop antireflux medication, whereas 10 underwent laparoscopic fundoplication within 12 months for a failed EsophyX procedure. Overall, the published literature suggests EsophyX is much less effective than any type of partial fundoplication,[4] and less than half of patients treated have objective evidence that reflux has been cured.

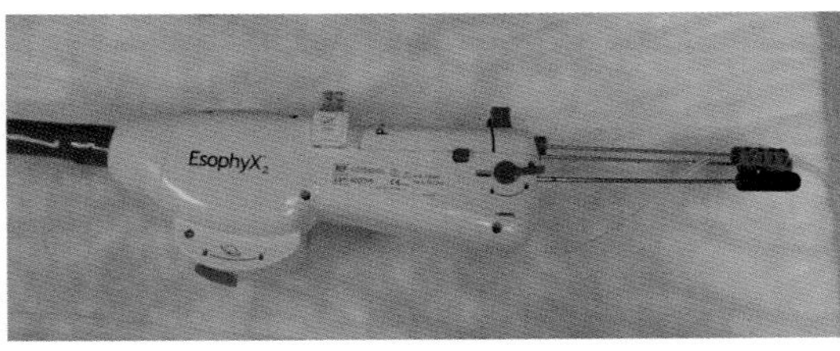

Figure 13.13 • Operating handle for the EsophyX device for endoluminal anterior partial fundoplication.

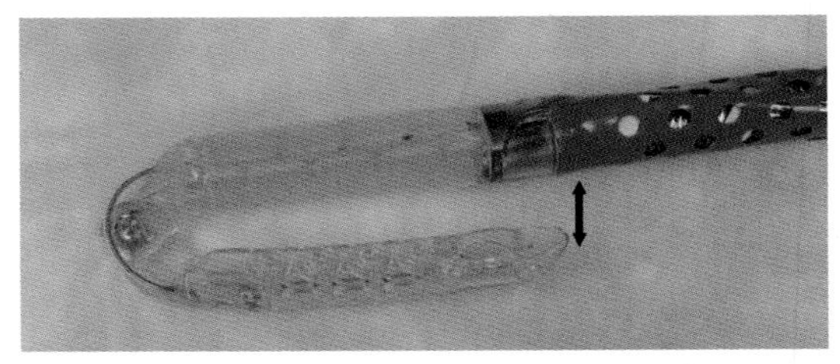

Figure 13.14 • Distal end of EsophyX device. The tip is sited within the stomach and the shaft in the distal oesophagus. The two components close together as indicated to allow the fasteners to be deployed.

A similar approach has also been pursued by Medigus (Omer, Israel), who developed a stapling endoscope for the construction of an anterior partial fundoplication.[182] However, clinical trial data are yet to be reported, and this device has not been commercialised. For now it still seems that a durable partial fundoplication cannot be reliably fashioned using an endoscopic approach. This could be because the endoscopic approaches are unable to repair a hiatus hernia and also fail to anchor the fundus to the diaphragm, both important steps for constructing a stable partial fundoplication.

Overview of endoscopic antireflux surgery

The newer procedures that aim to perform an anterior partial fundoplication appear to be based on more sound principles. However, the results remain disappointing, and this is probably because some key steps used routinely during antireflux surgery are still being ignored when undertaking this approach. It is hard to see how an endoscopic approach can be modified to include repair of a hiatus hernia or accurate anchorage of the fundoplication to the hiatal rim, and for these reasons endoscopic treatments are unlikely to offer a viable alternative to antireflux surgery, even in carefully selected subgroups of patients, in the near future.

Lessons can be learnt from the experience with failed endoscopic antireflux treatments. Before any new endoscopic or surgical treatment for reflux is made widely available, it should first be evaluated in well-designed clinical trials. An appropriate procedure must be as effective as a conventional fundoplication, it should apply the same principles that underpin an effective antireflux operation, and it should be equally safe or safer. Furthermore, surgeons will need to have an appropriate strategy to deal with patients who develop recurrent reflux after these procedures, and any procedure that makes a subsequent laparoscopic fundoplication procedure more difficult or more dangerous will be a problem, particularly if there is a substantial risk of the primary endoscopic procedure failing.

✔✔ None of the endoscopic approaches to the treatment of gastro-oesophageal reflux have achieved outcomes that are comparable to those of a surgical fundoplication, and some of the procedures that were initially applied enthusiastically have now been withdrawn from clinical use, either because of safety concerns or lack of efficacy, or both. For many of these procedures, this is not surprising, as the initial endoscopic procedures ignored the principles that underpin antireflux surgery, i.e. accentuation of the angle of His, and maintaining a close anatomical relationship between the fundus of the stomach and the intra-abdominal oesophagus.

Key points

- The treatment of reflux is usually incremental, commencing with various levels of medical measures. Surgery is reserved for patients with more severe disease, who either fail to respond adequately to medical treatment or who do not wish to take lifelong medication.
- It is apparent that a single management strategy is unlikely to be appropriate for all patients. Surgical therapy achieves better control of reflux in patients with moderate to severe reflux.
- Endoscopic findings and 24-hour pH studies have to be interpreted in the light of the patient's clinical presentation. A final recommendation for surgery must be based on all available clinical and objective information.
- Barrett's oesophagus alone is not an indication for antireflux surgery. Patients with Barrett's should be selected for surgery on the basis of their reflux symptoms and their response to medications, not simply because they have a columnar-lined oesophagus.
- The overwhelming majority of patients claim that the disadvantages of an antireflux operation (temporary dysphagia, early fullness, increased flatulence, and inability to belch and vomit) are far outweighed by the advantages of the operation.
- Endoscopy is a mandatory prerequisite before recommending antireflux surgery.
- The presence of weak peristaltic amplitudes or poor propagation of peristalsis is not a contraindication to antireflux surgery. Many surgeons recommend a tailored approach to patient selection by choosing a partial fundoplication in patients with poor peristalsis – there is no strong evidence to support this.
- Twenty-four-hour ambulatory pH monitoring is not sufficiently accurate to select patients for surgery, as up to 20% of patients who have oesophagitis and typical reflux symptoms would be unnecessarily excluded from antireflux surgery.
- Total fundoplications and partial fundoplications (whether anterior or posterior) probably all work in a similar fashion. No one procedure currently yields perfect results, i.e. 100% cure of reflux and no side-effects.
- The available evidence appears to support the view that the main difference in outcome between total and posterior fundoplication is in the wind-related problems.
- Reflux control is slightly better after total compared with anterior fundoplication, but this is offset by significantly less dysphagia, less epigastric bloating and better preservation of belching.
- The results of randomised trials of open versus laparoscopic surgery confirm advantages for the laparoscopic approach, albeit less dramatic than the advantages expected from the results of non-randomised studies.
- Most large series of laparoscopic procedures report the occurrence of paraoesophageal herniation following surgery, particularly in the immediate postoperative period. Routine hiatal repair has been shown to reduce the incidence by approximately 80%.
- None of the currently reported endoscopic procedures achieve the level of reflux control associated with fundoplication.

References

1. Watson DI, Lally CJ. Incidence of symptoms and use of medication for gastro-esophageal reflux in South Australia. World J Surg 2009;33:88–94.
2. Thompson WE, Heaton KW. Heartburn and globus in apparently healthy people. Can Med Assoc J 1982;126:46–8.
3. Lord RVN, Law MG, Ward RL, et al. Rising incidence of oesophageal adenocarcinoma in men in Australia. J Gastroenterol Hepatol 1998;13: 356–62.
4. Watson DI, Jamieson GG, Pike GK, et al. A prospective randomised double blind trial between laparoscopic Nissen fundoplication and anterior partial fundoplication. Br J Surg 1999;86:123–30.
   The first published randomised trial to compare an anterior partial fundoplication with the Nissen procedure.
5. Watson DI, Pike GK, Baigrie RJ, et al. Prospective double blind randomised trial of laparoscopic Nissen fundoplication with division and without division of short gastric vessels. Ann Surg 1997;226: 642–52.
   A randomised trial of 102 patients who underwent a total fundoplication with or without division of the short gastric vessels.
6. Ireland AC, Holloway RH, Toouli J, et al. Mechanisms underlying the antireflux action of fundoplication. Gut 1993;34:303–8.
7. Dent J. Australian clinical trials of omeprazole in the management of reflux oesophagitis. Digestion 1990;47:69–71.
8. Watson DI, Mathew G, Pike GK, et al. Comparison of anterior, posterior and total fundoplication using a viscera model. Dis Esophagus 1997;10:110–4.
9. Bate CM, Keeling PW, O'Morain C, et al. Comparison of omeprazole and cimetidine in reflux oesophagitis: symptomatic, endoscopic, and histological evaluations. Gut 1990;31:968–72.
10. Hetzel DJ, Dent J, Reed WD, et al. Healing and relapse of severe peptic esophagitis after treatment with omeprazole. Gastroenterology 1998;95:903–13.
11. Kuipers EJ, Lundell L, Klinkenberg-Knol EC, et al. Atrophic gastritis and *Helicobacter pylori* infection in patients with reflux esophagitis treated with omeprazole or fundoplication. N Engl J Med 1996;334:1018–22.
12. Driman DK, Wright C, Tougas G, et al. Omeprazole produces parietal cell hypertrophy and hyperplasia in humans. Dig Dis Sci 1996;41:2039–47.
13. Verlinden M. Review article: a role for gastrointestinal prokinetic agents in the treatment of reflux oesophagitis? Aliment Pharmacol Ther 1989;3:113–31.
14. Waring JP, Hunter JG, Oddsdottir M, et al. The preoperative evaluation of patients considered for laparoscopic antireflux surgery. Am J Gastroenterol 1995;90:35–8.
15. Francis DO, Goutte M, Slaughter JC, et al. Traditional reflux parameters and not impedance monitoring predict outcome after fundoplication in extraesophageal reflux. Laryngoscope 2011;121:1902–9.
16. Bischof G, Feil W, Riegler M, et al. Peptic esophageal stricture: is surgery still necessary? Wei Klin Wochenschr 1996;108:267–71.
17. Ratnasingam D, Irvine T, Thompson SK, et al. Laparoscopic antireflux surgery in patients with throat symptoms: a word of caution. World J Surg 2011;35:343–8.
18. Farrell TM, Smith CD, Metreveli RE, et al. Fundoplication provides effective and durable symptom relief in patients with Barrett's esophagus. Am J Surg 1999;178:18–21.
19. Ortiz EA, Martinez de Haro LF, Parrilla P, et al. Conservative treatment versus antireflux surgery in Barrett's oesophagus: long-term results of a prospective study. Br J Surg 1996;83:274–8.
20. Ortiz A, De Maro LT, Parrilla P, et al. 24-h pH monitoring is necessary to assess acid reflux suppression in patients with Barrett's oesophagus undergoing treatment with proton pump inhibitors. Br J Surg 1999;86:1472–4.
21. Sagar PM, Ackroyd R, Hosie KB, et al. Regression and progression of Barrett's oesophagus after antireflux surgery. Br J Surg 1995;82:806–10.
22. Gurski RR, Peters JH, Hagen JA, et al. Barrett's esophagus can and does regress after antireflux surgery: a study of prevalence and predictive features. J Am Coll Surg 2003;196:706–12.
23. Ackroyd R, Brown NJ, Davis MF, et al. Photodynamic therapy for dysplastic Barrett's oesophagus: a prospective, double blind, randomised, placebo controlled trial. Gut 2000;47:612–7.
24. Ackroyd R, Tam W, Schoeman M, et al. Prospective randomised controlled trial of argon plasma coagulation ablation versus endoscopic surveillance of Barrett's oesophagus in patients following antireflux surgery. Gastrointest Endosc 2004;59:1–7.
25. Goers TA, Leão P, Cassera MA, et al. Concomitant endoscopic radiofrequency ablation and laparoscopic reflux operative results in more effective and efficient treatment of Barrett esophagus. J Am Coll Surg 2011;213:486–92.
26. Bright T, Watson DI, Tam W, et al. Randomized trial of argon plasma coagulation vs. endoscopic surveillance for Barrett's oesophagus following antireflux surgery – late results. Ann Surg 2007;246: 1016–20.
27. Behar J, Sheahan DG, Biancani P. Medical and surgical management of reflux oesophagitis, a 38-month report on a prospective clinical trial. N Engl J Med 1975;293:263–8.

28. Spechler SJ. Comparison of medical and surgical therapy for complicated gastroesophageal reflux disease in veterans. N Engl J Med 1992;326:786–92.
The first large prospective randomised trial to compare medical with surgical therapy for gastro-oesophageal reflux.

29. Parrilla P, Martinez de Haro LF, Ortiz A, et al. Long-term results of a randomized prospective study comparing medical and surgical treatment of Barrett's esophagus. Ann Surg 2003;237:291–8.

30. Lundell L, Miettinen P, Myrvold HE, et al. Continued (5-year) followup of a randomized clinical study comparing antireflux surgery and omeprazole in gastroesophageal reflux disease. J Am Coll Surg 2001;192:172–81.

31. Lundell L, Miettinen P, Myrvold HE, et al. Long-term management of gastroesophageal reflux disease with omeprazole or open antireflux surgery: results of a prospective, randomized clinical trial. Eur J Gastroenterol Hepatol 2000;12:879–87.

32. Mehta S, Bennett J, Mahon D, et al. Prospective trial of laparoscopic Nissen fundoplication versus proton pump inhibitor therapy for gastroesophageal reflux disease: seven-year follow-up. J Gastrointest Surg 2006;10:1312–6.

33. Mahon D, Rhodes M, Decadt B, et al. Randomized clinical trial of laparoscopic Nissen fundoplication compared with proton-pump inhibitors for treatment of chronic gastro-oesophageal reflux. Br J Surg 2005;92:695–9.
The first randomised trial of proton-pump inhibitor versus laparoscopic antireflux surgery.

34. Anvari M, Allen C, Marshall J, et al. A randomized controlled trial of laparoscopic Nissen fundoplication versus proton pump inhibitors for treatment of patients with chronic gastroesophageal reflux disease: one-year follow-up. Surg Innov 2006;13:238–49.

35. Anvari M, Allen C, Marshall J, et al. A randomized controlled trial of laparoscopic Nissen fundoplication versus proton pump inhibitors for the treatment of patients with chronic gastroesophageal reflux disease (GERD): 3-year outcomes. Surg Endosc 2011;25:2547–54.

36. Goeree R, Hopkins R, Marshall JK, et al. Cost-utility of laparoscopic Nissen fundoplication versus proton pump inhibitors for chronic and controlled gastroesophageal reflux disease: a 3-year prospective randomized controlled trial and economic evaluation. Value Health 2011;14:263–73.

37. Lundell L, Attwood S, Ell C, et al. Comparing laparoscopic antireflux surgery with esomeprazole in the management of patients with chronic gastro-oesophageal reflux disease: a 3-year interim analysis of the LOTUS trial. Gut 2008;57:1207–13.
Largest randomised trial of medical versus surgical therapy for gastro-oesophageal reflux.

38. Attwood SE, Lundell L, Hatlebakk JG, et al. Medical or surgical management of GERD patients with Barrett's esophagus: the LOTUS trial 3-year experience. J Gastrointest Surg 2008;12:1646–54.

39. Lundell L, Miettinen P, Myrvold HE, et al. Comparison of outcomes twelve years after antireflux surgery or omeprazole maintenance therapy for reflux esophagitis. Clin Gastroenterol Hepatol 2009;7:1292–8.
Long-term results of a randomised trial of proton-pump inhibitor versus open antireflux surgery.

40. Spechler SJ, Lee E, Ahnen D, et al. Long-term outcome of medical and surgical therapies for gastroesophageal reflux disease. Follow-up of a randomized controlled trial. JAMA 2001;285:2331–8.
Longer-term follow-up from a randomised trial of medical versus surgical therapy.

41. Lundell L, Miettinen P, Myrvold HE, et al. Seven-year follow-up of a randomized clinical trial comparing proton-pump inhibition with surgical therapy for reflux oesophagitis. Br J Surg 2007;94:198–203.
Longer-term follow-up from a randomised trial of medical versus open surgical therapy.

42. Cookson R, Flood C, Koo B, et al. Short-term cost effectiveness and long-term cost analysis comparing laparoscopic Nissen fundoplication with proton-pump inhibitor maintenance for gastrooesophageal reflux disease. Br J Surg 2005;92:700–6.

43. Watson DI, Jamieson GG, Baigrie RJ, et al. Laparoscopic surgery for gastro-oesophageal reflux: beyond the learning curve. Br J Surg 1996;83:1284–7.

44. Ackroyd R, Watson DI, Games PA. Fizzy drinks following laparoscopic Nissen fundoplication: a cautionary tale of explosive consequences. Aust N Z J Surg 1999;69:887–8.

45. Gotley DC, Smithers BM, Rhodes M, et al. Laparoscopic Nissen fundoplication – 200 consecutive cases. Gut 1996;38:487–91.

46. Trus TL, Laycock WS, Branum G, et al. Intermediate follow-up of laparoscopic antireflux surgery. Am J Surg 1996;171:32–5.

47. Watson DI, Davies N, Devitt PG, et al. Importance of dissection of the hernial sac in laparoscopic surgery for very large hiatus hernias. Arch Surg 1999;134:1069–73.

48. Kauer WKH, Peters JH, DeMeester TR, et al. A tailored approach to antireflux surgery. J Thorac Cardiovasc Surg 1995;110:141–7.

49. Little AG. Gastro-oesophageal reflux and oesophageal motility diseases; who should perform antireflux surgery? Ann Chir Gynaecol 1995;84:103–5.

50. Beckingham IJ, Cariem AK, Bornman PC, et al. Oesophageal dysmotility is not associated with poor outcome after laparoscopic Nissen fundoplication. Br J Surg 1998;85:1290–3.

51. Baigrie RJ, Watson DI, Myers JC, et al. The outcome of laparoscopic Nissen fundoplication in patients with disordered pre-operative peristalsis. Gut 1997;40:381–5.

52. Rydberg L, Ruth M, Abrahamsson H, et al. Tailoring antireflux surgery: a randomized clinical trial. World J Surg 1999;23:612–8.

53. Chrysos E, Tsiaoussis J, Zoras OJ, et al. Laparoscopic surgery for gastroesophageal reflux disease patients with impaired esophageal peristalsis: total or partial fundoplication? J Am Coll Surg 2003;197:8–15.

54. Booth MI, Stratford J, Jones L, et al. Randomized clinical trial of laparoscopic total (Nissen) versus posterior partial (Toupet) fundoplication for gastro-oesophageal reflux disease based on preoperative oesophageal manometry. Br J Surg 2008;95(1):57–63.

55. Strate U, Emmermann A, Fibbe C, et al. Laparoscopic fundoplication: Nissen versus Toupet two-year outcome of a prospective randomized study of 200 patients regarding preoperative esophageal motility. Surg Endosc 2007;22:21–30.

56. Watson DI, Jamieson GG, Bessell JR, et al. Laparoscopic fundoplication in patients with an aperistaltic esophagus and gastroesophageal reflux. Dis Esophagus 2006;19:94–8.

57. Watson DI, Mathew G, Pike GK, et al. Efficacy of anterior, posterior and total fundoplication in an experimental model. Br J Surg 1998;85:1006–9.

58. Collard JM, De Koninck XJ, Otte JB, et al. Intrathoracic Nissen fundoplication: long-term clinical and pH-monitoring evaluation. Ann Thorac Surg 1991;51:34–8.

59. Watson A, Jenkinson LR, Ball CS, et al. A more physiological alternative to total fundoplication for the surgical correction of resistant gastro-oesophageal reflux. Br J Surg 1991;78:1088–94.

60. Watson DI, Baigrie RJ, Jamieson GG. A learning curve for laparoscopic fundoplication. Definable, avoidable, or a waste of time. Ann Surg 1996;224:198–203.

61. Nissen R. Eine einfache operation zur beeinflussung der refluxoesophagitis. Schweiz Med Wochenschr 1956;86:590–2.

62. DeMeester TR, Bonavina L, Albertucci M. Nissen fundoplication for gastroesophageal reflux disease. Evaluation of primary repair in 100 consecutive patients. Ann Surg 1986;204:9–20.

63. Watson DI, Jamieson GG, Devitt PG, et al. Paraoesophageal hiatus hernia: an important complication of laparoscopic Nissen fundoplication. Br J Surg 1995;82:521–3.

64. Donahue PE, Bombeck CT. The modified Nissen fundoplication – reflux prevention without gas bloat. Chir Gastroent 1977;11:15–27.

65. Rossetti M, Hell K. Fundoplication for the treatment of gastroesophageal reflux in hiatal hernia. World J Surg 1977;1:439–44.

66. Toupet A. Technique d'oesophago-gastroplastie avec phrenogastropexie appliquee dans la cure radicale des hernies hiatales et comme complement de l'operation d'Heller dans les cardiospasmes. Med Acad Chir 1963;89:374–9.

67. Lind JF, Burns CM, MacDougal JT. 'Physiological' repair for hiatus hernia – manometric study. Arch Surg 1965;91:233–7.

68. Belsey R. Mark IV, repair of hiatal hernia by the trans thoracic approach. World J Surg 1977;1:475–81.

69. Nguyen NT, Schauer PR, Hutson W, et al. Preliminary results of thoracoscopic Belsey Mark IV antireflux procedure. Surg Laparosc Endosc 1998;8:185–8.

70. Dor J, Himbert P, Paoli JM, et al. Treatment of reflux by the so-called modified Heller–Nissen technique. Presse Med 1967;75:2563–9.

71. Ludemann R, Watson DI, Game PA, et al. Laparoscopic total versus anterior 180 degree fundoplication – five year follow-up of a prospective randomized trial. Br J Surg 2005;92:240–3.

72. Watson DI, Jamieson GG, Lally C, et al. Multicentre prospective double blind randomized trial of laparoscopic Nissen versus anterior 90 degree partial fundoplication. Arch Surg 2004;139:1160–7.
Early outcomes from a multicentre randomised trial of anterior 90° vs. Nissen fundoplication.

73. Spence GM, Watson DI, Jamieson GG, et al. Single centre prospective randomized trial of laparoscopic Nissen versus anterior 90 degree partial fundoplication. J Gastrointest Surg 2006;10:698–750.

74. Cai W, Watson DI, Lally CJ, et al. Ten-year clinical outcome of a prospective randomized clinical trial of laparoscopic Nissen versus anterior 180° partial fundoplication. Br J Surg 2008;95:1501–5.
Longer-term follow-up from a randomised trial of anterior versus Nissen fundoplication.

75. Nijjar RS, Watson DI, Jamieson GG, et al. Five year follow-up of a multicentre double blind randomized clinical trial of laparoscopic Nissen vs. anterior 90° partial fundoplication. Arch Surg 2010;145:552–7.

76. Hill LD. An effective operation for hiatal hernia: an eight year appraisal. Ann Surg 1967;166:681–92.

77. Aye RW, Hill LD, Kraemer SJM, et al. Early results with the laparoscopic Hill repair. Am J Surg 1994;167:542–6.

78. Jobe BA, Horvath KD, Swanstrom LL. Postoperative function following laparoscopic Collis gastroplasty for shortened esophagus. Arch Surg 1998;133:867–74.

79. Swanstrom LL, Marcus DR, Galloway GQ. Laparoscopic Collis gastroplasty is the treatment of choice for the shortened esophagus. Am J Surg 1996;171:477–81.

80. Johnson AB, Oddsdottir M, Hunter JG. Laparoscopic Collis gastroplasty and Nissen fundoplication. A new technique for the management of esophageal foreshortening. Surg Endosc 1998;12:1055–60.

81. Bonavina L, DeMeester T, Fockens P, et al. Laparoscopic sphincter augmentation device eliminates reflux symptoms and normalizes esophageal acid exposure: one- and 2-year results of a feasibility trial. Ann Surg 2010;252:857–62.

82. Lipham JC, Demeester TR, Ganz RA, et al. The LINX® reflux management system: confirmed safety and efficacy now at 4 years. Surg Endosc 2012;26(10):2944–2949.

83. Rodriguez L, Rodriguez P, Gomez B, et al. Electrical stimulation therapy (EST) of the lower esophageal sphincter (LES) is successful in treating GERD in proton pump inhibitors (PPI) incomplete responders – post-hoc analysis of open-label prospective trial. Gastroenterology 2012;142(5):S-584–5.

84. DeMeester TR, Johnson LF, Kent AH. Evaluation of current operations for the prevention of gastro-esophageal reflux. Ann Surg 1974;180:511–25.

85. Thor KBA, Silander T. A long-term randomized prospective trial of the Nissen procedure versus a modified Toupet technique. Ann Surg 1989;210:719–24.

86. Walker SJ, Holt S, Sanderson CJ, et al. Comparison of Nissen total and Lind partial transabdominal fundoplication in the treatment of gastro-oesophageal reflux. Br J Surg 1992;79:410–4.

87. Laws HL, Clements RH, Swillies CM. A randomized, prospective comparison of the Nissen versus the Toupet fundoplication for gastroesophageal reflux disease. Ann Surg 1997;225:647–54.

88. Koch OO, Kaindlstorfer A, Antoniou SA, et al. Laparoscopic Nissen versus Toupet fundoplication: objective and subjective results of a prospective randomized trial. Surg Endosc 2012;26(2): 413–22.

89. Lundell L, Abrahamsson H, Ruth M, et al. Lower esophageal sphincter characteristics and esophageal acid exposure following partial or 360° fundoplication: results of a prospective, randomized clinical study. World J Surg 1991;15:115–21.

90. Lundell L, Abrahamsson H, Ruth M, et al. Long-term results of a prospective randomized comparison of total fundic wrap (Nissen–Rossetti) or semifundoplication (Toupet) for gastro-oesophageal reflux. Br J Surg 1996;83:830–5.

91. Mardani J, Lundell L, Engström C. Total or posterior partial fundoplication in the treatment of GERD: results of a randomized trial after 2 decades of follow-up. Ann Surg 2011;253:875–8.
Longer-term follow-up from a randomised trial of Nissen versus posterior partial fundoplication.

92. Zornig C, Strate U, Fibbe C, et al. Nissen vs. Toupet laparoscopic fundoplication. Surg Endosc 2002;16:758–66.

93. Guérin E, Bétroune K, Closset J, et al. Nissen versus Toupet fundoplication: results of a randomized and multicenter trial. Surg Endosc 2007;21: 1985–90.

94. Khan MA, Smythe A, Globe J, et al. Randomized controlled trial of laparoscopic Nissen versus Lind fundoplication for gastro-oesophageal reflux disease. Scand J Gastroenterol 2009;44:269–75.

95. Shaw JM, Bornman PC, Callanan MD, et al. Long-term outcome of laparoscopic Nissen and laparoscopic Toupet fundoplication for gastroesophageal reflux disease: a prospective, randomized trial. Surg Endosc 2010;24:924–32.

96. Baigrie RJ, Cullis SN, Ndhluni AJ, et al. Randomized double-blind trial of laparoscopic Nissen fundoplication versus anterior partial fundoplication. Br J Surg 2005;92:819–23.
A large randomised trial of anterior versus Nissen fundoplication.

97. Cao Z, Cai W, Qin M, et al. Randomized clinical trial of laparoscopic anterior 180° partial versus 360° Nissen fundoplication: 5-year results. Dis Esophagus 2012;25(2):114–20.

98. Raue W, Ordemann J, Jacobi CA, et al. Nissen versus Dor fundoplication for treatment of gastroesophageal reflux disease: a blinded randomized clinical trial. Dig Surg 2011;28:80–6.

99. Hagedorn C, Jonson C, Lonroth H, et al. Efficacy of an anterior as compared with a posterior laparoscopic partial fundoplication: results of a randomized, controlled clinical trial. Ann Surg 2003;238:189–96.

100. Engström C, Lönroth H, Mardani J, et al. An anterior or posterior approach to partial fundoplication? Long-term results of a randomized trial. World J Surg 2007;31:1221–5.

101. Engström C, Ruth M, Lönroth H, et al. Manometric characteristics of the gastroesophageal junction after anterior versus posterior partial fundoplication. Dis Esophagus 2005;18:31–6.

102. Khan M, Smythe A, Globe J, et al. Randomized controlled trial of laparoscopic anterior versus posterior fundoplication for gastro-oesophageal reflux disease. Aust N Z J Surg 2010;80:500–5.

103. Chen Z, Thompson SK, Jamieson GG, et al. Anterior 180 degree partial fundoplication – a 16 year experience with 548 patients. J Am Coll Surg 2011;212:827–34.

104. Hunter JG, Swanstrom L, Waring JP. Dysphagia after laparoscopic antireflux surgery. The impact of operative technique. Ann Surg 1996;224:51–7.

105. Dallemagne B, Weerts JM, Jehaes C, et al. Causes of failures of laparoscopic antireflux operations. Surg Endosc 1996;10:305–10.

106. Luostarinen M, Koskinen M, Reinikainen P, et al. Two antireflux operations: floppy versus standard Nissen fundoplication. Ann Med 1995;27:199–205.

107. Luostarinen ME, Isolauri JO. Randomized trial to study the effect of fundic mobilization on long-term results of Nissen fundoplication. Br J Surg 1999;86:614–8.

108. O'Boyle CJ, Watson DI, Jamieson GG, et al. Division of short gastric vessels at laparoscopic Nissen fundoplication – a prospective double blind randomized trial with five year follow-up. Ann Surg 2002;235:165–70.

109. Yang H, Watson DI, Lally CJ, et al. Randomized trial of division versus non-division of the short gastric vessels during laparoscopic Nissen fundoplication – 10 year outcomes. Ann Surg 2008;247:38–42.

Long-term follow-up from a randomised trial of Nissen fundoplication with or without division of the short gastric blood vessels.

110. Blomqvist A, Dalenback J, Hagedorn C, et al. Impact of complete gastric fundus mobilization on outcome after laparoscopic total fundoplication. J Gastrointest Surg 2000;4:493–500.

111. Mardani J, Lundell L, Lönroth H, et al. Ten-year results of a randomized clinical trial of laparoscopic total fundoplication with or without division of the short gastric vessels. Br J Surg 2009;96:61–5.

112. Engström C, Jamieson GG, Devitt PG, et al. Meta-analysis of two randomized controlled trials to identify long-term symptoms after division of short gastric vessels during Nissen fundoplication. Br J Surg 2011;98:1063–7.

Meta-analysis of original data from two randomised trials of division versus no division of the short gastric vessels during Nissen fundoplication. Vessel division is associated with significantly more abdominal bloating symptoms.

113. Farah JF, Grande JC, Goldenberg A, et al. Randomized trial of total fundoplication and fundal mobilization with or without division of short gastric vessels: a short-term clinical evaluation. Acta Cir Bras 2007;22:422–9.

114. Kösek V, Wykypiel H, Weiss H, et al. Division of the short gastric vessels during laparoscopic Nissen fundoplication: clinical and functional outcome during long-term follow-up in a prospectively randomized trial. Surg Endosc 2009;23:2208–13.

115. Chrysos E, Tzortzinis A, Tsiaoussis J, et al. Prospective randomized trial comparing Nissen to Nissen–Rossetti technique for laparoscopic fundoplication. Am J Surg 2001;182:215–21.

116. Geagea T. Laparoscopic Nissen's fundoplication: preliminary report on ten cases. Surg Endosc 1991;5:170–3.

117. Dallemagne B, Weerts JM, Jehaes C, et al. Laparoscopic Nissen fundoplication: preliminary report. Surg Laparosc Endosc 1991;1:138–43.

118. Kelly J, Watson DI, Chin K, et al. Laparoscopic Nissen fundoplication – clinical outcomes at 10 years. J Am Coll Surg 2007;205:570–5.

119. Cowgill SM, Gillman R, Kraemer E, et al. Ten-year follow up after laparoscopic Nissen fundoplication for gastroesophageal reflux disease. Am Surg 2007;73:748–52.

120. Luostarinen M, Isolauri J, Laitinen J, et al. Fate of Nissen fundoplication after 20 years. A clinical, endoscopical, and functional analysis. Gut 1993;34:1015–20.

121. Watson DI, Chan ASL, Myers JC, et al. Illness behaviour influences the outcome of laparoscopic antireflux surgery. J Am Coll Surg 1997;184:44–8.

122. Rattner DW, Brooks DC. Patient satisfaction following laparoscopic and open antireflux surgery. Arch Surg 1995;130:289–94.

123. Peters JH, Heimbucher J, Kauer WKH, et al. Clinical and physiological comparison of laparoscopic and open Nissen fundoplication. J Am Coll Surg 1995;180:385–93.

124. Laine S, Rantala A, Gullichsen R, et al. Laparoscopic vs conventional Nissen fundoplication. A prospective randomized study. Surg Endosc 1997;11:441–4.

125. Franzen T, Anderberg B, Tibbling L, et al. A report from a randomized study of open and laparoscopic 360° fundoplication. Surg Endosc 1996;10:582 (Abstract).

126. Heikkinen T-J, Haukipuro K, Koivukangas P, et al. Comparison of costs between laparoscopic and open Nissen fundoplication: a prospective randomized study with a 3-month follow-up. J Am Coll Surg 1999;188:368–76.

127. Perttila J, Salo M, Ovaska J, et al. Immune response after laparoscopic and conventional Nissen fundoplication. Eur J Surg 1999;165:21–8.

128. Chrysos E, Tsiaoussis J, Athanasakis E, et al. Laparoscopic vs open approach for Nissen fundoplication. Surg Endosc 2002;16:1679–84.

129. Bais JE, Bartelsman JFWM, Bonjer HJ, et al. Laparoscopic or conventional Nissen fundoplication for gastro-oesophageal reflux disease: randomised clinical trial. Lancet 2000;355:170–4.

130. Luostarinen M, Vurtanen J, Koskinen M, et al. Dysphagia and oesophageal clearance after laparoscopic versus open Nissen fundoplication. A randomized, prospective trial. Scand J Gastroenterol 2001;36:565–71.

131. Nilsson G, Larsson S, Johnsson F. Randomized clinical trial of laparoscopic versus open fundoplication: blind evaluation of recovery and discharge period. Br J Surg 2000;87:873–8.

132. Håkanson BS, Thor KB, Thorell A, et al. Open vs laparoscopic partial posterior fundoplication. A prospective randomized trial. Surg Endosc 2007;21:289–98.

133. Draaisma WA, Rijnhart-de Jong HG, Broeders IA, et al. Five-year subjective and objective results of laparoscopic and conventional Nissen fundoplication: a randomized trial. Ann Surg 2006;244:34–41.

134. Draaisma WA, Buskens E, Bais JE, et al. Randomized clinical trial and follow-up study of cost-effectiveness of laparoscopic versus conventional Nissen fundoplication. Br J Surg 2006;93:690–7.

135. Franzén T, Anderberg B, Wirén M, et al. Long-term outcome is worse after laparoscopic than after conventional Nissen fundoplication. Scand J Gastroenterol 2005;40:1261–8.

136. Nilsson G, Wenner J, Larsson S, et al. Randomized clinical trial of laparoscopic versus open fundoplication for gastro-oesophageal reflux. Br J Surg 2004;91:552–9.

137. Salminen PT, Hiekkanen HI, Rantala AP, et al. Fundoplication: a prospective randomized study with an 11-year follow-up. Ann Surg 2007;246:201–6.
Long-term follow-up from a randomised trial of laparoscopic versus open Nissen fundoplication.

138. Ackroyd R, Watson DI, Majeed AW, et al. Randomized clinical trial of laparoscopic versus open fundoplication for gastro-oesophageal reflux disease. Br J Surg 2004;91:975–82.

139. Broeders JA, Rijnhart-de Jong HG, Draaisma WA, et al. Ten-year outcome of laparoscopic and conventional Nissen fundoplication: randomized clinical trial. Ann Surg 2009;250:698–706.
Long-term follow-up from a randomised trial of laparoscopic versus open Nissen fundoplication demonstrating less surgical reintervention following laparoscopic surgery.

140. Salminen P, Hurme S, Ovaska J. Fifteen-year outcome of laparoscopic and open Nissen fundoplication: a randomized clinical trial. Ann Thorac Surg 2012;93(1):228–33.

141. Bloechle C, Mann O, Gawad KA, et al. Gastrooesophageal reflux disease. Lancet 2000;356:69.

142. deBeaux AC, Watson DI, Jamieson GG. Gastrooesophageal reflux disease. Lancet 2000;356:71–2.

143. Watson DI, Mitchell PC, Game PA, et al. Pneumothorax during laparoscopic dissection of the oesophageal hiatus. Aust N Z J Surg 1996;66:711–2.

144. Stallard N. Pneumomediastinum during laparoscopic Nissen fundoplication. Anaesthesia 1995;50:667–8.

145. Jamieson GG, Watson DI, Britten-Jones R, et al. Laparoscopic Nissen fundoplication. Ann Surg 1994;220:137–45.

146. Munro W, Brancatisano R, Adams IP, et al. Complications of laparoscopic fundoplication: the first 100 patients. Surg Laparosc Endosc 1996;6:421–3.

147. Baigrie RJ, Watson DI, Game PA, et al. Vascular perils during laparoscopic dissection of the oesophageal hiatus. Br J Surg 1997;84:556–7.

148. Johansson B, Glise H, Hallerback B. Thoracic herniation and intrathoracic gastric perforation after laparoscopic fundoplication. Surg Endosc 1995;9:917–8.

149. Watson DI, Jamieson GG, Mitchell PC, et al. Stenosis of the esophageal hiatus following laparoscopic fundoplication. Arch Surg 1995;130:1014–6.

150. Mitchell PC, Jamieson GG. Coeliac axis and mesenteric arterial thrombosis following laparoscopic Nissen fundoplication. Aust N Z J Surg 1994;64:728–30.

151. Medina LT, Vientimilla R, Williams MD, et al. Laparoscopic fundoplication. J Laparoendosc Surg 1996;6:219–26.

152. Schauer PR, Meyers WC, Eubanks S, et al. Mechanisms of gastric and esophageal perforations during laparoscopic Nissen fundoplication. Ann Surg 1996;223:43–52.

153. Swanstrom LL, Pennings JL. Safe laparoscopic dissection of the gastroesophageal junction. Am J Surg 1995;169:507–11.

154. Collet D, Cadiere GB. Conversions and complications of laparoscopic treatment of gastroesophageal reflux disease. Am J Surg 1995;169:622–6.

155. Hinder RA, Filipi CJ, Wetscher G, et al. Laparoscopic Nissen fundoplication is an effective treatment for gastroesophageal reflux disease. Ann Surg 1994;220:472–83.

156. Firoozmand E, Ritter M, Cohen R, et al. Ventricular laceration and cardiac tamponade during laparoscopic Nissen fundoplication. Surg Laparosc Endosc 1996;6:394–7.

157. Viste A, Horn A, Lund-Tonnessen S. Reactive pleuropericarditis following laparoscopic fundoplication. Surg Laparosc Endosc 1997;7:206–8.

158. Viste A, Vindenes H, Gjerde S. Herniation of the stomach and necrotizing chest wall infection following laparoscopic Nissen fundoplication. Surg Endosc 1997;11:1029–31.

159. Wetscher GJ, Glaser K, Wieschemeyer T, et al. Tailored antireflux surgery for gastroesophageal reflux disease: effectiveness and risk of post-operative dysphagia. World J Surg 1997;21:605–10.

160. Collard JM, Romagnoli R, Kestens PJ. Reoperation for unsatisfactory outcome after laparoscopic antireflux surgery. Dis Esophagus 1996;9:56–62.

161. Watson DI, Jamieson GG, Game PA, et al. Laparoscopic reoperation following failed antireflux surgery. Br J Surg 1999;86:98–101.

162. McKenzie T, Esmore D, Tulloh B. Haemorrhage from aortic wall granuloma following laparoscopic Nissen fundoplication. Aust N Z J Surg 1997;67:815–6.

163. Farlo J, Thawgathurai D, Mikhail M, et al. Cardiac tamponade during laparoscopic Nissen fundoplication. Eur J Anaesthesiol 1998;15:246–7.

164. Schorr RT. Laparoscopic upper abdominal operations and mesenteric infarction. J Laparoendosc Surg 1995;5:389–91.

165. Torquati A, Houston HL, Kaiser J, et al. Long-term follow-up study of the Stretta procedure for the treatment of gastroesophageal reflux disease. Surg Endosc 2004;18:1475–9.

166. Johnson DA, Ganz R, Aisenberg J, et al. Endoscopic implantation of enteryx for treatment of GERD: 12-month results of a prospective, multicenter trial. Am J Gastroenterol 2003;98:1921–30.

167. Tam WC, Holloway RH, Dent J, et al. Impact of endoscopic suturing of the gastroesophageal

junction on lower esophageal sphincter function and gastroesophageal reflux in patients with reflux disease. Am J Gastroenterol 2004;99:195–202.

168. Hogan WJ. Clinical trials evaluating endoscopic GERD treatments: is it time for a moratorium on the clinical use of these procedures? Am J Gastroenterol 2006;101:437–9.

169. Cadière GB, Rajan A, Rqibate M, et al. Endoluminal fundoplication (ELF) – evolution of EsophyX, a new surgical device for transoral surgery. Minim Invasive Ther Allied Technol 2006;15:348–55.

170. Triadafilopoulos G, DiBaise JK, Nostrant TT, et al. The Stretta procedure for the treatment of GERD: 6 and 12 month follow-up of the U.S. open label trial. Gastrointest Endosc 2002;55:149–56.

171. Corley DA, Katz P, Wo JM, et al. Improvement of gastresophageal reflux symptoms after radiofrequency energy: a randomized, sham-controlled trial. Gastroentrology 2003;125:668–76.

A randomised trial of sham endoscopy versus endoscopic application of radiofrequency energy to the gastro-oesophageal junction.

172. Devière J, Costamagna G, Neuhaus H, et al. Nonresorbable copolymer implantation for gastroesophageal reflux disease: a randomized sham-controlled multicenter trial. Gastroenterology 2005;128:532–40.

173. Noh KW, Loeb DS, Stockland A, et al. Pneumomediastinum following Enteryx injection for the treatment of gastroesophageal reflux disease. Am J Gastroenterol 2005;100:723–6.

174. Tintillier M, Chaput A, Kirch L, et al. Esophageal abscess complicating endoscopic treatment of refractory gastroesophageal reflux disease by Enteryx injection: a first case report. Am J Gastroenterol 2004;99:1856–8.

175. Fockens P, Bruno MJ, Gabbrielli A, et al. Endoscopic augmentation of the lower esophageal sphincter for the treatment of gastroesophageal reflux disease: multicenter study of the Gatekeeper Reflux Repair System. Endoscopy 2004;36:682–9.

176. Abou-Rebyeh H, Hoepffner N, Rösch T, et al. Long-term failure of endoscopic suturing in the treatment of gastroesophageal reflux: a prospective follow-up study. Endoscopy 2005;37:213–6.

177. Schwartz MP, Wellink H, Gooszen HG, et al. Endoscopic gastroplication for the treatment of gastro-oesophageal reflux disease: a randomised, sham-controlled trial. Gut 2007;56:20–8.

A randomised trial of sham endoscopy versus endoscopic mucosal suturing at the gastro-oesophageal junction.

178. Rothstein R, Filipi C, Caca K, et al. Endoscopic full-thickness plication for the treatment of gastroesophageal reflux disease: a randomized, sham-controlled trial. Gastroenterology 2006;131:704–12.

A randomised trial of sham endoscopy versus endoscopic full-thickness plication of the gastro-oesophageal junction.

179. Cadière GB, Buset M, Muls V, et al. Antireflux transoral incisionless fundoplication using EsophyX: 12-month results of a prospective multicenter study. World J Surg 2008;32:1676–88.

180. Cadière GB, Van Sante N, Graves JE, et al. Two-year results of a feasibility study on antireflux transoral incisionless fundoplication using EsophyX. Surg Endosc 2009;23:957–64.

181. Hoppo T, Immanuel A, Schuchert M, et al. Transoral incisionless fundoplication 2.0 procedure using EsophyX for gastroesophageal reflux disease. J Gastrointest Surg 2010;14:1895–901.

182. Kauer WK, Roy-Shapira A, Watson D, et al. Preclinical trial of a modified gastroscope that performs a true anterior fundoplication for the endoluminal treatment of gastroesophageal reflux disease. Surg Endosc 2009;23:2728–31.

14

Treatment of the complications of gastro-oesophageal reflux disease and failed gastro-oesophageal surgery

Robert Mason

Introduction

Gastro-oesophageal reflux affects up to a quarter of the UK population on a regular basis. Most will not seek medical help and self-medicate. Of those who do see a doctor the vast majority will be well controlled by medical therapy – invariably proton-pump inhibitors. It has been calculated that only 1% of patients with gastro-oesophageal reflux disease (GORD) will develop complications of the reflux. These complications are consequent on damage to the mucosa resulting in erosive oesophagitis with, rarely, a peptic oesophageal ulcer, a peptic stricture or Barrett's oesophagus (see Chapter 15). The vast majority of sufferers of GORD have non-erosive reflux disease (NERD) and never develop either erosive oesophagitis or Barrett's oesophagus.[1]

There are two main treatments for GORD. These are medical therapy with proton-pump inhibitors or surgical therapy based on either a total or partial fundoplication. Comparative studies suggest there is little to choose between the two therapeutic arms in either the control of symptoms or prevention of complications. This is well documented in the results of the multicentre LOTUS trial, comparing esomeprazole and laparoscopic antireflux surgery, with good control of symptoms and microscopic oesophagitis in over 85% of cases in both arms out to 5 years.[2,3]

In recent years there has been a significant increase in the use of fundoplication based on the laparoscopic approach. This is claimed to be a one-off long-term treatment that removes the need for expensive long-term ingestion of proton-pump inhibitors. However, it is recognised that with time the use of these drugs does increase in patients who have had a successful initial surgical outcome, reaching 25% at 10 years.[4,5]

In the USA, the number of antireflux operations increased by 260% between 1993 and 2000 but decreased by 40% between 2000 and 2006.[6] Similar trends have been seen in Europe, particularly in Sweden. The reasons are unclear but may reflect disappointing long-term results for surgery, with a significant proportion of patients back on medical therapy as described above and recognition of the complications, which although rare can have a serious impact on a young, previously fit patient.

Gastro-oesophageal reflux results from failure of the lower oesophageal sphincter to either provide a mechanical barrier (volume/supine refluxers) or which relaxes inappropriately, usually secondary to gaseous distension of the gastric fundus (upright refluxers). These differences can have an effect on the outcome of antireflux surgery whereas defective oesophageal motility, other than undiagnosed achalasia, does not.[7,8]

Complications of GORD

Complications arise from damage caused by the refluxate to the squamous mucosa of the oesophagus. The contents of the refluxate may include any combination of acid and/or 'bile' (duodenogastric contents). Chronic exposure of the oesophageal mucosa to this fluid in patients with an intact stomach causes inflammation, can result in erosive oesophagitis with ulceration and subsequent peptic stricture, and in some results in metaplastic change and the development of Barrett's oesophagus. It appears that acid alone is the principal factor in determining the severity of oesophagitis, whereas in patients experiencing symptoms who are on long-term proton-pump inhibitors weak acid or bile is implicated.[9,10]

Short oesophagus

A complication of chronic reflux that promotes much debate among upper gastrointestinal (GI) surgeons is the short oesophagus. This is claimed to be a complication of prolonged reflux damage and fibrosis, and is manifested by an inability to mobilise the oesophagogastric junction at surgery to allow 2–3 cm of oesophagus below the hiatus. Whether this exists in reality is contentious. In this author's experience it is very rare, although it may have been more prevalent 30–40 years ago in the pre-antisecretory era. By opening the hiatus and fully mobilising the oesophagus, the oesophagus can always be brought down without tension.

Those who recognise the complication advocate a Collis gastroplasty to lengthen the oesophagus through either an open abdominal or laparoscopic approach. It may provide a better outcome in such patients when compared with fundoplication alone.[11] In this procedure a 40 F bougie is passed into the stomach and kept on the lesser curve. A neo-oesophagus is created using a circular and linear cutting stapler and a loose wrap performed using the mobilised stomach (**Fig. 14.1**). This has the potential to leave a tube of acid-secreting stomach above the wrap, with consequent complications of bleeding, ulceration and stenosis. It has been used in revisional surgery, where mobilisation of the gastro-oesophageal junction below the diaphragm has proven difficult. In experienced hands the results are reported to be good.[12]

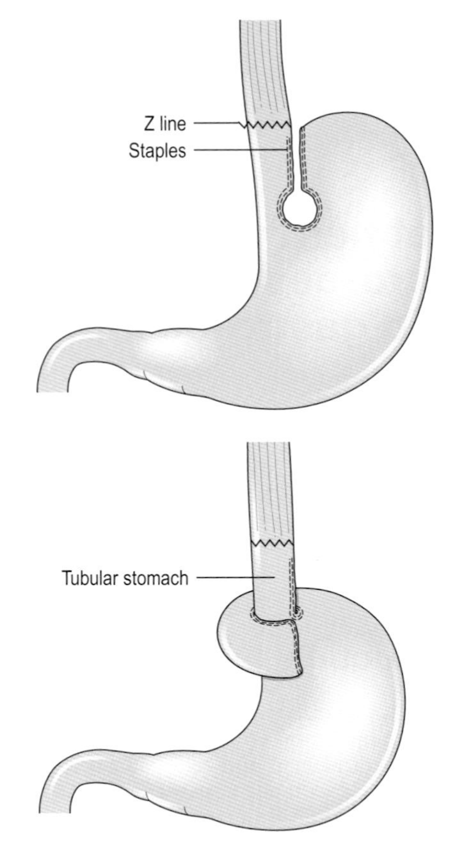

Figure 14.1 • A Collis gastroplasty. Stapled lines shown with Z line above the wrap.

Gastrointestinal haemorrhage

The treatment of erosive oesophagitis is medical with proton-pump inhibitors in the first instance, with excellent healing rates, although double-dose treatment may be required with maintenance therapy after healing has been achieved.[13] To attribute gastrointestinal haemorrhage to erosive oesophagitis is a matter of exclusion after full endoscopic examination as it is not a common cause of significant bleeding except in those with a tendency to bleeding, usually as a result of other medication they are taking.

In rare cases a true peptic ulcer can arise in an area of oesophagitis or Barrett's oesophagus. Such an ulcer can erode into blood vessels and bleed. This can be controlled endoscopically by injection of the ulcer base with adrenaline and application of clips or a heater probe. In rare cases where the bleeding cannot be controlled, embolisation can help and possibly the use of a Sengstaken tube. Surgery will be difficult as it requires oversewing of the bleeding vessel or possible resection through a left thoracoabdominal approach. In all cases of ulceration the surrounding mucosa and ulcer margins should be biopsied to exclude Barrett's oesophagus, dysplasia and malignancy when the acute episode has passed.

Peptic oesophageal stricture

The incidence of symptomatic stricture is extremely low in the pantheon of reflux disease. The management involves endoscopy and biopsy to exclude serious pathology followed by optimum acid inhibition with proton-pump inhibitors and H_2-receptor antagonists and gentle dilatation with an endoscopic balloon (**Fig. 14.2**). The diameter is dependent on the size of the stricture but it is better to undertake sequential dilatation starting with a 10-mm balloon rather than use too big a balloon and risk splitting the oesophagus.

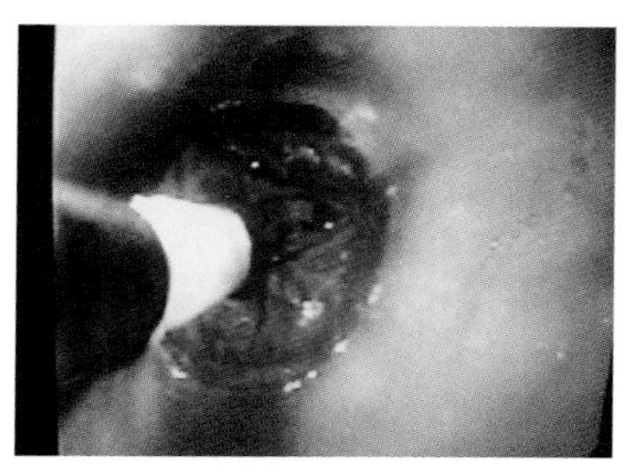

Figure 14.2 • Endoscopic balloon dilatation of peptic stricture.

Box 14.1 • Algorithm for the management of recalcitrant peptic oesophageal strictures

1. Repeat graded dilatation
2. Injection of steroid (laser short stricture – Schatski ring)
3. Removable or biodegradable stent
4. Resect

The risk of perforation is of the order of 2–3%. This should be recognised at the time and treated conservatively with nil by mouth, intravenous proton-pump inhibitors and antibiotics plus placement of a nasojejunal tube under screening for feeding. Success can be achieved in over 90% of cases with conservative management. If the perforation is not recognised and the patient develops sepsis then a more aggressive approach is required, including drainage and surgical repair. Such patients are best referred to specialist centres with full intensive care and interventional radiological support.[14,15] The use of self-expanding plastic stents in such perforations shows promise but can cause problems and is best avoided. Any stent used in this context must be removable.

Patients with symptomatic peptic strictures will often require repeat dilatation to maintain swallowing. In such cases injection of steroids can be beneficial and division of a tight band-type stricture with a laser can reduce the frequency of dilatation.[16] The use of self-expanding plastic stents is controversial and in resistant strictures only removable stents (plastic) or the new biodegradable stents should be used.[17] The patient with a stricture resistant to these treatments may require surgical resection. Such cases may be technically difficult as there has been transmural inflammation or perforation and an open approach is recommended. An algorithm is shown in Box 14.1.

Failed antireflux surgery

Failure may be due to persistence or recurrence of reflux symptoms, development of new symptoms or complications of the surgical procedure. The incidence of complications[17–19] is listed in Table 14.1.

Table 14.1 • Complications of antireflux surgery

Pneumothorax		2%
Paraoesophageal hernia		7%
Dysphagia – Slipped wrap, tight wrap, tight hiatus	early late	34% 6%
Perforated oesophagus		1%
Bloating/diarrhoea		30%

Complications and failures tend to occur soon after laparoscopic surgery and later after open surgery.

As described above, the success rate for fundoplication in controlling symptoms is in the region of 85% using accepted criteria for surgical success – volume reflux, failed medical treatment, etc.[2–5] This implies that 15% fail and with time even successful initial surgery results in 25% of patients subsequently requiring regular medication.

It is now recognised that the type of wrap (partial or total) does not have a long-term effect on dysphagia, although total fundoplication may give better control of reflux symptoms whereas partial fundoplication has less dysphagia in the short term, although this difference disappears with time.[20,21]

Investigation of the failed antireflux operation

In all cases of failed surgery it is crucial to go through the history carefully and then fully investigate the patient. The patient must then undergo full investigation, including endoscopy, barium swallow and meal, computerised tomography (CT) scan with contrast and repeat physiology tests when indicated.

Endoscopy

Endoscopy is important to exclude any new pathology, especially when the original surgery was undertaken for Barrett's oesophagus. As antireflux surgery has not been shown to prevent progression of Barrett's, awareness of the risk of malignant change must be high. In addition, endoscopy will show if a wrap has become disrupted or slipped down on to the stomach with gastric mucosa above the wrap. It is not reliable in demonstrating the position of the wrap in relation to the diaphragm or whether a stricture is at the hiatus or wrap.

Barium studies

Barium studies provide important information about both anatomy and function. A swallow can

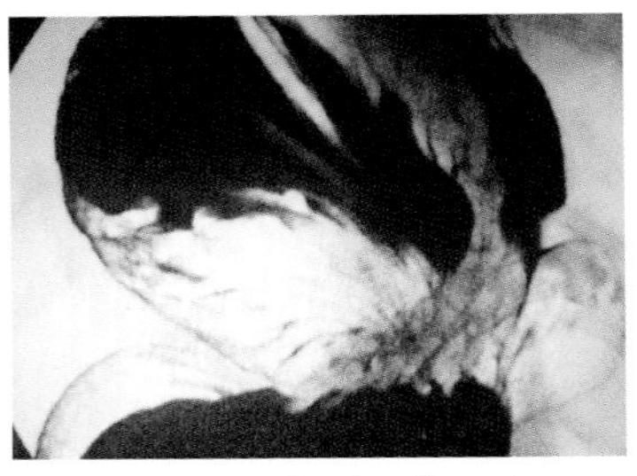

Figure 14.3 • Barium study of a slipped wrap.

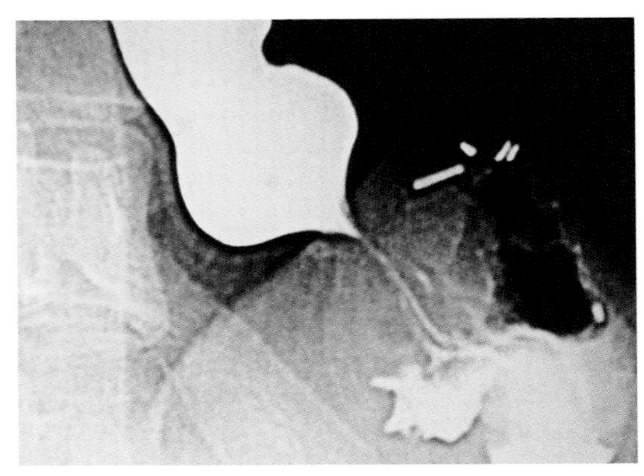

Figure 14.4 • Barium study of dysphagia due to a tight wrap.

demonstrate the pattern of obstruction and its relation to the diaphragm. It can also demonstrate the integrity of a wrap and slippage into the chest (**Figs 14.3** and **14.4**), which is not infrequently associated with volvulus (**Fig. 14.5**). It is also important to look at the gastric component of the study to visualise gastric emptying and pyloric function.

Computerised tomography

CT scanning with contrast should be undertaken in all cases where malignancy is suspected with endoluminal ultrasound scan if there is doubt. It is also invaluable where there is a large intrathoracic stomach to display the anatomy, especially if the repair is to be undertaken using the transabdominal approach (**Fig. 14.6**). CT is almost invariably contributory in difficult revisional cases.

Oesophageal physiology tests

Repeat oesophageal physiology and in particular oesophageal impedance can be very revealing in failed surgery, especially if it was not undertaken prior to original surgery. The missed diagnosis of achalasia will invariably result in dysphagia, as will scleroderma where the oesophagus is amotile. There is no evidence, however, that normal but low-amplitude motility affects outcome, and high-amplitude waves may be associated with a tight wrap.[8]

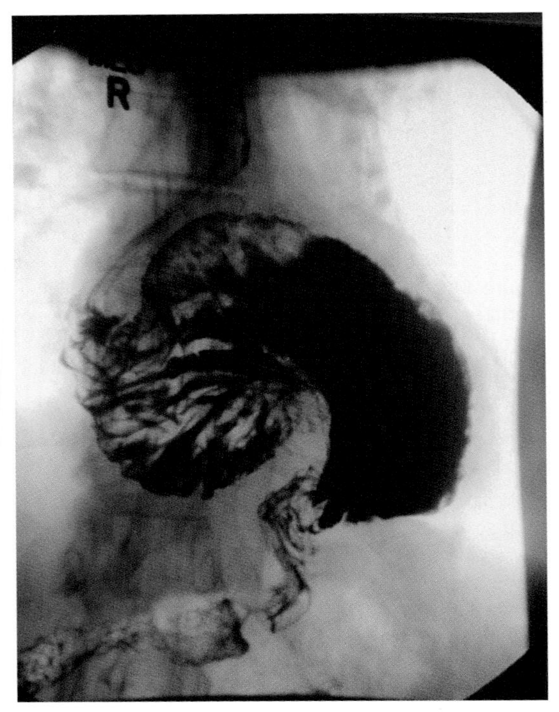

Figure 14.5 • Barium study of gastric volvulus with large hiatal hernia.

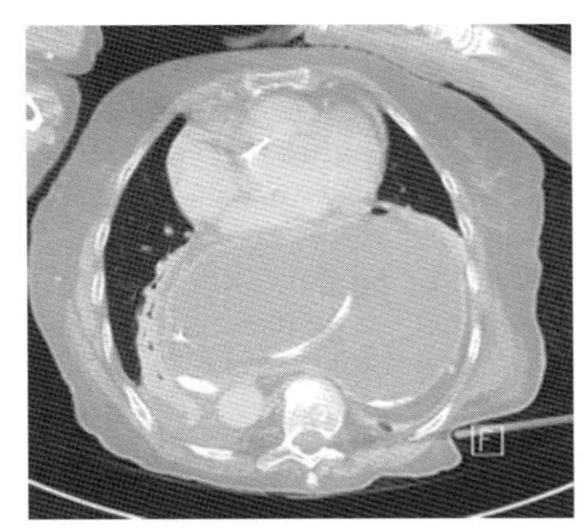

Figure 14.6 • CT scan of gastric volvulus.

The results of 24-hour pH monitoring post-fundoplication are very interesting.[22] The usual pattern is that there is no measurable reflux in spite of symptoms that seem classical of reflux. This relates to the observation that many patients undergoing revisional surgery for recurrent symptoms have a wrap that is in good position and is intact. The cause of the symptoms is therefore unclear and caution must be expressed on the successful outcome of re-operation. When the pH studies are positive and there is good symptom correlation and positive DeMeester score, this will usually be associated with wrap disruption and a better outcome can be expected with revision.

Management of failure after antireflux surgery

Failure will be discussed on the basis of the clinical problem that arises from 'failure'. It should be recognised that some patients will actually have a persistence of symptoms that they had prior to surgery and that these symptoms were not actually related to their identified reflux. The importance of a careful history that takes into account the patient's preoperative history, the symptoms with which they have re-presented and the time course of development of these symptoms cannot be overemphasised.

Recurrence of reflux symptoms

Recurrence of symptoms as described earlier is more common than generally recognised and a significant proportion of patients (25%) are back on medication post-surgery, although their symptoms are better controlled. It is wise to repeat the physiology studies in such patients to identify those who have true reflux, especially if considering revisional surgery.[23]

The reasons for this recurrence of symptoms include wrap disruption, wrap slippage and migration into the chest. The latter is more frequent when at the first operation there was a large hiatal defect, which was not closed properly with sutures, and if the sac was not excised from the chest or the repair was associated with tension (**Fig. 14.7**). Closure of a large hiatus with removal of the sac can be difficult, especially when undertaken laparoscopically, and if problems arise this should lead to conversion to open surgery. An alternative is to close the hiatus with a mesh, preferably from behind the oesophagus. Good results have been reported using this technique but caution is needed as the mesh can erode the oesophagus and cause dense strictures at the hiatus.[23,24] Removal will invariably require open surgery, usually via a thoracoabdominal incision with an oesophagogastrectomy. The use of man-made products to cover the hiatus adjacent to the oesophagus should be avoided if at all possible.

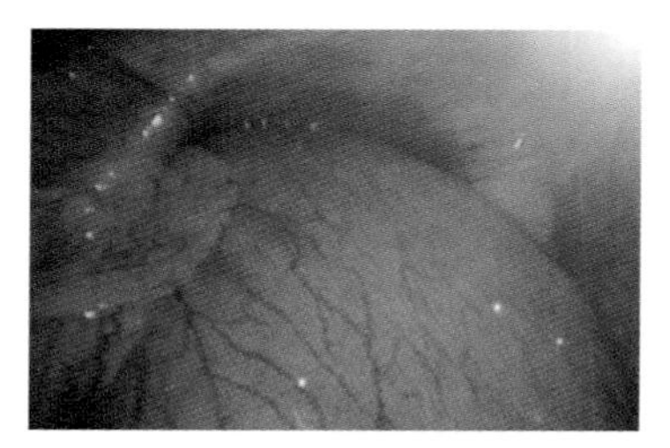

Figure 14.7 • Laparoscopic view of wrap migrated into the chest.

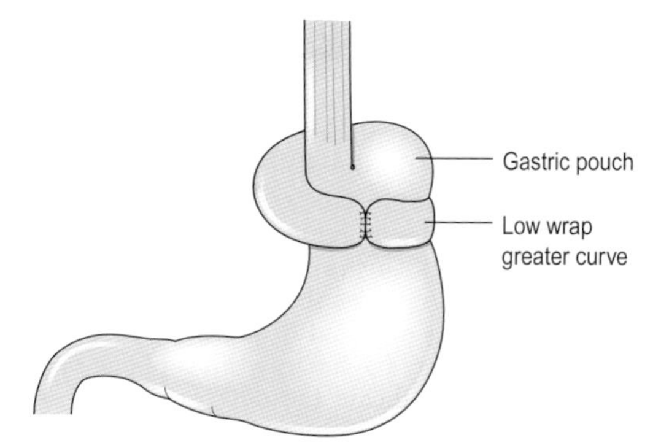

Figure 14.8 • Diagram of a 'bad wrap' where the greater curve is used rather than fundus.

Failure of the symptoms to improve after surgery questions the original diagnosis and may be associated with a sensitive oesophagus. It can be related to a 'bad' operation when the wrong part of the stomach is brought up (**Fig. 14.8**). This can produce the equivalent of a gastric band as used in bariatric surgery. Such patients often experience significant weight loss in the postoperative period and require revisional surgery.

Persistence of preoperative symptoms

Persistence of symptoms suggests that the original diagnosis was at fault. Review of preoperative 24-hour pH and oesophageal manometry together with a repeat study may reveal underlying motility disorders such as achalasia, lack of symptom correlation and low DeMeester scores. Such patients tend to be upright refluxers or if the original studies were negative may represent 'functional heartburn'.[25] Taking down the wrap in the absence of dysphagia is unlikely to benefit the patient and is only a last resort. Other causes of pain must be sought and 24-hour pH study on and off full-dose medical treatment can be revealing.

Dysphagia

Dysphagia tends to occur early following laparoscopic surgery and late following open surgery. It can be an immediate complication in the first 24 hours and, if total, requires immediate return to theatre as the wrap may have slipped or twisted. Redoing the wrap or converting to a partial wrap will lead to resolution.

Dysphagia persisting beyond 2 months may be due to a pre-existing motility disorder, an over-tight wrap, scarring in the hiatus or over-tight repair of the hiatus. If in doubt, especially in cases where fluids only can be taken, early barium studies can be very helpful,[26] revealing migrated or slipped wraps or strictures at the hiatus (Figs 14.3 and 14.4). If the stenosis is thought to be due to stricturing of the hiatus then care should be taken with dilatation as the oesophageal wall can be compressed against a hard fibrous band and the result is invariably poor (**Fig. 14.9**). The solution to this is re-operation and incision of the fibrous hiatal ring to release the oesophagus. It is important to visualise and avoid injury to the inferior phrenic vein when undertaking this procedure. This procedure can be achieved laparoscopically in most cases.

When dysphagia arises after a period of normal swallowing this may be due to wrap slippage or migration but may indicate the development of malignancy, especially if the operation was performed for Barrett's oesophagus. The first investigation is endoscopy (**Fig. 14.10**), biopsy of any suspicious lesion and balloon dilatation of the wrap up to 20 mm with an endoscopic balloon dilatator. Barium studies and CT are also indicated as wrap migration into the chest may not be obvious on endoscopy (**Fig. 14.11**).

The incidence of dysphagia is initially less when a partial wrap is performed, in contrast to a full 360° Nissen fundoplication. The use of a partial fundoplication is increasing, with no apparent reduction in efficacy in the control of reflux.[20,21] Certainly, in patients with pre-existing motility disorders such as scleroderma, or as part of surgery for achalasia, a partial wrap should be undertaken or dysphagia is likely.

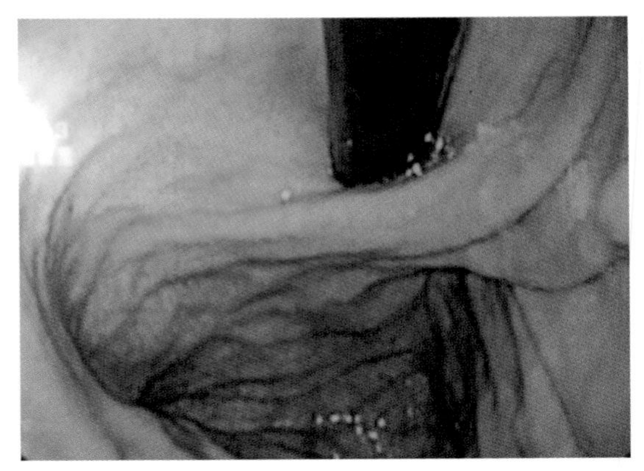

Figure 14.9 • Balloon dilatation of a tight hiatal ring demonstrating the resistant short stricture characteristic of this complication.

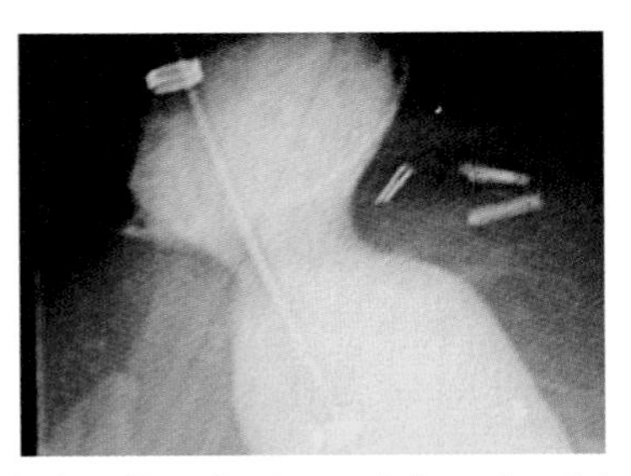

Figure 14.10 • Retroflection and view of partial fundoplication on endoscopy.

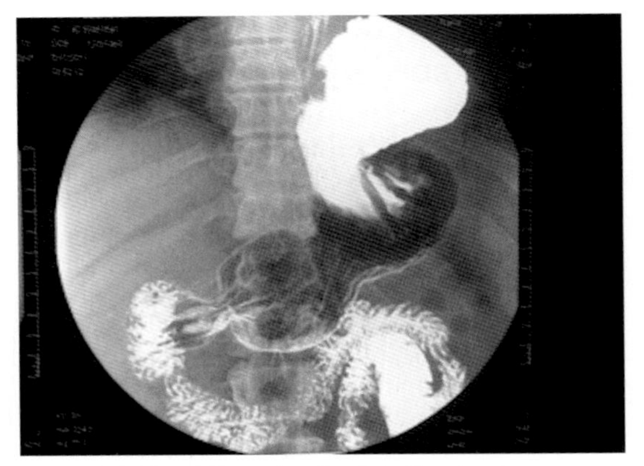

Figure 14.11 • Wrap migration into the chest.

Other symptoms

Gas bloat and change in bowel habit often indicate a functional gastrointestinal disorder that has either been exacerbated by the surgery or has arisen de novo. In some series the incidence of these complications can be as high as 60%, with half arising de novo. Such patients tend to be air swallowers and re-operation should be avoided at all costs and medical management undertaken. A not infrequent complication of surgery at the gastro-oesophageal junction is damage to the vagus nerve, especially the anterior vagus, which may influence gastric emptying. In such cases, poor emptying will precipitate GORD and will resolve with pyloric dilatation. Functional solid and liquid emptying studies will confirm this and should be undertaken if formal surgery on the stomach is considered. Trial of dilatation of the pylorus with a 20-mm balloon can be very instructive. Surgery in such cases would involve an antrectomy and Roux-en-Y anastomosis.

Revisional surgery following failed antireflux surgery

Before embarking on revisional surgery it is crucial to gather all the above information and have detailed consultations with the patient on what can be expected to be achieved. There are situations such as a tight hiatus, bad wrap or slippage into the chest (whether the whole stomach as a volvulus or a rolling component) in which there is either a significant risk of complications or a good chance of a successful outcome where surgery can be recommended. This includes missed motility disorders in which conversion to a partial wrap and myotomy, if appropriate, can improve symptoms.

Care should be taken in recommending re-operation in patients with persistent or recurrent symptoms in whom the investigations reveal an intact wrap in a good position and normal physiological studies. However, if re-operation is undertaken for the correct reasons then the outcome is generally good, although the outcome is worse if re-operation is for dysphagia.[12,27]

This should not be undertaken by an occasional surgeon or by one who is unfamiliar with entering the chest. The most frequently used procedure is revision of the fundoplication, either redoing a 360° wrap or converting it to a partial wrap, together with appropriate hiatal repair (**Figs 14.12** and **14.13**). This can be undertaken laparoscopically, especially if the previous procedure was laparoscopic, but should be converted to open surgery if any difficulty is encountered.

The principles are to take the whole wrap down and return the anatomy to normal prior to undertaking a re-fundoplication. This enables good visualisation of the crura and hiatus, and must be associated with mobilisation of the oesophagus while preserving the vagi. Great care must be undertaken to avoid opening the oesophagus and stomach, and placement of a small-diameter endoscope into the stomach enables accurate identification of the structures and also enables leak testing to identify small defects. A guide to the wrap is the previous sutures and lifting these with forceps will often reveal the wrap.

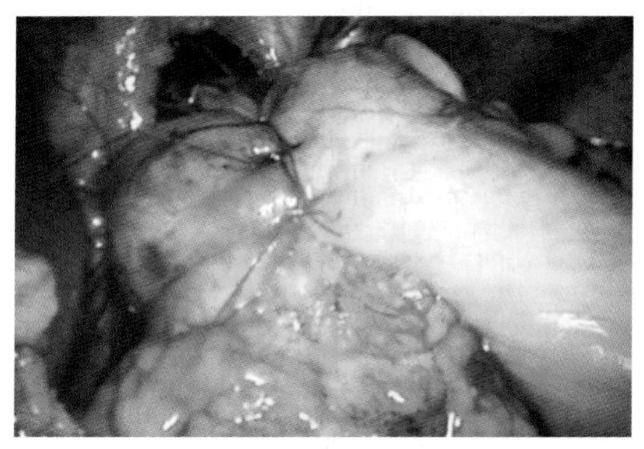

Figure 14.12 • Revision with 360° wrap.

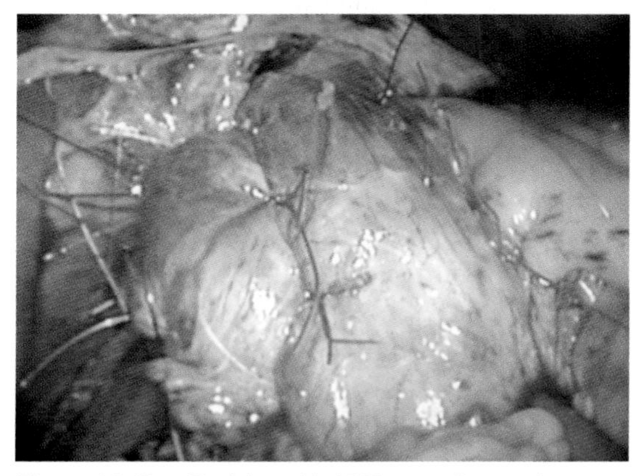

Figure 14.13 • Revision with 270° wrap. Sutures between wrap and right crus are clearly visualised.

The author's preferred approach is an open operation through a bilateral subcostal incision using an Omnitract retractor. If there are dense adhesions the oesophagus can be approached over the top of the left lobe of the liver, which can then be mobilised.

This approach makes reduction of a stomach that has slipped into the chest easier. The sac can be reduced by blunt dissection from the front of the hiatus, dividing the peritoneum with a diathermy point and extending this to the right and left, thus exposing the crura. The sac should be fully excised (**Fig 14.14**).

Posterior repair of the hiatus can be achieved by placing non-absorbable sutures in the left crus and bringing them behind the oesophagus to place in the right crus. Usually, three well-placed sutures are enough to close the hiatus without tension. This invariably enables avoidance of the use of mesh. Full mobilisation of the fundus and short gastric vessels enables a loose 360° or 270° wrap to be performed. On completion of the wrap, it is sutured to the right crus with two or three non-absorbable sutures (Fig. 14.13).

In cases associated with gastric volvulus, the author adds a tube gastrostomy on the greater curve to fix the stomach in three places – gastrostomy, hiatus and duodenum. This avoids any need for a nasogastric

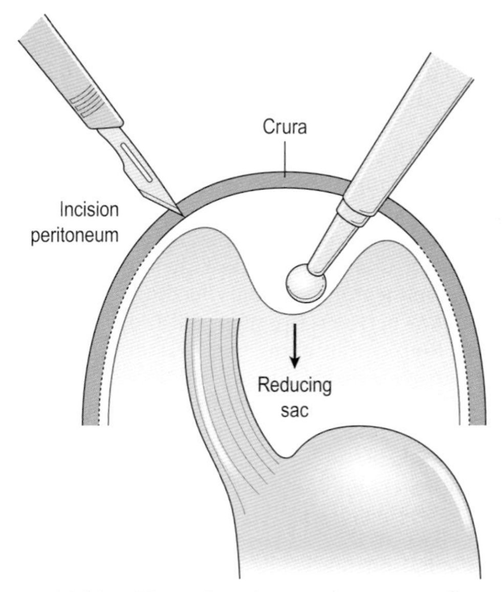

Figure 14.14 • Dissection of sac and exposure of crura in revision of large hiatal defect.

tube and by leaving it in place for 3 weeks fixes the stomach and prevents any recurrence.

It is reasonable to have one attempt at repairing and revising a wrap. Further operations may well result in a devitalised gastro-oesophageal zone necessitating oesophagogastric resection via a left thoracoabdominal approach with a 25-mm stapled anastomosis at the aortic arch.[28] The gastric tube is based on the right gastroepiploic artery and should be no more than 3 cm wide. Unless there is previous peptic ulceration, a pyloroplasty is not needed and the addition of a wrap at the anastomosis does not protect from reflux. If the stomach is not suitable then a short-segment colonic interposition is an alternative approach. The functional result of such a procedure will never be 'normal'.

In cases with a failed second operation, further surgery should only be undertaken if there are major nutritional or quality-of-life issues and a second specialist opinion should be sought. In such cases the options will rest between a subtotal gastrectomy and Roux-en-Y anastomosis if the problem is reflux and resection if a there is a persistent stricture that is leading to inability to eat.

Complex revisional surgery

Such patients fall into three distinct categories: those with oesophageal occlusion; those with a cervical oesophagostomy and gastrostomy following salvage surgery for failed resection for cancer or Boerhaave's syndrome; and the late complications following previous surgery for oesophageal atresia. These cases must be managed in specialist units with full access to advanced imaging, thoracic, microvascular and upper GI surgeons, and full ITU back-up.

Oesophageal occlusion usually results from ingestion of caustic fluids with either complete occlusion of the oesophagus from the pharynx or a long tight complex stricture.[29] Rare causes include epidermolysis bullosa.[30] In such cases the pharynx is also involved with inflammation and fibrosis and patients are unable to swallow their own saliva and have permanent gastrostomy feeding. A colonic interposition between the pharynx and stomach or a jejunal loop can in many cases restore swallowing, although pharyngeal fibrosis inhibits the initiation of swallowing. If the stricture is high with a relatively normal oesophagus below, then a pharyngoplasty can help.

It is now recognised that in cases of failed oesophageal resection with tube necrosis of major anastomotic breakdown, resection of the conduit with cervical oesophagostomy and stapling off the distal end can be life saving. Similar oesophageal resection or exclusion can have benefits in Boerhaave's syndrome with oesophageal necrosis and mediastinitis.[31] Such patients require reconstruction to restore continuity when they have recovered. This can usually be achieved by the use of either a colonic interposition or a long 'supercharged' jejunal Roux-en-Y loop.[32,33]

If possible, the author prefers the colon in the first instance, using the transverse and descending colon based on the ascending branch of the left colic artery. An angiogram CT scan should be performed prior to surgery to ensure a good anastomosis at the splenic flexure. The colon can be brought up either substernally or subcutaneously in unfit patients. A sternal split is preferred together with clearing of the anterior mediastinum of fat and thymus, and mobilising the left brachiocephalic vein. This removes any compression on the conduit at the thoracic inlet, which is the major reason for failure. If a 'blind' retrosternal tunnel is used then the manubrium and sternoclavicular joint must be removed or compression and venous infarction will result. The author prefers not to use the right colon as it is more bulky and more difficult to straighten out at the hepatic flexure. A short length of terminal ileum should be used to anastomose to the oesophagus if the right colon has to be used.

In cases where the colon is unavailable, a supercharged jejunal loop can be used. In order to reach the neck, the proximal part of the loop will be ischaemic and requires 'supercharging' by a microvascular anastomosis between a mesenteric artery and usually the left internal mammary artery and a venous anastomosis to any suitable vein (**Figs 14.15** and **14.16**).

In a series of 25 consecutive patients (seven supercharged jejunum and 18 colonic interpositions), 75% are able to maintain oral nutrition and 20% require nocturnal jejunostomy nutritional supplementation. Mortality was 4% but morbidity was 57%, emphasising the need to centralise such cases.

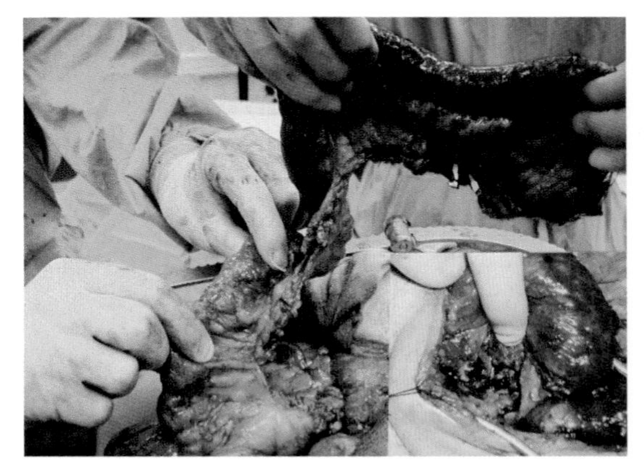

Figure 14.15 • A long supercharged Roux loop showing the long mesentery and dusky appearance at the top end.

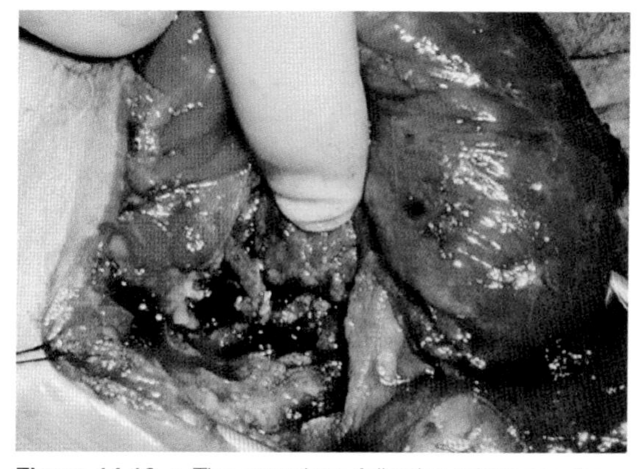

Figure 14.16 • The same loop following microvascular anastomosis in the neck and the well-vascularised bowel.

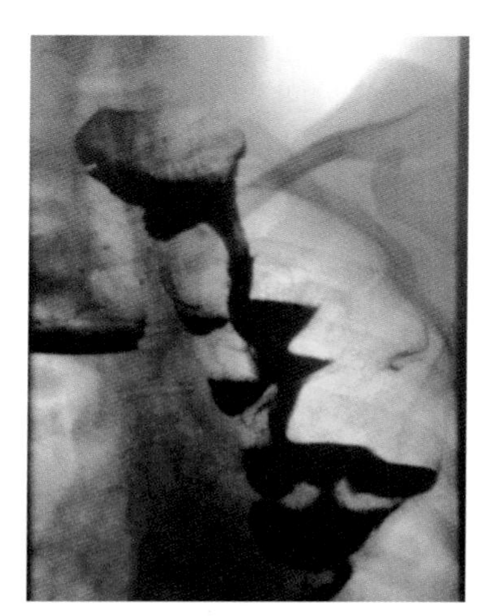

Figure 14.17 • A contrast swallow demonstrating redundant colonic loops in the left chest.

There are now an increasing number of patients in their thirties who had successful surgery for oesophageal atresia in infancy. This was invariably a colonic interposition via the left chest with multiple neck and thoracic operations. In such cases presenting with difficulty in swallowing, it is crucial to investigate thoroughly prior to considering any reconstruction to determine accurately the site of obstruction. This can be at the root of the neck, which bulges on swallowing, in redundant colonic loops in the chest, or at the level of the diaphragm where a fibrotic stricture causes a mechanical obstruction and proximal dilatation. Investigation includes endoscopy, barium studies and contrast-enhanced CT scanning (**Fig. 14.17**).

The most common causes for difficulty in swallowing are redundant colonic loops and strictures at the diaphragm.[33,34,35] A long left thoracoabdominal approach gives the best access, and it is crucial to identify the vascular pedicle at an early stage and preserve it at all costs. The diaphragm is split to the hiatus, the cologastric anastomosis taken down, redundant colon excised with a harmonic scalpel keeping to the bowel wall, preserving the vascular arcade and re-anastomosis of the colon to stomach. The diaphragm is closed without any compression at the new pseudo-hiatus. Such patients will require jejunostomy feeding for some time.

If the problem occurs in the neck, excision of the manubrium and left costoclavicular joint and pexy of the redundant colon may help. The colon can be resected in the left chest with primary anastomosis, again taking extra care to preserve the vascular arcade.

It cannot be overstressed that a conservative approach is best as such patients have a life expectancy of many decades, and a realistic discussion regarding outcome should take place at the first consultation. Taking such an approach can lead to good results and quality of life.

Summary

Gastro-oesophageal reflux disease is a common condition, which in the majority of cases can be managed by appropriate antisecretory medication. In a small proportion significant complications such as erosive disease, stricture and Barrett's oesophagus occur. They can usually be managed with medical or endoscopic treatment, but in resistant cases of stricture a graded approach of increasing proton-pump inhibitors, repeat dilatation, steroid injection and surgery may be required. Stents are best avoided.

A cautious approach to surgery for reflux should be employed, especially in patients whose symptoms are well controlled on medication, as success of only 85% can be expected with surgery. Surgery does, however, offer good results in patients in whom medical treatment fails to control symptoms or in whom there is a significant volume reflux problem.

In cases of failed surgery, a thorough reinvestigation of the patient is mandatory before considering revision. Revisional surgery should be undertaken by surgeons who are expert in the field and involves returning the anatomy to normal prior to repeating either partial or total fundoplication with proper crural repair. Failure of such surgery may lead to the need for resection, with all that entails.

In cases of complex revisional and reconstructive surgery, early referral to a specialist multidisciplinary team is mandatory.

Key points

- Both antisecretory medication and fundoplication are effective treatments of gastro-oesophageal reflux disease.
- Complications (severe erosive oesophagitis and peptic stricture) are rare and can usually be managed by optimising medical therapy and endoscopic therapy with dilatation, and in severe cases removable or absorbable stents.
- Laparoscopic fundoplication is an effective operation for GORD but has a failure rate of 15%, with up to 25% taking medication with time.
- All cases of failed surgery should be thoroughly investigated before any revisional surgery is contemplated.
- Revisional surgery should be avoided in patients who have persistent or recurrent symptoms with normal physiology and intact wrap.
- Patients who benefit most from revisional surgery are those with recurrent symptoms and abnormal physiology due to a disrupted wrap. Results are less satisfactory if the reason for revision is dysphagia.
- Revisional surgery should involve taking the original procedure down completely before undertaking a new loose fundoplication and hiatal repair with the wrap tension free below the hiatus.
- Although revisional surgery is possible laparoscopically in many cases, any surgeon undertaking such procedures must be able to convert to open operation, enter the chest and be able to resect if necessary.
- Specialist management is mandatory in patients with oesophageal occlusion or following failed resection, or who are having complications following previous surgery for atresia. Such patients require complex and often repeated surgery.

References

1. Fass R, Ofman JJ. Gastroesophageal reflux disease – should we adopt a new conceptual framework? Am J Gastroenterol 2002;97:1901–9.
2. Fiocca R, Mastracci L, Engstrom C, et al. Long-term outcome of microscopic esophagitis in chronic GERD patients treated with esomeprazole or laparoscopic antireflux surgery in the LOTUS trial. Am J Gastroenterol 2010;105:1015–23.
3. Galmiche JP, Hatlebakk J, Attwood S, et al. Laparoscopic antireflux surgery vs esomeprazole treatment for chronic GERD: the LOTUS randomised clinical trial. JAMA 2011;305:1969–77.
   A randomised study demonstrating the equal efficacy of medical and surgical treatment of GORD.
4. Broeders JA, Rijnhart-de Jong HJ, Draaisma WA, et al. Ten-year outcome of laparoscopic and conventional Nissen fundoplication. Ann Surg 2009;250:698–706.
5. Kelly JJ, Watson DI, Chin KF, et al. Laparoscopic Nissen fundoplication: clinical outcomes at 10 years. J Am Coll Surg 2007;205:570–5.
6. Wang YR, Dempsey DT, Richter JE. Trends and perioperative outcomes of inpatient antireflux surgery in the United States 1993–2006. Dis Esophagus 2011;24:215–23.
7. Zingg U, Smith L, Carney N, et al. The influence on outcome of indications for antireflux surgery. World J Surg 2010;34:2813–20.
8. Broeders JA, Sportel IG, Jamieson GG, et al. Impact of ineffective motility and wrap type on dysphagia after laparoscopic fundoplication. Br J Surg 2011;98:1414–21.
9. Richter JE. Role of the gastric refluxate in gastroesophageal reflux disease: acid, weak acid and bile. Am J Med Sci 2009;338:89–95.
10. Brillantins A, Monaco L, Schettmo M, et al. Prevalence of pathological duodenogastric reflux and the relationship between duodenogastric and duodenogastroesophageal reflux in chronic gastroesophageal reflux disease. Eur J Gastroenterol Hepatol 2008;20:1136–43.
11. Nason KS, Luketich JD, Awais O, et al. Quality of life after Collis gastroplasty for short esophagus in patients with paraesophageal hernia. Ann Thorac Surg 2011;92:1854–61.
12. Awais O, Luketich JD, Schuchert MJ, et al. Reoperative antireflux surgery for failed fundoplication: an analysis of outcomes in 275 patients. Ann Thorac Surg 2011;92:1083–9.
    An extensive experience of revisional surgery with good outcomes. Good guidance for those undertaking these procedures.

13. Edwards SJ, Lind T, Lundell L, et al. Systematic review: standard- and double-dose proton pump inhibitors for the healing of severe erosive oesophagitis – a mixed treatment comparison of randomized controlled trials. Aliment Pharmacol Ther 2009;30:547–56.
14. Kuppasamy HK, Hubka M, Felisky CD, et al. Evolving management strategies in oesophageal perforation: surgeons using non-operative techniques to improve outcome. J Am Coll Surg 2011;213: 164–71.
15. Søreide JA, Viste A. Esophageal perforation: diagnostic workup and clinical decision making in the first 24 hours. Scand J Trauma Resusc Emerg Med 2011;19:66.
An excellent overview of the problem of perforation with guidance for management.
16. De Wijkerslooth LR, Vleggaar FP, Siersema PD. Endoscopic management of difficult or recurrent esophageal strictures. Am J Gastroenterol 2011;106:2080–91.
This gives an excellent overview of the management of recalcitrant oesophageal strictures with a management plan that is evidence based.
17. Repici A, Vieggaar FP, Hassan C, et al. Efficacy and safety of biodegradable stents for refractory benign oesophageal strictures. The BEST study. Gastrointest Endosc 2010;72:927–34.
18. Watson DI, de Beaux AC. Complications of laparoscopic antireflux surgery. Surg Endosc 2001;15:344–52.
19. Richter JE. Let the patient beware: the evolving truth about laparoscopic antireflux surgery. Am J Med 2003;114:71–3.
A cautionary note before recommending surgery. Should be part of preoperative consent.
20. Nijjar RS, Watson DI, Jamieson GG, et al. Five year followup of a multicentre, double blinded randomized clinical trial of laparoscopic Nissen vs anterior 90 degree partial fundoplication. Arch Surg 2010;145:552–7.
21. Mardani J, Lundell L, Engstrom C. Total or posterior partial fundoplication in the treatment of GERD: results of a randomised trial after 2 decades of followup. Ann Surg 2011;253:875–8.
Demonstrates that the type of fundoplication does not matter.
22. Thompson SK, Jamieson GG, Myers JC, et al. Recurrent heartburn after laparoscopic fundoplication is not always recurrent reflux. J Gastrointest Surg 2007;11:642–7.
23. Antoniou SA, Koch OO, Antoniou GA, et al. Mesh reinforced hiatal hernia repair: a review on the effect on postoperative dysphagia and recurrence. Langenbecks Arch Surg 2012;397:19–27.
24. Soricelli E, Basso N, Genco A, et al. Long term results of hiatal hernia mesh repair and antireflux laparoscopic surgery. Surg Endosc 2009;23: 2499–504.
25. Thompson SK, Cai W, Jamieson GG, et al. Recurrent symptoms after fundoplication with a negative pH study – recurrent reflux or functional heartburn? J Gastrointest Surg 2009;13:54–60.
26. Tsunoda S, Jamieson GG, Devitt PG, et al. Early reoperation after laparoscopic fundoplication: the importance of routine postoperative contrast studies. World J Surg 2010;34:79–84.
27. Lamb PJ, Myers JC, Jamieson GG, et al. Longterm outcomes of revisional surgery following laparoscopic fundoplication. Br J Surg 2009;96:391–7.
Demonstrates that revisional surgery can be beneficial if done for the correct reasons.
28. Forshaw MJ, Gossage JA, Ockrim J, et al. Left thoracoabdominal oesophagogastrectomy: still a valid operation for carcinoma of the distal oesophagus and oesophagogastric junction. Dis Esophagus 2006;19:340–5.
29. Ananthakrishnan N, Kate V, Parthasarathy G. Therapeutic options for management of pharyngo-oesophageal corrosive strictures. J Gastrointest Surg 2011;15:566–75.
Demonstrates the problems with corrosive strictures from an area of high prevalence, which unfortunately is becoming more common in the UK.
30. Elton C, Marshall RE, Hibbert J, et al. Pharyngogastric colonic interposition for total oesophageal occlusion in epidermolysis bullosa. Dis Esophagus 2000;13:175–7.
31. Barkley C, Orringer MB, Iannettoni MD, et al. Challenges in reversing esophageal discontinuity operations. Ann Thorac Surg 2003;76:989–94.
An extensive experience of an uncommon and varied problem. Should be read by anyone wanting to undertake such operations.
32. Dowson HM, Strauss D, Ng R, et al. The acute management and surgical reconstruction following failed esophagectomy in malignant disease of the esophagus. Dis Esophagus 2007;20:135–40.
33. Khan AZ, Nikolopous I, Botha AJ, et al. Substernal long segment left colon interposition for oesophageal replacement. Surgeon 2008;6:54–6.
34. Strauss DC, Forshaw MJ, Tandon RC, et al. Surgical management of colonic redundancy following esophageal replacement. Dis Esophagus 2008;21:E1–5.
35. Dhir R, Sutcliffe RP, Rohatgi A, et al. Surgical management of late complications after colonic interposition for esophageal atresia. Ann Thorac Surg 2008;86:1965–7.

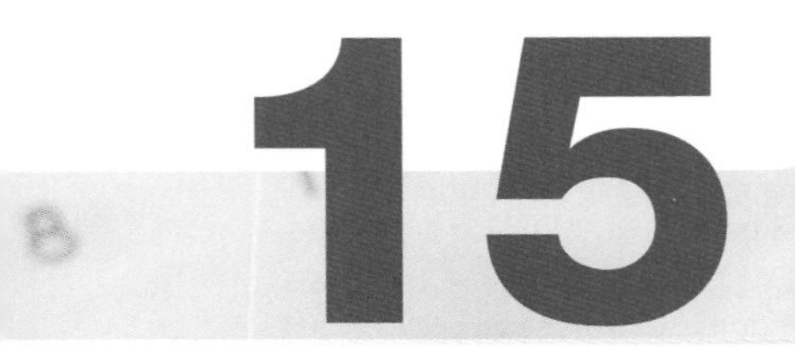

15 Barrett's oesophagus

Max Almond
Hugh Barr
Janusz Jankowski

Definition

Barrett's oesophagus is a change in any portion of the normal squamous oesophageal epithelium to a metaplastic columnar epithelium that is visible endoscopically and can be confirmed or corroborated histologically.[1,2] There are three histologically distinct types of columnar metaplasia: intestinal (IM), cardiac (CM) and fundic. In the USA, unlike the UK and Japan, the diagnosis of Barrett's oesophagus requires the identification of intestinalisation characterised by the presence of goblet cells. However, the UK definition considers that Barrett's oesophagus is analogous to a 'columnar lined oesophagus' and does not require identification of goblet cells due to fears that sampling bias could lead to under-diagnosis and potentially exclude patients from surveillance programmes. It has been reported that a minimum of eight biopsies are required to confidently exclude intestinal metaplasia – if only four biopsies are taken the diagnostic yield is only 35%.[3]

Occasionally, biopsies will be histologically diagnostic for Barrett's oesophagus in that they contain a native oesophageal gland or, more usually, a duct from these glands in close juxtaposition to metaplastic mucosa. However, the superficial nature of most biopsies makes this unusual. More typically, columnar epithelium is endoscopically recognisable but must be correlated with the location from which the biopsy is taken, as intestinal-type mucosa may also be found at the gastric cardia and fundus. Histologically, these biopsies can only be said to be corroborative of an endoscopic diagnosis of Barrett's oesophagus. Thus Barrett's oesophagus is a clinicopathological diagnosis.

Epidemiology

The exact population prevalence of Barrett's oesophagus is unclear. Data described in post-mortem and endoscopic series range from 0.9% to 5.6% depending on the precise definition used and the type of study.[4–7] It is likely that the true prevalence in the West is around 2%. When extrapolated to the UK and US populations, conservative estimates of prevalence are 1 million and 4 million affected individuals, respectively.[8] There is also some evidence that the incidence of Barrett's oesophagus in the West is increasing by up to 2% per year.[5,9–11] Data from the Netherlands demonstrated an increase in the number of cases of Barrett's oesophagus despite a decrease in the number of endoscopies being performed over the same period, suggesting a true increase in incidence.[11]

✔✔ A population-based study recruited a representative sample of 1000 people from two communities in northern Sweden to undergo upper endoscopy and confirmed the presence of intestinal metaplasia in 1.6% of the population studied.[9]

The incidence of Barrett's oesophagus increases with age, the mean age at diagnosis being approximately 62 years for men and 68 years for women.

It predominantly affects Caucasians[12] and is more common in men than women, with a ratio of approximately 1.7:1.[13]

The risk of developing Barrett's is related to increased frequency and duration of reflux symptoms.[14] This appears to correlate with the well-known association between increased frequency, duration and severity of reflux symptoms, and increased risk of adenocarcinoma of the oesophagus. The incidence of Barrett's oesophagus in patients with symptomatic gastro-oesophageal reflux disease (GORD) is between 5% and 12%.[9,15] Evidence from one case series suggests that more than 60% of patients with Barrett's oesophagus develop the condition secondary to chronic GORD, although other causes of oesophagitis, including non-steroidal anti-inflammatory drugs (NSAIDs), chemotherapy and viral infections are also associated with the disease. It does raise an intriguing possibility that a smaller proportion of patients can develop Barrett's de novo in the absence of obvious symptomatic or perhaps even pathological reflux. Therefore, other factors that may catalyse changes at the oesophagogastric junction (OGJ) are obesity and cigarette smoking,which have been identified as risk factors for both Barrett's oesophagus and progression to malignancy.[16]

A Swedish case–control study demonstrated that patients with recurrent reflux symptoms, when compared with asymptomatic patients, had an odds ratio of 7.7 for oesophageal adenocarcinoma and 2.0 for adenocarcinoma of the gastric cardia. Patients with severe long-standing symptoms had an odds ratio of 43.5 and 4.4 for oesophageal and cardia adenocarcinoma, respectively.[17]

Endoscopic assessment

Barrett's oesophagus has a classical appearance at oesophagogastroduodenoscopy (OGD). There is proximal displacement of the squamocolumnar junction, which in normal circumstances lies at the proximal limit of the linear gastric mucosal folds. 'Salmon pink' columnar mucosa is seen in the distal oesophagus arising from the OGJ, often with characteristic tongue extensions and/or columnar islands.

Proximal extension above the OGJ should be measured and documented, taking care to accurately identify any sliding hiatus hernia that may confuse this measurement. It is crucial that biopsies originate from the oesophagus to prevent misclassification of cardiac intestinal metaplasia as Barrett's oesophagus.

✔ The 'Prague C and M criteria', defined by an International Working Group on Barrett's oesophagus, offers a validated method of disease classification based on endoscopic appearance.[18]

The extent of circumferential involvement (C value) in centimetres from the OGJ should be recorded, as should the maximum length (M value) of the Barrett's segment, including tongue extensions but excluding isolated 'islands'. These criteria have been shown to have a high degree of reliability between different endoscopists. The use of the terms long-segment Barrett's (>3 cm) and short-segment Barrett's (<3 cm) should now be discouraged.

It is crucial to make a thorough and systematic inspection of the mucosa in order to identify any macroscopic neoplastic disease. Water or 1% acetylcysteine should be used to remove blood, saliva and refluxate from the oesophagus, and sufficient insufflation should be ensured to clearly visualise any mucosal abnormalities. Particular care must be taken to identify the OGJ in patients with a hiatus hernia as it is easy to miss the distal extent of a Barrett's segment in these patients. Clinicians should be aware that at endoscopic inspection most areas of early neoplasia and cancer are detected in an area around the 2 to 4 o'clock position in the endoscopist's view.[19]

✔ Despite meticulous inspection during white light video endoscopy, recognition of dysplasia and intramucosal cancer is difficult and subjective, even for experienced endoscopists. Guidelines therefore recommend that quadrantic biopsies are taken every 2 cm of Barrett's oesophagus in addition to further biopsies from any areas of visible mucosal abnormality.[1] Currently, the use of jumbo biopsy forceps is not recommended routinely.

This rigorous biopsy protocol, which is often poorly adhered to outside of specialist centres, samples less than 5% of the mucosa and may miss up to 57% of dysplasia.[20,21] Advanced endoscopic imaging techniques may allow targeted biopsies from high-risk areas, improving diagnostic yield (Table 15.1).[22–26] Potentially, these imaging tools may also facilitate targeted endoscopic resection of high-grade dysplasia (HGD) and intramucosal cancer.

Pathophysiology of Barrett's oesophagus and progression to adenocarcinoma

It is currently believed that Barrett's metaplasia develops as a mucosal 'adaptive' response to increased cell loss as a result of chronic inflammation, secondary to GORD. Oesophageal squamous epithelium is highly sensitive to acid, alkaline and biliary reflux, which all cause inflammation, with cell loss, necrosis and ulceration. There is strong evidence

Table 15.1 • Advanced endoscopic imaging modalities being investigated for use in Barrett's oesophagus surveillance programmes and for facilitation of targeted endoscopic resection

Imaging modality	Concept	Reference
White light endoscopy		
High-resolution magnification endoscopy (HRME)	Greater magnification and resolution than normal endoscopy allowing more detailed visualisation of the mucosa	May et al. (2004)[137]
Chromoendoscopy	Topical application of dyes improves visualisation of mucosal surfaces. Examples: methylene blue – absorbed with different patterns into different types of mucosa; indigo carmine – accumulates in mucosal fissures accentuating surface topography	Canto et al. (2006)[138]
Optical endoscopy		
Autofluorescence imaging (AFI)	Short-wavelength light causes excitation of endogenous biological tissues with subsequent release of longer wavelength fluorescent light	Kara et al. (2005)[139]
Narrow-band imaging (NBI)	Narrow-bandwidth green and blue light (with exclusion of red light) only superficially penetrates mucosa, improving visualisation of mucosal microvasculature and surface morphology	Curvers et al. (2008)[25]
Confocal microscopy (CM)	Real-time magnification of the mucosa up to 1000-fold enables visualisation of cellular structures	Dunbar and Canto (2010)[22]
Elastic scattering spectroscopy (ESS)	Elastic scattering of white light generates real-time morphological information about the size and shape of the cell nuclei and the degree of cellular crowding in the mucosa and submucosa	Qiu et al. (2010)[23]
Trimodal imaging	Incorporates HRME, AFI and NBI in a single endoscope with ability to switch between modalities during procedure	Curvers et al. (2010, 2011)[140,141]
Molecular imaging	Fluorescently tagged molecular probes bind selectively to metaplastic or dysplastic cells	Bird-Lieberman et al. (2012)[142]

that the site of origin of Barrett's metaplasia is a progenitor stem cell located in the submucosal oesophageal gland ducts, following demonstration that a *p16* point mutation originating in microdissected squamous duct tissue was also present in adjoining metaplastic crypts.[27] Duodenal and gastric reflux-induced ulceration and inflammation is believed to induce tumour suppressor gene mutations, typically *p53* and *p16*, in some of the stem cell populations located in oesophageal gland squamous ducts, which are present throughout the entire length of the oesophagus. Following this initiation phase, multiple distinct clones of metaplastic tissue compete to colonise the oesophagus, creating a mosaic pattern of clones across the segment. Clonal expansion of populations with greater selective advantage, such as ability to survive in a markedly acid- or bile-rich environment, leads to dominant and widespread clones. Once initiated, the promotion and propagation of metaplastic clones is dependent on the surrounding microenvironment, particularly the presence of a chronic inflammatory cell infiltrate, characterised by T lymphocytes, and cytokines such as interleukin-1, tumour necrosis factor-α and transforming growth factor-β. These lead to an increase in cyclo-oxygenase-2, c-*myc* and cyclin D1, which increase proliferation and decrease apoptosis, and a reduction in E-cadherin, with resultant loss of cell adhesion and localisation of β-catenin to the nucleus.[28] These molecular changes underlie the progression of Barrett's oesophagus to cancer via the metaplasia–dysplasia–adenocarcinoma sequence (see **Fig. 15.1**).

The presence of dysplasia is regarded as the best marker for malignant transformation in the epithelium. Dysplasia is classified histologically: HGD is diagnosed when there are distinct cytological changes, particularly nuclear pleomorphism and loss of crypt architecture. Low-grade dysplasia (LGD) is more difficult to classify; there is loss of cellular differentiation

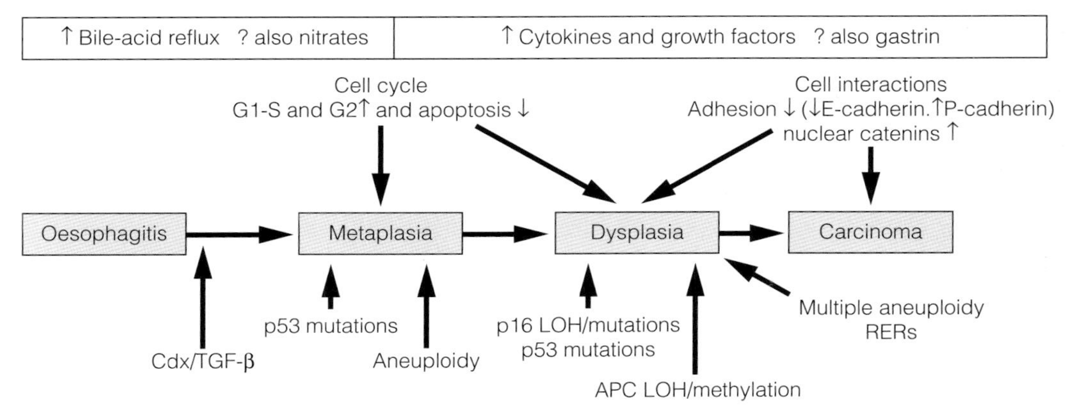

Figure 15.1 • The metaplasia–dysplasia–adenocarcinoma sequence. There are histological stages of progression (shaded rectangles representing the clonal expansion of competing stem cells). In addition there are structural genetic changes in the form of mutations (vertical arrows) and environmental changes (white rectangles) driving cell cycle and cell adhesion biological sequelae. APC, adenomatous polyposis coli gene; Cdx, CauDal protein gene; LOH, loss of heterozygosity; RERs, random errors of replication; TGF-β, transforming growth factor-β. Adapted from Jankowski J, Harrison RF, Perry I et al. Barrett's metaplasia. Lancet 2000; 356:2079–85. With permission from Elsevier.

and loss of goblet cells but with milder changes than those seen in HGD. Intramucosal cancer is said to have occurred when there is invasion through the basement membrane into the lamina propria. The term carcinoma in situ has been abandoned.

Although traditionally thought of as an acquired condition, genetic factors may play a part in a small proportion of patients with Barrett's metaplasia, as family and twin studies suggest a subgroup of individuals with a strong familial tendency to Barrett's oesophagus.[29,30] A family in the UK has been identified with a male index case with oesophageal adenocarcinoma, three brothers with Barrett's-associated cancer or HGD, and six children with Barrett's oesophagus.[31] Linkage studies are being undertaken in order to further our understanding of this genetic inheritance. However, there are data to suggest Barrett's is a polygenic disease with multiple contributing genes acting together.

Several studies have used a candidate gene approach to attempt to identify genetic variants in inflammatory and DNA repair pathways that could account for host susceptibility. Furthermore, results from ongoing genome-wide association studies of Barrett's oesophagus and oesophageal adenocarcinoma will direct further study towards particular loci of interest in the future.

Risk of cancer and mortality in Barrett's oesophagus

Barrett's oesophagus is accepted as a significant risk factor for adenocarcinoma of the oesophagus, although the risk of progression to adenocarcinoma and the risk of disease-specific mortality is low. A large number of studies have estimated the risk of adenocarcinoma arising from Barrett's oesophagus, with very variable results.[32–42] Former studies included small numbers of patients and were likely subject to publication bias, with results only being published if they showed a high incidence of cancer, leading to an overestimate of risk.[43] Recently, two large population-based cohort studies have reported much lower annual rates of progression to adenocarcinoma (0.12–0.13% per year) than in former series (Table 15.2). It should be noted that these figures exclude carcinomas of the gastric cardia and also do not reflect progression to HGD. In addition, the two studies used different approaches to select patients with Barrett's oesophagus. The study by Hvid-Jensen et al.[33] identified patients with intestinal metaplasia (IM) from the Danish National Pathology Registry without corroboration with endoscopic findings. Therefore, potentially, patients may have been included who had a diagnosis of cardiac IM rather than true Barrett's oesophagus, producing an incorrect denominator and leading to a slight underestimate of the risk of disease progression. Bhat et al.[32] included patients with columnar-lined oesophagus (CLO) at endoscopy (although the validated Prague system was not used), which was corroborated histologically, and demonstrated an increased risk of progression in patients who had IM confirmed histologically at index endoscopy, compared to those with CLO without IM. This finding is in keeping with previous studies demonstrating a higher risk of disease progression in patients with confirmed IM.[1,44,45]

Table 15.2 • Studies reporting the incidence of oesophageal adenocarcinoma in Barrett's oesophagus

Reference	Patients	Mean follow-up (years)	Total follow-up (patient years)	Annual risk of progression to cancer
Bhat et al. (2011)[32]	8522	7.0	59784	0.13%
	3179*	–	23417*	0.04%*
	3917†	–	28323†	0.23%†
Hvid-Jensen et al. (2011)[33]	11028	5.2 (median)	67105	0.12%

Unless stated, figures represent annual risk of progression for non-dysplastic intestinal metaplasia. Figures from Bhat et al. are divided into patients where IM was absent following index biopsy (*) and patients who had IM identified on index biopsy (†). The presence or absence of IM was unknown for 1426 patients.

Previous studies have, however, suggested a significant geographical variation in the incidence of carcinoma arising in Barrett's oesophagus in Western countries, with incidence rates in the UK almost double those in the USA.[46] It is also worth noting that the population demographic in Denmark differs somewhat from the USA and UK, where rates of obesity are significantly higher and where a greater proportion of men, who are at higher risk of malignant progression, develop Barrett's oesophagus.

✔✔ A Danish population-based case–control study identified 11 028 patients from the national pathology registry with a diagnosis of intestinal metaplasia following oesophageal biopsy.[33] Patients were followed for a median of 5.2 years. Compared to the general population, patients with Barrett's oesophagus were found to have a relative risk of 11.3 for developing adenocarcinoma with an annual risk of 0.12%. Only 7.6% of the total oesophageal adenocarcinomas diagnosed nationwide over the study period had a previous diagnosis of Barrett's oesophagus.

A recent meta-analysis reported a pooled estimate of the annual risk of cancer progression in non-dysplastic Barrett's of 0.39% per year. Importantly, only eight of 47 studies that met all three quality criteria were included in this analysis; inclusion of the remaining studies significantly increased this figure.[35] The risk in the UK following a meta-analysis is indicated as closer to 1%, higher than is reported in the USA.[46]

✔ It is important to appreciate that while patients with Barrett's oesophagus have an increased relative risk of adenocarcinoma, the majority of patients will die from other causes. A UK study has demonstrated an increase in both overall mortality rate and oesophageal cancer mortality rate in Barrett's patients compared with the age- and sex-matched general population. However, only 10% of deaths were due to oesophageal cancer, while 49% were due to cardiorespiratory disease, especially ischaemic heart disease and bronchopneumonia, and 18% of deaths were due to other cancers.[47]

Natural history of dysplasia in Barrett's oesophagus

When considering the natural history of dysplasia in Barrett's oesophagus we must remember that in addition to potential problems with length of follow-up and sampling error at endoscopy, there is considerable inter- and intra-observer variation among experienced pathologists in the histological diagnosis of dysplasia. While pathologists can demonstrate acceptable levels of agreement in distinguishing HGD combined with carcinoma from no dysplasia combined with indefinite and low-grade dysplasia (kappa values of 0.8), there are much poorer levels of agreement in distinguishing between the four groups: indefinite for dysplasia, LGD, HGD and carcinoma (intra-observer kappa values of 0.43–0.64).[48] Pathologists find it particularly difficult to separate inflammation in Barrett's oesophagus from LGD. In this situation pathologists should be encouraged to make use of the indefinite for dysplasia category: such a diagnosis does not mean that the pathologist is uncertain, but rather that it is not possible, with confidence, to exclude LGD in inflamed material. The diagnosis of HGD has serious implications for patient management and the diagnosis should be confirmed by two expert pathologists.

✔✔ A systematic review involving a total of 1488 patients with Barrett's oesophagus reported that LGD was present at initial endoscopy in 169 patients (11%) and HGD in 18 patients (1.2%); 1301 (87%) had metaplasia with no dysplasia.[49]

Low-grade dysplasia

The natural history of LGD is not fully understood and reported rates of regression/progression vary considerably, reflecting the diagnostic difficulties discussed above. Sharma et al.[50] followed 156 patients for a mean of 4.1 years and reported progression to HGD or cancer in 13%, regression in 66% and stable LGD in 21%. A more recent prospective cohort study of 713 Barrett's patients, including 111 with LGD, reported that compared to non-dysplastic disease, LGD was a significant risk factor for progression to HGD or adenocarcinoma (relative risk (RR) 9.7; 95% confidence interval (CI) 4.4–21.5).[51] Similarly, in their large population-based study, Hvid-Jensen et al.[33] reported that the relative risk of oesophageal cancer among those who had LGD at baseline, as compared to those without LGD at baseline, was 4.8 (95% CI 2.6–8.8). The annual risk of progression to HGD or cancer was found to be 1.27% for those with LGD at baseline. Bhat et al.[32] reported a hazard ratio of 5.67% (95% CI 3.77–8.33) for patients with LGD compared to no dysplasia. However, a recent study by Wani et al.,[52] which followed up 210 patients with Barrett's oesophagus with or without LGD for a mean of 6.2 years, found no associations of presence of prevalent, incident or persistent LGD, or the extent of LGD, with progression rates.

Bergman and colleagues recently demonstrated that LGD is over-diagnosed by non-specialist pathologists and argued that its true significance might have been underestimated by many reported series.[53] In their study, 1198 patients underwent Barrett's surveillance at six non-specialist hospitals, identifying 147 (12.5%) patients with LGD. However, only eight (0.7%) patients were deemed to have LGD following histological review by two external expert gastrointestinal pathologists. The majority of diagnoses were reclassified as non-dysplastic Barrett's oesophagus. During a mean follow-up period of 51 months, 42% of patients with LGD diagnosed by consensus expert pathologists demonstrated progression to either carcinoma or HGD, and 2.2% regressed to non-dysplastic Barrett's oesophagus.[53]

✓ The natural history of LGD is still not fully understood and there is wide variation in reported rates of progression to HGD or cancer. However, it appears that the majority of patients with LGD diagnosed without consensus pathology reporting will either remain stable or regress to to Barrett's metaplasia without dysplasia (BM). The majority of evidence from large recent trials reports that the presence of LGD at baseline endoscopy increases the relative risk of progression compared to patients with non-dysplastic disease (RR 4.8–9.7). The misdiagnosis of non-dysplastic Barrett's oesophagus or oesophagitis as LGD may have led to a widespread under-recognition of the true risk of LGD.

High-grade dysplasia

Studies reporting the natural history of HGD have also reported widely differing results. Reid et al.[54] followed 76 patients for 5 years and reported that 59% developed adenocarcinoma. In a study of 100 patients with HGD, 66 of whom underwent surveillance, 3 of 24 patients (13%) with focal HGD and 17 of 42 patients (40%) with diffuse HGD developed carcinoma after a mean follow-up of 41 and 23 months, respectively.[55]

An important question to consider is what proportion of patients with a diagnosis of HGD who undergo oesophagectomy have an occult cancer detected in the resected specimen? Table 15.3 shows reported rates in the literature of 0–73%: overall the rate appears to be approximately 40%.[56–72] Patients with visible, nodular HGD appear at greatest risk of harbouring coexisting cancer.[73,74] This emphasises the fact that patients with HGD may be harbouring an undetected cancer and confirms the need for complete staging in these patients.

Given that endotherapy is becoming a recognised treatment option for focal intramucosal cancers (T1a), a more pertinent question to ask might be: what is the prevalence of submucosal invasive cancer at oesophagectomy for HGD? The majority of studies in Table 15.3 make no attempt to separate intramucosal cancer (IMC) from more advanced lesions; however, some more recent reports suggest that rates of *invasive* cancer (submucosa or beyond) are considerably lower than 40%. Wang et al.[71] retrospectively assessed 60 patients (41 with preoperative HGD and 19 with preoperative IMC) who underwent oesophagectomy. The overall rate of submucosal cancer was 6.7%, with a rate of 5% in patients with preoperative HGD and 11% in patients with preoperative IMC. Only one patient (1.7%) had nodal metastasis. Another recent study found the rate of invasive adenocarcinoma (excluding IMC) in association with Barrett's HGD to be 11.7% (8/68), with 5.9% having occult cancer.[75]

Although some HGD may be stable or even regress, between 15% and 59% will progress to adenocarcinoma over 5 years. However, if detailed biopsy mapping endoscopies showed no previous HGD (prevalent HGD), then the detection of new HGD (incident HGD) is associated with a risk of subsequent progression to cancer of only between

Table 15.3 • Studies reporting the incidence of adenocarcinoma in resected specimens following oesophagectomy for high-grade dysplasia

Reference	Patients with high-grade dysplasia	Invasive cancer at postoperative histology	Percentage
Altorki et al. (1991)[57]	8	4	50
Pera et al. (1992)[58]	18	9	50
Streitz et al. (1993)[59]	9	2	22
Levine et al. (1993)[56]	7	0	0
Peters et al. (1994)[60]	9	5	56
Edwards et al. (1996)[61]	11	8	73
Rice et al. (1997)[62]	16	6	38
Collard et al. (1997)[63]	12	4	33
Ferguson and Naunheim (1997)[64]	15	8	53
Cameron and Carpenter (1997)[65]	19	2	11
Falk et al. (1999)[66]	28	10	36
Headrick et al. (2002)[67]	54	19	35
Tseng et al. (2003)[68]	60	18	30
Sujendran et al. (2005)[69]	17	11	65
Reed et al. (2005)[70]	49	18	37
Wang et al. (2009)[71]	41	16 (14 IMC; 2 inv. ca.)	39% (34% IMC, 5% inv. ca.)
Nasr and Schoen (2011)[72]	68	12 (4 IMC; 8 inv. ca.)	17.6 (5.9 IMC; 11.7 inv. ca.)
Total	**441**	**152**	**34**

IMC, intramucosal cancer; inv. ca., invasive cancer (denotes invasion into submucosa or beyond).

3% and 5% per year.[73,76] This area is being actively discussed in the Barrett's Dysplasia and Cancer Taskforce (BAD CAT) group.

Risk factors for progression to cancer

The length of Barrett's segment has been shown to be a significant risk factor for progression to cancer, a doubling of length increasing the risk 1.7-fold.[77] The extent of HGD and/or LGD also appears to be a risk factor for progression to adenocarcinoma.[55,78]

Importantly, in a prospective longitudinal cohort study, individuals with Barrett's oesophagus who were regularly taking aspirin or other NSAIDs were found to have a significantly lower 5-year cumulative incidence of adenocarcinoma compared with individuals not taking NSAIDs (6.6% and 14.3%, respectively), suggesting that this may be an effective chemotherapeutic intervention.[79] An ongoing phase III multicentre randomised controlled trial (RCT), the AspECT trial (Aspirin and Esomeprazole Chemoprevention in Barrett's Metaplasia), designed to test this hypothesis is due to report in 2016. The primary aim of this study is to determine whether acid suppression with proton-pump inhibition (high dose vs. low dose) with or without aspirin can reduce mortality or the conversion from Barrett's metaplasia to HGD or adenocarcinoma. Both high- and low-dose acid suppression are being investigated as there remains doubt about the optimal dose of proton-pump inhibitor (PPI) to use, especially given the fact that Barrett's mucosa is relatively insensitive, thus rendering symptoms unreliable. There is an argument that incomplete acid suppression might increase the risk of cancer by exposing the mucosa to short pulses of acid, thus stimulating the proliferation of abnormal cells. In contrast, there is some epidemiological evidence that high-dose proton-pump inhibition might increase the risk of cancer as bile acid might become cytotoxic at neutral pH. In addition, there have been fears that PPI-induced hypergastrinaemia could stimulate hyperproliferation of Barrett's epithelium.[80,81] Although this risk is yet to be evaluated in vivo, it appears more likely that gastrin induces epithelial restitution in Barrett's oesophagus, without stimulation of clonal expansion or disease progression.[82]

AspECT is the world's largest chemopreventive RCT of Barrett's oesophagus. It aims to decrease cancer conversion by 35% and cardiac deaths by 20%. The premise is that the shared cardiac and cancer susceptibility could be addressed by a joint chemoprevention regimen in order to prevent premature death.

Screening for Barrett's oesophagus and adenocarcinoma using molecular markers

It is accepted that GORD is a significant risk factor for the development of adenocarcinoma, with a well-known Swedish case–control study demonstrating a 44-fold increased relative risk in individuals with frequent heartburn of greater than 20 years' duration.[17] This has led to the suggestion that screening individuals with chronic reflux symptoms to detect Barrett's oesophagus and cancer may be of benefit. However, it is important to appreciate two flaws in this concept: firstly, approximately 40% of individuals with cancer in the series mentioned above denied frequent heartburn; secondly, a significant proportion of individuals with Barrett's oesophagus are asymptomatic. In addition, Barrett's patients experience less heartburn and use PPIs less frequently compared with controls.[2,83,84]

The endoscopic screening of individuals with chronic reflux symptoms to detect either Barrett's or cancer is not currently recommended in the UK or USA.[1,2] This is because of the low absolute risk of developing adenocarcinoma in individuals with chronic reflux, combined with the knowledge that most individuals with Barrett's oesophagus die from causes other than oesophageal cancer. There are also concerns about the cost-effectiveness and invasiveness of endoscopy as a screening tool.

Several attempts have been made to develop a scoring system using patient demographics and symptoms to predict the presence of Barrett's oesophagus for screening purposes.[85,86] However, interest in these risk prediction strategies has declined due to inability to generate sufficient sensitivity and specificity.

It is hoped that future non-invasive molecular screening tests might be developed to detect patients with Barrett's oesophagus who display phenotypes that could act as markers of disease progression. Promising techniques include DNA microarrays (measuring genome-wide alterations in DNA copy number), single nucleotide polymorphism (SNP) arrays (detecting allelic imbalances) and measurement of hyperproliferation, which occurs as a sequel of genetic mutation.

Mutations in the *p53* tumour suppressor gene are widely found in dysplastic Barrett's oesophagus and oesophageal cancer. Younes et al.[87] found *p53* mutation in 9% of Barrett's patients with LGD, 55% of patients with HGD and 87% of patients with carcinoma: no patients without dysplasia had a *p53* mutation. Importantly, in a further study, 56% of patients with LGD and *p53* mutation progressed to HGD or carcinoma, whereas no patient with LGD without *p53* mutation progressed.[88] Similarly, Reid et al.[89] demonstrated that loss of heterozygosity of gene 17 (*p53*) was found in 6% of patients without dysplasia, 20% of patients with LGD and 57% of patients with HGD. Patients with loss of heterozygosity had a 16-fold increased risk of cancer after 3 years. These results have led to the suggestion that the subgroup of patients with low-grade or indefinite dysplasia and *p53* mutation should be subjected to more rigorous surveillance protocols. However, it is important to remember that not all oesophageal adenocarcinomas express *p53*, and patients without expression can progress to cancer.

Other markers that have been identified as conferring a high risk of progression are *p16* mutations,[90] cyclin D1 overexpression,[91] flow cytometry abnormalities such as aneuploidy and increase in the G2/tetraploidy fraction of DNA content,[92] and reduced expression of E-cadherin, with resultant loss of cell adhesion and localisation of β-catenin to the nucleus.[93]

Several clinical trials are under way, including the Chemoprevention of Premalignant Intestinal Neoplasia (ChOPIN) trial and the Barrett's Oesophagus Screening Trial (BEST2) trial, which aim to explore non-invasive methods of screening for malignant progression. ChOPIN aims to detect a panel of predictive serum biomarkers, whereas BEST2 is a case–control trial investigating the potential of a non-endoscopic immunocytological device (Cytosponge).[94,95] This trial requires patients to swallow a small capsule that dissolves into a 3-cm sponge in the stomach and is then withdrawn through the oesophagus. Oesophageal cells are assessed for a range of predictive biomarkers, including TFF3 positivity (the principal end-point) as well as ploidy, Mcm2, cyclin A, TP53 and methylation. Cost data and the impact of screening on psychosocial well-being are also being evaluated. It is hoped that non-invasive screening tests such as these could enable safe, accurate and cost-effective population-based screening in the future.

✔ There are currently no validated biomarkers for prognostic evaluation of Barrett's metaplasia ready for clinical use other than the presence or absence of dysplasia, especially HGD, as determined by histopathological assessment. A multicentre case–control study (BEST2) is currently under way, aiming to demonstrate potential for screening using a non-endoscopic Cytosponge test; however, a large RCT will be required before this test can be considered for use in clinical practice.

Surveillance of non-dysplastic disease

Surveillance biopsies should be taken from all four quadrants of the oesophagus at 2-cm intervals in addition to any areas of mucosal abnormality, as described previously (see 'Endoscopic assessment').

The central concept of surveillance is that regular endoscopic examination and biopsy will allow the detection of cancer at an early asymptomatic stage, thereby resulting in better treatment outcomes. Several small retrospective studies have demonstrated a survival benefit associated with surveillance-detected cancers.[59,60,96–98] However, other series have failed to support these findings.[99] These studies may be subject to both selection bias and length bias, concerns that prompted the ongoing Barrett's Oesophagus Surveillance Study (BOSS), which aims to define the objective value of endoscopic surveillance and the most appropriate surveillance protocol. BOSS randomises patients with at least 1 cm of circumferential or 2 cm non-circumferential Barrett's oesophagus to either endoscopic surveillance with protocol biopsy[1] (n = 1250) or endoscopy at the time of need (n = 1250), the latter group being discharged unless they develop new symptoms or alarming symptoms.

Clearly, surveillance is only appropriate for patients who are suitable for treatment of detected lesions, either HGD or cancer, and traditionally, as this was limited to oesophagectomy, this meant that individuals had to be of a relatively young age and lacking in any significant comorbidity. However, with the development of endoscopic techniques for mucosal ablation and resection, surveillance may be appropriate for an additional cohort of patients.

There are a number of disadvantages and limitations to surveillance programmes. In addition to the physical and psychological burden imposed on patients, it must be remembered, and communicated to patients at enrolment, that surveillance does not guarantee to detect all cancers (due to sampling error and limitations of current endoscopic imaging techniques) or to offer a cure for all detected cancers.

✔ Current UK guidelines suggest that individuals with Barrett's oesophagus without dysplasia should undergo surveillance endoscopy every 2 years – this is based on a mathematical model that assumes the risk of developing adenocarcinoma in Barrett's oesophagus is approximately 1% per annum. Recent evidence suggests that rates of malignant progression may be significantly lower than previously reported, thus questioning the rationale for surveillance of patients with non-dysplastic disease. Outcomes of the BOSS trial are awaited; however, it is possible that future recommendations may require additional risk factors (segment length >3 cm, history of dysplasia, molecular markers of high risk) to prompt surveillance, as opposed to the current policy of surveillance for all-comers.

Future surveillance strategies could use genomics and/or molecular profiling to predict patients at higher risk of malignant progression. Such strategies could enable individualised surveillance policies, ensuring those at genuine risk of progression are monitored and removing the psychological burden of serial endoscopies for those with a diminutive risk of disease progression.

✔ One of the fundamental goals of translational research in Barrett's oesophagus is to distinguish the small number of patients who will progress to oesophageal adenocarcinoma from the majority who will not.

Effect of medical therapy and antireflux surgery

It has been shown that long-term acid suppression with PPIs can lead to an improvement in Barrett's metaplasia. A study of 23 patients following a regimen of omeprazole 40 mg daily for 2 years demonstrated a significant reduction in the length of columnar mucosa, an increase in squamous islands within the columnar epithelium and a reduction in the proportion of sulphomucin-rich intestinal metaplasia.[100] More recently, a study of 188 patients followed for up to 13 years (mean 5 years) reported development of squamous islands in 48% of patients, although the mean length of Barrett's segment was not reduced and no patients regressed to squamous mucosa.[101]

✔✔ A randomised double-blind trial of omeprazole 80 mg daily versus ranitidine 300 mg daily in patients with proven Barrett's oesophagus and gastro-oesophageal reflux disease demonstrated a reduction in the length and surface area of columnar metaplasia in the omeprazole group but not in the ranitidine group. Both treatments successfully controlled reflux symptoms.[102]

The effect of antireflux surgery on Barrett's metaplasia has proved a controversial subject. Selected series have demonstrated regression in Barrett's length in 14–35% of patients, with complete regression of LGD in 44–93% of patients.[103–105] However, the RCT evidence has not supported these findings, at best demonstrating a reduction in Barrett's length without achieving complete regression of dysplasia.[105] In addition, studies have failed to show an absolute reduction in rates of oesophageal adenocarcinoma following antireflux surgery.

Currently there are no RCTs comparing laparoscopic fundoplication (the favoured method of antireflux surgery) with PPI therapy to assess the effect on malignant progression in Barrett's oesophagus. The numbers of patients required, due to low progression rates, would probably make such a study impracticable. In addition, any benefits of antireflux surgery would need to be tempered by the potential morbidity and economic implications of prophylactic surgery.

✔✔ A meta-analysis comparing the reported incidence of adenocarcinoma in Barrett's patients after antireflux surgery with patients treated medically found no statistically significant difference in the incidence rates of 3.8 and 5.3 per 1000 patient years, respectively.[106] A recent systematic review reported a statistically significant lower incidence of adenocarcinoma after antireflux surgery compared with medical therapy (2.8 vs. 6.3 per 1000 patient years, $P = 0.03$); however, when uncontrolled case series were excluded and the analysis was confined to randomised trials and cohort studies there was no significant difference between the two treatments (4.4 vs. 6.5 per 1000 patient years, $P = 0.32$).[49] Accordingly, at present there is insufficient evidence to recommend antireflux surgery over proton-pump inhibition as a cancer-preventing procedure.

Endotherapy

Endotherapy, including endoscopic resection and ablative therapies, is indicated in selected patients with HGD, intramucosal cancer (T1a) and early submucosal cancers (T1b). The potential role of endotherapy in early oesophageal cancer, including the important diagnostic role of endoscopic resection, is addressed in Chapter 6 and so will not be discussed further here.

Endotherapies offer an attractive alternative to radical surgery in terms of reduced mortality and morbidity, with excellent short-term results, but long-term efficacy remains unclear.

Endoscopic resection

Endoscopic mucosal resection aims to remove the mucosa and submucosa down to the muscularis and for this reason the term endoscopic resection (ER) is now preferred. ER is indicated for removal of focal HGD. Piecemeal resection is required for lesions greater than 2 cm, with meticulous care being taken to ensure completeness of excision. Complications are uncommon – bleeding (3%) and perforation (0.1–5%) – and most can be managed endoscopically.[107]

ER has been shown to achieve remission in 82.5–95% of patients with HGD, but may be associated with metachronous lesions or disease recurrence in up to 14% of patients within 12 months, and 21.5% of patients over 5 years.[108–111] Factors associated with recurrence include piecemeal resection, long-segment Barrett's oesophagus (>5 cm), delayed treatment of HGD (>10 months), multifocal disease and omission of adjuvant ablative therapy.[108] Recurrent disease necessitates re-treatment, which can be successful and provide long-term disease control but which may have higher complication rates.

Several trials have reported circumferential ER for removal of widespread multifocal disease; however, this practice has led to high rates of post-treatment stricture formation (17–26%) and higher rates of perforation (3%) and is therefore not widely recommended.[112,113]

Endoscopic ablation

Endoscopic ablation techniques include: thermal methods, such as argon-beam plasma photocoagulation (APC), multipolar electrocautery (MPEC), laser therapy and cryotherapy; chemical methods, such as photodynamic therapy (PDT); and radiofrequency ablation (RFA).

RFA and PDT deliver an even distribution of treatment over a consistent therapeutic depth and can be readily applied to large areas of circumferential disease. Both have been shown to be highly efficacious at eradicating dysplastic Barrett's oesophagus.[114–124] However, RFA is now widely regarded as the first-line therapy due to its relative ease of administration, more favourable side-effect profile and low rates of recurrent dysplasia.[123]

✔✔ Shaheen et al.[115] randomised 127 patients with dysplastic Barrett's oesophagus in a 2:1 ratio to receive either RFA or sham procedure. Complete eradication of LGD occurred in 90.5% (ablation group) compared to 22.7% (control group) ($P < 0.001$) at 1 year. Complete eradication of HGD occurred in 81.0% (ablation group) versus 19.0% (control group) ($P < 0.001$). RFA decreased both the likelihood of disease progression (3.6% vs. 16.3%, $P = 0.03$) and cancer (1.2% vs. 9.3%, $P = 0.045$). Recent follow-up data after 3 years have shown that this effect is durable.[114]

There is RCT evidence supporting the efficacy of both MPEC and APC for treatment of dysplastic Barrett's although, compared to RFA, these techniques are less user-friendly for treating large Barrett's segments and treatment depths are less consistent. In addition, they may be more likely to be complicated by strictures and the development of buried glandular mucosa beneath neosquamous epithelium.[125] Currently these techniques are favoured for 'touch-up' therapy in patients with small patches of persistent metaplasia following previous RFA treatments. An RCT comparing the two thermal techniques, MPEC and APC, found no significant advantage with either technique.[125]

Management of LGD

The detection of LGD should prompt a course of high-dose acid suppression with a PPI for 8–12 weeks followed by repeat endoscopy with extensive biopsies. If LGD persists then surveillance endoscopy should be repeated at 6-monthly intervals and the patient should remain on a PPI. If regression to metaplasia without dysplasia occurs on two consecutive examinations then the surveillance interval may return to 2-yearly.[1]

Endoscopic treatment of LGD is controversial and is not supported by current UK guidelines based on a number-needed-to-treat analysis. However, simple surveillance of LGD is not universally supported and there is growing backing for early intervention.

The likely significant over-diagnosis of LGD in routine clinical practice may account for low reported rates of disease progression and supports the widely recommended policy of close surveillance, without endoscopic therapy. However, an alternative option might be for referral of all histology slides showing suspected LGD for specialist consensus reporting, with subsequent endoscopic treatment for confirmed cases of LGD. This approach would have considerable economic and practical implications and is not currently feasible in the UK.

Management of HGD

The detection of HGD has serious implications for the patient and should be considered a malignant lesion. The diagnosis should always be confirmed by a second expert pathologist and all cases should be discussed in a multidisciplinary meeting for consideration of both endoscopic and surgical treatments. The diagnosis of HGD is usually an indication to end surveillance and patients should be fully informed of the significance of the diagnosis and of the pros and cons of the different treatment options.

Following referral to specialist centres patients with HGD should be re-biopsied using a Seattle biopsy protocol: quadrantic biopsies every 1 cm with further targeted biopsies from suspicious areas. A large number of samples should be taken – up to 84 biopsies from a single patient have been reported.[56] Patients should be carefully staged, including use of diagnostic ER, and patients with nodular disease should be considered at particular risk of harbouring occult invasive disease.[73,74]

Falk et al.[66] demonstrated that 38% of cancers were missed when taking quadrantic biopsies every 2 cm from patients with HGD. Jumbo biopsy forceps made little difference to detection rates (67% vs. 62%). Similarly, Cameron and Carpenter[65] found 2 of 19 (10.5%) unsuspected adenocarcinomas following quadrantic 2-cm biopsies in patients who subsequently underwent oesophagectomy. Reid et al.[126] compared a quadrantic 2-cm biopsy protocol to biopsies taken at 1-cm intervals in 45 patients diagnosed with HGD who subsequently developed cancer. The 2-cm protocol missed 50% of the cancers that were detected by the 1-cm protocol in Barrett's segments 2 cm or more without visible lesions. This more intensive biopsy regimen is recommended in patients with HGD, at 3-monthly intervals. However, it is important to consider that Barrett's adenocarcinomas may still be missed in up to 29% of cases.[127]

The choice of intervention in patients with HGD remains a controversial subject. Traditionally, individuals who were fit enough were recommended to undergo oesophagectomy while endoscopic techniques were reserved for those unfit for resection. However, with increasing evidence of therapeutic benefit, endoscopic therapy is now considered by many to be first-line treatment ahead of oesophagectomy in fit patients, provided they have been adequately staged.

Most units favour a policy of focal lesion resection using ER followed by ablation of the entire Barrett's segment using RFA to destroy the neoplastic field change in adjacent metaplasia. ER improves histological assessment and aids detection of occult adenocarcinoma,[128,129] but the need for subsequent ablation of the surrounding non-dysplastic Barrett's oesophagus is controversial. There are no RCTs addressing this directly; however, there is some evidence to suggest lower recurrence rates if ER is used in conjunction with whole segment ablation.[44,66]

The decision between endotherapy and oesophagectomy is controversial and dependent on patient comorbidity and the nature of the disease: HGD versus intramucosal cancer; unifocal versus multifocal; long- versus short-segment Barrett's; presence or absence of lymphovascular invasion; and grade of differentiation. Endotherapy can effectively eradicate HGD, with low rates of disease recurrence in the medium term (long-term data awaited).[114,115,130] In addition, any recurrent disease can usually be managed endoscopically, or if necessary surgically, without excess mortality.[131,132] However, advocates of surgery point to the risk of occult adenocarcinoma, particularly in nodular disease, and the possible risk of under-staging of disease using a non-operative approach. In addition, there is evidence that prophylactic oesophagectomy in HGD is associated with a lower risk of operative mortality than routine oesophagectomy as patients are typically younger with fewer comorbidities, and have not undergone neoadjuvant therapy.[68]

Patients must be informed of the need for lifelong surveillance (including biopsy) following endotherapy, even in cases of complete response, to ensure the absence of long-term recurrence and the identification of buried glandular elements that may retain malignant potential. Surveillance after oesophagectomy is not routine as recurrence rates are low, although Barrett's-associated adenocarcinoma above the gastric conduit has been described.

The Surveillance Epidemiology and End Results (SEER) database of the US National Cancer Institute found no difference in survival between patients with HGD or stage 1 (T1N0M0) tumours treated by endoscopic therapy compared to radical surgery.[133,134] However, most studies directly comparing radical surgery and endoscopic therapy have been severely limited by selection bias.[133–135] Well-designed multicentre randomised trials are awaited.

✔ There are no randomised trials comparing surgery and endotherapy in the management of HGD and these studies should be undertaken as a matter of urgency. Endotherapy is a viable treatment option for patients with HGD, with close surveillance, early endoscopic treatment of recurrence, and progression to oesophagectomy if indicated. A recent Cochrane review was unable to recommend either surgery or endotherapy as first-line treatment in HGD due to the paucity of high-level evidence and the multitude of contributing factors.[136]

Conclusion

In the last 5 years we have come a considerable way in the improved understanding and treatment of Barrett's oesophagus. We have two strategies for the prevention of cancer, namely chemoprevention and surveillance, that are being tested in two of the world's largest randomised trials. Furthermore, non-endoscopic molecular-based screening tests have now entered clinical trials. Finally, there is strong evidence to support the efficacy of several minimally invasive endoscopic therapies. However, long-term follow-up data are awaited, and randomised studies are required to compare endotherapy to oesophagectomy in the setting of HGD and intramucosal oesophageal cancer.

Key points

- The incidence of Barrett's adenocarcinoma is increasing and is especially high in the UK.
- The exact prevalence of Barrett's oesophagus is unclear but is probably around 2%. Most patients with Barrett's oesophagus are undetected in the community.
- Barrett's metaplasia develops as a mucosal 'adaptive' response as a result of chronic inflammation, secondary to gastro-oesophageal reflux disease. There is strong evidence that the site of origin of Barrett's metaplasia is a progenitor stem cell located in the submucosal oesophageal gland ducts.
- The development of adenocarcinoma in Barrett's oesophagus is thought to follow a progressive sequence from intestinal metaplasia to low-grade dysplasia (LGD) to high-grade dysplasia (HGD) and finally to cancer. The presence of dysplasia is currently the best marker for malignant transformation in the epithelium.
- There is considerable inter- and intra-observer variation among experienced pathologists in the histological diagnosis of dysplastic Barrett's oesophagus.
- Most Barrett's epithelium is stable and will not undergo malignant transformation. The risk of neoplastic progression in non-dysplastic disease appears lower than previously reported. Oesophageal adenocarcinoma is an uncommon cause of death in persons with Barrett's oesophagus.

- Ninety to ninety-five per cent of oesophageal adenocarcinoma arises in patients who have no prior diagnosis of Barrett's oesophagus.
- The AspECT cancer prevention trial is the world's largest trial in this area and aims to decrease cancer by 35%.
- A randomised double-blind study has confirmed that acid suppression with a proton-pump inhibitor induces a partial regression of the columnar-lined segment.
- At present there is insufficient evidence to recommend antireflux surgery over proton-pump inhibition as a cancer-preventing procedure.
- Patients with intestinal metaplasia should have regular surveillance endoscopy and biopsy at 2-yearly intervals and should remain on a proton-pump inhibitor.
- Patients who have a surveillance-detected cancer survive longer following surgery than patients who develop symptomatic cancers.
- The detection of HGD is an indication to end surveillance.
- Patients with HGD should be adequately staged, including the use of endoscopic resection where appropriate.
- Endotherapy for HGD should involve endoscopic resection of focal HGD lesions followed by whole Barrett's segment ablation using radiofrequency ablation to destroy the malignant field change.
- Randomised trials are required to compare the efficacy of endotherapy versus oesophagectomy in the setting of HGD; however, both appear viable treatment options.

References

1. Watson A, Heading RC, Shepherd NA. A Report of the Working Party of the British Society of Gastroenterology. Guidelines for the diagnosis and management of Barrett's columnar-lined oesophagus. 2005.
2. Wang KK, Sampliner RE. Practice Parameters Committee of the American College of Gastroenterology. Updated guidelines 2008 for the diagnosis, surveillance and therapy of Barrett's esophagus. Am J Gastroenterol 2008;103(3):788–97.
3. Harrison R, Perry I, Haddadin W, et al. Detection of intestinal metaplasia in Barrett's esophagus: an observational comparator study suggests the need for a minimum of eight biopsies. Am J Gastroenterol 2007;102(6):1154–61.
4. Rex DK, Cummings OW, Shaw M, et al. Screening for Barrett's esophagus in colonoscopy patients with and without heartburn. Gastroenterology 2003;125(6):1670–7.
5. Vakil N, van Zanten SV, Kahrilas P, et al. Global Consensus Group. The Montreal definition and classification of gastroesophageal reflux disease: a global evidence-based consensus. Am J Gastroenterol 2006;101(8):1900–20. quiz 1943.
6. Cameron AJ, Zinsmeister AR, Ballard DJ, et al. Prevalence of columnar-lined (Barrett's) esophagus. Comparison of population-based clinical and autopsy findings. Gastroenterology 1990;99(4):918–22.
7. Cameron AJ, Lomboy CT. Barrett's esophagus: age, prevalence, and extent of columnar epithelium. Gastroenterology 1992;103(4):1241–5.
8. Jankowski J, Barr H, Wang K, et al. Diagnosis and management of Barrett's oesophagus. Br Med J 2010;341:4551.
9. Ronkainen J, Aro P, Storskrubb T, et al. Prevalence of Barrett's esophagus in the general population: an endoscopic study. Gastroenterology 2005;129(6):1825–31.
   This population-based study recruited a representative sample of 1000 people from two communities in northern Sweden to undergo upper endoscopy and confirmed the presence of intestinal metaplasia in 1.6% of the population studied.
10. Gerson LB, Banerjee S. Screening for Barrett's esophagus in asymptomatic women. Gastrointest Endosc 2009;70(5):867–73.
11. van Soest EM, Dieleman JP, Siersema PD, et al. Increasing incidence of Barrett's oesophagus in the general population. Gut 2005;54(8):1062–6.
12. Spechler SJ, Zeroogian JM, Antonioli DA, et al. Prevalence of metaplasia at the gastro-oesophageal junction. Lancet 1994;344(8936):1533–6.
13. Caygill CP, Watson A, Reed PI, et al. UK National Barrett's Oesophagus Registry (UKBOR) and the 27 Participating Centres. Characteristics and regional variations of patients with Barrett's oesophagus in the UK. Eur J Gastroenterol Hepatol 2003;15(11):1217–22.
14. Eisen GM, Sandler RS, Murray S, et al. The relationship between gastroesophageal reflux disease and its complications with Barrett's esophagus. Am J Gastroenterol 1997;92(1):27–31.

15. Winters Jr. C, Spurling TJ, Chobanian SJ, et al. Barrett's esophagus. A prevalent, occult complication of gastroesophageal reflux disease. Gastroenterology 1987;92(1):118–24.
16. Smith KJ, O'Brien SM, Smithers BM, et al. Interactions among smoking, obesity, and symptoms of acid reflux in Barrett's esophagus. Cancer Epidemiol Biomarkers Prev 2005;14(11, Pt 1):2481–6.
17. Lagergren J, Bergstrom R, Lindgren A, et al. Symptomatic gastroesophageal reflux as a risk factor for esophageal adenocarcinoma. N Engl J Med 1999;340(11):825–31.
18. Sharma P, Dent J, Armstrong D, et al. The development and validation of an endoscopic grading system for Barrett's esophagus: the Prague C & M criteria. Gastroenterology 2006;131(5):1392–9.
19. Curvers WL, Bansal A, Sharma P, et al. Endoscopic work-up of early Barrett's neoplasia. Endoscopy 2008;40(12):1000–7.
20. Singh R, Ragunath K, Jankowski J. Barrett's esophagus: diagnosis, screening, surveillance, and controversies. Gut Liver 2007;1(2):93–100.
21. Vieth M, Ell C, Gossner L, et al. Histological analysis of endoscopic resection specimens from 326 patients with Barrett's esophagus and early neoplasia. Endoscopy 2004;36(9):776–81.
22. Dunbar KB, Canto MI. Confocal laser endomicroscopy in Barrett's esophagus and endoscopically inapparent Barrett's neoplasia: a prospective, randomized, double-blind, controlled, crossover trial. Gastrointest Endosc 2010;72(3):668.
23. Qiu L, Pleskow DK, Chuttani R, et al. Multispectral scanning during endoscopy guides biopsy of dysplasia in Barrett's esophagus. Nat Med 2010;16(5):603–6.
24. Kara MA, Smits ME, Rosmolen WD, et al. A randomized crossover study comparing light-induced fluorescence endoscopy with standard videoendoscopy for the detection of early neoplasia in Barrett's esophagus. Gastrointest Endosc 2005;61(6):671–8.
25. Curvers W, Baak L, Kiesslich R, et al. Chromoendoscopy and narrow-band imaging compared with high-resolution magnification endoscopy in Barrett's esophagus. Gastroenterology 2008;134(3):670–9.
26. Thomas T, Singh R, Ragunath K. Trimodal imaging-assisted endoscopic mucosal resection of early Barrett's neoplasia. Surg Endosc 2009;23(7):1609–13.
27. Leedham SJ, Preston SL, McDonald SA, et al. Individual crypt genetic heterogeneity and the origin of metaplastic glandular epithelium in human Barrett's oesophagus. Gut 2008;57(8):1041–8.
28. Jankowski JA, Harrison RF, Perry I, et al. Barrett's metaplasia. Lancet 2000;356(9247):2079–85.
29. Cameron AJ, Lagergren J, Henriksson C, et al. Gastroesophageal reflux disease in monozygotic and dizygotic twins. Gastroenterology 2002;122(1):55–9.
30. Mohammed I, Cherkas LF, Riley SA, et al. Genetic influences in gastro-oesophageal reflux disease: a twin study. Gut 2003;52(8):1085–9.
31. Groves C, Jankowski J, Barker F, et al. A family history of Barrett's oesophagus: another risk factor? Scand J Gastroenterol 2005;40(9):1127–8.
32. Bhat S, Coleman HG, Yousef F, et al. Risk of malignant progression in Barrett's esophagus patients: results from a large population-based study. J Natl Cancer Inst 2011;103(13):1049–57.
33. Hvid-Jensen F, Pedersen L, Drewes AM, et al. Incidence of adenocarcinoma among patients with Barrett's esophagus. N Engl J Med 2011;365(15):1375–83.
This Danish population-based case–control study is the largest study following patients with intestinal metaplasia. Over a median of 5.2 years, patients with IM were found to have a relative risk of 11.3 for developing adenocarcinoma with an annual risk of just 0.12%. Only 7.6% of the total oesophageal adenocarcinomas diagnosed nationwide over the study period had a previous diagnosis of Barrett's oesophagus.
34. Sikkema M, de Jonge PJ, Steyerberg EW, et al. Risk of esophageal adenocarcinoma and mortality in patients with Barrett's esophagus: a systematic review and meta-analysis. Clin Gastroenterol Hepatol 2010;8(3):235–44.
35. Yousef F, Cardwell C, Cantwell MM, et al. The incidence of esophageal cancer and high-grade dysplasia in Barrett's esophagus: a systematic review and meta-analysis. Am J Epidemiol 2008;168(3):237–49.
36. Robertson CS, Mayberry JF, Nicholson DA, et al. Value of endoscopic surveillance in the detection of neoplastic change in Barrett's oesophagus. Br J Surg 1988;75(8):760–3.
37. Miros M, Kerlin P, Walker N. Only patients with dysplasia progress to adenocarcinoma in Barrett's oesophagus. Gut 1991;32(12):1441–6.
38. Iftikhar SY, James PD, Steele RJ, et al. Length of Barrett's oesophagus: an important factor in the development of dysplasia and adenocarcinoma. Gut 1992;33(9):1155–8.
39. Wright TA, Gray MR, Morris AI, et al. Cost effectiveness of detecting Barrett's cancer. Gut 1996;39(4):574–9.
40. Drewitz DJ, Sampliner RE, Garewal HS. The incidence of adenocarcinoma in Barrett's esophagus: a prospective study of 170 patients followed 4.8 years. Am J Gastroenterol 1997;92(2):212–5.
41. Katz D, Rothstein R, Schned A, et al. The development of dysplasia and adenocarcinoma during endoscopic surveillance of Barrett's esophagus. Am J Gastroenterol 1998;93(4):536–41.
42. Hage M, Siersema PD, van Dekken H, et al. Oesophageal cancer incidence and mortality in

patients with long-segment Barrett's oesophagus after a mean follow-up of 12.7 years. Scand J Gastroenterol 2004;39(12):1175–9.

43. Shaheen NJ, Crosby MA, Bozymski EM, et al. Is there publication bias in the reporting of cancer risk in Barrett's esophagus? Gastroenterology 2000;119(2):333–8.

44. Das D, Ishaq S, Harrison R, et al. Management of Barrett's esophagus in the UK: overtreated and underbiopsied but improved by the introduction of a national randomized trial. Am J Gastroenterol 2008;103(5):1079–89.

45. Cook MB, Wild CP, Everett SM, et al. Risk of mortality and cancer incidence in Barrett's esophagus. Cancer Epidemiol Biomarkers Prev 2007;16(10):2090–6.

46. Jankowski JA, Provenzale D, Moayyedi P. Esophageal adenocarcinoma arising from Barrett's metaplasia has regional variations in the west. Gastroenterology 2002;122(2):588–90.

47. Moayyedi P, Burch N, Akhtar-Danesh N, et al. Mortality rates in patients with Barrett's oesophagus. Aliment Pharmacol Ther 2008;27(4):316–20.

48. Montgomery E, Bronner MP, Greenson JK, et al. Are ulcers a marker for invasive carcinoma in Barrett's esophagus? Data from a diagnostic variability study with clinical follow-up. Am J Gastroenterol 2002;97(1):27–31.

49. Chang EY, Morris CD, Seltman AK, et al. The effect of antireflux surgery on esophageal carcinogenesis in patients with Barrett esophagus: a systematic review. Ann Surg 2007;246(1):11–21.

A systematic review that failed to demonstrate a lower incidence of adenocarcinoma after antireflux surgery compared with medical therapy after excluding uncontrolled case series from analysis.

50. Sharma P, Falk GW, Weston AP, et al. Dysplasia and cancer in a large multicenter cohort of patients with Barrett's esophagus. Clin Gastroenterol Hepatol 2006;4(5):566–72.

51. Sikkema M, Looman CW, Steyerberg EW, et al. Predictors for neoplastic progression in patients with Barrett's esophagus: a prospective cohort study. Am J Gastroenterol 2011;106(7):1231–8.

52. Wani S, Falk GW, Post J, et al. Risk factors for progression of low-grade dysplasia in patients with Barrett's esophagus. Am J Gastroenterol 2011 Oct; 141(4):1179–86.

53. Curvers WL, ten Kate FJ, Krishnadath KK, et al. Low-grade dysplasia in Barrett's esophagus: overdiagnosed and underestimated. Am J Gastroenterol 2010;105(7):1523–30.

54. Reid BJ, Levine DS, Longton G, et al. Predictors of progression to cancer in Barrett's esophagus: baseline histology and flow cytometry identify low- and high-risk patient subsets. Am J Gastroenterol 2000;95(7):1669–76.

55. Buttar NS, Wang KK, Sebo TJ, et al. Extent of high-grade dysplasia in Barrett's esophagus correlates with risk of adenocarcinoma. Gastroenterology 2001;120(7):1630–9.

56. Levine DS, Haggitt RC, Blount PL, et al. An endoscopic biopsy protocol can differentiate high-grade dysplasia from early adenocarcinoma in Barrett's esophagus. Gastroenterology 1993;105(1):40–50.

57. Altorki NK, Sunagawa M, Little AG, et al. High-grade dysplasia in the columnar-lined esophagus. Am J Surg 1991;161(1):97–100.

58. Pera M, Trastek VF, Carpenter HA, et al. Barrett's esophagus with high-grade dysplasia: an indication for esophagectomy? Ann Thorac Surg 1992;54(2):199–204.

59. Streitz Jr JM, Andrews Jr CW, Ellis Jr FH. Endoscopic surveillance of Barrett's esophagus. Does it help? J Thorac Cardiovasc Surg 1993;105(3):383–8.

60. Peters JH, Clark GW, Ireland AP, et al. Outcome of adenocarcinoma arising in Barrett's esophagus in endoscopically surveyed and nonsurveyed patients. J Thorac Cardiovasc Surg 1994;108(5):813–22.

61. Edwards MJ, Gable DR, Lentsch AB, et al. The rationale for esophagectomy as the optimal therapy for Barrett's esophagus with high-grade dysplasia. Ann Surg 1996;223(5):585–91.

62. Rice TW, Adelstein DJ, Zuccaro G, et al. Advances in the treatment of esophageal carcinoma. Gastroenterologist 1997;5(4):278–94.

63. Collard JM, Romagnoli R, Hermans BP, et al. Radical esophageal resection for adenocarcinoma arising in Barrett's esophagus. Am J Surg 1997;174(3):307–11.

64. Ferguson MK, Naunheim KS. Resection for Barrett's mucosa with high-grade dysplasia: implications for prophylactic photodynamic therapy. J Thorac Cardiovasc Surg 1997;114(5):824–9.

65. Cameron AJ, Carpenter HA. Barrett's esophagus, high-grade dysplasia, and early adenocarcinoma: a pathological study. Am J Gastroenterol 1997;92(4):586–91.

66. Falk GW, Rice TW, Goldblum JR, et al. Jumbo biopsy forceps protocol still misses unsuspected cancer in Barrett's esophagus with high-grade dysplasia. Gastrointest Endosc 1999;49(2):170–6.

67. Headrick JR, Nichols 3rd FC, Miller DL, et al. High-grade esophageal dysplasia: long-term survival and quality of life after esophagectomy. Ann Thorac Surg 2002;73(6):1697–703.

68. Tseng EE, Wu TT, Yeo CJ, et al. Barrett's esophagus with high grade dysplasia: surgical results and long-term outcome – an update. J Gastrointest Surg 2003;7(2):164–71.

69. Sujendran V, Sica G, Warren B, et al. Oesophagectomy remains the gold standard for treatment of high-grade dysplasia in Barrett's oesophagus. Eur J Cardiothorac Surg 2005;28(5):763–6.

70. Reed MF, Tolis Jr. G, Edil BH, et al. Surgical treatment of esophageal high-grade dysplasia. Ann Thorac Surg 2005;79(4):1110–5.

71. Wang VS, Hornick JL, Sepulveda JA, et al. Low prevalence of submucosal invasive carcinoma at esophagectomy for high-grade dysplasia or intramucosal adenocarcinoma in Barrett's esophagus: a 20-year experience. Gastrointest Endosc 2009;69(4):777–83.

72. Nasr JY, Schoen RE. Prevalence of adenocarcinoma at esophagectomy for Barrett's esophagus with high grade dysplasia. J Gastrointest Oncol 2011;2(1):34–8.

73. Konda VJ, Ross AS, Ferguson MK, et al. Is the risk of concomitant invasive esophageal cancer in high-grade dysplasia in Barrett's esophagus overestimated? Clin Gastroenterol Hepatol 2008;6(2):159–64.

74. Tharavej C, Hagen JA, Peters JH, et al. Predictive factors of coexisting cancer in Barrett's high-grade dysplasia. Surg Endosc 2006;20(3):439–43.

75. Boustany NN, Crawford JM, Manoharan R, et al. Analysis of nucleotides and aromatic amino acids in normal and neoplastic colon mucosa by ultraviolet resonance Raman spectroscopy. Lab Invest 1999;79(10):1201–14.

76. Schnell TG, Sontag SJ, Chejfec G, et al. Long-term nonsurgical management of Barrett's esophagus with high-grade dysplasia. Gastroenterology 2001;120(7):1607–19.

77. Menke-Pluymers MB, Hop WC, Dees J, et al. Risk factors for the development of an adenocarcinoma in columnar-lined (Barrett) esophagus. The Rotterdam Esophageal Tumor Study Group. Cancer 1993;72(4):1155–8.

78. Srivastava A, Hornick JL, Li X, et al. Extent of low-grade dysplasia is a risk factor for the development of esophageal adenocarcinoma in Barrett's esophagus. Am J Gastroenterol 2007;102(3):483–94.

79. Vaughan TL, Dong LM, Blount PL, et al. Non-steroidal anti-inflammatory drugs and risk of neoplastic progression in Barrett's oesophagus: a prospective study. Lancet Oncol 2005;6(12):945–52.

80. Abdalla SI, Lao-Sirieix P, Novelli MR, et al. Gastrin-induced cyclooxygenase-2 expression in Barrett's carcinogenesis. Clin Cancer Res 2004;10(14):4784–92.

81. Haigh CR, Attwood SE, Thompson DG, et al. Gastrin induces proliferation in Barrett's metaplasia through activation of the CCK2 receptor. Gastroenterology 2003;124(3):615–25.

82. Obszynska JA, Atherfold PA, Nanji M, et al. Long-term proton pump induced hypergastrinaemia does induce lineage-specific restitution but not clonal expansion in benign Barrett's oesophagus in vivo. Gut 2010;59(2):156–63.

83. Trimble KC, Pryde A, Heading RC. Lowered oesophageal sensory thresholds in patients with symptomatic but not excess gastro-oesophageal reflux: evidence for a spectrum of visceral sensitivity in GORD. Gut 1995;37(1):7–12.

84. de Jonge PJ, Steyerberg EW, Kuipers EJ, et al. Risk factors for the development of esophageal adenocarcinoma in Barrett's esophagus. Am J Gastroenterol 2006;101(7):1421–9.

85. Gerson LB, Edson R, Lavori PW, et al. Use of a simple symptom questionnaire to predict Barrett's esophagus in patients with symptoms of gastroesophageal reflux. Am J Gastroenterol 2001;96(7):2005–12.

86. Locke GR, Zinsmeister AR, Talley NJ. Can symptoms predict endoscopic findings in GERD? Gastrointest Endosc 2003;58(5):661–70.

87. Younes M, Lebovitz RM, Lechago LV, et al. p53 protein accumulation in Barrett's metaplasia, dysplasia, and carcinoma: a follow-up study. Gastroenterology 1993;105(6):1637–42.

88. Younes M, Ertan A, Lechago LV, et al. p53 protein accumulation is a specific marker of malignant potential in Barrett's metaplasia. Dig Dis Sci 1997;42(4):697–701.

89. Reid BJ, Prevo LJ, Galipeau PC, et al. Predictors of progression in Barrett's esophagus II: baseline 17p (p53) loss of heterozygosity identifies a patient subset at increased risk for neoplastic progression. Am J Gastroenterol 2001;96(10):2839–48.

90. Wong DJ, Paulson TG, Prevo LJ, et al. p16 (INK4a) lesions are common, early abnormalities that undergo clonal expansion in Barrett's metaplastic epithelium. Cancer Res 2001;61(22):8284–9.

91. Bani-Hani K, Martin IG, Hardie LJ, et al. Prospective study of cyclin D1 overexpression in Barrett's esophagus: association with increased risk of adenocarcinoma. J Natl Cancer Inst 2000;92(16):1316–21.

92. Menke-Pluymers MB, Mulder AH, Hop WC, et al. Dysplasia and aneuploidy as markers of malignant degeneration in Barrett's oesophagus. The Rotterdam Oesophageal Tumour Study Group. Gut 1994;35(10):1348–51.

93. Bailey T, Biddlestone L, Shepherd N, et al. Altered cadherin and catenin complexes in the Barrett's esophagus–dysplasia–adenocarcinoma sequence: correlation with disease progression and dedifferentiation. Am J Pathol 1998;152(1):135–44.

94. Kadri S, Lao-Sirieix P, Fitzgerald RC. Developing a nonendoscopic screening test for Barrett's esophagus. Biomark Med 2011;5(3):397–404.

95. Kadri SR, Lao-Sirieix P, O'Donovan M, et al. Acceptability and accuracy of a non-endoscopic screening test for Barrett's oesophagus in primary care: cohort study. Br Med J 2010;341:c4372.

96. van Sandick JW, van Lanschot JJ, Kuiken BW, et al. Impact of endoscopic biopsy surveillance of Barrett's oesophagus on pathological stage and clinical outcome of Barrett's carcinoma. Gut 1998;43(2):216–22.

97. Fountoulakis A, Zafirellis KD, Dolan K, et al. Effect of surveillance of Barrett's oesophagus on the clinical outcome of oesophageal cancer. Br J Surg 2004;91(8):997–1003.

98. Corley DA, Levin TR, Habel LA, et al. Surveillance and survival in Barrett's adenocarcinomas: a population-based study. Gastroenterology 2002;122(3):633–40.

99. Wong T, Tian J, Nagar AB. Barrett's surveillance identifies patients with early esophageal adenocarcinoma. Am J Med 2010;123(5):462–7.

100. Gore S, Healey CJ, Sutton R, et al. Regression of columnar lined (Barrett's) oesophagus with continuous omeprazole therapy. Aliment Pharmacol Ther 1993;7(6):623–8.

101. Cooper BT, Chapman W, Neumann CS, et al. Continuous treatment of Barrett's oesophagus patients with proton pump inhibitors up to 13 years: observations on regression and cancer incidence. Aliment Pharmacol Ther 2006;23(6):727–33.

102. Peters FT, Ganesh S, Kuipers EJ, et al. Endoscopic regression of Barrett's oesophagus during omeprazole treatment; a randomised double blind study. Gut 1999;45(4):489–94.
A blinded randomised trial showing that acid suppression can result in alterations in Barrett's metaplasia.

103. Hofstetter WL, Peters JH, DeMeester TR, et al. Long-term outcome of antireflux surgery in patients with Barrett's esophagus. Ann Surg 2001;234(4):532–9.

104. O'Riordan JM, Byrne PJ, Ravi N, et al. Long-term clinical and pathologic response of Barrett's esophagus after antireflux surgery. Am J Surg 2004;188(1):27–33.

105. Rees JR, Lao-Sirieix P, Wong A, et al. Treatment for Barrett's oesophagus. Cochrane Database Syst Rev 2011;1:004060.

106. Corey KE, Schmitz SM, Shaheen NJ. Does a surgical antireflux procedure decrease the incidence of esophageal adenocarcinoma in Barrett's esophagus? A meta-analysis. Am J Gastroenterol 2003;98(11):2390–4.
A meta-analysis demonstrating no difference between the incidence rates of adenocarcinoma in patients with Barrett's oesophagus treated medically or following antireflux surgery.

107. Peters FP, Kara MA, Curvers WL, et al. Multiband mucosectomy for endoscopic resection of Barrett's esophagus: feasibility study with matched historical controls. Eur J Gastroenterol Hepatol 2007;19(4):311–5.

108. Pech O, Behrens A, May A, et al. Long-term results and risk factor analysis for recurrence after curative endoscopic therapy in 349 patients with high-grade intraepithelial neoplasia and mucosal adenocarcinoma in Barrett's oesophagus. Gut 2008;57(9):1200–6.

109. ASGE Technology Committee, Kantsevoy SV, Adler DG, Conway JD, et al. Endoscopic mucosal resection and endoscopic submucosal dissection. Gastrointest Endosc 2008;68(1):11–8.

110. Ciocirlan M, Lapalus MG, Hervieu V, et al. Endoscopic mucosal resection for squamous premalignant and early malignant lesions of the esophagus. Endoscopy 2007;39(1):24–9.

111. Inoue H, Fukami N, Yoshida T, et al. Endoscopic mucosal resection for esophageal and gastric cancers. J Gastroenterol Hepatol 2002;17(4):382–8.

112. Ell C, May A, Pech O, et al. Curative endoscopic resection of early esophageal adenocarcinomas (Barrett's cancer). Gastrointest Endosc 2007;65(1):3–10.

113. Seewald S, Akaraviputh T, Seitz U, et al. Circumferential EMR and complete removal of Barrett's epithelium: a new approach to management of Barrett's esophagus containing high-grade intraepithelial neoplasia and intramucosal carcinoma. Gastrointest Endosc 2003;57(7):854–9.

114. Shaheen NJ, Overholt BF, Sampliner RE, et al. Durability of radiofrequency ablation in Barrett's esophagus with dysplasia. Gastroenterology 2011;141(2):460–8.
Follow-up report of patients with dysplastic Barrett's oesophagus treated using RFA. The study demonstrated that the effect of RFA was durable after 3 years.

115. Shaheen NJ, Sharma P, Overholt BF, et al. Radiofrequency ablation in Barrett's esophagus with dysplasia. N Engl J Med 2009;360(22):2277–88.
This RCT compared RFA to sham procedure in the management of dysplastic Barrett's oesophagus. Complete eradication of LGD occurred in 90.5% (ablation group) compared to 22.7% (control group) ($P < 0.001$) at 1 year. Complete eradication of HGD occurred in 81.0% (ablation group) versus 19.0% (control group) ($P < 0.001$). RFA decreased both the likelihood of disease progression (3.6% vs. 16.3%, $P = 0.03$) and cancer (1.2% vs. 9.3%, $P = 0.045$).

116. Overholt BF, Wang KK, Burdick JS, et al. Five-year efficacy and safety of photodynamic therapy with Photofrin in Barrett's high-grade dysplasia. Gastrointest Endosc 2007;66(3):460–8.

117. Ragunath K, Krasner N, Raman VS, et al. Endoscopic ablation of dysplastic Barrett's oesophagus comparing argon plasma coagulation and photodynamic therapy: a randomized prospective trial assessing efficacy and cost-effectiveness. Scand J Gastroenterol 2005;40(7):750–8.

118. Biddlestone LR, Barham CP, Wilkinson SP, et al. The histopathology of treated Barrett's esophagus: squamous reepithelialization after acid suppression and laser and photodynamic therapy. Am J Surg Pathol 1998;22(2):239–45.

119. Overholt BF, Lightdale CJ, Wang KK, et al. Photodynamic therapy with porfimer sodium for ablation of high-grade dysplasia in Barrett's

esophagus: international, partially blinded, randomized phase III trial. Gastrointest Endosc 2005;62(4):488–98.

120. Bulsiewicz WJ, Shaheen NJ. The role of radiofrequency ablation in the management of Barrett's esophagus. Gastrointest Endosc Clin North Am 2011;21(1):95–109.
121. Herrero LA, van Vilsteren FG, Pouw RE, et al. Endoscopic radiofrequency ablation combined with endoscopic resection for early neoplasia in Barrett's esophagus longer than 10 cm. Gastrointest Endosc 2011;73(4):682–90.
122. Lyday WD, Corbett FS, Kuperman DA, et al. Radiofrequency ablation of Barrett's esophagus: outcomes of 429 patients from a multicenter community practice registry. Endoscopy 2010;42(4):272–8.
123. Semlitsch T, Jeitler K, Schoefl R, et al. A systematic review of the evidence for radiofrequency ablation for Barrett's esophagus. Surg Endosc 2010;24(12):2935–43.
124. van Vilsteren FG, Pouw RE, Seewald S, et al. Stepwise radical endoscopic resection versus radiofrequency ablation for Barrett's oesophagus with high-grade dysplasia or early cancer: a multicentre randomised trial. Gut 2011;60(6):765–73.
125. Sharma P, Wani S, Weston AP, et al. A randomised controlled trial of ablation of Barrett's oesophagus with multipolar electrocoagulation versus argon plasma coagulation in combination with acid suppression: long term results. Gut 2006;55(9):1233–9.
126. Reid BJ, Blount PL, Feng Z, et al. Optimizing endoscopic biopsy detection of early cancers in Barrett's high-grade dysplasia. Am J Gastroenterol 2000;95(11):3089–96.
127. Williams VA, Watson TJ, Herbella FA, et al. Esophagectomy for high grade dysplasia is safe, curative, and results in good alimentary outcome. J Gastrointest Surg 2007;11(12):1589–97.
128. Hull MJ, Mino-Kenudson M, Nishioka NS, et al. Endoscopic mucosal resection: an improved diagnostic procedure for early gastroesophageal epithelial neoplasms. Am J Surg Pathol 2006;30(1):114–8.
129. Moss A, Bourke MJ, Hourigan LF, et al. Endoscopic resection for Barrett's high-grade dysplasia and early esophageal adenocarcinoma: an essential staging procedure with long-term therapeutic benefit. Am J Gastroenterol 2010;105(6):1276–83.
130. Pouw RE, Wirths K, Eisendrath P, et al. Efficacy of radiofrequency ablation combined with endoscopic resection for Barrett's esophagus with early neoplasia. Clin Gastroenterol Hepatol 2010;8(1):23–9.
131. Badreddine RJ, Prasad GA, Wang KK, et al. Prevalence and predictors of recurrent neoplasia after ablation of Barrett's esophagus. Gastrointest Endosc 2010;71(4):697–703.
132. Pech O, May A, Rabenstein T, et al. Endoscopic resection of early oesophageal cancer. Gut 2007;56(11):1625–34.
133. Das A, Singh V, Fleischer DE, et al. A comparison of endoscopic treatment and surgery in early esophageal cancer: an analysis of surveillance epidemiology and end results data. Am J Gastroenterol 2008;103(6):1340–5.
134. Allum WH, Blazeby JM, Griffin SM, et al. Guidelines for the management of oesophageal and gastric cancer. Gut 2011;60(11):1449–72.
135. Prasad GA, Wang KK, Buttar NS, et al. Long-term survival following endoscopic and surgical treatment of high-grade dysplasia in Barrett's esophagus. Gastroenterology 2007;132(4):1226–33.
136. Bennett C, Green S, Barr H, et al. Surgery versus radical endotherapies for early cancer and high grade dysplasia in Barrett's oesophagus. Cochrane Database Syst Rev 2010;(5): CD007334.
137. May A, Gunter E, Roth F, et al. Accuracy of staging in early oesophageal cancer using high resolution endoscopy and high resolution endosonography: a comparative, prospective, and blinded trial. Gut 2004;53(5):634–40.
138. Canto MI, Kalloo A. Chromoendoscopy for Barrett's esophagus in the twenty-first century: to stain or not to stain? Gastrointest Endosc 2006;64(2):200–5.
139. Kara MA, Peters FP, Ten Kate FJ, et al. Endoscopic video autofluorescence imaging may improve the detection of early neoplasia in patients with Barrett's esophagus. Gastrointest Endosc 2005;61(6):679–85.
140. Curvers WL, Herrero LA, Wallace MB, et al. Endoscopic tri-modal imaging is more effective than standard endoscopy in identifying early-stage neoplasia in Barrett's esophagus. Gastroenterology 2010;139(4):1106–14.
141. Curvers WL, van Vilsteren FG, Baak LC, et al. Endoscopic trimodal imaging versus standard video endoscopy for detection of early Barrett's neoplasia: a multicenter, randomized, crossover study in general practice. Gastrointest Endosc 2011;73(2):195–203.
142. Bird-Lieberman EL, Neves AA, Lao-Sirieix P, et al. Molecular imaging using fluorescent lectins permits rapid endoscopic identification of dysplasia in Barrett's esophagus. Nat Med 2012;18(2):315–21.
143. Rice TW, Falk GW, Achkar E, et al. Surgical management of high-grade dysplasia in Barrett's esophagus. Am J Gastroenterol 1993;88(11):1832–6.

16

The management of achalasia and other motility disorders of the oesophagus

Derek Alderson

Introduction

Most patients who turn out to have oesophageal motor disorders undergo endoscopy and/or contrast radiology to make sure that their dysphagia is not due to cancer or their chest pain to gastro-oesophageal reflux disease. While these tests can provide the diagnosis, they are often normal, leading to specific investigation of oesophageal motor function. Modified barium swallows to look at solid bolus transit using bread or marshmallow can provide added qualitative information. Radionuclide transit does much the same in a semiquantitative way, but the mainstay of specialised investigation is oesophageal manometry.

For many years oesophageal manometry was done using water-perfused systems that were difficult to set up and with many technical constraints. These were gradually replaced by solid-state pressure transducers.With further miniaturisation and developments in computer software, thin catheters containing multiple pressure recording transducers (high-resolution manometry) have become widely available, leading to novel ways of displaying pressure information as isobaric contour plots using colour gradations to indicate different pressures (high-resolution oesophageal pressure topography). The latter systems have disclosed considerable new information about oesophageal motor disturbances, resulting in new criteria (Chicago classification, Table 16.1) to define these disorders.[1] Further details of manometry techniques are described in Chapter 12 and manometry of a normal swallow is shown in Fig. 12.1.

Achalasia

Background

The term 'achalasia' comes from Greek, meaning 'failure to relax'. It was first used by Sir Arthur Hurst early in the 20th century, although the clinical features were first described in 1697 by Thomas Willis. It is conventionally defined by the absence of peristalsis (this does not mean the absence of contractions) in association with a lower oesophageal sphincter (LOS) that fails to relax completely. High-resolution pressure topography recognises this classic type (type I) but also considers two other types of achalasia, where there can be either pan-oesophageal pressurisation to more than 30 mmHg with at least 20% of swallows (type II) or preserved fragments of distal peristaltic activity or premature (spastic) contractions with at least 20% of swallows (type III).[2] These last two types probably represent the entity usually referrred to as 'vigorous achalasia' when seen on conventional manometry. Primary or idiopathic achalasia needs to be considered separately from secondary achalasia. While symptoms may be similar, the presence of a specific aetiology can influence management. These secondary causes are discussed later in this chapter.

Primary achalasia

This is an uncommon condition with an incidence in the Western world that is probably less than 1 case per 100 000 people per year.[3] It is due to progressive loss of ganglion cells in the myenteric plexus

Table 16.1 • The Chicago classification of oesophageal motility

Diagnosis	Criteria
Achalasia type I	Classic achalasia: mean IRP>upper limit of normal, 100% failed peristalsis
Achalasia type II	Achalasia with oesophageal compression: mean IRP>upper limit of normal, no normal peristalsis, pan-oesophageal pressurisation with ≥20% of swallows
Achalasia type III	Mean IRP>upper limit of normal, no normal peristalsis, preserved fragments of distal peristalsis or premature (spastic) contractions with ≥20% of swallows
Oesophagogastric junction outflow obstruction	Mean IRP>upper limit of normal, some instances of intact peristalsis or weak peristalsis with small breaks such that the criteria for achalasia are not met
Distal oesophageal spasm	Normal mean IRP, ≥20% premature contractions
Hypercontractile oesophagus	At least one swallow DCI>8000 mmHg • s • cm with single peaked or multipeaked contraction
Absent peristalsis	Normal mean IRP, 100% of swallows with failed peristalsis
Weak peristalsis with large peristaltic defects	Mean IRP<15 mmHg and >20% swallows with large breaks in the 20 mmHg isobaric contour (>5 cm in length)
Weak peristalsis with small peristaltic defects	Mean IRP<15 mmHg and >30% swallows with small breaks in the 20 mmHg isobaric contour (2–5 cm in length)
Frequent failed peristalsis	>30%, but <100% of swallows with failed peristalsis
Rapid contractions with normal	Rapid contraction with ≥20% of swallows, DL>4.5 s
Hypertensive peristalsis (nutcracker oesophagus)	Mean DCI>5000 mmHg • s • cm, but not meeting criteria for hypercontractile oesophagus

DCI, distal contractile integral; DL, distal latency; IRP, integrated relaxation pressure.

of unknown cause. The neural loss is somewhat selective as there is particularly severe loss of inhibitory nitrergic neurotransmission.[4,5] This process is often accompanied by an inflammatory infiltrate that has led to many theories regarding aetiology. While there is circumstantial evidence of viral exposure and autoimmune phenomena, neither provides a satisfactory explanation for all patients.[5]

Clinical features

The disease is most common in middle life, but can occur at any age. It typically presents with dysphagia and characteristically this affects fluids as well as solids. Symptom severity varies from day to day and patients often develop tricks to assist oesophageal emptying, such as Valsalva manoeuvres or air swallowing. Many admit to having been 'slow eaters' for many years. In patients who have remained untreated for many years, regurgitation is frequent and there may be overspill into the trachea, especially at night. In the early stages, achalasia may present with retrosternal discomfort and this may lead to a mistaken diagnosis of gastro-oesophageal reflux disease (GORD). Chest pain is common in achalasia and particularly so in those individuals said to have 'vigorous achalasia'.

There are few physical signs that point specifically to any underlying motility disorder, including achalasia. There are two important areas of physical examination that should be carefully evaluated as positive findings will play an important part in management. A careful examination of the respiratory system is essential. Recurrent chest infections due to episodes of aspiration from an oesophagus that is unable to clear itself may lead to acute and chronic signs as pulmonary performance deteriorates. It is not rare for these patients to be labelled as asthmatic. The other important area is to make a careful assessment of the patient's nutritional state. Insidious nutritional failure is easily missed in patients with a long history, although it is rare to see this in achalasia, where regular filling of the oesophagus with food and an upright posture eventually create a hydrostatic pressure that will overcome the LOS, allowing the oesophagus to partially empty.

Investigations

Most patients with dysphagia are offered endoscopy as their first investigation. While achalasia may be suspected at endoscopy by finding a tight cardia and food residue in the oesophagus, early or vigorous achalasia is easily missed as the oesophagus is not dilated and still contracts.

Barium radiology may show hold-up in the distal oesophagus, dilatation of the oesophageal body, peristaltic dysfunction and a tapering stricture in the distal oesophagus, often described as a 'bird's beak'. The gastric gas bubble is usually absent, because most patients cannot swallow air through their non-relaxing LOS. It should, however, be emphasised that, like endoscopy, these typical features of well-developed achalasia are often absent and radiology is frequently passed as normal.

A firm diagnosis can only be made by oesophageal manometry. High-resolution techniques suggest that conventional manometry, however, only diagnoses about a quarter of patients with achalasia on the basis of the classic features of a hypertensive lower oesophageal sphincter that does not relax completely on swallowing, aperistalsis of the oesophageal body and a raised resting pressure in the oesophagus (**Fig. 16.1**). The other two variants can be separated by the Chicago classification and this may be clinically relevant. Limited evidence suggests that patients with type II achalasia with pan-oesophageal pressurisation do respond well to treatment, but this seems not to be the case for type III.[2]

Treatment

Most patients with achalasia respond well to treatment. There is no reliable drug therapy. Patients can be treated by endoscopic botulinum toxin injection into the LOS, but the two main methods are forceful (pneumatic) dilatation of the cardia and operative cardiomyotomy. Very rarely, patients require oesophagectomy.

Botulinum toxin injection

This involves the injection of 100 units of botulinum toxin into the LOS.

✔✔ Whether a single treatment or multiple treatments is performed, only about a third of patients experience marked improvement in symptoms 1 year after the last treatment.[6–9]

When compared to pneumatic dilatation in a randomised trial, only 32% of patients who had received botulinum toxin were in symptomatic remission after a year compared to 70% after dilatation.[7] A Cochrane review published in 2006 came to the conclusion that botulinum toxin injection was inferior to pneumatic dilatation at 6 months.[10]

It is for this reason that botulinum toxin should be reserved for frail patients with major comorbidities.

Pneumatic dilatation

This involves stretching the cardia with a balloon to disrupt the muscle and render it less competent. The treatment was first described by Plummer in 1908. Many varieties of balloon have been described, but nowadays plastic balloons with a precisely controlled external diameter are used. If the pressure in the balloon is too high the balloon is designed to split along its length rather than expand further. Balloons of 30–40 mm diameter are available and are inserted over a guidewire.

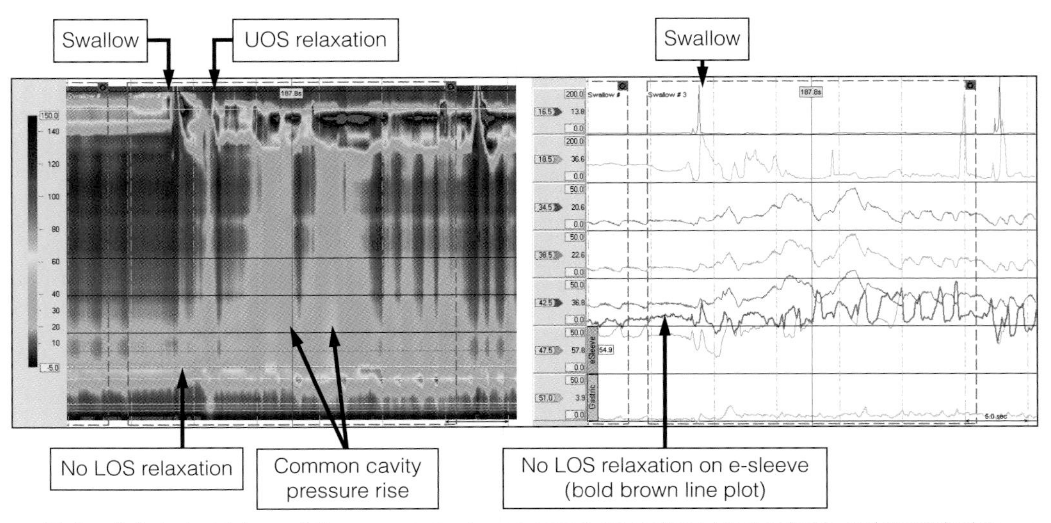

Figure 16.1 • Achalasia. High-resolution manometry from a patient presenting with dysphagia and regurgitation. The swallow is followed by a 'common cavity' rise in oesophageal pressure indicating filling. LOS relaxation is absent and there is a positive oesophagogastric pressure gradient. Upper oesophageal sphincter (UOS) relaxation shortly after the swallow was related to regurgitation of oesophageal contents.

Perforation is the major complication. With a 30-mm balloon, the incidence of perforation should be <0.5%. The risk of perforation increases with the bigger balloons and they should be used cautiously for progressive dilatation over a period of weeks.

✔✔ Forceful dilatation produces good to excellent relief of symptoms for more than a year in 70–90% of patients.[9,11,12]

There is wide variation in the incidence of GORD (between 4% and 40%) after successful dilatation, which reflects method of assessment (symptomatic versus endoscopic), the number of repeat dilatations and the length of follow-up.[13–15] In most patients, however, this can usually be controlled satisfactorily with a proton-pump inhibitor.

Cardiomyotomy

This operation is generally associated with Heller, who first carried it out in 1913. Heller's original description involved a double myotomy on the anterior and posterior walls at the cardia, but over the years a single anterior cardiomyotomy has become widely used, often in conjunction with an anterior partial fundoplication (Heller–Dor operation). Cardiomyotomy involves cutting the muscle of the lower oesophagus and cardia. The major complication is gastro-oesophageal reflux and this is less problematic by limiting the incision so that it does not extend for more than 1 cm on to the stomach and including a prophylactic antireflux operation.

✔✔ In a small randomised trial, the addition of a Dor fundoplication reduced acid reflux documented by pH study from 48% to 9% at 6 months.[16]

It is customary to perform a partial rather than a total fundoplication in this situation because of the risk of causing dysphagia in the presence of an aperistaltic oesophagus. The proximal extent of the myotomy does not seem to matter provided that the obstructing segment is divided and this is easily determined by intraoperative endoscopy. Heller's myotomy is ideally suited to a minimal access approach and although it can be undertaken by thoracoscopy or laparoscopy, the latter approach seems far more popular.

✔✔ There is some variation in success rates that mainly reflects the proportion of patients with marked oesophageal dilatation and the length of follow-up in different case series. In the normal calibre oesophagus or where dilatation is minimal, cardiomyotomy is successful in more than 80% of patients.[13,17,18]

✔ The impact of previous treatments on the safety and efficacy of subsequent surgery is unclear. Two large European case series involving nearly 350 patients (including more than 80 patients who had undergone previous botulinum toxin injection or pneumatic dilatation) came to different conclusions regarding the likelihood of perforation at laparoscopic surgery.[19,20]

✔✔ Three randomised trials have compared balloon dilatation with surgical cardiomyotomy. Two found the surgical technique to be more effective in relieving dysphagia and one found no difference.[21,22]

The two trials that claimed a difference are open to major criticism, not least because both were statistically underpowered. In the trial published by Csendes et al. in 1981,[21] a superior result in favour of surgery in terms of relieving dysphagia needs to be balanced against a higher rate of reflux. In addition, the pneumatic dilatation was of very short duration and there is no doubt that the results in that arm of the study were inferior to those achieved subsequently with more modern balloons. A trial in Sweden with 51 patients included a routine partial fundoplication as part of the surgery and found more treatment failures in the dilatation arm. A pan-European study involving over 200 patients found no difference in success rates at 2 years (dilatation 86% and cardiomyotomy 90% success).[23]

A number of studies have used decision analysis (Markov modelling) techniques to identify optimal treatment strategies in the absence of a large number of randomised trials.

✔ When the outcome difference was expressed as quality-adjusted life years (QALYs), dilatation and surgery were equally effective.[24] Similar analyses examining cost-effectiveness tend to favour pneumatic dilatation.[25–27]

For these reasons, patient preference and levels of local expertise should be the main determinants in selecting treatment.

Revisional procedures and oesophagectomy

Failure to relieve dysphagia is usually because the myotomy is too short. The diagnosis is generally made on a contrast swallow but repeat manometry may be necessary. Balloon dilatation can be undertaken and there is no convincing evidence that this is more hazardous after a previous failed cardiomyotomy. The alternative is a redo operation conducted by thoracoscopy if the first attempt was laparoscopic or vice versa. Recurrent dysphagia is occasionally due to a slipped wrap and if symptoms are sufficiently troublesome, this should be surgically corrected.

Chest pain after surgery is more difficult to diagnose and manage. Some of these patients will have symptomatic gastro-oesophageal reflux, but chest pain related to swallowing and obstruction may not seem very different to heartburn for some patients. In type III achalasia, chest pain related to powerful simultaneous contractions can still persist after successful cardiomyotomy and is probably the main symptom that is associated with a poor result in these patients. Careful re-evaluation is necessary, potentially involving endoscopy, contrast radiology, manometry and 24-hour pH studies. A therapeutic trial of a proton-pump inhibitor may be worthwhile as well as being diagnostic. The addition of a fundoplication, where this was not done at the original operation, merits consideration in patients who are intolerant of proton-pump inhibitors. In other circumstances, unless a clear mechanical problem can be demonstrated (e.g. wrap disruption), revisional surgery is best avoided.

In a small proportion of patients, presentation is with a hugely dilated, flaccid oesophagus, and symptoms and signs of aspiration. Some patients also develop this as a late complication of previous treatment. While standard first-line treatments can be attempted, they often provide only very short-term relief of symptoms. Stapled cardioplasty to create a wide anastomosis between the oesphagus and the stomach may be an alternative, and this can be supplemented by antrectomy and Roux-en-Y reconstruction to minimise reflux, although the small case series describing these operations deal only with short-term outcomes.

✔ Oesophagectomy (ideally with vagal nerve preservation) may be the only solution.[28]

✔✔ Primary achalasia is associated with a small increase in risk of developing squamous cell carcinoma of the oesophagus, presumably as a result of chronic inflammation related to food retention and fermentation. Most large studies estimate the increased risk to be about 30- to 40-fold.[29–32] A Swedish study also highlighted a 10-fold increased risk of adenocarcinoma in men with achalasia.[33]

Secondary achalasia

In South America, chronic infection with the parasite *Trypanosoma cruzi* causes Chagas' disease, which has marked similarities to achalasia. The oesophagus becomes dilated ('megaoesophagus') and tortuous with a persistent retention oesophagitis due to fermentation of food residues. A severe cardiomyopathy is the main cause of death in these patients but some do require oesophagectomy.[34]

Pseudo-achalasia is an achalasia-like disorder that is usually produced by adenocarcinomas at the cardia or by any other tumour in the oesophageal wall at that level (e.g. gastrointestinal stromal tumours). While it seems attractive to suppose that the structural abnormalities related to these neoplasms must interfere with local neurotransmitters, pseudo-achalasia is sometimes also seen in patients with cancers outside the oesophagus (e.g. lung, pancreas), suggesting a paraneoplastic process.[35]

Secondary achalasia occasionally follows antireflux surgery. Provided there was preoperative evidence of peristalsis and this is not simply a case of misdiagnosis, the condition probably represents a wrap that is too tight for that patient. Interestingly, endoscopy is usually normal and manometry is required to establish that this is the problem. Truncal vagotomy is also recognised as a rare cause of secondary achalasia, but this can probably be condemned to history now.

Diffuse oesophageal spasm

This is a rare condition of unknown cause characterised clinically by episodes of severe chest pain and/or dysphagia.[36] The upper oesophagus covered by striated muscle is usually unaffected, in contrast to the lower two-thirds, where there is pronounced muscular thickening. Chest pain can be very severe and often occurs in isolation at night. Sometimes chest pain and dysphagia occur at the same time. Many patients undergo detailed assessment for cardiac causes of chest pain or reflux disease.

The diagnosis is rarely made by endoscopy or contrast radiology. Corkscrew oesophagus on a barium swallow is the exception rather than the rule. Diffuse oesophageal spasm is defined by conventional manometry as the presence of two or more non-peristaltic sequences in a series of 10 wet swallows, but high-resolution techniques suggest that this is inadequate (Table 16.1). In many patients, abnormal contractions are characterised by multipeaked waves of increased duration and amplitude[37] (**Fig. 16.2**) exceeding 300 mmHg on conventional studies or 8000 mmHg • s • cm as defined by high-resolution pressure topography (hypercontractile or jackhammer oesophagus). It is evident that not all abnormal contractions produce a symptomatic event, but all symptomatic events are associated with abnormal manometric appearances.[38]

These patients develop considerable thickening of the muscular wall of the oesophagus and treatment is usually directed towards this. Short-acting nitrates, calcium-channel blockers, phosphodiesterase inhibitors and botulinum injection have all been used to provide some patients with a degree of relief

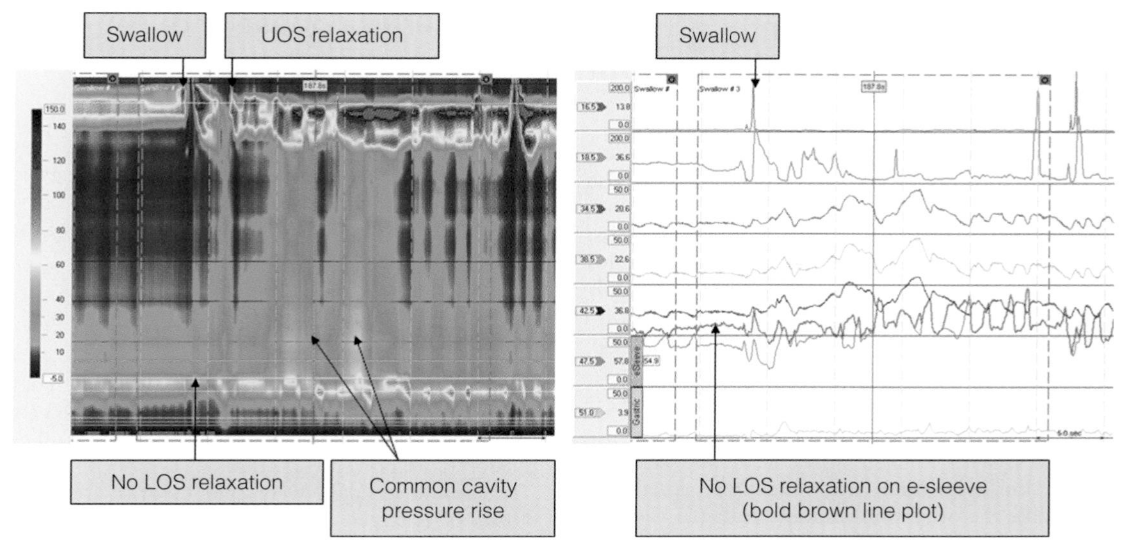

Figure 16.2 • Diffuse oesophageal spasm. High-resolution manometry from a patient presenting with dysphagia and chest pain. The swallow is followed by simultaneous, repetitive contractions in the mid-distal smooth muscle oesophagus. LOS relaxation is preserved. Note that the sequential simultaneous contractions first in the middle and distal segments of the oesophagus and then LOS make it appear as if there is progressive peristalsis on the conventional line plots (dotted arrow). Repetitive contractions are seen clearly on both.

from mild symptoms, but there is no evidence that any specific drug treatment will reliably prevent attacks or provide sustained relief from symptoms. A careful explanation of the cause of their symptoms and reassurance will often suffice for patients with mild symptoms, as there is no real evidence that this is a progressive condition in the majority.

✔ A small number of patients have very severe symptoms and long oesophageal myotomy provides good symptomatic improvement in about 80% of patients.[39]

It seems important that the myotomy should encompass the entire length of the manometric abnormality, so most surgeons advocate that this should be from the aortic arch down to within a few centimetres of the oesophagogastric junction. There is no consensus regarding the need to cross the cardia and incorporate an antireflux procedure. The operation is generally completed thoracoscopically.

Oesophagogastric junction outflow obstruction and non-specific oesophageal motor disorders

A number of 'conditions' can be identified by oesophageal manometry. Often, the correlation between manometric abnormalities and symptoms is poor. Inevitably, patients undergoing the test have some oesophageal symptoms that have initiated the investigation in the first place and it is tempting to imply a causal relationship.

Nutcracker oesophagus merely refers to high-amplitude contractions (>180 mmHg) with normal peristalsis during standard manometry and undoubtedly some of these patients can be re-classified by high-resolution techniques. So-called 'hypertensive LOS' (on the basis of a resting pressure >45 mmHg) used to be diagnosed when the sphincter was thought to still exhibit normal relaxation and there was normal peristalsis. The ability of high-resolution pressure topography to separate effects of the lower sphincter from the diaphragmatic crura has shed new light on this phenomenon, implying that in a proportion of such patients the true functional obstruction is at the diaphragm and not the sphincter, potentially related to the presence of a sliding hiatus hernia. Non-specific motor disorders cover a ragbag of manometric abnormalities that lie outside the normal ranges covered by conventional or high-resolution manometry. Many patients with reflux disease will have one or more of these abnormalities and treatment should be directed towards their reflux disease. Inevitably, most patients with a non-specific manometric abnormality have oesophageal symptoms, but correlation with these manometric abnormalities is poor. Great care should be exercised in labelling patients with a manometric diagnosis.[40] There is virtually no evidence that any of these abnormalities responds to a specific treatment.

Oesophageal motor disturbances and autoimmune disease

Systemic sclerosis, polymyositis, dermatomyositis, systemic lupus erythematosus, polyarteritis nodosa and rheumatoid disease can all be associated with oesophageal dysmotility. The condition of most clinical relevance is systemic sclerosis. It is rare for the oesophageal involvement to occur as an early feature in any of these conditions.

Systemic sclerosis

This condition has characteristic cutaneous appearances, with thickening, oedema and sclerosis of the skin associated with subcutaneous calcinosis. Unlike the other autoimmune collagen vascular disorders, visceral involvement is unusual except for the oesophagus, which is affected in up to 80% of patients. The striated muscle of the oesophagus is unaffected and there is smooth muscle atrophy involving the LOS. Peristalsis is weak and reflux common. The spectrum of oesophageal symptoms is wide, from mild to severe dysphagia with regurgitation and aspiration, as well as reflux symptoms related to the LOS defect and poor clearance. Endoscopy, barium radiology and manometry are used as appropriate to understand the extent of disease in individual patients.

Treatment usually centres around reflux symptoms and the management of complications such as stricture development. Most patients are adequately managed by proton-pump inhibitors and antireflux surgery is only rarely required.

Polymyositis and dermatomyositis

Both of these conditions predominantly affect skeletal muscle and the most common clinical problems occur in the pharynx and at the level of the upper oesophageal sphincter. Up to 60% of patients have a swallowing problem and aspiration is a real concern. Dietary modification may be necessary to minimise this risk. Investigation is only needed to exclude other common causes of oropharyngeal dysphagia.

Systemic lupus erythematosus

Oesophageal involvement is rare, compared to the many other organs involved, including other parts of the gastrointestinal tract. The clinical spectrum is similar to that seen in systemic sclerosis and similar management approaches are therefore recommended.

Polyarteritis nodosa and rheumatoid disease

While many patients with these conditions have non-specific motor disorders on manometry, very few are symptomatic. Dysphagia in the rheumatoid patient may be related to arthritis in the cricoarytenoid joints and stricture in the upper third of the oesophagus has been reported.

Oesophageal diverticula

These can occur anywhere in the oesophagus. They are either congenital (rare) or acquired. In the case of the latter, they are described as traction (rare) or pulsion (common) diverticula.

Traction diverticula were said to arise from the effects of enlarged mediastinal lymph glands (particularly due to tuberculosis) and this was meant to account for the predominant location in the upper half of the oesophagus. Malignant mediastinal nodes, however, rarely cause these diverticula and with the reduction in tuberculosis, it is clear that most mid-oesophageal diverticula are of the pulsion type.

Pulsion diverticula, therefore, occur anywhere in the oesophagus but are most common in the lower half. Those that occur near the diaphragm are called epiphrenic diverticula. Most of these occur just above the diaphragm and for some reason tend to arise from the posterolateral wall of the oesophagus on the right.

> ✔ All pulsion diverticula represent the effects of an underlying motor disturbance where normally coordinated peristaltic activity is inconsistent and where a degree of functional distal obstruction is present.[41] Achalasia and diffuse oesophageal spasm can both lead to diverticulum formation and identifying the underlying motor abnormality may be important in management.[42]

Clinical features

Symptoms largely reflect the extent to which the diverticulum causes pressure effects and the disorder that gave rise to the diverticulum. Chest pain and/or dysphagia bring most diverticula to light, but large diverticula can be complicated by inflammation, fistula formation, perforation and neoplastic change.

Diagnosis

Most are discovered at endoscopy or in a barium swallow during investigation of the patient with chest pain or a swallowing problem. A large diverticulum containing food is sometimes picked up on a chest X-ray. Manometry may be necessary to characterise the motor abnormality, when symptoms are severe enough to warrant intervention.

Treatment

Small diverticula require no treatment in their own right and management should be directed towards the underlying motor disturbance. When the diverticulum itself is perceived to contribute to symptoms, surgery is aimed at correction of the motor disorder and excision of the diverticulum. There are three elements to consider: removal of the diverticulum with secure closure of the oesophagus, correction of distal obstruction by a myotomy of appropriate length and the need for an associated antireflux procedure. Good historical results with open surgery have largely been replicated by stapled excision and closure of the oesophagus with myotomy and a partial fundoplication using minimal access approaches.

Acknowledgements

All high-resolution manometry figures were kindly supplied by Dr Mark Fox.

Key points

- High-resolution pressure topography is likely to supplant conventional manometry.
- Achalasia is an uncommon disorder that generally responds well to treatment by either pneumatic dilatation or surgery.
- Surgery and pneumatic dilatation appear equally effective in relieving dysphagia and improving quality of life in achalasia.
- Botulinum toxin injection for achalasia should be reserved for patients with significant comorbidities.
- Diffuse oesophageal spasm usually presents with chest pain. It is difficult to diagnose because symptoms are intermittent.
- A long myotomy may be indicated in patients with very severe diffuse oesophageal spasm but most patients should be treated non-surgically.
- Oesophageal involvement occurs in a variety of autoimmune disorders. It is particularly common in systemic sclerosis (affected in 80% of cases).
- The vast majority of oesophageal diverticula are of the pulsion type and arise within or proximal to an area of oesophageal motor disturbance.
- Treatment of oesophageal diverticula is aimed at identifying and treating the underlying motility disorder. Additional diverticulectomy is only indicated when it contributes to symptoms.
- Non-specific manometric abnormalities are not diagnoses. The correlation with symptoms is poor. Patients should not be labelled with a manometric diagnosis. Many have underlying reflux and treatment of this is often effective.

References

1. Bredenoord AJ, Fox M, Kahrilas PJ, et al. Chicago classification criteria of esophageal motility disorders defined in high resolution esophageal pressure topography. Neurogastroenterol Motil 2012;24(Suppl. 1):57–65.
2. Pandolfino JE, Kwiatek NA, Nealis T, et al. Achalasia: a new clinically relevant classification by high resolution manometry. Gastroenterology 2008;135:1526–33.
3. Podas T, Eaden J, Mayberry M, et al. Achalasia: a critical review of epidemiological studies. Am J Gastroenterol 1998;93(12):2345–7.
4. Mearin F, Mourelle M, Guarner F, et al. Patients with achalasia lack nitric oxide synthase in the gastro-oesophageal junction. Eur J Clin Invest 1993;23:724–8.
5. Kraichely RE, Farrugia G. Achalasia: physiology and etiopathogenesis. Dis Esophagus 2006;19:213–23.
6. Pasricha PJ, Ravich WJ, Hendrix TR, et al. Intrasphincteric botulinum toxin for the treatment of achalasia. N Engl J Med 1995;322:774–8.
7. Fishman VM, Parkman HP, Schiano TD, et al. Symptomatic improvement in achalasia after botulinum toxin injection into the lower oesophageal sphincter. Am J Gastroenterol 1996;91:1724–30.
8. Gordon JM, Eaker EY. Prospective study of oesophageal botulinum toxin injection in high-risk achalasia patients. Am J Gastroenterol 1997;92:1812–7.

9. Vaezi MF, Richter JE, Wilcox CM, et al. Botulinum toxin versus pneumatic dilatation in the treatment of achalasia: a randomised trial. Gut 1999;44:231–9.
A small study, with no CONSORT diagram to explain recruitment and randomisation, and no power calculation.

10. Leyden JE, Moss AC, MacMathuna P. Endoscopic pneumatic dilatation versus botulinum toxin injection in the management of primary achalasia. Cochrane Database Syst Rev 2006;18:CD005046.
A careful overview of the relative merits of the two techniques. Nothing has changed in the last few years.

11. Kadakia SC, Wong RKH. Graded pneumatic dilatation using Rigiflex achalasia dilators in patients with primary oesophageal achalasia. Am J Gastroenterol 1993;88:34–8.

12. Annese V, Basciani M, Perri F, et al. Controlled trial of botulinum toxin injection versus placebo and pneumatic dilatation in achalasia. Gastroenterology 1996;111:1418–24.

13. Vela MF, Richter JE, Khandwala F, et al. The long-term efficacy of pneumatic dilatation and Heller myotomy for the treatment of achalasia. Clin Gastroenterol Hepatol 2006;4:580–7.

14. Zerbib F, Thetiot V, Benajah DA, et al. Repeated pneumatic dilatations as long-term maintenance therapy for esophageal achalasia. Am J Gastroenterol 2006;101:692–7.

15. Leeuwenburgh I, Van Dekken H, Scholten P, et al. Oesophagitis is common in patients with achalasia after pneumatic dilatation. Aliment Pharmacol Ther 2006;23:1197–203.

16. Richards WO, Torquati A, Holzman MD, et al. Heller myotomy versus Heller myotomy with Dor fundoplication for achalasia: a prospective randomized double-blind clinical trial. Ann Surg 2004;240:405–12.
A small study from a centre with a number of publications on achalasia. Compare this with their own results in earlier studies.

17. Sharp KW, Khaitan L, Scholz S, et al. 100 consecutive minimally invasive Heller myotomies: lessons learned. Ann Surg 2002;235:631–8.

18. Costantini M, Zaninotto G, Guirolli E, et al. The laparoscopic Heller–Dor operation remains an effective treatment for esophageal achalasia at a minimum 6-year follow-up. Surg Endosc 2005;19:345–51.
The most useful recent article describing long-term outcomes, highlighting the paucity of data in relation to all achalasia treatments.

19. Bonavina L, Incarbone R, Reitano M, et al. Does previous endoscopic treatment affect the outcome of laparoscopic Heller myotomy? Ann Chir 2000;125:45–9.

20. Portale G, Costantini M, Rizzetto C, et al. Long-term outcome of Heller–Dor surgery for esophageal achalasia: possible detrimental role of previous endoscopic treatment. J Gastrointest Surg 2005;9:1332–9.

21. Csendes A, Velasco N, Braghetto J, et al. A prospective randomized study comparing forceful dilatation and oesophagomyotomy in patients with achalasia of the oesophagus. Gastroenterology 1981;80:789–95.
An important study and clearly the first true comparison. It is inevitably open to criticism, mainly regarding the method of pneumatic dilatation. The late follow-up paper from the same group is worth reading.

22. Kostic S, Kjellin A, Ruth M, et al. Pneumatic dilatation or laparoscopic cardiomyotomy in the management of newly diagnosed achalasia. Results of a randomised controlled trial. World J Surg 2007;31:470–8.

23. Boeckxstaens GE, Annese V. Bruley des Varannes S, et al. Pneumatic dilatation versus laparoscopic Heller's myotomy for idiopathic achalasia. N Engl J Med 2011;364:1807–16.
The first adequately powered and generalisable study, showing no important differences.

24. Urbach DR, Hansen PD, Khajanchee YS, et al. A decision analysis of the optimal initial approach to achalasia: laparoscopic Heller myotomy with partial fundoplication, thoracoscopic Heller myotomy, pneumatic dilatation or botulinum toxin injection. J Gastrointest Surg 2001;5:192–205.

25. O'Connor JB, Singer ME, Imperiale TF, et al. The cost-effectiveness of treatment strategies for achalasia. Dig Dis Sci 2002;47:1516–25.

26. Kostic S, Johnsson E, Kjellin A, et al. Health economic evaluation of therapeutic strategies in patients with idiopathic achalasia: results of a randomized trial comparing pneumatic dilatation with laparoscopic cardiomyotomy. Surg Endosc 2007;21:1184–9.

27. Karanicolas PJ, Smith SE, Inculet RI, et al. The cost of laparoscopic myotomy versus pneumatic dilatation for esophageal achalasia. Surg Endosc 2007;21:1198–206.

28. Devaney EJ, Lannettoni MD, Orringer MB, et al. Esophagectomy for achalasia: patient selection and clinical experience. Ann Thorac Surg 2001;72:854–8.
A highly informative case series that highlights the problems faced in dealing with end-stage disease.

29. Meijssen MA, Tilanus HW, van Blankenstein M, et al. Achalasia complicated by oesophageal squamous cell carcinoma: a prospective study in 195 patients. Gut 1992;33:155–8.

30. Aggestrup S, Holm JC, Sorensen HR. Does achalasia predispose to cancer of the esophagus? Chest 1992;102:1013–6.

31. Streitz Jr JM, Ellis Jr FH, Gibb SP, et al. Achalasia and squamous cell carcinoma of the esophagus: analysis of 241 patients. Ann Thorac Surg 1995;59:1604–9.

32. Sandler RS, Nyren O, Ekbom A, et al. The risk of esophageal cancer in patients with achalasia. A population-based study. JAMA 1995;274:1359–62.

33. Zendehdel K, Nyren O, Edberg A, et al. Risk of esophageal adenocarcinoma in achalasia patients, a retrospective cohort study in Sweden. Am J Gastroenterol 2011;106(1):57–61.
34. Pinotti HW. A new approach to the thoracic esophagus by the abdominal trans-diaphragmatic route. Langenbecks Arch Chir 1983;359:229–35.
35. Portale G, Costantini M, Zaninotto G, et al. Pseudoachalasia: not only esophago-gastric cancer. Dis Esophagus 2007;20:168–72.
36. Osgood H. A peculiar form of oesophagismus. Boston Med Surg J 1889;120:401–5.
37. Richter JE, Bradley LA, Castell DO. Esophageal chest pain: current controversies in pathogenesis, diagnosis and therapy. Ann Intern Med 1989;110:66–78.
38. Barham CP, Gotley DC, Fowler A. Diffuse oesophageal spasm: diagnosis by ambulatory 24 hour manometry. Gut 1997;41:151–5.
The first study to characterise diffuse oesophageal spasm in this way. It emphasises the importance of manometric abnormality and symptom correlation.
39. Leconte M, Douard R, Gaudric M, et al. Functional results after extended myotomy for diffuse oesophageal spasm. Br J Surg 2007;94:1113–8.
40. Hsi JJ, O'Connor MK, Kang YW, et al. Nonspecific motor disorder of the esophagus: a real disorder or a manometric curiosity? Gastroenterology 1993;104:1281–4.
41. Kaye MD. Oesophageal motor dysfunction in patients with diverticula of the mid-thoracic oesophagus. Thorax 1974;29:666–72.
42. Di Marino AJ, Cohen S. Characteristics of lower esophageal sphincter function in symptomatic diffuse esophageal spasm. Gastroenterology 1974;66:1–6.

17

Paraoesophageal hernia and gastric volvulus

Nathan W. Bronson
Kyle A. Perry
John G. Hunter

Introduction

Paraoesophageal hiatal hernia is a relatively rare condition comprising approximately 15% of hiatal hernias. This condition was first identified on post-mortem examination in 1903,[1] and on upper gastrointestinal contrast radiography by Akerlund et al. in 1926.[2] Since that time, the importance of these hernias has been recognised because of the resulting life-threatening complications including gastrointestinal bleeding, iron deficiency anaemia, gastric volvulus with subsequent strangulation and perforation.[3] Management of paraoesophageal hernias has changed considerably since the development of laparoscopic repair and several areas of controversy remain as this technique continues to evolve.

Epidemiology

Hiatal hernias occur in approximately 10% of the population, with approximately 15% of these being paraoesophageal hernias.[4] Risk factors for hiatal hernias include age greater than 50, body mass index greater than 25 kg/m^2 and male gender.[5] There is also a familial occurrence that confers a 20-fold increased risk in younger siblings of children with a hiatal hernia.[6]

Anatomy and natural history

The oesophagus enters the abdomen via the oesophageal hiatus of the diaphragm, which is comprised of the limbs of the right diaphragmatic crus,[7] although varying degrees of contribution of the left crus are often present. Although not anatomically correct, descriptions of hiatal dissection and repair, including those presented here, typically refer to these limbs as the right and left diaphragmatic crura or pillars. The intra-abdominal oesophagus is anchored to the diaphragm by the phreno-oesophageal ligament, which maintains the position of the squamocolumnar junction within or slightly distal to the diaphragmatic hiatus and prevents displacement of the stomach through the diaphragm.[8]

Derangements in the normal anatomy of the gastro-oesophageal junction and oesophageal hiatus allow herniation of the stomach through this opening into the thoracic cavity. The aetiology of these hernias is often unclear. Hiatal hernias are rare in Asian and African populations, and are more common in conditions of increased intra-abdominal pressure, such as obesity and pregnancy. Hiatal hernias are classified as types I–IV, with types II–IV representing forms of paraoesophageal hernia (**Fig. 17.1**). This nomenclature is slightly confusing, as giant hiatal hernias may appear to be a sliding or paraoesophageal hiatal hernia depending on the patient position. We prefer to use the term 'giant hiatal hernias' for the large hernias that are usually classified as type III and IV paraoesophageal hernia.

Most hiatal hernias (90%) are type I, or sliding, hernias in which the gastric cardia herniates upwards with proximal migration of the lower oesophageal sphincter into the thorax. The phreno-oesophageal ligament is attenuated, but remains intact.[9] The term 'sliding hiatal hernia' is applied here because the gastric wall comprises a portion of the

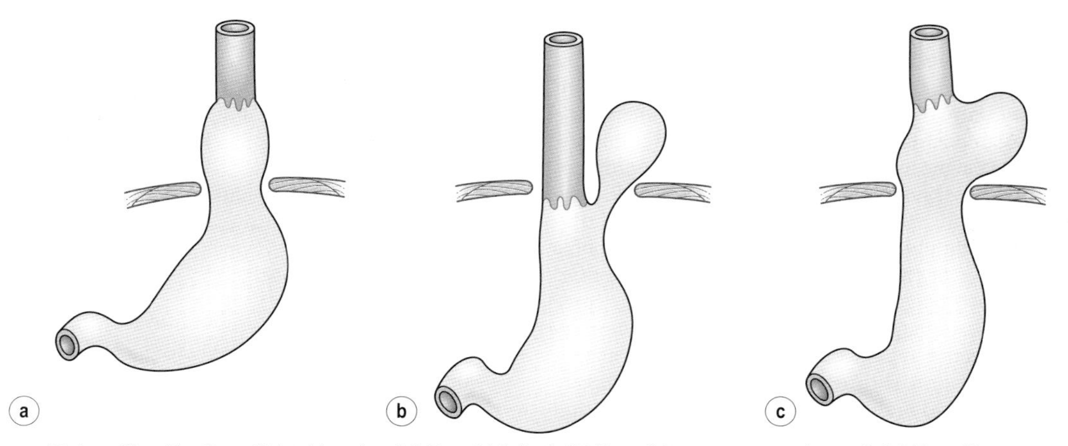

Figure 17.1 • Classification of hiatal hernias. **(a)** Type I (sliding). **(b)** Type II (true paraoesophageal). **(c)** Type III (combined).

hernia sac, analogous to retroperitoneal structures in sliding inguinal hernias.

Type II (true paraoesophageal) hiatal hernias are less common, constituting about 3% of hiatal hernias. In this type of hernia, the gastro-oesophageal junction remains anchored in its normal position, and the gastric fundus herniates through an enlarged hiatus. This defect is very rare because most paraoesophageal hernias evolve directly from type I (sliding hiatal hernia) to type III (mixed paraoesophageal hernia).

Type III (combined) hiatal hernias involve elements of both type I and II hernias, and represent the majority of paraoesophageal hernias presenting for surgical repair. These hernias result from enlargement of a type I hernia defect, to allow cephalad migration of the stomach in response to the transdiaphragmatic pressure gradient. There is a true hernia sac present with fundic herniation and proximal migration of the gastro-oesophageal junction into the thorax. This type of hernia is associated with laxity of the elements that retain normal gastric position, and the natural history is to progress to complete gastric herniation, with the appearance of an upside-down intrathoracic stomach on contrast radiography.[10] This increased gastric mobility predisposes patients to gastric volvulus, which we will address in detail later in this chapter.

Type IV hiatal hernia refers to a large hernia defect with other viscera or abdominal organs contained within the hernia sac. The transverse colon is the most common other structure found in these hernias. Splenic herniation is rare.

As with all hernias, the natural history of paraoesophageal hernia is progressive enlargement over time. Early in their course some are clinically silent, but most people have gastro-oesophageal reflux symptoms, which may have been treated with medical therapy or not at all. By the time the hernia grows large enough to allow a paraoesophageal hernia of the stomach, a cardio-oesophageal angle is often recreated, which may cause reflux symptoms to wane as the paraoesophageal herniation recreates a more competent antireflux valve.[11] The term 'giant paraoesophageal hiatal hernia' refers to defects in which at least half of the stomach is located within the thorax on contrast radiography, the hernia measures at least 6 cm in length on preoperative endoscopy, or a distance between the crura of at least 5 cm is noted on intraoperative inspection.[12,13] These hernias are repaired using the same principles required for all paraoesophageal hernias, but the large hernia sac and propensity for oesophageal shortening make these cases especially challenging.

Presentation and diagnosis

Approximately half of all paraoesophageal hernias are clinically silent and become apparent on imaging studies obtained for another reason. Symptomatic hernias may present with epigastric or chest pain, heartburn, postprandial fullness, regurgitation or dysphagia. Many of the signs and symptoms are non-specific and may mimic those of acute myocardial infarction, gastric ulcer or pneumonia. Type II hernias typically present without reflux symptoms, whereas type III hernias most typically present with postprandial chest pain with or without reflux symptoms (e.g. heartburn, dysphagia, regurgitation). Others present with iron deficiency anaemia secondary to chronic blood loss from erosions of the gastric mucosa caused by repeated movement across the hiatus, a phenomenon originally described by Collis in 1961,[14] or from an ulcer at the level of the diaphragm, described by Cameron from the Mayo Clinic.[15,16]

In the acute setting of foregut obstruction, chest X-ray typically demonstrates a retrocardiac air–fluid level and often a second one below the diaphragm. A barium study will reveal obstruction at the level of the volvulus and can be used as a confirmatory study in this setting if the diagnosis remains uncertain. In the setting of ischaemia, the presentation is one of septic shock, with epigastric pain and resultant multiorgan system dysfunction. It should be emphasised that the catastrophic presentations of paraoesophageal hernia are quite rare.

Several tests may be used to classify the hernia, degree of gastro-oesophageal reflux and oesophageal motility prior to elective repair. Barium swallow may suggest the presence of a shortened oesophagus and classify the hernia to aid in decision-making, especially in frail patients with asymptomatic hernias. Manometry is useful in identifying oesophageal motility disorders, which may preclude the use of full fundoplication, but may not be technically possible due to difficulties positioning the catheter beyond the lower oesophageal sphincter. Upper gastrointestinal (GI) endoscopy is required to inspect for gastric ischaemia, ulceration or erosion. If a gastric ulcer is present, elective surgery should be delayed until after the ulcer is healed, or at least 6 weeks of proton-pump inhibitor treatment.

Operative indications

It has been generally accepted that reasonable surgical candidates should undergo repair regardless of symptoms. This recommendation is based on early series that showed an increased mortality after emergency surgery of 30% compared to 1% in elective cases. In 1967, Skinner and Belsey found that 6 of 21 patients with a known diagnosis of paraoesophageal hernia died from complications of their hernia when followed conservatively for 5 years.[12]

More recent studies have suggested differences in both the natural history of the disease and operative outcomes. Allen et al. followed 23 patients who refused operative repair of paraoesophageal hernias for a median follow-up of 78 months without development of any life-threatening complications.[17] Others have advocated that asymptomatic or minimally symptomatic paraoesophageal hernias may be managed by a strategy of 'watchful waiting', with emergency surgery required in only 1.2% of cases and an operative mortality of 5.4% in this setting.[18]

✔ The current recommendation is that all type II hernias should be repaired, and consideration should be given to type III hernias regardless of symptoms. However, in the case of an elderly, frail patient with significant comorbidities it may be appropriate to decide on a course of watchful waiting due to increased risks associated with surgical repair in these patients.

Operative approaches

Principles of paraoesophageal hernia repair

The repair of paraoesophageal hernias may be approached via thoracotomy, laparotomy or laparoscopy. The principles of proper surgical repair are the same with each approach:[19–21]

1. Complete excision of the hernia sac.
2. Reduction of the herniated stomach and 2–3 cm of distal oesophagus into the abdominal cavity.
3. Repair of the diaphragmatic hiatus.

Transthoracic repair

Traditionally, transthoracic repair of paraoesophageal hernias has been advocated. Approaching these via thoracotomy provides excellent visualisation of the hernia sac from within the mediastinum and allows extensive oesophageal mobilisation under direct vision. However, this approach is rarely used any more because it has been associated with longer hospital stay and increased incisional discomfort. Blind reduction of the stomach also leaves the potential for recurrence of organoaxial rotation leading to postoperative intra-abdominal gastric volvulus.

Transabdominal repair

Paraoesophageal hernias may be approached via laparotomy, which provides most general surgeons with a familiar anatomical orientation, allows placement of the stomach in its proper orientation, and does not require single-lung ventilation or placement of an intercostal drain. Disadvantages include compromised ability to mobilise the oesophagus and perform oesophageal lengthening (Collis gastroplasty) when necessary.

Laparoscopic repair

Since its introduction by Cuschieri et al. in 1992,[22] laparoscopic paraoesophageal hernia repair has gained popularity and proven to be feasible, safe and effective.[23–30] Laparoscopy provides an attractive option because it combines some of the advantages of both thoracotomy (access to the hiatus and ability to perform extensive mobilisation of the oesophagus under direct vision) and laparotomy (lower morbidity and no need for single-lung ventilation or postoperative chest tube). Further, this minimally invasive approach may be better suited for the elderly patients in whom this disease most commonly occurs. This is a technically challenging operation that requires advanced laparoscopic skills, but when performed properly, carries a recurrence rate similar to the open approach.[31]

Set-up and port placement

The patient is placed in the supine split-leg position under general anaesthesia. Intravenous antibiotics are given, and sequential compression devices and a Foley catheter are placed. The operating surgeon stands between the patient's legs, with the first assistant positioned on the patient's left side.

A total of five trocars are used (**Fig. 17.2**). Peritoneal access is gained using a Veress needle, and an 11-mm trocar is placed just left of the midline, 15 cm caudal to the xyphoid process. Two ports are placed in the left subcostal position, a 12-mm trocar 12 cm lateral to the xyphoid process, and a 5-mm trocar 8 cm further to the left. Finally, two 5-mm ports are placed along the right costal margin, one in the subxyphoid position and the second approximately 10 cm lateral. A Nathenson liver retractor is used to retract the left lobe of the liver and expose the oesophageal hiatus.

Reduction of hernia sac and fundic mobilisation

The stomach is gently reduced from the hernia sac (**Fig. 17.3**) and the left diaphragmatic pillar is identified. The dissection is carried out along the left crus between the endothoracic fascia and the hernia sac. After the anterior phreno-oesophageal membrane is divided using ultrasonic dissection, the stomach is retracted to the left to expose the right crus. The pars flaccida of the lesser omentum is divided and the dissection continues along the right crus to the decussation of the crura. The gastrosplenic omentum is then divided using ultrasonic dissection, and the short gastric vessels are divided all the way up to the cephalad extent of the stomach. Division of the posterior gastric attachments creates a retro-oesophageal window through which a Penrose drain is passed around the oesophagus to allow caudal

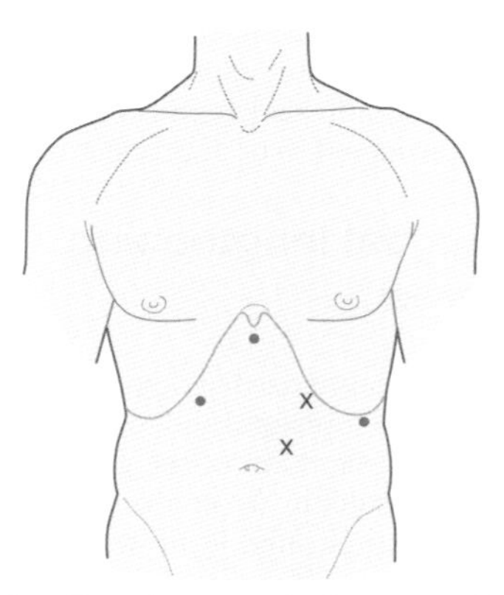

Figure 17.2 • Port placement for laparoscopic paraoesophageal hernia repair.

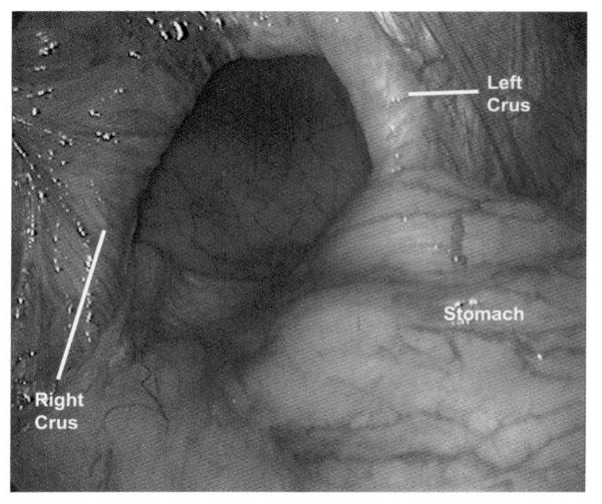

Figure 17.3 • A large paraoesophageal hernia with the stomach reduced into the abdomen prior to beginning the dissection.

retraction on the oesophagus and create exposure for the mediastinal dissection. Dissection proceeds from right to left, and the sac is opened to reveal a plane between the peritoneal sac and the mediastinum. Careful blunt and ultrasonic dissection develops this plane, with care taken to identify and preserve the vagal trunks and the peritoneal coverage of the crura, which aids in a second crural closure. With gentle retraction, the sac can be slowly mobilised out of the mediastinum and reduced into the abdominal cavity. Most surgeons excise and remove the hernia sac, but excessive fastidiousness in this exercise risks injury to the vagi as they course in close apposition to the hernia sac in the epiphrenic fat. We usually remove the majority of the sac, including all sac and epiphrenic fat on the left side of the oesophagus, well away from the vagal trunks and the end branches of the left gastric artery.

Assessment of oesophageal length

When the hernia sac is completely reduced from the mediastinum, it is imperative to have at least 2.5 cm of tension-free intra-abdominal oesophageal length. If a shortened oesophagus is identified an extensive circumferential mobilisation of the intrathoracic oesophagus is performed, which usually provides the desired oesophageal length. True shortened oesophagus is rare but a wedge gastroplasty can be performed over a 48 French bougie. A point is marked 3 cm below the angle of His, and a transverse staple line is created with two or three applications of a linear endoscopic stapler inserted via the left upper quadrant trocar. When the oesophageal dilator is reached, a vertical staple line created along the bougie creates a 3–4 cm neo-oesophagus, and the gastric wedge is removed from the abdomen.[32]

Crural dissection and repair

After complete reduction of the hernia sac and identification of an adequate length of intra-abdominal oesophagus, attention is turned to the crural closure. This is performed using interrupted, pledgeted, braided non-absorbable suture such as 0 silk (**Fig. 17.4**). It is frequently beneficial to reduce pneumoperitoneum pressure to 7 cm to close large diaphragmatic defects that are held open by the pneumoperitoneum. Once closed, the adequacy of closure may be tested by the passage of a 56–60 French Maloney dilator, which should completely fill the new hiatal aperture. If the diaphragmatic repair appears to be 'pinching' the oesophagus with the dilator in place, a suture is removed. Conversely, if the closure is loose, the dilator is withdrawn into the upper oesophagus and another suture is added. In addition to suture repair, we have advocated the use of biological mesh for reinforcement of the crural repair. A 3 cm×5 cm U-shaped piece of bioprosthetic mesh is fixed in place overlying the repair. Rather than struggle with difficult suture angles, or risking an intrathoracic injury by using hernia tacks to hold the mesh in place, we 'glue' the mesh to the diaphragm with tissue sealant (**Fig. 17.5**).

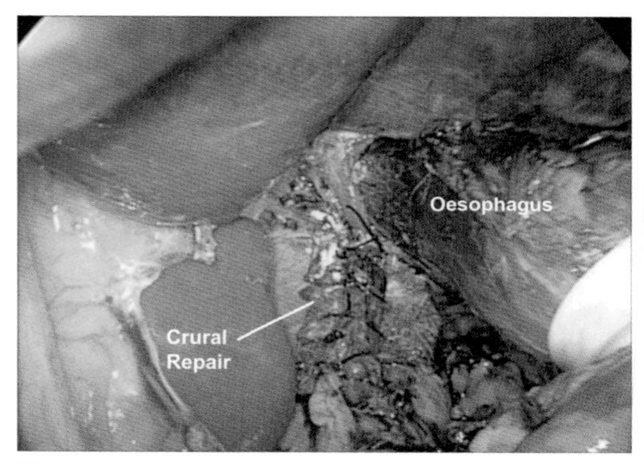

Figure 17.4 • Completed crural repair.

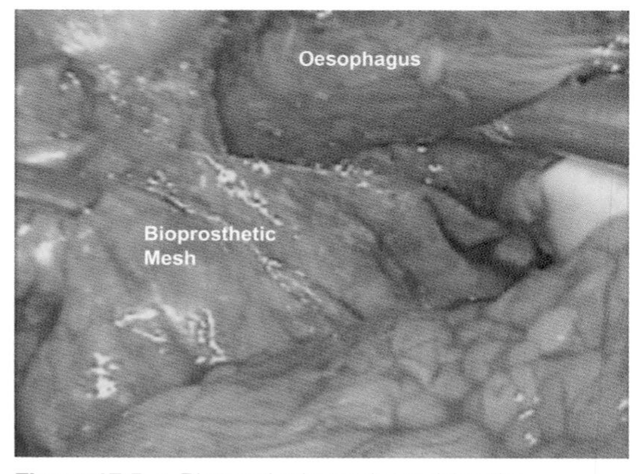

Figure 17.5 • Bioprosthetic mesh overlying the completed crural repair.

Fundoplication

After the completion of the crural repair, we routinely perform an antireflux procedure because failure to do so has been associated with a 20–40% rate of postoperative reflux and preoperative testing cannot successfully predict postoperative reflux.[33–37] A Nissen fundoplication is performed unless the patient has a known history of severe oesophageal dysmotility, necessitating a partial fundoplication. A floppy Nissen is performed by passing the fundus of the stomach behind the oesophagus. When a wedge gastroplasty is performed, the staple line is apposed to the stomach wall and the most cephalad stitch of the fundoplication is placed on the true oesophagus above the neo-oesophagus, ensuring that no gastric mucosa lies above the wrap. The fundoplication is created using three 2/0 silk or braided nylon sutures incorporating the stomach and oesophagus with each 'bite'. An additional suture may be placed from the posterior portion of the wrap to the oesophagus.

Current controversies in paraoesophageal hernia management

Although many centres have adopted laparoscopic paraoesophageal hernia repair as their primary treatment approach, several technical considerations draw debate. These include methods to minimise hernia recurrence following laparoscopic paraoesophageal hernia repair, oesophageal lengthening procedures, and prosthetic reinforcement of the crural repair.

Recurrence rate

As with any hernia repair, recurrence is a well-known complication of paraoesophageal hernia surgery. Early studies demonstrated a higher rate of recurrence in the laparoscopic approach as compared to the open approach,[26] but after the introduction of mesh crural reinforcement and oesophageal lengthening when indicated, the rate of recurrence for laparoscopic paraoesophageal hernia repair decreased[31] and is now considered to be equivalent to open repair.

Oesophageal lengthening procedures

Most surgeons today agree that oesophageal shortening can result from oesophageal inflammation in the setting of proximal migration of the gastro-oesophageal junction. This results in tension on the hiatal repair, which has been implicated in up to 33% of surgical failures after open and laparoscopic repairs.[38–41]

Short oesophagus has been recognised and studied for several decades, with the Collis gastroplasty described for its treatment in 1957.[40] Although preoperative testing can show the position of the gastro-oesophageal junction and suggest the presence of shortened oesophagus, these tests cannot reliably predict difficulty reducing the stomach to its anatomical position without tension intraoperatively.[42] Currently, shortened oesophagus is defined as the inability to gain 2.5–3 cm of tension-free intra-abdominal oesophagus following mediastinal dissection.

Oesophageal tension due to shortened length favours hernia recurrence by cephalad migration of the fundoplication through the crural repair. Ten per cent of paraoesophageal hernia repairs require a lengthening procedure and their use is mandatory in cases when adequate tension-free oesophageal length cannot be obtained from mediastinal dissection alone. The wedge gastroplasty and fundoplication has demonstrated improved resolution of symptoms as compared to fundoplication alone in the repair of type II–IV hernias, while maintaining no difference in hospital length of stay or overall quality of life.[43]

Prosthetic crural reinforcement

The high recurrence rate of laparoscopic paraoesophageal hernia repair led to the development of pledgeted suture repairs and synthetic or bioprosthetic mesh repairs. Three prospective studies showed decreased recurrence rates when prosthetic crural reinforcement was performed compared to primary repair.

Two prospective randomised trials have evaluated synthetic mesh reinforcement. One showed a decreased recurrence rate with polytetrafluoroethylene reinforcement of the crural repair[44] and another showed similar results with prolene mesh reinforcement of the hiatus.[45] However, movement of the mesh along the oesophagus with each respiration can cause serious and significant complications such as mesh erosion, ulceration, stricture and dysphagia.[46–49] Occasionally, these complications can be so severe as to necessitate oesophagectomy or gastrectomy,[49] and as a result the use of synthetic mesh has fallen out of favour and should be avoided.

Two studies have evaluated the rate of recurrence after repair with bioprosthetic mesh in a multicentre, prospective, randomised fashion. The first, published in 2006, showed a significant reduction in early recurrence following bioprosthetic mesh repair, without increased dysphagia or impaired quality of life compared to those with primary crural repair.[50] This study was limited by rather short-term follow-up of only 6 months, so a second study was performed of the same patient population at 5-year follow-up.[51] By 5 years, there was no difference in recurrence rate by either upper GI swallow study or symptoms, and there were no complications related to the mesh. Accordingly, bioprosthetic mesh reinforcement appears to be safe, but it may not change the long-term rate of recurrence. No study to date has prospectively compared the numerous types of bioprosthetic mesh in paraoesophageal hernia repair.

Acute gastric volvulus

Gastric volvulus, first described by Berti in 1896,[52] is the rotation of the stomach more than 180° around a fixed axis of rotation. Gastric strangulation from acute gastric volvulus is a dreaded complication of paraoesophageal hernia and it remains the driving force for recommending elective repair of asymptomatic hernias. Gastric strangulation occurs in up to 28% of cases of acute gastric volvulus,[53] and may progress to gastric necrosis, perforation and severe sepsis leading to cardiovascular collapse if it is not diagnosed quickly and managed aggressively.

Frequency and mechanism

The true incidence of gastric volvulus remains unknown, but it affects males and females equally. Approximately 20% of cases occur in infants and young children, with the remainder occurring in adults older than 50 years of age.

The anatomical classification of gastric volvulus is based on the axis of rotation (**Fig. 17.6**). **Organoaxial**

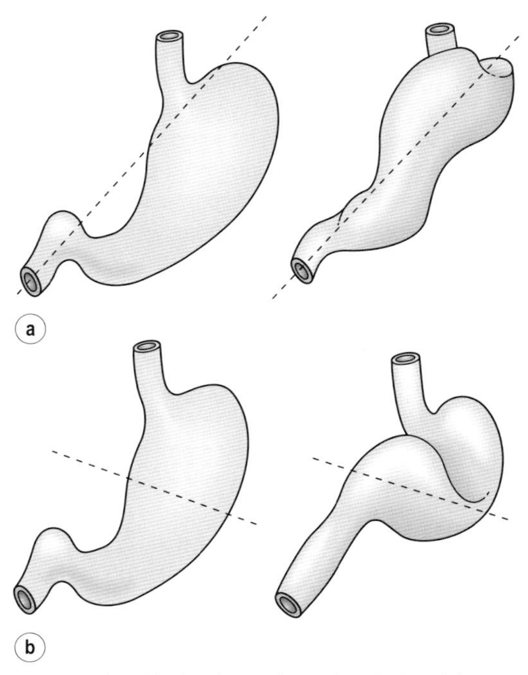

Figure 17.6 • Mechanisms of gastric volvulus. **(a)** Organoaxial rotation. **(b)** Mesentericoaxial rotation.

volvulus is the most common type, and it accounts for almost all cases of acute gastric volvulus. This involves rotation of the stomach around the anatomical (longitudinal) axis, represented as a line drawn from the cardia to the pylorus,[10] frequently resulting in gastric strangulation. In **mesoentericoaxial volvulus**, the antrum of the stomach rotates anteriorly and superiorly around a transverse axis that extends from the mid-lesser curvature to the mid-greater curvature.[10] The rotation is typically incomplete and results in intermittent gastric obstruction, rather than acute strangulation.

Presentation and diagnosis

Acute gastric volvulus typically presents with a history of dysphagia and high gastric obstruction. In 1904, Borchardt described the classic symptom triad of severe epigastric pain, retching and inability to vomit, and inability to pass a nasogastric tube.[54] Patients may also present with severe chest pain and minimal abdominal findings as the incarcerated segment is often located within the chest.[53]

The clinical history and a plain chest radiograph are usually sufficient for diagnosis. The X-ray shows a retrocardiac air–fluid level, often with a second air–fluid level present below the diaphragm. In cases where the diagnosis remains in question, barium swallow is diagnostic and will show an obstruction at the level of the volvulus, or computed tomography of the chest will demonstrate the presence of the stomach within the chest and no oral contrast past the level of the diaphragm.

Management

Once the diagnosis has been made, intravenous fluid resuscitation should be initiated and an attempt made at gastric decompression with a nasogastric tube. If successful, this results in rapid symptom improvement, and allows time for intravenous fluid resuscitation prior to surgical repair. If nasogastric decompression is unsuccessful, the patient must be taken to the operating room immediately for emergency operative repair.

Surgical repair of gastric volvulus may be approached via thoracotomy, laparotomy or laparoscopy. The principles of repair include reduction of the hernia, release of the volvulus, debridement of all non-viable tissue, hiatal closure and anterior gastropexy or fundoplication to prevent recurrent volvulus. In cases where nasogastric decompression can be achieved preoperatively and adequate intravenous fluid resuscitation accomplished, most can be managed laparoscopically. In the setting of acute peritonitis or gastric distention that cannot be relieved by decompression, laparotomy or thoracotomy would be the preference of most surgeons. In high-risk patients deemed unfit for a laparoscopic or open approach, several authors have proposed the use of endoscopic reduction with gastropexy performed via either one or two percutaneous endoscopic gastrostomy tubes.

Key points

- Paraoesophageal hernias comprise approximately 15% of hiatal hernias and, of these, type III hernias most commonly present for surgical repair.
- Paraoesophageal hernias should be repaired in symptomatic patients with reasonable surgical risk to prevent the development of potentially life-threatening complications.
- Watchful waiting is an acceptable management strategy in most asymptomatic individuals, especially the elderly or those with significant comorbidities.
- Laparoscopic paraoesophageal hernia repair is safe and effective in the management of paraoesophageal hernias and is the operative approach of choice.
- Shortened oesophagus is defined as the inability to gain at least 2.5 cm of intra-abdominal oesophagus after standard mediastinal dissection. This can be managed in most cases by extensive mediastinal dissection and oesophageal mobilisation. A lengthening procedure is indicated when sufficient length cannot be produced by dissection alone.
- Bioprosthetic mesh reinforcement of the crural closure decreases the rate of early recurrence and can be performed safely but may not affect long-term recurrence rates. Other mesh reinforcement should be avoided.
- Acute gastric volvulus is a serious complication of paraoesophageal hernias that requires aggressive management to avoid life-threatening complications of gastric strangulation, infarction and perforation.
- When gastric decompression of acute gastric volvulus can be obtained preoperatively, most operative repairs can be completed laparoscopically. However, in cases with acute peritonitis an open approach via laparotomy or thoracotomy is required.

References

1. Andrew L. The height of the diaphragm in relation to the position of certain abdominal viscera. Lancet 1903;1:790.
2. Akerlund A, Onnell H, Key E. Hernia diaphragmatica hiatus oesophagei vom anatomischen und rontgenologischen gesichtspunct. Acta Radiol 1926;6:3–22.
3. Ellis Jr FH, Crozier RE, Shea JA. Paraesophageal hiatus hernia. Arch Surg 1986;121(4):416–20.
4. Hill LD, Tobias JA. Paraesophageal hernia. Arch Surg 1968;96(5):735–44.
5. Menon S, Trugdill N. Risk factors in the aetiology of hiatus hernia: a meta-analysis. Eur J Gastroenterol Hepatol 2011;23:133–8.
6. Carre IJ, Johnston BT, Thomas PS, et al. Familial hiatal hernia in a large five generation family confirming true autosomal dominant inheritance. Gut 1999;45(5):649–52.
7. Marchand P. The anatomy of esophageal hiatus of the diaphragm and the pathogenesis of hiatus herniation. J Thorac Surg 1959;37(1):81–92.
8. Kahrilas PJ, Wu S, Lin S, et al. Attenuation of esophageal shortening during peristalsis with hiatus hernia. Gastroenterology 1995;109(6):1818–25.
9. Skinner DB, Roth JLA, Sullivan BH, editors. Gastroenterology. 4th ed. Philadelphia: W.B. Saunders; 1985.
10. Kahrilas PJ, Speiss AE, editors. The Esophagus. 3rd ed Philadelphia: Lippincott, Williams & Wilkins; 1999.
11. Wo JM, Branum GD, Hunter JG, et al. Clinical features of type III (mixed) paraesophageal hernia. Am J Gastroenterol 1996;91(5):914–6.
12. Skinner DB, Belsey RH. Surgical management of esophageal reflux and hiatus hernia. Long-term results with 1,030 patients. J Thorac Cardiovasc Surg 1967;53(1):33–54.
13. Treacy PJ, Jamieson CG. An approach to the management of paraesophageal hiatus hernias. Aust N Z J Surg 1987;57:813–7.
14. Collis JL. A review of surgical results in hiatus hernia. Thorax 1961;16:114–9.
15. Cameron AJ. Incidence of iron deficiency anemia in patients with large diaphragmatic hernia. A controlled study. Mayo Clin Proc 1976;51(12):767–9.
16. Cameron AJ, Higgins JA. Linear gastric erosion A lesion associated with large diaphragmatic hernia and chronic blood loss anemia. Gastroenterology 1986;91(2):338–42.
17. Allen MS, Trastek VF, Deschamps C, et al. Intrathoracic stomach. Presentation and results of operation. J Thorac Cardiovasc Surg 1993;105(2):253–9.
18. Stylopoulos N, Gazelle GS, Rattner DW. Paraesophageal hernias: operation or observation? Ann Surg 2002;236(4):492–501.
19. Edye M, Salky B, Posner A, et al. Sac excision is essential to adequate laparoscopic repair of paraesophageal hernia. Surg Endosc 1998;12(10):1259–63.
20. Patel HJ, Tan BB, Yee J, et al. A 25-year experience with open primary transthoracic repair of paraesophageal hiatal hernia. J Thorac Cardiovasc Surg 2004;127(3):843–9.
21. Watson DI, Davies N, Devitt PG, et al. Importance of dissection of the hernial sac in laparoscopic surgery for large hiatal hernias. Arch Surg 1999;134(10):1069–73.
22. Cuschieri A, Shimi S, Nathanson LK. Laparoscopic reduction, crural repair, and fundoplication of large hiatal hernia. Am J Surg 1992;163(4):425–30.
23. Diaz S, Brunt LM, Klingensmith ME, et al. Laparoscopic paraesophageal hernia repair, a challenging operation: medium-term outcome of 116 patients. J Gastrointest Surg 2003;7(1):59–67.
24. Edye MB, Canin-Endres J, Gattorno F, et al. Durability of laparoscopic repair of paraesophageal hernia. Ann Surg 1998;228(4):528–35.
25. Gantert WA, Patti MG, Arcerito M, et al. Laparoscopic repair of paraesophageal hiatal hernias. J Am Coll Surg 1998;186(4):428–33.
26. Hashemi M, Peters JH, DeMeester TR, et al. Laparoscopic repair of large type III hiatal hernia: objective follow-up reveals high recurrence rate. J Am Coll Surg 2000;190(5):553–61.
27. Horgan S, Eubanks TR, Jacobsen G, et al. Repair of paraesophageal hernias. Am J Surg 1999;177(5):354–8.
28. Mattar SG, Bowers SP, Galloway KD, et al. Long-term outcome of laparoscopic repair of paraesophageal hernia. Surg Endosc 2002;16(5):745–9.
29. Schauer PR, Ikramuddin S, McLaughlin RH, et al. Comparison of laparoscopic versus open repair of paraesophageal hernia. Am J Surg 1998;176(6):659–65.
30. Wiechmann RJ, Ferguson MK, Naunheim KS, et al. Laparoscopic management of giant paraesophageal herniation. Ann Thorac Surg 2001;71(4):1080–7.
31. Zehetner J, Demeester SR, Ayazi S, et al. Laparoscopic versus open repair of paraesophageal hernia: the second decade. J Am Coll Surg 2011;212(5):813–20.
32. Terry ML, Vernon A, Hunter JG. Stapled-wedge Collis gastroplasty for the shortened esophagus. Am J Surg 2004;188(2):195–9.
33. Behrns KE, Schlinkert RT. Laparoscopic management of paraesophageal hernia: early results. J Laparoendosc Surg 1996;6(5):311–7.
34. Trus TL, Bax T, Richardson WS, et al. Complications of laparoscopic paraesophageal hernia repair. J Gastrointest Surg 1997;1(3):221–8.

35. Casabella F, Sinanan M, Horgan S, et al. Systematic use of gastric fundoplication in laparoscopic repair of paraesophageal hernias. Am J Surg 1996;171(5):485–9.
36. Lal DR, Pellegrini CA, Oelschlager BK. Laparoscopic repair of paraesophageal hernia. Surg Clin North Am 2005;85(1):105–18.
37. Swanstrom LL, Jobe BA, Kinzie LR, et al. Esophageal motility and outcomes following laparoscopic paraesophageal hernia repair and fundoplication. Am J Surg 1999;177(5):359–63.
38. DePaula AL, Hashiba K, Bafutto M, et al. Laparoscopic reoperations after failed and complicated antireflux operations. Surg Endosc 1995; 9(6):681–6.
39. Ellis Jr FH, Gibb SP, Heatley GJ. Reoperation after failed antireflex surgery. Review of 101 cases. Eur J Cardiothorac Surg 1996;10(4):225–32.
40. Collis JL. An operation for hiatus hernia with short oesophagus. Thorax 1957;12(3):181–8.
41. Jobe BA, Horvath KD, Swanstrom LL. Postoperative function following laparoscopic Collis gastroplasty for shortened esophagus. Arch Surg 1998;133(8):867–74.
42. Gastal OL, Hagen JA, Peters JH, et al. Short esophagus: analysis of predictors and clinical implications. Arch Surg 1999;134(6):633–8.
43. Nason KS, Luketich JD, Awais O, et al. Quality of life after Collis gastroplasty for short esophagus in patients with paraesophageal hernia. Ann Thorac Surg 2011;92(5):1854–61.
44. Frantzides CT, Madan AK, Carlson MA, et al. A prospective, randomized trial of laparoscopic polytetrafluoroethylene (PTFE) patch repair vs simple cruroplasty for large hiatal hernia. Arch Surg 2002;137(6):649–52.
45. Kamolz T, Granderath FA, Bammer T, et al. Dysphagia and quality of life after laparoscopic Nissen fundoplication in patients with and without prosthetic reinforcement of the hiatal crura. Surg Endosc 2002;16(4):572–7.
46. Granderath FA, Kamolz T, Schweiger UM, et al. Impact of laparoscopic Nissen fundoplication with prosthetic hiatal closure on esophageal body motility: results of a prospective randomized trial. Arch Surg 2006;141(7):625–32.
47. Paul MG, DeRosa RP, Petrucci PE, et al. Laparoscopic tension-free repair of large paraesophageal hernias. Surg Endosc 1997;11(3):303–7.
48. Tatum RP, Shalhub S, Oelschlager BK, et al. Complications of PTFE mesh at the diaphragmatic hiatus. J Gastrointest Surg 2008;12(5):953–7.
49. Stadlhuber RJ, Sherif AE, Mittal SK, et al. Mesh complications after prosthetic reinforcement of hiatal closure: a 28-case series. Surg Endosc 2009;23(6):1219–26.
50. Oelschlager BK, Pellegrini CA, Hunter J, et al. Biologic prosthesis reduces recurrence after laparoscopic paraesophageal hernia repair: a multicenter, prospective, randomized trial. Ann Surg 2006;244(4):481–90.
51. Oelschlager BK, Pellegrini CA, Hunter JG, et al. Biologic prosthesis to prevent recurrence after laparoscopic paraesophageal hernia repair: long-term follow-up from a multicenter, prospective, randomized trial. J Am Coll Surg 2011;213:461–8.
52. Berti A. Singulare attortigliamento dele'esofago col duodeno seguita da rapida morte. Gazz Med Ital 1896;9:139.
53. Carter R, Brewer 3rd. LA, Hinshaw DB. Acute gastric volvulus. A study of 25 cases. Am J Surg 1980;140(1):99–106.
54. Borchardt M. Aus Pathologie und therapie des magenvolvulus. Arch Klin Chir 1904;74:243.

18

Benign ulceration of the stomach and duodenum and the complications of previous ulcer surgery

John Wayman

Introduction

The role of the surgeon in the management of peptic ulcer disease has changed in the last few decades. Since the introduction of effective acid antisecretories and greater understanding of *Helicobacter pylori* (HP), the role of the surgeon has become limited to the management of occasional resistant ulcers, emergency management of complicated ulcer disease and management of the consequences of previous ulcer surgery.

Management of refractory peptic ulceration

Endoscopic confirmation

Gastric and duodenal ulcers may be considered 'refractory' to medical treatment if there is no sign of significant healing by 12 and 8 weeks, respectively. Gastric ulcers must be carefully re-biopsied as there is a risk that an apparently benign gastric ulcer is in fact an early malignancy. Direct endoscopic inspection, adequate tissue biopsy and expert histological interpretation are essential to identify dysplasia, neoplasia or other more uncommon mucosal disease. Repeat endoscopy to confirm healing and re-biopsy are mandatory for all gastric ulcers but probably unnecessary for duodenal ulcers if symptoms have resolved. Persistent duodenal ulceration should be re-biopsied for similar, albeit less likely, reasons given above to identify the several neoplastic, infectious and inflammatory conditions that can mimic peptic ulcer disease. Assuming that the diagnosis of peptic ulcer is correct, there are three main causes to consider: that HP has not been eradicated, that there are other factors inhibiting ulcer healing or that there is a state of acid hypersecretion (Zollinger–Ellison syndrome). Having examined all of these factors, true 'refractory' ulcers have become rare.

Confirmation of persistent *Helicobacter* infection

Multiple non-invasive diagnostic tests for *Helicobacter* are available, including carbon isotope (^{13}C or ^{14}C) urea breath test, serological enzyme-linked immunosorbent assay or the monoclonal antibody faecal antigen test. At endoscopy, biopsy material can be analysed by a rapid functional assay of urease activity as well as histological analysis. Several drugs, including proton-pump inhibitors, bismuth and antibiotics, temporarily suppress HP and may render functional assays falsely negative. The sensitivity of any test may be less following treatment when the inoculum is reduced. For tests relying on functional assay of endoscopic biopsy tissue, the sensitivity may be enhanced post-treatment by using more than one biopsy and, since there may be proximal migration of the infection, analysis of biopsies from both the antrum and body of the stomach. More elaborate immunohistochemistry using polyclonal antisera to HP can improve sensitivity and the polymerase chain reaction allows detection of the presence of HP DNA in the absence of viable bacteria.

✔ In clinical practice, the urea breath test is considered the most reliable tool for assessing HP status post-treatment.[1]

Failure of HP eradication may be due to antibiotic resistance or non-compliance. The former may be overcome by appropriate modification of the antibiotic regimen, occasionally even using bacteriological culture to help direct treatment.

Non-HP-related refractory ulceration

Ingestion of non-steroidal anti-inflammatory drugs (NSAIDs) should be re-evaluated. Surreptitious aspirin ingestion has been observed and if suspected can be established by assay of plasma salicylate levels. Any other factor that may be facilitating ulceration and impairing healing, such as intercurrent disease and smoking, should be sought and eliminated where possible. Diseases associated with peptic ulceration are chronic liver disease, hyperparathyroidism and chronic renal failure, particularly during dialysis and after successful transplantation. Smokers are more likely to fail both medical and, indeed, surgical ulcer treatment. Smoking impairs the therapeutic effects of antisecretories, may stimulate pepsin secretion and promotes reflux of duodenal contents into the stomach. Smoking increases the harmful effects of HP, and increases the production of free radicals, endothelin and platelet-activating factor. Smoking also affects the mucosal protective mechanisms by decreasing gastric mucosal blood flow and inhibiting gastric prostaglandin generation and the secretion of gastric mucous, salivary epidermal growth factor, duodenal mucosal bicarbonate and pancreatic bicarbonate.[2] Stopping smoking is an important, yet often ignored, first step to allow effective ulcer treatment.

A diagnosis of Zollinger–Ellison should be suspected in cases of *Helicobacter*-negative, non-NSAID-induced refractory ulceration and especially where there is ulceration of the second part of the duodenum or large confluent ulcers in the duodenum. Hypergastrinaemia should be excluded prior to a decision to treat a refractory ulcer.

Where no cause for persistent ulceration can be found it may be necessary for the patient to take long-term antisecretory drugs. Alternatively, elective surgery may be considered in this group of patients. The risks of complications of persistent ulcer disease, the degree of disability experienced by patients and their fitness for surgery should all be considered in the decision of whether or not to operate.

Elective surgery for peptic ulceration

Surgery for peptic ulcer disease evolved around the concept of acid reduction either by resection of most of the parietal cell mass, vagal denervation of the parietal cells or resection of the antral gastrin-producing cells. The balance lay in minimising the chance of ulcer recurrence while at the same time trying to avoid the symptomatic and metabolic sequelae of the procedure that would affect patients for the rest of their life.

The trend by the mid-1970s was towards highly selective vagotomy (HSV) or proximal gastric vagotomy, which denervated the parietal cell mass but left the antrum and pylorus innervated and so allowed a gastric-emptying pattern that, while not completely normal, did not require a drainage procedure. This was the first ulcer procedure that did not involve bypass, destruction or removal of the pylorus, and as a result has significantly fewer side-effects than other ulcer operations. The main concern with this operation, whether for duodenal or gastric ulcer, has been the recurrence rate. In the best hands recurrence rates of 5–10% have been achieved.

Anterior seromyotomy with posterior truncal vagotomy probably denervates the proximal stomach more consistently. This proved that the posterior vagal trunk can be divided and the patient not experience significant diarrhoea, provided the pylorus is intact and innervated. Some surgeons advocated the use of truncal vagotomy and antrectomy, suggesting that this operation is the most effective for reducing acid secretion and has a very low recurrence rate of about 1%. The procedure was subsequently modified to a selective vagotomy and antrectomy, leaving the hepatic and coeliac fibres of the vagi intact. This did reduce the incidence of side-effects, especially diarrhoea, though dumping was still a problem. Bile gastritis and oesophagitis were also troublesome side-effects unless a Roux-en-Y reconstruction was used, though recurrent stomal ulceration was then more frequent unless a more extensive gastric resection was performed. The perfect ulcer operation has remained elusive and there is none that has no side-effects or risks.

Operations for refractory duodenal ulcers

There is no good evidence on which to base the decision of operation in cases of resistant ulceration in the modern era. Intuitively, one might predict a poor result with HSV alone since its success rate historically was less than that of modern medical treatment. It seems likely that resection of the antral gastrin-producing mucosa and either resection or vagal denervation of the parietal cell mass is necessary. The operations that could be considered include the following:

- **Selective vagotomy and antrectomy.** Selective denervation is preferred because of a lower incidence of side-effects. It is not an easy procedure; in particular, the dissection around the lower oesophagus and cardia has to be done very carefully. The vagotomy should be performed before the resection and tested intraoperatively. The reconstruction should either

be a gastroduodenal (Billroth I) anastomosis or a Roux-en-Y gastrojejunostomy. The latter is associated with fewer problems with bile reflux into the gastric remnant and oesophagus, but a higher risk of stomal ulceration and so at least a two-thirds gastrectomy is advised.
- **Subtotal gastrectomy**. Removal of a large part of the parietal cell mass is sound in theory and indeed ulcer recurrence after this operation is unusual. However, there is an incidence of postprandial symptoms, and in particular epigastric discomfort and fullness that can limit calorie intake. Importantly, there is a high incidence of long-term nutritional and metabolic sequelae that require lifelong surveillance and can be difficult to prevent, although this is mainly in women.
- **Pylorus-preserving gastrectomy**. This operation involves highly selective vagotomy with resection of about 50% of the parietal cell mass and the antral mucosa, but preserving the pyloric mechanism and the vagus nerves to the distal antrum and pylorus. There is some evidence that this may be a superior technique with fewer sequelae compared to the traditional approaches.[3] Comparable results of the technique used in the context of treatment of early gastric cancer confirm a good long-term functional result.[4]

Operations for refractory gastric ulcers

There are no reliable data on which to base a recommendation for surgical treatment of refractory gastric ulcers. HSV is not recommended for prepyloric ulcers since they follow the same pattern as described for duodenal ulceration. The choice of operation for a more proximal ulcer, often along the lesser curve and often associated with atrophic gastritis, is between excision of the ulcer with HSV or partial gastrectomy. The recurrence rate is higher after HSV/excision, but the operative mortality is lower and side-effects fewer after this procedure.

Laparoscopic peptic ulcer surgery

Interest in minimally invasive procedures has led to many publications proving the feasibility of laparoscopic definitive ulcer operations. The indications and considerations for elective laparoscopic peptic ulcer surgery should be exactly the same as for open procedures. The choice of approach must be a technical decision related to the expertise and experience of the operator: there is an insufficient evidence base to recommend one approach over another.

Zollinger–Ellison syndrome (ZES)

Refractory peptic ulceration should raise the suspicion of ZES. Alternatively, the syndrome may present with diarrhoea and weight loss and a third present with oesophagitis only. The disease may present more dramatically with perforation, haemorrhage, oesophageal stricture, jejunal or anastomotic ulceration. The condition should be suspected particularly when a duodenal ulcer coexists with primary hyperparathyroidism or metastatic adenocarcinoma of unknown origin. The aims of treatment are control of gastric acid hypersecretion and, where possible, removal of the underlying tumour itself to prevent metastatic disease. Since the introduction of adequate medical acid suppression the former aim is no longer the primary concern of the surgeon.

Pathology

Although originally described as a pancreatic endocrine tumour, the definition has also come to include extrapancreatic gastrin-secreting tumours. The majority of tumours lie within an area defined by the junction of the cystic and common bile ducts superiorly, the junction of the second and third portions of the duodenum inferiorly, and the junction of the neck and body of the pancreas medially: the 'gastrinoma triangle of Stabile'[5] (**Fig. 18.1**). Where the condition is due to a pancreatic tumour, in two-thirds of cases the tumour will be multifocal within the pancreas.[6] At least two-thirds will be histologically malignant. One-third will already have demonstrable metastases by the time of diagnosis.[7] The most common extrapancreatic site is in the wall of the

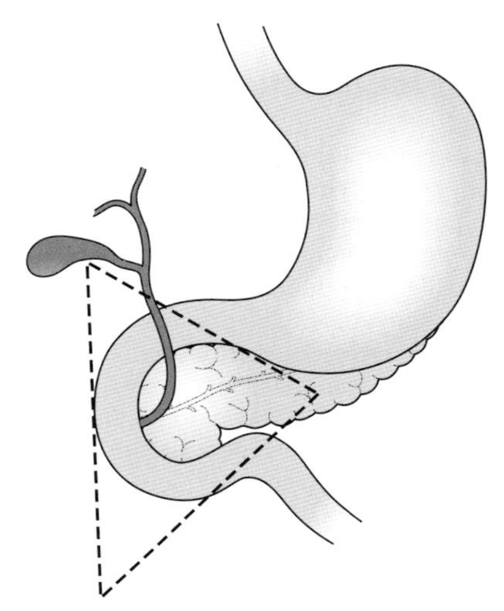

Figure 18.1 • Gastrinoma triangle of Stabile et al.[5]

duodenum. Less frequently (6–11% of cases) ectopic gastrinoma tissue has been identified in the liver, common bile duct, jejunum, omentum, pylorus, ovary and heart.[8] These extrapancreatic tumours rarely metastasise to the liver and, even though they do metastasise just as frequently to regional lymph nodes, they tend to have a better prognosis than primary pancreatic tumours.

One-quarter of patients with ZES have other endocrine tumours as part of a familial multiple endocrine neoplasia (MEN-1) syndrome, particularly hyperparathyroidism.[7] This group of patients has a much worse prognosis than sporadic ZES, in part due to the multifocal nature of the disease.

Diagnosis

Diagnosis may be confirmed by paradoxical fasting hypergastrinaemia associated with gastric acid hypersecretion. Hypergastrinaemia may be expected to occur in cases of achlorhydria such as ingestion of antisecretory drugs, postvagotomy, pernicious anaemia, atrophic gastritis, antral G-cell hyperplasia or gastric outlet obstruction. Hypergastrinaemia is also associated with a retained antrum after a Billroth II/Polya-type gastrectomy where a small cuff of antrum has been included in the 'duodenal' closure (if a retained antrum is suspected, technetium pertechnetate scan may be useful in identifying the antral mucosa). If there is diagnostic uncertainty or the basal serum gastrin level is marginal, dynamic assay of serum gastrin following secretin (or alternatively calcium or glucagon) provocation may be required. Gastrin response to a standard meal helps to differentiate hypergastrinaemia due to antral G-cell hyperplasia, which will result in an increase in serum gastrin levels, while no response would be expected in cases of gastrinoma. Serum chromogranin A, a non-specific marker for neuroendocrine tumours, should also be measured.[9]

Tumour localisation

Tumours may be localised initially by computed tomography (CT). This may also identify metastatic disease. Endoscopic ultrasound (EUS) is highly accurate in the localisation of pancreatic tumours and gastrinomas in the duodenal wall as small as 4mm. Octreotide scan and selective arterial secretagogue injection (SASI) testing are the most reliable approaches to localising gastrinomas. Liver metastases can frequently be detected by conventional imaging, but octreotide scan has proved a more sensitive investigation that may prevent unnecessary surgical exploration. SASI involves selective catheterisation of the feeding arteries of the duodenum and pancreas and the hepatic veins. Secretin is injected in turn into the splenic, gastroduodenal (GDA) and superior mesenteric (SMA) arteries. Corresponding hepatic venous gastrin levels are measured and allow identification of the main feeding vessel. More precise localisation can be achieved by more peripheral cannulation of the SMA and GDA or different points along the splenic artery. The test has greater than 90% sensitivity and specificity for preoperative tumour localisation.[10]

Surgery for ZES

The surgical management of ZES is characterised by controversy and little evidence. Historically, the debate centred around the radicality of surgical approaches to eliminate end organ acid production such as total gastrectomy. This is generally accepted, as unnecessary given that adequate acid suppression can usually be achieved with proton-pump inhibitors (PPIs), albeit at much higher doses than those usually recommended. How aggressively surgery should be pursued for the gastrinoma itself became the next area of controversy. With adequate acid suppression, patients may be rendered asymptomatic and the natural history of the gastrinoma tended to one of only very slow progression. Nevertheless, 60–90% of gastrinomas are reported to be malignant and some do have a more aggressive course. It became more acceptable to consider resection, as 30–50% with sporadic disease may be cured or at least have a reduced rate of development of liver metastases. Whether that should be local enucleation or a wider resection remains controversial. In the past many would say that patients with MEN-1 and those with liver metastases should not be treated surgically. Nevertheless, impressive results have been reported even in the former group and there is evidence that surgical resection of metastatic liver disease does offer long-term survival, even where resection may be incomplete. One of the largest series has shown that surgical exploration and resection resulted in excellent long-term results, with a 15-year disease-related survival rate of 98% compared to 74% for non-operated cases.[11]

Surgical exploration when preoperative investigations have failed to precisely localise a tumour is now a less frequent problem, particularly in specialist centres with access to SASI and octreotide scan. Nevertheless, a laparotomy will detect a third more gastrinomas than even octreotide scan. If surgical exploration is performed then the pancreas must be mobilised along its entire length, inspected, palpated and if the facilities are available re-scanned intraoperatively by endoluminal or standard ultrasound. Palpation of the duodenal wall will identify 61% of duodenal gastrinomas. Duodenal transillumination by endoscopy will improve detection to 84% and duodenotomy identifies the remaining cases.[12] If no gastrinoma is found in the usual locations, other ectopic sites should be examined carefully. Resection of these primary ectopic tumours can sometimes lead to durable biochemical cures. Gastrinomas may be identified in 96% of surgical explorations if these approaches are adopted.[11] With the use of SASI in particular, though a tumour cannot be precisely localised, it may be sufficiently 'narrowed down' to allow a limited pancreatic and/or duodenal resection.[10] The intraoperative secretin test in which gastrin levels in response to secretin are measured before and after resection can be useful in assessing the effectiveness of resection.

Emergency management of complicated peptic ulcer disease

Although very few patients now require elective surgery, the number who require surgery for the complications of peptic ulcer disease has remained constant for many years.

Perforation

A number of factors associated with poor outcome in perforated peptic ulcer have been identified: delay in diagnosis, coexistent medical illness, shock on admission, leucocytosis and age over 75. A delay in treatment of greater than 24 hours is associated with a sevenfold increase in mortality, threefold risk of morbidity and a twofold increase in hospital stay. The elderly are particularly vulnerable and often more difficult to diagnose because of poorly localised symptoms and signs and fewer preceding symptoms. The principles of treatment of peptic ulcer perforation involve resuscitation, control of contamination and prevention of recurrence.

✔✔ Careful resuscitation and perioperative optimisation play a significant role in reducing morbidity and mortality associated with perforated peptic ulcer disease.[13]

Conservative management

Study of the natural history of perforated peptic ulcers suggests that they frequently seal spontaneously by omentum or adjacent organs and that, particularly when this occurs rapidly, contamination can be minimal. Taylor showed that the mortality in his series of patients with peptic ulcer disease was half that of the contemporary (pre-1946) reported mortality for perforation treated surgically.[14] Conservative treatment today consists of parenteral broad-spectrum antibiotics, intravenous acid antisecretories, intravenous fluid resuscitation and nasogastric aspiration. In addition, water-soluble meal and limited follow-through is recommended to confirm that the leak has sealed. CT is becoming increasingly used in the diagnosis of acute abdominal pain and the degree of fluid contamination may also serve as a useful guide as to whether peritoneal lavage or drainage is necessary.

✔ The conservative approach may be particularly appropriate in patients under 70, whose comorbidity (recent myocardial infarction, severe chronic obstructive pulmonary disease, etc.) place them at high operative risk. Sometimes, where there is some delay in presentation and patients exhibit an already improving clinical picture with minimal abdominal signs, conservative treatment is likely to be successful. Such an approach, however, requires careful interval assessment by an experienced surgeon with a low threshold for performing surgery if clinical improvement is not apparent, both to confirm the diagnosis and oversew an unsealed perforation. Small series have demonstrated low, comparable mortality for the conservative approach with conversion to operation of around 20–30%. Those that failed conservative treatment were more often over 70 years of age.[15–17]

Surgery

In most cases the treatment of choice for patients with perforation of the duodenum is still laparotomy, peritoneal lavage and simple closure of perforation, usually by pedicled omental patch repair (**Fig. 18.2**). The routine use of drains is unnecessary and may in fact increase morbidity. This simple treatment is safe and effective in the long term, when combined with pharmacological acid suppression. Ninety per cent of perforations are associated with HP infection,[18] and HP eradication further significantly reduces the risk of ulcer recurrence.[19]

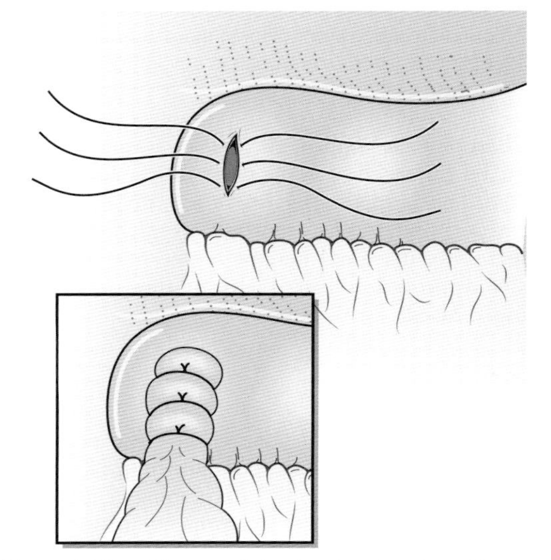

Figure 18.2 • Closure of duodenal perforation with pedicled omental patch.

In cases of 'giant' perforation, where the defect measures 2.5 cm or more, partial gastrectomy with closure of the duodenal stump should be considered (see also management of bleeding from giant duodenal ulcer below). Alternatively, in situations where the clinical situation or expertise dictates more expeditious surgery, the duodenal perforation should be closed as well as possible around a large Foley or T-tube catheter to create a controlled fistula. This can be combined with venting gastrototomy and feeding jejunostomy.[20] The advances in understanding of the medical treatment of peptic ulcer disease together with the decrease in experience of elective antiulcer surgery have made the argument for definitive ulcer surgery in the emergency setting almost untenable.

Although laparoscopic treatment of peptic ulcer perforation was first reported in 1990[21] and many excellent series have been reported since, a European population study demonstrated that the proportion of cases performed laparoscopically is as low as 6%,[22] and even in centres with a specialist interest in laparoscopic surgery the proportion of cases completed laparoscopically is less than 50%.[23]

✔✔ There are several series that show favourable results with the laparoscopic approach,[24] but there are very few prospective studies.[25] Shock, delayed presentation, confounding medical condition, age greater than 70 years, poor laparoscopic expertise and ASA grade are risk factors for open conversion and for poorer outcome.[26] In 'low-risk' patients the laparoscopic approach may have significant advantages. For higher-risk patients (prolonged perforation for >24 h, shock on admission and confounding medical conditions) there is no evidence that the laparoscopic approach is advantageous.

Whatever the approach, basic surgical tenets must be observed: careful preparation for theatre with timely expeditious operation involves thorough peritoneal lavage and secure closure of the defect. Any marginal benefit of the minimally invasive approach is lost if any of these tenets are compromised.

Bleeding

Management of acute haemorrhage from peptic ulceration of the stomach and duodenum has been revolutionised by rapidly developing endoscopic technology and expertise. The principle of successful management is by prompt resuscitation, accurate endoscopic diagnosis and the timely application of appropriate therapy.

Medical therapy

✔✔ Although there is evidence that proton-pump inhibitors given pre-endoscopy reduce the incidence of endoscopic findings of stigmata of recent haemorrhage and the need for endoscopic intervention, there is no evidence that this or any other specific pre-endoscopy medical intervention has any effect on overall morbidity, mortality, or specifically the risk of re-bleeding or need for surgery.[27]

✔✔ There is compelling evidence that proton-pump inhibitors given after endoscopic control of bleeding are beneficial. A randomised controlled study (n=240) from Hong Kong has demonstrated a significant reduction in re-bleeding following endoscopic treatment with a protocol of intravenous omeprazole (omeprazole 80 mg i.v. bolus followed by 8 mg/h infusion for 72 hours).[28] This is supported by meta-analysis of subsequent studies.[29]

✔✔ Meta-analysis of randomised, double-blinded trials with tranexamic acid reveals no significant difference in the incidence of re-bleeding but an increase in complications related to therapy such as stroke, myocardial infarction, deep vein thrombosis and pulmonary embolism.[30]

Somatostatin decreases gastric acid and pepsin secretion. Nevertheless, there is no proven benefit of somatostatin or its analogue (octreotide) in the management of active non-variceal upper gastrointestinal bleeding. Prostaglandin E_2 and its analogue (misoprostol) inhibit gastric acid production, stimulate mucosal perfusion, and promote bicarbonate and mucus secretion. Small studies to date have demonstrated no benefit of stopping acute bleeding or preventing re-bleeding.

Endoscopic therapy

The various techniques of endoscopic haemostasis have dramatically reduced the need for emergency surgery for bleeding due to peptic ulceration.

✔✔ Meta-analysis suggests that endoscopic therapy reduces the mortality of acute upper gastrointestinal bleed in patients' active bleeding or non-bleeding visible vessel by avoiding the often considerable morbidity or mortality of emergency surgery.[31]

✔ Ulcers with a clean base or non-protuberant pigmented dot in an ulcer bed, which are at low risk of re-bleeding, do not require endoscopic treatment. For all others, including those who have active bleeding or non-bleeding visible vessels or have adherent blood clot, endoscopic treatment should be given.[32]

Injection with 4–16 mL 1:10 000 adrenaline around the bleeding point and then into the bleeding vessel achieves haemostasis in up to 95% of cases. Additional injection with sclerosants (sodium tetradecyl sulphate, polidoconal, ethanolamine) or absolute alcohol does not confer additional benefit and may cause perforation. Fibrin glue and thrombin may be more effective, but they are not widely available.

Techniques used commonly are the heater probe, multipolar coagulation (BICAP) and argon plasma coagulation. There is no strong evidence to recommend one thermal haemostasis technique over another.

Mechanical clips have had variable success reported when compared with other techniques. This may reflect the technical difficulties with their placement. In certain situations, such as active bleeding from a large vessel, they may be particularly useful.

✔✔ There is strong evidence that, for patients at higher risk of re-bleeding, treatment by a combination of two different modalities is more beneficial than relying on one modality alone.[33] The commonest combination is likely to be adrenaline injection and heater probe application.

There is no evidence to support a repeat endoscopy unless there is a suggestion of further active bleeding or it is felt that the initial endoscopic treatment was suboptimal. Nevertheless, some clinicians do choose to re-evaluate higher risk cases after 24–48 hours and consider further endoscopic treatment.

✔✔ If there is evidence of re-bleeding following endoscopic treatment, unless there is evidence of haemodynamic instability or the ulcer size was greater than 2 cm, a further attempt at endoscopic control is recommended.[34]

Surgery

Operative or radiological intervention is mandatory if initial control of bleeding is not possible endoscopically. Further intervention should also still be considered if re-bleeding occurs following initially successful endoscopic treatment. Re-bleeding may be observed directly endoscopically or indirectly by continuing haematemesis, or the continuing need for transfusion. If there is doubt as to whether re-bleeding has occurred, a check endoscopy should be performed before subjecting a patient to surgery.

Surgical intervention should be anticipated where there is a significant risk of re-bleeding. Various scoring criteria have been suggested to predict risk of significant re-bleeding and death; one commonly used is the Rockall system (Table 18.1). In addition, the size of the ulcer (particularly >2 cm) and its proximity to major vessels, such as the gastroduodenal ulcer on the posterior inferior wall of the duodenal bulb and the left gastric artery high on the lesser curve of the stomach, suggest a high risk of massive bleeding.

Bleeding duodenal ulcer

The first step is to make a longitudinal duodenotomy immediately distal to the pyloric ring. Haemostasis can be initially achieved by digital pressure. While it may be necessary to extend the duodenotomy through the pyloric ring, the pylorus should be preserved if at all possible. Older texts frequently assume that vagotomy is an integral part of ulcer surgery and recommend a larger pyloroduodenotomy, but this is usually not necessary. The stomach and duodenum should be cleared of blood and clots using suction to obtain optimal view of the bleeding site. If access is still difficult, kocherisation of the duodenum may help, along with drawing up of the posterior duodenal mucosa using Babcock's forceps.

Table 18.1 • Rockall scoring system for risk of re-bleeding and death after admission to hospital for acute gastrointestinal bleeding

	Score			
Variable	**0**	**1**	**2**	**3**
Age	<60	60–79	>80	
Shock	No shock	Pulse >100 BP >100	Pulse >100 BP <100	
Comorbidity	None		Cardiac failure, IHD, major comorbidity	Renal failure, liver failure, disseminated malignancy
Diagnosis	Mallory–Weiss tear, no lesion, no SRH	All other diagnoses	Malignancy of upper GI tract	
Major SRH	None or dark spot		Blood in upper GI tract, adherent clot, visible or spurting vessel	

A total score of >3 is associated with good prognosis; <8 is associated with high risk of death.
BP, blood pressure; GI, gastrointestinal; IHD, ischaemic heart disease; SRH, stigmata of recent haemorrhage.

The actively bleeding or exposed vessel should be secured. Points of note in securing the vessel are the limited access, the proximity of underlying structures such as the common bile duct and the tough fibrous nature of the base of a chronic ulcer. In view of these problems, a small, heavy, round-bodied or taper-cut semicircular needle with 0 or No. 1 suture material should be used. The argument of absorbable versus non-absorbable sutures is irrelevant: the sutures probably slough off as the ulcer heals. Securing bleeding from the gastroduodenal artery may involve a horizontal mattress 'U-stitch' to incorporate posterior and medial perforating vessels (**Fig. 18.3**).

The duodenotomy may be closed longitudinally. If vagotomy has been performed the pyloric ring should be divided and the duodenotomy closed transversely to create a Heineke–Mikulicz pyloroplasty (**Fig. 18.4a**). If transverse closure is difficult because of the length of the duodenotomy, longitudinal closure may be performed and a gastrojejunostomy considered. Alternatively, a Finney pyloroplasty may be fashioned (**Fig. 18.4b**).

In a giant ulcer, the first part of the duodenum may be virtually destroyed and, once opened, impossible to close. In this situation it is necessary to proceed to partial gastrectomy. The right gastric and right gastroepiploic arteries are divided. The stomach is disconnected from the duodenum by a combination of blunt and sharp dissection. Antrectomy is perfomed and continuity restored by a gastrojejunostomy. The duodenal stump can then be closed. Although this can be achieved by pinching the second part of the duodenum away from the ulcer to allow conventional closure, this is probably more safely achieved by the technique of Nissen (**Fig. 18.5**). The duodenal stump is drained by either a tube or Foley catheter either through the duodenal suture line or more securely though the healthy sidewall of the second part of the duodenum (**Fig. 18.6**).

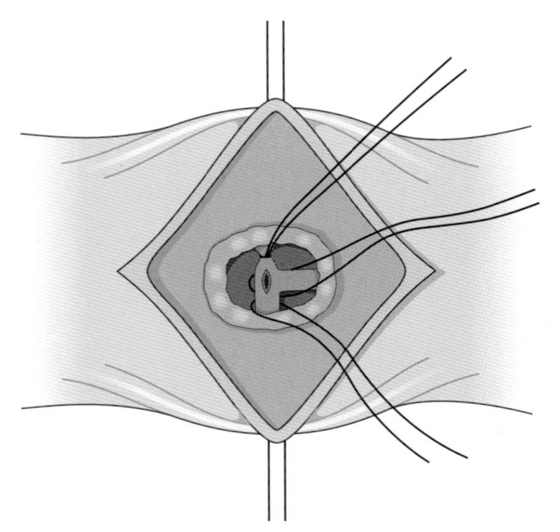

Figure 18.3 • Suture control of bleeding from gastroduodenal artery illustrating the 'U-stitch' incorporating any perforating vessels.

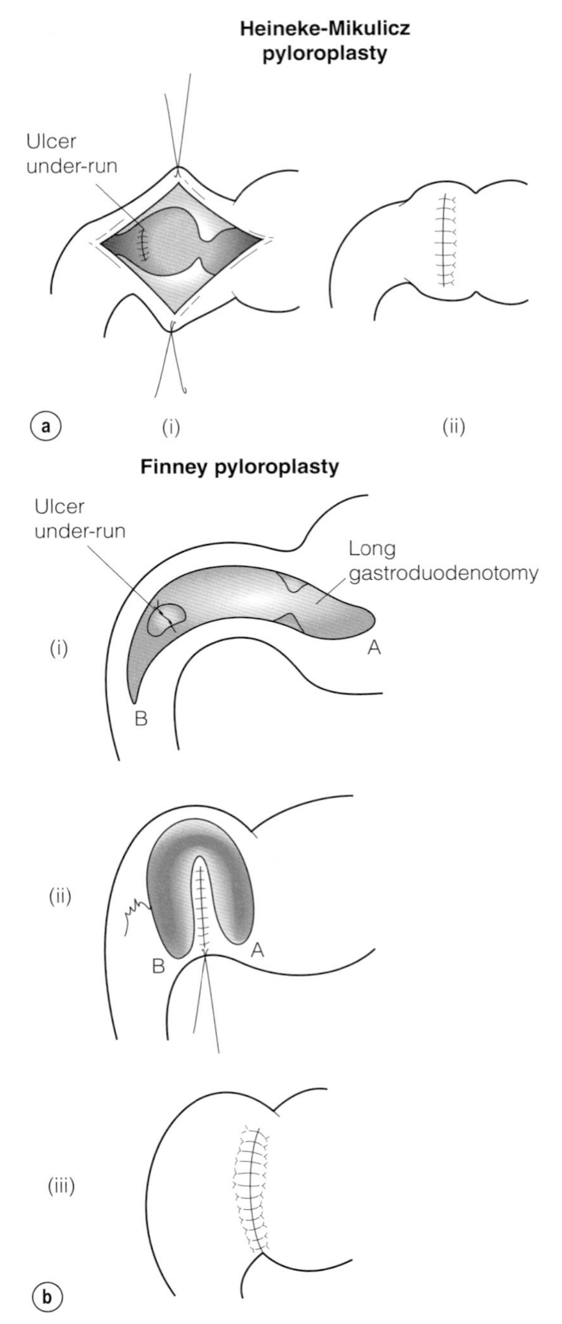

Figure 18.4 • **(a)** Heineke–Mikulicz pyloroplasty. **(b)** Finney pyloroplasty.

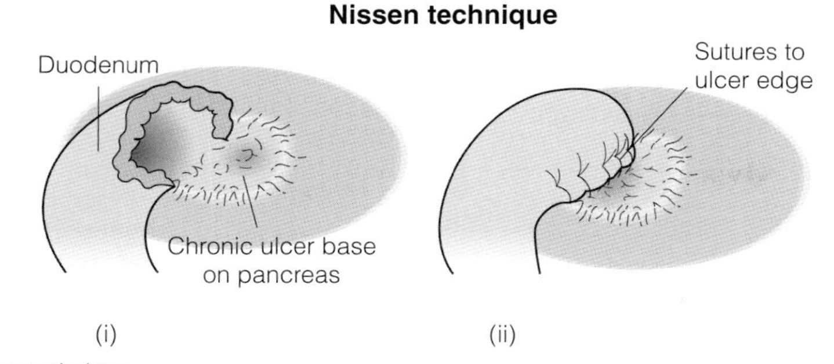

Figure 18.5 • Nissen technique.

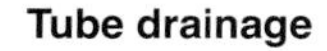

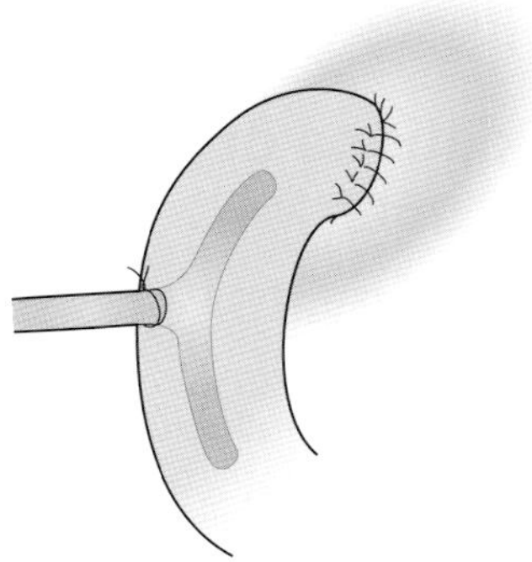

Figure 18.6 • Duodenal drainage following partial gastrectomy for duodenal ulcer.

Long-term acid suppression is required postoperatively. With the advent of proton-pump inhibitors and the recognition of the role of HP, vagotomy should have no part of surgery for bleeding duodenal ulceration.

Bleeding gastric ulcer

The precise site of bleeding should already have been identified endoscopically. If not, intraoperative endoscopy and careful palpation of the stomach for induration should identify the site of the bleeding ulcer. If there is still doubt a generous incision should be made across the pylorus and duodenum, followed by a more proximal gastrotomy if the source of bleeding is still not clear. Most chronic gastric ulcers are at the incisura or in the antrum. The traditional treatment for such ulcers that fail endoscopic therapy is partial gastrectomy. Some groups have advocated simple under-running of bleeding gastric ulcers. While this may be appropriate in selected cases with small bleeding gastric ulcers such as the Dieulafoy lesion, the only randomised trial to date (n=129) suggests that this 'conservative' approach has a higher mortality and is more likely to result in re-bleeding if used unselectively.[35]

For proximal gastric ulcers, typically those high on the lesser curve eroding through into the left gastric artery, the choice of operation lies between total gastrectomy or local excision of the lesser curve (Pauchet's manoeuvre). Frequently such limited procedures involve as much mobilisation of the stomach as total gastrectomy. There is no evidence to recommend one approach over another, though the experience of the surgeon is a major factor in the decision-making process.

Interventional radiology

There are no randomised controlled trials comparing surgery with transcatheter arterial embolisation as salvage treatment following endoscopy. Despite this, in some centres, interventional radiology has become the 'gold standard' intervention following failed endoscopy. Loffroy et al. looked at 15 studies that included 819 patients who had had failed endoscopic control of bleeding; 93% of cases were reported to have 'technical success'.[36] Of these, 67% had immediate cessation of bleeding. Of those that continued to bleed after initial treatment, half responded to a second embolisation. Overall, 20% of patients underwent salvage surgery. The overall mortality in these series was 28%. This seems disappointing and no better than one might expect from a series of bleeders salvaged by surgery. In fact, there was a wide variation between reported mortality in the series, which may indicate different levels of expertise, and case selection. The series were also collected over a 17-year period, during which time there has been considerable improvement in radiological technique. There have been two small retrospective comparisons involving a total of 161 patients.[37,38] They showed that although the radiologically treated patients tended to be older and less fit, they had a comparable (26% vs. 21%) or lower (3% vs. 14%) mortality compared with the surgically treated group.

✔ With a limited evidence base it seems that angiography is a reasonable option where the expertise and facilities are readily available, particularly if the surgery itself is deemed high risk.[36,37]

Pyloric stenosis

Gastric outlet obstruction can result from peptic ulcer disease of the duodenum or pre-pyloric region. It is a condition usually associated with chronic relapsing ulceration and is now fairly uncommon in the Western world.

Resuscitation and medical therapy

Initial management should consist of aggressive parenteral fluid and biochemical restoration with nutritional and vitamin supplementation as necessary. Nasogastric intubation with a wide-bore tube allows gastric washout of undigested food and so reduces antral stimulation. Aggressive parenteral antisecretory therapy and *Helicobacter pylori* eradication, if appropriate, are used. In cases where the obstruction has been due to oedema and spasm, the situation can be expected to resolve once medical treatment has healed the ulcer.[39] Dietary changes to decrease the fibre content while providing a high calorie and protein intake are important until ulcer healing has occurred. In cases where the obstruction is due to fibrosis and cicatrisation of a pyloric ulcer, some form of intervention will be necessary.

Endoscopic treatment

The group of patients who develop gastric outflow obstruction are generally elderly with established comorbidities and tolerate major surgery poorly. As a result, minimally invasive approaches such as endoscopic management are often more appropriate in the first instance. Initial reports of successful resolution of pyloric stenosis following endoscopic balloon dilatation were challenged due to the relatively high number of cases that ultimately required open surgery. Nevertheless, this remains a useful first-line endoscopic procedure that can be repeated on several occasions with good long-term results in up to 80% of patients.[40]

✔ Only if a combination of intensive medical treatment and repeated dilatation fails to reopen the gastric outlet is surgery indicated.[40]

Surgery

There are no published series that prove which procedure achieves the best results in this situation. Initial fears about the capacity of a large atonic stomach to resume function have not been realised. The operation with least complications is simple pyloroplasty (or gastroenterostomy where the inflammation around the pylorus is particularly intense), with the use of long-term medical acid suppression. Antrectomy and selective vagotomy or subtotal gastrectomy are more aggressive alternatives less likely to result in re-stenosis, but with a higher mortality and incidence of both short- and long-term side-effects.

Laparoscopic highly selective vagotomy with balloon dilatation has been attempted with some success in cases of pyloric stenosis. This has not been proven to be superior to dilatation and long-term acid suppression. Laparoscopic truncal vagotomy and gastroenterostomy has proven to be a technically feasible solution with good symptomatic, sustained response.[41]

Complications of previous ulcer surgery

Although elective surgery for benign ulcer disease is now rare, there remains a large cohort of patients operated on prior to the mid-1980s with a variety of surgical procedures, of whom a small percentage will develop further symptoms, some of which may be severely disabling. Although numerous clinical syndromes have been well described (Box 18.1), patients presenting with pure syndromes are uncommon. The majority presents with a mixed picture, but usually have a dominant symptom complex suggesting one main problem. This needs to be elucidated by a careful and detailed history of the clinical events occurring during a bad attack.

Box 18.1 • Post-peptic ulcer surgery sequelae

Pathophysiological problems

- Gastro-oesophageal reflux
- Recurrent ulcer
- Enterogastric reflux
- Dumping
- Reactive hypoglycaemia
- Diarrhoea
- Malabsorption

Mechanical problems

- Loop obstruction
- Small stomach syndrome
- Bezoars

Other sequelae

- Cholelithiasis
- Carcinoma

Preoperative evaluation

Endoscopy

Endoscopic examination is essential, and as with patients after previous antireflux surgery, it should be carried out by the surgeon considering any revisional procedure. The exact anatomy, size of the gastric remnant, size and position of any drainage procedure, the presence of enterogastric reflux of bile, recurrent ulceration, the general state of the gastric mucosa, and the presence of a hiatus hernia and/or reflux oesophagitis can be assessed. All abnormalities should be biopsied. All patients should be assessed for the presence of HP.

Radiology

Barium meal examination of the stomach is a useful adjunct where the anatomy remains unclear.

Gastric-emptying studies

Gastric-emptying studies may occasionally be useful. Barium meal examination may show rapid emptying of the contrast from the stomach and may demonstrate gross intestinal hurry with the meal reaching the caecum within a short time of leaving the stomach. Gastric emptying is, however, best studied using a radioactively labelled meal, either liquid or solid. In general, the radioactive liquid meals are easier to interpret than solid meals. The normal measured indices such as 10-minute emptying, the $T_{1/2}$ and the percentage retention after 60 minutes are often used in assessment. However, after gastric surgery these indices can be misleading as the patients often show a fast initial emptying component followed by a slower component.

Other tests

Congo red for the evaluation of the completeness of vagotomy and dumping provocation tests are now seldom performed. Oesophageal function tests will be required in those patients suspected of having gastro-oesophageal reflux. Enterogastric reflux can be assessed using the hepatobiliary dimethylacetanilide iminodiacetic acid (HIDA) scan. Bacterial overgrowth can be diagnosed by aspiration and culture of jejunal contents or by the [^{14}C]glycocholate breath test.

Various nutritional indices, including weight, serum albumin, transferase and corrected serum calcium concentration, should be measured in all patients. In selected patients full assessment for metabolic bone disease should be undertaken, especially in postmenopausal women. A full haematological survey should be carried out including measurement of serum iron, iron-binding capacity, folate and vitamin B_{12} levels.

Enterogastric reflux

Reflux of alkaline duodenal content into the stomach occurs following surgery that damages, bypasses or removes the pylorus. Enterogastric reflux is more common after gastrectomy where reconstruction as a Billroth II gastrojejunostomy has been carried out.

The symptoms consist of persistent epigastric discomfort, sometimes made worse by eating and frequently associated with intermittent vomiting of bile-stained fluid or food mixed with bile, usually occurring within 90 minutes of a meal. Some patients become malnourished because of inadequate food intake, and anaemia develops in about a quarter of the patients as a result of chronic blood loss from the associated gastritis. Gastro-oesophageal reflux disease may also develop.

Endoscopy shows a diffuse gastritis with an oedematous hyperaemic friable mucosa and frequently superficial erosions. Endoscopic biopsy shows typical histological features including foveolar hyperplasia, glandular cystification, oedema of the lamina propria and vasocongestion of the mucosal capillaries, all in association with inflammatory cell infiltration.

Medical treatment

Cholestyramine has been shown to be an effective bile-acid-binding agent in vitro, although the results of several therapeutic trials have been disappointing. Antacids containing aluminium hydroxide have also been studied because of their bile-acid-binding capacity but the results have been equally unimpressive. In clinical trials sucralfate has been shown to reduce the inflammation within the gastric mucosa but this has not been associated with any improvement in symptoms. Prokinetic agents have also been used to improve clearance of the refluxate from the stomach, and the occasional patient may respond. These agents may, however, worsen dumping and diarrhoea. Ursodeoxycholic acid has been shown in one study to almost abolish the nausea and vomiting associated with enterogastric reflux and to significantly decrease the intensity and frequency of pain.

Surgical treatment

In patients with a previous truncal vagotomy and drainage, reversal of the drainage procedure can be undertaken provided at least 1 year has elapsed from the original operation. This is based on the premise that the stomach will regain some of its lost motility during this time. In fact, more than half of the patients with truncal vagotomy probably did not require a drainage procedure in the first place. Improvement or complete relief usually follows closure of gastrojejunostomy for enterogastric reflux and bile vomiting in the vast majority of patients. The risks of gastric stasis are minimal and conversion to a pyloroplasty should be avoided.

Reconstruction of the pylorus after pyloroplasty is a relatively straightforward operation. Having cleared the anteropyloroduodenal segment of all adhesions, the scar of the previous pyloroplasty is accurately opened. The pyloric ring is palpated and the scarred ends freshened if necessary. One approach is to make a small antral gastrotomy to allow the insertion of a size 12 or 14 Hegar dilator through the area of the pyloric reconstruction into the duodenum. Using a double-ended monofilament suture the pyloric ring is accurately opposed around the Hegar dilator before reapproximating the duodenum and antrum using a continuous serosubmucosal technique. Withdrawal of the Hegar dilator allows fingertip palpation of the reconstructed pylorus prior to closure of the antral gastrotomy. The overall results of pyloric reconstruction show that 80% of patients gain a satisfactory or good result,[42] although in one study only half of the patients with enterogastric reflux had a satisfactory or good response.[43]

If enterogastric reflux is not relieved, then the duodenal switch operation would seem an appropriate further remedial procedure for patients whose symptoms necessitate further surgery[44] (**Fig. 18.7**). Recent experience with this has shown good results, although acid suppression is needed to prevent jejunal ulceration.[45]

In patients who have had a gastric resection or in those with a gastrojejunostomy with pyloric stenosis, a Roux limb (approximately 45 cm in length) would seem an appropriate revisional procedure (with antrectomy in patients with pyloric stenosis). The procedure, however, does carry risks, as it is ulcerogenic because it diverts the buffering effect of upper gastrointestinal contents away from the gastroenteric anastomosis. The second problem is the development of delayed gastric emptying of solid food, producing a symptom complex of satiety, epigastric pain and non-bilious vomiting that has been termed the 'Roux syndrome'. Although many patients will demonstrate objective evidence of delayed gastric emptying of solids, this is usually of little or no clinical consequence except in a minority. The Roux syndrome is more likely to develop in patients who demonstrate delay in gastric emptying of solids prior to construction of the Roux limb and those who have a large residual gastric pouch. A completion vagotomy at the time of revisional surgery may make these symptoms more likely. Where these conditions exist, the operative procedure required is a more extensive gastric resection. The entire anastomosis should be resected to leave a small gastric pouch, and the Roux limb should be anastomosed to the stomach as an end-to-side Polya-type gastrojejunostomy. In those patients who develop severe symptoms from the Roux syndrome postoperatively, then the treatment is near-total resection of the gastric remnant with a Polya-type gastrojejunostomy.

Roux diversion will control enterogastric reflux in over 70% of patients. Recurrent jejunal ulcers can be avoided by checking and if necessary completing the truncal vagotomy as part of the operative procedure. More commonly, today, one would consider relying on long-term treatment with proton-pump inhibitors rather than perhaps risking further side-effects of vagotomy.

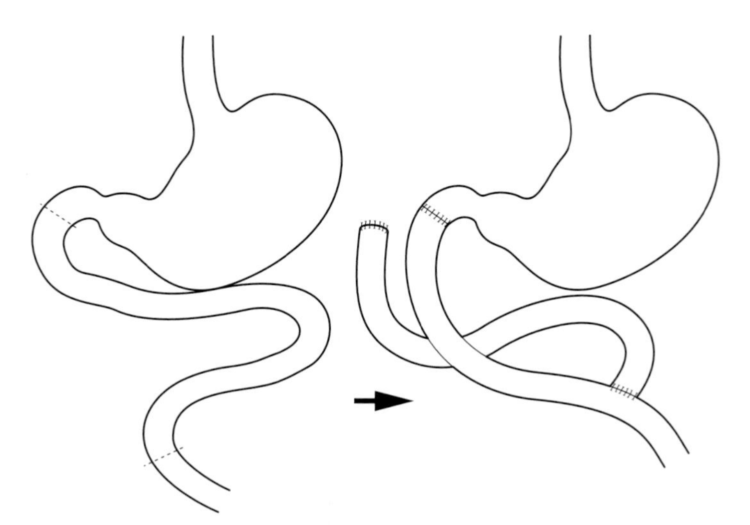

Figure 18.7 • Pylorus-preserving Roux loop – the duodenal switch operation.

Chronic afferent loop syndrome

The afferent loop syndrome can only occur after gastrojejunostomy or a Billroth II-type reconstruction after partial gastrectomy. The condition is caused by intermittent postprandial obstruction of the afferent limb of the gastrojejunostomy. The clinical picture is very similar to that produced by enterogastric reflux (Table 18.2). The problem is rarely encountered if surgeons use a short afferent jejunal loop. The obstruction may be due to anastomotic kinking, adhesions, internal herniation, volvulus of the afferent limb or obstruction of the gastrojejunal stoma itself (**Fig. 18.8**). Once diagnosed, the treatment is always surgical. Conversion to a Billroth I anastomosis or a Roux-en-Y reconstruction of the afferent limb both produce good results.

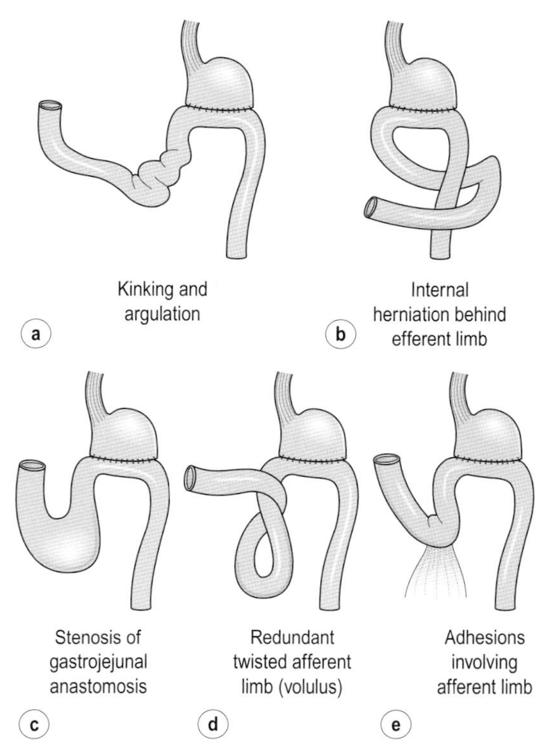

Figure 18.8 • Causes of afferent limb syndrome.

Dumping

The literature shows a considerable variability in the incidence of dumping after each procedure due at least partly to variations in definitions of the syndrome. A significant number of patients will develop dumping-type symptoms in the early period after their initial gastric operation but the majority have sufficient reserve to adjust to the changes without developing severe sequelae.

The symptoms of early dumping can be divided into vasomotor and gastrointestinal, as shown in Box 18.2. In a severe attack, the vasomotor symptoms are usually experienced by the patient towards the end of a meal or within 15 minutes of finishing, and the gastrointestinal symptoms develop a little later, but usually within 30 minutes after eating.

Early dumping is associated with rapid gastric emptying leading to hyperosmolar jejunal content causing massive fluid shifts from the extracellular space into the lumen. This is associated with a significant fall in plasma volume. It is also known that plasma concentrations of several gut regulatory peptides are elevated in patients with the dumping syndrome, but it is not clear whether this is coincidental or causative. Late dumping symptoms are the result of reactive hypoglycaemia. Taking a careful history, delineating the vasomotor and gastrointestinal components, usually makes the diagnosis of the dumping syndrome. Where there is any doubt, the patient should be encouraged to keep a diary card recording the foods eaten and the symptoms that develop thereafter. A provocative test for assessing dumping syndrome can be used to confirm clinical suspicion. This test is a modification of the oral glucose tolerance test and involves the ingestion of 50 or 75 g glucose in solution after an overnight fast. Immediately before and up to 180 min after ingestion of this solution, the blood glucose concentration, haematocrit, pulse rate and blood pressure are measured at 30-min intervals. The provocative test is considered positive if late (120–180 min) hypoglycaemia occurs, or if an early (30 min) increase in haematocrit of more than 3% occurs. The best predictor of dumping syndrome seems to be a rise in the pulse rate of more than 10 b.p.m. after 30 min.[46]

Table 18.2 • Differentiation between the chronic afferent loop syndrome and enterogastric reflux

Chronic afferent loop syndrome	Enterogastric reflux
Meal-related pain – relieved by vomiting	Constant pain (worsened by eating) – not relieved by vomiting
Vomitus contains bile	Vomitus contains bile and food
Vomiting projectile	Vomiting non-projectile
Rarely associated with bleeding/anaemia	Bleeding/anaemia found in 25% of patients

Box 18.2 • Symptoms of dumping

Vasomotor (early dumping)
- Palpitations
- Flushings
- Sweating
- Headache
- Weakness
- Faintness
- Anxiety

Gastrointestinal (early dumping)
- Vomiting
- Belching
- Fullness
- Colic
- Borborygmi
- Diarrhoea

Hypoglycaemia (late dumping)
- Perspiration
- Palpitations
- Hunger
- Weakness
- Confusion
- Tremor
- Syncope

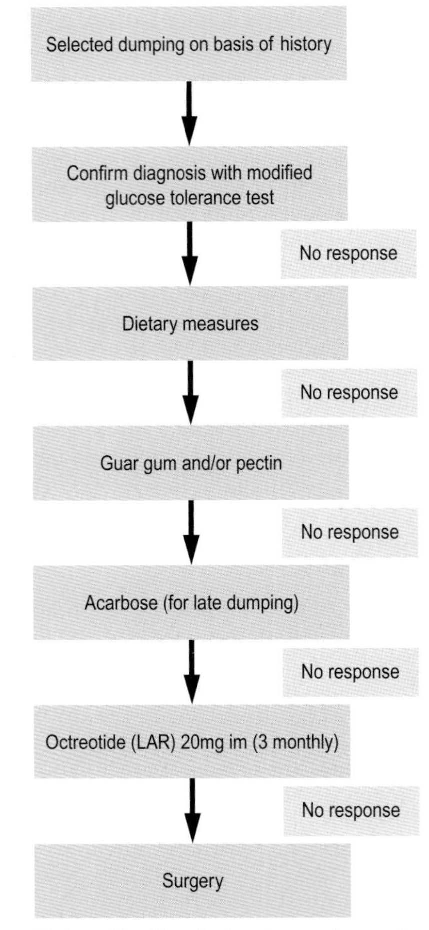

Figure 18.9 • Algorithm for treating postoperative dumping. Adapted from Tack J, Arts J, Caenepeel P et al. Pathophysiology, diagnosis and management of postoperative dumping syndrome. Nat Rev Gastroenterol Hepatol 2009; 6(10):583–90.

Medical treatment

The majority of patients displaying the dumping syndrome can be managed satisfactorily by dietary manipulation. Reducing the carbohydrate content and restricting fluid intake with meals will help many of these patients. Avoiding extra salt and eating more frequent small meals may also be required. Lying down after eating helps to slow gastric emptying and may minimise symptoms. Guar gum, a vegetable fibre, is known to reduce postprandial hyperglycaemia in both normal and diabetic patients. In a small study of postgastric surgery patients it has been shown to prevent the dumping syndrome and increase food tolerance in the majority of patients.[47] Pectin also delays gastric emptying but may precipitate diarrhoea. The use of acarbose, an alpha-glycoside hydrolase inhibitor, interferes with carbohydrate absorption and has been shown to help in patients with late dumping. Octreotide, given subcutaneously prior to eating, has been shown to significantly reduce or abolish the symptoms of dumping.[48] The use of short-acting octreotide was quite troublesome for patients and only around half saw long-term benefit.[49] Encouraging results have been seen with a longer-acting repeatable (LAR) formulation of octreotide, which only needs administration once a month, rather than with each meal.[50]

An algorithm for the treatment of postoperative dumping is shown in **Fig. 18.9.**[51]

Surgical treatment

For patients with truncal vagotomy and drainage procedures, taking down the gastrojejunostomy[52] should cure or improve dumping in over 80% of patients. Reconstruction of the pylorus produces similar results.[53] After gastrectomy, a number of procedures have been advocated for dumping. The simplest and probably the best is to convert the drainage procedure to a 45-cm Roux-en-Y gastrojejunostomy. The delay in liquid emptying after this procedure is thought to be due to myoelectrical abnormalities within the Roux limb itself, causing a degree of retrograde contraction. The delay in emptying of solids is probably a result of the vagotomy leading to a degree of gastric atony and loss of the antral propulsive force to propel solid food into the small intestine. Reversal of the proximal 10 cm of the jejunal limb to create an antiperistaltic interposition is unnecessary and may lead to further stasis and dilatation of the interposed segment. This will worsen any symptoms of gastric retention. The interposition of a segment of upper jejunum between the gastric remnant and the duodenum has been advocated. Both isoperistaltic and antiperistaltic interpositions have been used, but these procedures can be associated with serious complications, and the long-term success rate is variable.[54]

Diarrhoea

Alteration in bowel habit occurs in the majority of patients who undergo truncal vagotomy and in most this is a change from constipation to a more regular habit with one or two motions per day. However, 11% of patients following truncal vagotomy and pyloroplasty had continuous diarrhoea that significantly interfered with their lifestyle.[55] A further 20% of patients will have episodic attacks of diarrhoea more than once a week.

The aetiology of postvagotomy diarrhoea remains poorly understood. Gastric stasis, abnormal small-bowel motility, and impaired biliary and pancreatic function have all been incriminated. Malabsorption, bacterial colonisation of the proximal small bowel, and increased faecal excretion of bile salts and acid may all be contributing factors. Patients who have had a cholecystectomy are more likely to develop postvagotomy diarrhoea and have a particularly severe form.

Diarrhoea may be a component of the dumping syndrome, especially in patients after gastrectomy, but in many postvagotomy patients it is unassociated with dumping. The stool consistency varies from watery to soft, and in its severe form may be explosive in onset without warning, thus leading to incontinence. Patients may be unable to distinguish between the urge to pass flatus and a bowel motion. Occasionally symptoms will be so pronounced that weight loss and malnutrition become apparent.

Investigation of these patients includes the measurement of faecal fats, faecal elastase and vitamin B_{12} level. A barium enema or colonoscopy should be carried out to rule out disorders of the colon, and if bacterial overgrowth is suspected the diagnosis may be confirmed by bacteriological examination of jejunal aspirates or by using the [^{14}C]glycocholate breath test.

Medical treatment

The treatment of postvagotomy diarrhoea begins with dietary manipulation, and in particular the avoidance of refined carbohydrates and foods with a high fluid content. Restriction of fluid intake with meals is occasionally of benefit. Cholestyramine taken morning and evening may be of benefit, especially in patients who have also had a cholecystectomy. There are, however, long-term complications such as megaloblastic anaemia due to folate deficiency in patients on long-term cholestyramine therapy. Codeine and loperamide may also be useful.

Surgical treatment

Closure of a gastrojejunostomy will improve or cure diarrhoea in 80% of patients. A similar improvement is seen with reconstruction of the pylorus. Various intestinal interpositions to act as an intestinal brake have been advocated. The use of a 10-cm antiperistaltic jejunal segment placed 100 cm distal to the duodenojejunal junction has been described. The reversed segment produces a delay in the passage of contents through the small bowel. Many report poor results with these types of operation. The operation that has proved effective is the reverse distal ileal onlay graft, which creates a passive non-propulsive segment.[56]

Small stomach syndrome

This only occurs after a high subtotal gastrectomy in which 80–90% of the stomach is removed and is very unusual. Typically this leads to epigastric and retrosternal discomfort after ingesting food due to rapid gastric distention and is often accompanied by nausea, hiccoughing, increased flatulence and early satiety. Non-operative treatment consists of frequent small meals, antispasmodics, and mineral and vitamin replacement. Patients may also require fine-bore nasoenteric nutritional supplementation. In a small number of patients with uncontrollable symptoms, surgery may have to be considered. The reservoir jejunal interposition described by Cuschieri, a modification of the Hunt–Lawrence, is probably the procedure of choice.[54] Long-term follow-up of these patients is required as there is a tendency for the jejunal limb to elongate over several years and this can lead to stasis and ulceration.

Key points

- *Helocobacter pylori* infection and NSAID use remain the primary risk factors for peptic ulcer disease. Smoking increases the risk of complications from peptic ulcer disease and prevents effective healing.
- Gastric and duodenal ulcers are considered 'refractory' to medical treatment if there is no sign of significant healing by 12 and 8 weeks, respectively. Refractory ulceration should prompt biopsy from the ulcer margin, re-evaluation of *Helicobacter* eradication and assessment for other underlying causes.
- A diagnosis of Zollinger–Ellison syndrome (ZES) should be suspected in cases of *Helicobacter pylori*-negative, non-NSAID-induced refractory ulceration, especially when there is ulceration of the second part of the duodenum or large confluent ulcers in the duodenum.
- Management of the gastrinoma of ZES follows a similar treatment algorithm to other gastro-entero-hepatic neuroendocrine tumours and involves an aggressive approach to surgical resection. One-quarter of patients with ZES have familial multiple endocrine neoplasia (MEN-1) syndrome.
- Delay in diagnosis, coexistent medical illness, shock on admission, leucocytosis and age over 75 are associated with poor outcome in perforated peptic ulcer disease.
- In 'low-risk' patients with perforated peptic ulcer, the laparoscopic approach has advantages.
- Endoscopic therapy reduces the mortality of patients with acute active upper gastrointestinal bleeding or a non-bleeding visible vessel. A combination of two different endoscopic modalities is more successful than unimodality treatment.
- Proton-pump inhibitors given after endoscopic control of high-risk peptic ulcer bleeding improve outcomes.
- Only if a combination of intensive medical treatment and dilatation fails to reopen the gastric outlet is surgery indicated for benign pyloric stenosis.
- Problems related to previous upper GI surgery are infrequent, but logical, simple measures can improve symptoms significantly if a careful history is elicited and a treatment algorithm is followed for the dominant problem.
- After antrectomy or other forms of partial gastrectomy, diversion of bile and pancreatic secretion is best carried out with a 45-cm Roux loop.

References

1. Mégraud F, Lehours P. *Helicobacter pylori* detection and antimicrobial susceptibility testing. Clin Microbiol Rev 2007;20(2):280–322.
2. Eastwood GL. Is smoking still important in the pathogenesis of peptic ulcer disease? J Clin Gastroenterol 1997;25(Suppl. 1):S1–7.
3. Lu YF, Zhang XX, Zhao G, et al. Gastroduodenal ulcer treated by pylorus and pyloric vagus preserving gastrectomy. World J Gastroenterol 1999;5(2):156–9.
4. Park do J, Lee HJ, Jung HC, et al. Clinical outcome of pylorus-preserving gastrectomy in gastric cancer in comparison with conventional distal gastrectomy with Billroth I anastomosis. World J Surg 2008;32(6):1029–36.
5. Stabile BE, Morrow DJ, Passaro Jr E. The gastrinoma triangle: operative implications. Am J Surg 1984;147(1):25–31.
6. Ellison EH, Wilson SD. The Zollinger–Ellison syndrome: re-appraisal and evaluation of 260 registered cases. Ann Surg 1964;160:512–20.
7. Zollinger RM, Ellison EC, O'Darisio TM, et al. Thirty years of experience with gastrinoma. World J Surg 1984;8:427–35.
8. Wu PC, Alexander HR, Bartlett DL, et al. A prospective analysis of the frequency, location, and curability of ectopic (nonpancreaticoduodenal, nonnodal) gastrinoma. Surgery 1997;122(6):1176–82.
9. Ramage JK, Davies AHG, Ardill J, et al. Guidelines for the management of gastroenteropancreatic neuroendocrine (including carcinoid) tumours. Gut 2005;54:1–16.
10. Imamura M, Komoto I, Ota S. Changing treatment strategy for gastrinoma in patients with Zollinger–Ellison syndrome. World J Surg 2006;30:1–11.
11. Norton JA, Fraker DL, Alexander HR, et al. Surgery increases survival in patients with gastrinoma. Ann Surg 2006;244(3):410–9.

12. Norton JA. Intraoperative methods to stage and localize pancreatic and duodenal tumors. Ann Oncol 1999;10(Suppl. 4):182–4.

13. Møller MH, Adamsen S, Thomsen RW, et al., on behalf of the Peptic Ulcer Perforation (PULP) trial group. Multicentre trial of a perioperative protocol to reduce mortality in patients with peptic ulcer perforation. Br J Surg 2011;98:802–10.
This study describes a multimodality multidisciplinary perioperative protocol for resuscitation and treatment of sepsis in patients with perforated duodenal ulcers. It suggests a significant reduction in mortality. Although this study has demonstrated impressive results, it is not a controlled study and relies on reference to historical outcomes. It also adopts several measures at once, including the principles of the surviving sepsis campaign and goal-directed therapy, making it difficult to distil the precise interventions that made a difference. The authors themselves acknowledge that their study design inherently places a spotlight on this group of patients and it is impossible to know whether it was simply the increased 'attention' to this group rather than any particular element of the protocol that was responsible for the outcome.

14. Taylor H. Aspiration treatment of perforated ulcers. Lancet 1951;1:7–12.

15. Gul YA, Shine MF, Lennon F. Non-operative management of perforated duodenal ulcer. Irish J Med Sci 1999;168(4):254–6.

16. Crofts TJ, Park KGM, Steele RJC, et al. A randomised trial of nonoperative treatment for perforated peptic ulcer. N Engl J Med 1989;320(15):970–3.

17. Donovan AJ, Berne TV, Donovan JA. Perforated duodenal ulcer: an alternative therapeutic plan. Arch Surg 1998;133(11):1166–71.

18. Mihmanli M, Isgor A, Kabukcuoglu F, et al. The effect of *H. pylori* in perforation of duodenal ulcer. Hepatogastroenterology 1998;45(23):1610–2.

19. Ng EKW, Lam YH, Sung JJY, et al. Eradication of HP prevents recurrence of ulcer after simple closure of duodenal ulcer perforation: randomised controlled trial. Ann Surg 2000;231:153–8.

20. Herrod PJ, Kamali D, Pillai SC. Triple-ostomy: management of perforations to the second part of the duodenum in patients unfit for definitive surgery. Ann R Coll Surg Engl 2011;93(7):e122–4.

21. Mouret P, Francois Y, Vagnal J, et al. Laparoscopic treatment of perforated peptic ulcer. Br J Surg 1990;77:1006.

22. Sommer T, Elbroend H, Friis-Andersen H. Laparoscopic repair of perforated ulcer in Western Denmark – a retrospective study. Scand J Surg 2010;99:119–21.

23. Critchley AC, Phillips AW, Bawa SM, et al. Management of perforated peptic ulcer in a district general hospital. Ann R Coll Surg Engl 2011;93(8):615–9.

24. Bertleff MJ, Lange JF. Laparoscopic correction of perforated peptic ulcer: first choice? A review of literature. Surg Endosc 2010;24(6):1231–9.
This paper analysed the results of 36 studies of various designs involving 2788 patients. It found a conversion rate of 12.4%. The laparoscopic approach was associated with less postoperative pain, lower morbidity, less mortality and shorter hospital stay. By contrast, the open group had significantly shorter operation times and lower rate of recurrent leakage.

25. Sanabria A, Villegas MI, Morales Uribe CH. Laparoscopic repair for perforated peptic ulcer disease. Cochrane Database Syst Rev 2005;(4): CD004778.
This Cochrane review, updated in 2010, concluded that the data available at that time (just three randomised trials of acceptable quality) do not support laparoscopic over open surgery. Although there was a trend towards decrease in septic complications, wound infection, ileus, deep vein thrombosis and mortality in favour of the laparoscopic approach, there was a trend in favour of open surgery with respect to intra-abdminal abscess formation and re-operation.

26. Lunevicius R, Morkevicius M. Systematic review comparing laparoscopic and open repair for perforated peptic ulcer. Br J Surg 2005;92(10):1195–207.
This systematic review of 25 studies identified shock, delayed presentation (>24 hours), confounding medical condition, age >70 years, poor laparoscopic expertise and ASA Grade III–IV as risk factors for conversion to open surgery and postoperative morbidity.

27. Sreedharan A, Martin J, Leontiadis GI, et al. Proton pump inhibitor treatment initiated prior to endoscopic diagnosis in upper gastrointestinal bleeding. Cochrane Database Syst Rev 2010;(7):CD005415.
This paper examines the evidence for giving PPIs before endoscopy in cases of upper GI bleeding. Looking at six randomised controlled trials involving 2223 patients there was no difference in outcome but the studies themselves were weak. The authors recommend a pragmatic approach to using PPIs before endoscopy, particularly if endoscopy is likely to be delayed. One of the problems with this type of study is that the patient population studied is, by definition, a heterogeneous group and, while one might intuitively expect a similar response to that seen in post-endoscopy use of PPIs in a high-risk subgroup,[27] studies have perhaps not been powered to identify such an effect.

28. Lau JYW, Sung JJY, Lee KKC, et al. Effect of intravenous omeprazole on recurrent bleeding after endoscopic treatment of bleeding peptic ulcers. N Engl J Med 2000;343:310–6.
This study is a double blind randomised design and, unlike previous reports, included only patients at high risk of re-bleed. It found a reduction in rate of re-bleeding if intravenous omeprazole was given after endoscopy and endoscopic treatment. Previous studies that had not excluded cases at low risk of re-bleed (the great majority), probably for statistical reasons, failed to demonstrate an effect.

29. Leontiadis GI, Sreedharan A, Dorward S, et al. Systematic reviews of the clinical effectiveness and cost-effectiveness of proton pump inhibitors in acute upper gastrointestinal bleeding. Health Technol Assess 2007;11(51):iii–iv,1–164.

30. Gluud LL, Klingenberg SL, Langholz E. Tranexamic acid for upper gastrointestinal bleeding. Cochrane Database Syst Rev 2012;(1):CD006640.
This review looked at seven randomised double blind trials of tranexamic acid in cases of acute upper GI bleeding. The trials did not really reflect modern clinical practice, with studies published from 1973 and the most recent in 2001. They variously use tranexamic acid with placebo and acid antisecretories. No significant differences were found between tranexamic acid and placebo on bleeding, surgery or transfusion requirements, nor between tranexamic acid compared with cimetidine or lansoprazole.

31. Cook DJ, Guyatt GH, Salena BJ, et al. Endoscopic therapy for acute non-variceal upper gastrointestinal hemorrhage: a meta-analysis. Gastroenterology 1992;102:139–48.
This paper studied 30 randomised controlled trials evaluating haemostatic endoscopic treatments. Endoscopic therapy significantly reduced rates of re-bleeding, need for surgery and mortality in patients with high-risk endoscopic features of active bleeding or non-bleeding visible vessels. Re-bleeding was rare in patients with ulcers containing flat pigmented spots or adherent clots regardless of endoscopic treatment.

32. Palmer K, Nairn M, Guideline Development Group. Management of acute gastrointestinal blood loss: summary of SIGN guidelines. Br Med J 2008; 337:a1832.

33. Vergara M, Calvet X, Gisbert JP. Epinephrine injection versus epinephrine injection and a second endoscopic method in high risk bleeding ulcers. Cochrane Database Syst Rev 2007;(2):CD005584.
This meta-analysis looked at 18 randomised prospective studies involving 1868 patients. It found reductions in re-bleeding (18.5% vs. 10%), need for emergency surgery (10.8% vs. 6.7%) and mortality (4.7% vs. 2.5%) if more than one endoscopic method was used to secure haemostasis at the initial endoscopy.

34. Lau JYW, Sung JJY, Lam YH, et al. Endoscopic retreatment compared with surgery in patients with recurrent bleeding after initial endoscopic control of bleeding ulcers. N Engl J Med 1999;340:751–6.
This study from Hong Kong compared the outcome of patients who re-bleed following initial endoscopic haemostasis: 48 were randomised to a further endoscopic treatment and 44 directly to surgery. Although hypotension at randomisation and an ulcer size larger than 2 cm predicted a poor outcome with endoscopic re-treatment, overall a seond attempt at endoscopic treatment proved safe with no increased mortality, fewer complications and spared 73% of cases an operation.

35. Poxon VA, Keighley MR, Dykes PW, et al. Comparison of minimal and conventional surgery in patients with bleeding peptic ulcer: a multicentre trial. Br J Surg 1991;78(11):1344–5.

36. Loffroy R, Rao P, Ota S, et al. Embolization of acute nonvariceal upper gastrointestinal hemorrhage resistant to endoscopic treatment: results and predictors of recurrent bleeding. Cardiovasc Intervent Radiol 2010;33:1088–100.

37. Ripoll C, Banares R, Beceiro I, et al. Comparison of transcatheter arterial embolization and surgery for treatment of bleeding peptic ulcer after endoscopic treatment failure. J Vasc Interv Radiol 2004;15:447–50.

38. Eriksson LG, Ljungdahl M, Sundbom M, et al. Transcatheter arterial embolization versus surgery in the treatment of upper gastrointestinal bleeding after therapeutic endoscopy failure. J Vasc Interv Radiol 2008;19(10):1413–8.

39. Cherian PT, Cherian S, Singh P. Long-term follow-up of patients with gastric outlet obstruction related to peptic ulcer disease treated with endoscopic balloon dilatation and drug therapy. Gastrointest Endosc 2007;66(3):491–7.

40. Shabbir J, Durrani S, Ridgway PF, et al. Proton pump inhibition is a feasible primary alternative to surgery and balloon dilatation in adult peptic pyloric stenosis (APS): report of six consecutive cases. Ann R Coll Surg Engl 2006;88(2):174–5.

41. Kim SM, Song J, Oh SJ, et al. Comparison of laparoscopic truncal vagotomy with gastrojejunostomy and open surgery in peptic pyloric stenosis. Surg Endosc 2009;23(6):1326–30.

42. Koruth NM, Krukowski ZH, Matheson N. Pyloric reconstruction. Br J Surg 1985;72:808–10.

43. Martin CJ, Kennedy T. Reconstruction of the pylorus. World J Surg 1985;6:221–5.

44. DeMeester TR, Fuchs KH, Ball CS, et al. Experimental and clinical results with proximal end-to-end duodenojejunostomy for pathological duodenogastric reflux. Ann Surg 1987;206:414–26.

45. Strignano P, Collard JM, Michel JM, et al. Duodenal switch operation for pathologic transpyloric duodenogastric reflux. Ann Surg 2007;245(2):247–53.

46. van der Kleij FG, Vecht J, Lamers CB, et al. Diagnostic value of dumping provocation in patients after gastric surgery. Scand J Gastroenterol 1996;31:1162–6.

47. Harju E, Larmi TKI. Efficacy of guar gum in preventing the dumping syndrome. J Parent Enter Nutr 1983;7:470–2.

48. Primrose JN, Johnston D. Somatostatin analogue SMS 201-995 (octreotide) as a possible solution to the dumping syndrome after gastrectomy or vagotomy. Br J Surg 1989;76:140–4.

49. Didden P, Penning C, Masclee AA. Octreotide therapy in dumping syndrome: analysis of long-term results. Aliment Pharmacol Ther 2006;24(9):1367–75.
50. Arts J, Caenepeel P, Bisschops R, et al. Efficacy of the long-acting repeatable formulation of the somatostatin analogue octreotide in postoperative dumping. Clin Gastroenterol Hepatol 2009;7(4):432–7.
51. Tack J, Arts J, Caenepeel P, et al. Pathophysiology, diagnosis and management of postoperative dumping syndrome. Nat Rev Gastroenterol Hepatol 2009;6(10):583–90.
52. McMahon MJ, Johnston D, Hill GT, et al. Treatment of severe side effects after vagotomy and gastroenterostomy by closure of gastroenterostomy without pyloroplasty. Br Med J 1978;1:7–8.
53. Cheadle WG, Baker PR, Cuschieri A. Pyloric reconstruction for severe vasomotor dumping after vagotomy and pyloroplasty. Ann Surg 1985;202:568–72.
54. Cuschieri A. Long term evaluation of a reservoir jejunal interposition with an isoperistaltic conduit in the management of patients with a small stomach syndrome. Br J Surg 1982;69:386–8.
55. Cuschieri A. Isoperistaltic and antiperistaltic jejunal interposition for the dumping syndrome. A comparative study. J R Coll Surg Edinb 1977;22:319–42.
56. Cuschieri A. Surgical management of severe intractable postvagotomy diarrhoea. Br J Surg 1986;73:981–4.

19

Oesophageal emergencies

Jon Shenfine
S. Michael Griffin

Introduction

This chapter focuses on the diagnosis and management of injuries to the oesophagus from a variety of different insults from within and/or without, resulting in a spectrum of oesophageal damage. Most clinicians gain limited exposure to patients with oesophageal trauma due to its rarity and, as a result, misdiagnosis, incorrect investigations and inappropriate management are common. The difficulty in accessing the oesophagus, its unusual blood supply, the lack of a strong serosal layer and the proximity of vital structures also make clinicians wary. The lack of clinical experience is compounded by the lack of an evidence base for management, with published literature limited to observational studies. Yet the management of such injuries is actually straightforward to a clinician who regularly accesses the oesophagus and is familiar with the basic principles, developed by oesophageal surgeons of the past, to minimise morbidity and mortality. Hopefully, the outcomes from these injuries will improve with the changes in the structure of the service for patients with upper gastrointestinal disease and the provision of dedicated multidisciplinary specialist units with the inherent knowledge and skills to deal with them. This chapter will attempt to deal with perforations of the oesophagus as a grouped entity but will cover foreign body impaction and caustic injuries to the oesophagus separately.

Perforation of the oesophagus

The availability of upper gastrointestinal endoscopy and associated instrumentation has resulted in an increase in iatrogenic trauma, which now accounts for the majority of oesophageal injuries. The rare, eponymous Boerhaave syndrome of spontaneous perforation of the oesophagus occurs in the absence of pre-existing pathology and minor differences in management can lead to major outcome improvements. Penetrating and blunt injuries to the oesophagus are similarly uncommon and misdiagnosis often compounds any injury.

Aetiology and pathophysiology

Iatrogenic perforation of the oesophagus

Iatrogenic damage to the oesophagus leading to full-thickness disruption occurs from within in 60–70% of cases, such as during endoscopic instrumentation, or from without, such as during para-oesophageal surgery. Although flexible video endoscopy is safe and has almost totally replaced rigid oesophagoscopy (0.03% perforation risk compared to 0.11% for rigid endoscopy), the dramatic increase in the number of examinations performed has led to an increase in the number of associated injuries. Intubation of the oesophagus can cause proximal perforation with risk increased by hyper-extension of the neck and the presence of arthritic cervical osteophytes or an oesophageal diverticulum. However, in 75–90% of diagnostic cases, trauma is sustained to the distal oesophagus, often in conjunction with an abnormality (Table 19.1). Therapeutic endoscopy carries a significantly higher perforation risk (200-fold), around 5%, that is further increased in patients who have received prior

Table 19.1 • Risk of iatrogenic oesophageal disruption through instrumentation

Medical instrumentation	Percentage risk of iatrogenic oesophageal disruption
Dilatation	0.5
Dilatation for achalasia	2
Endoscopic thermal therapy	1–2
Treatment of variceal bleeding	1–6
Endoscopic laser therapy	1–5
Photodynamic therapy	5
Stent placement	5–25

radiotherapy or chemotherapy (as the majority of therapeutic endoscopy is for palliation). Dilatation accounts for the majority of injuries and with a lower risk of perforation when placing self-expanding metal stents. Benign pneumatic dilatation for achalasia carries a higher risk than graded dilatation, due to higher pressures and large balloon size.[1] Transoesophageal echocardiography carries risk not only for perforation during blind placement but also when placed for perioperative monitoring due to pressure necrosis. Similarly, any intubation such as placement of a nasogastric tube or inadvertent oesophageal placement of an endotracheal tube may all cause direct trauma. A case review of 75 patients with iatrogenic perforation of the oesophagus reported a not insubstantial overall mortality rate of 19%. Prevention is therefore the best solution, with increasing awareness and training likely to reduce the incidence.[2]

Spontaneous perforation of the oesophagus

Boerhaave's syndrome is characterised by barogenic oesophageal injury leading to immediate and gross gastric content contamination of the pleural cavity. However, various degrees of damage and contamination are possible. As a result, a number of clinical terms have evolved to describe these events: this text will only use the term 'spontaneous perforation of the oesophagus', with the term 'disruption' used to describe the 'process' of perforation. Spontaneous perforation of the oesophagus is most accurately defined as complete disruption of the oesophageal wall occurring in the absence of pre-existing pathology. Since the oesophagus possesses no serosa, transgression of oesophagogastric contents leads rapidly to chemical and septic mediastinitis. In 80–90% of cases, this disruption is associated with a sudden rise in intra-abdominal pressure, most usually as a result of retching or vomiting; however, blunt trauma, weight-lifting, parturition, defecation, the Heimlich manoeuvre or status epilepticus have all been cited as causal factors. Although vomiting is commonplace, spontaneous oesophageal perforation is not, which suggests that other as yet unidentified factors may be important, such as pre-existing anatomical or pathological abnormalities. However, an underlying pathology is identified in only 10–20% of cases, such as malignancy, peptic ulceration or infection (as such not truly spontaneous perforation). A common misconception is that Mallory–Weiss tears represent part of the spectrum of spontaneous perforation but it is likely that these mucosal injuries reflect 'shearing' rather than 'barogenic' trauma.[3] Equally, eosinophilic oesophagitis has also been associated with an increased risk of both mucosal tears and full-thickness perforation either spontaneously induced by vomiting to dislodge impacted food or following endoscopic procedures.[4]

Spontaneous perforations are usually single, longitudinal, 1–8 cm long and occur most commonly in the left posterolateral position above the oesophagogastric junction. Barogenic pleural disruption occurs instantly but may also occur later through gastric acid erosion, exacerbated by negative intrathoracic pressure. Caucasian males are predominantly affected, in a ratio of 4:1, which may reflect a predisposition to alcohol ingestion, overindulgence and vomiting rather than a true gender variation.

Penetrating injuries

Penetrating injuries to the oesophagus usually occur in conjunction with serious injuries to surrounding viscera so are easily missed. Associated delay and contamination greatly increase morbidity and mortality so any penetrating transcervical or transmediastinal injury, especially when gunshot derived, should raise suspicion of oesophageal trauma.

Blunt trauma

Blunt oesophageal trauma is extremely uncommon, almost exclusively occurring in high-impact injuries and associated with more immediately life-threatening airway or cardiopulmonary damage. Impaction of the neck or upper chest on the steering wheel in high-velocity road traffic accidents or extreme 'whiplash' flexion–extension can injure the cervical oesophagus. Rapid deceleration can lead to traction laceration of the thoracic oesophagus at fixed points (such as the cricoid, carina or pharyngo-oesophageal junction) or barogenic damage can occur after a sudden rise in intra-abdominal pressure from compression against a closed glottis or as a secondary event following interruption of vascular supply.

Clinical presentation

Clinical features depend on the cause, site and duration from injury. Most full-thickness, iatrogenic trauma is recognised immediately or at least there is a high index of suspicion. In contrast, the presentation of a patient with spontaneous perforation of the oesophagus can be maze-like.

> ✔ The classical Mackler triad of sudden, 'dramatic' chest pain following an episode of raised intra-abdominal pressure, usually vomiting, and the development of subcutaneous emphysema is surprisingly uncommon, present in only 7 of 51 patients (14%) in one large case series.[5,6] As such, the classical presentation is not necessarily the common presentation.

As a result, in spontaneous perforation, the diagnostic error is high, with only 5% of cases diagnosed at presentation. This leads to diagnostic delay of greater than 12 hours in the majority of cases.[7] It may be that less than 35% of cases are correctly diagnosed pre-mortem[8] (Box 19.1). As time passes, the critical condition of the patient further obscures relevant clinical features and the pursuit of incorrect investigations makes the diagnosis even more elusive.

Depending on the aetiology and amount of contamination, pain may be severe, constant, retrosternal or epigastric, distressing, exacerbated by movement and poorly relieved by narcotics or relatively mild. Dysphagia and odynophagia are common. Patients can be tachypnoeic and may sit up to splint their diaphragm. Abdominal pain or tenderness are not uncommon and can lead to a negative laparotomy.[6] Similarly, subcutaneous emphysema takes time to develop; mediastinal emphysema precedes this and may be visible on a plain chest radiograph. With time the negative intrathoracic pressure draws air, food and fluids into the mediastinum and pleural cavities and a chemical pleuromediastinitis develops. A low-grade pyrexia ensues, and a sympathetic nervous system response develops with pallor, sweating, peripheral circulatory shutdown, tachycardia, tachypnoea and overt haemodynamic shock, which worsens as the systemic inflammatory response gives way to sepsis. Within 24–48 hours cardiopulmonary embarrassment and collapse develop as a consequence of overwhelming bacterial mediastinitis and septic shock. The combination of chest pain and shock may inappropriately, but all too commonly lead to a cardiological referral. Survival is dependent on the evacuation of the contamination, from the mediastinal and pleural cavities at the earliest possible opportunity.[9] Systemic effects are less common when the cervical oesophagus is damaged, with neck pain, torticollis, dysphonia, cervical dysphagia, hoarseness and subcutaneous emphysema predominating.

Penetrating oesophageal trauma manifests in the same pattern but a high index of suspicion based on the likely tract of the insult is essential for diagnosis. Any deep penetrating transcervical or transmediastinal injury, especially gunshot derived, should be deemed suspect for oesophageal trauma. In contrast, except in the most violent of circumstances, blunt trauma rarely causes oesophageal injury but in high impact events a high index of suspicion should be exercised and injury actively excluded.

Box 19.1 • Common misdiagnoses for spontaneous perforation of the oesophagus

Medical
- Myocardial infarction
- Pericarditis
- Spontaneous pneumothorax
- Pneumonia
- Oesophageal varices/Mallory–Weiss tear

Surgical
- Peritonitis
- Acute pancreatitis
- Perforated peptic ulcer
- Renal colic
- Aortic aneurysm (dissection/leak)
- Biliary colic
- Mesenteric ischaemia

Investigations

Plain radiography

The typical findings on plain chest radiography are subtle – dependent on the site and the time interval following the insult. These are documented in Box 19.2 and **Fig. 19.1**. A plain abdominal radiograph may help to exclude a perforated intra-abdominal viscus.[7]

Contrast radiography

Oral water-soluble contrast radiography ascertains the site, the degree of containment and the degree of drainage of the perforation (**Fig. 19.2**). Aqueous agents are rapidly absorbed, do not exacerbate inflammation and have minimal tissue effects. However, false-negative results in 27–66% and the limited applicability to a collapsed, unwell patient have downgraded their usefulness.

Box 19.2 • Typical chest radiograph findings in spontaneous perforation of the oesophagus

- Pleural effusion
- Pneumomediastinum
- Subcutaneous emphysema
- Hydropneumothorax
- Pneumothorax
- Collapse/consolidation

Upper gastrointestinal endoscopy

Endoscopic assessment excludes the diagnosis if normal, influences management if underlying pathology is discovered and facilitates the placement of a nasojejunal tube to allow enteral feeding. Risks are minimised using modern, flexible videoscopes together with fluoroscopic guidance, but should only be performed by a highly experienced endoscopist conversant with the consequences of their actions (**Figs 19.3** and **19.4**). Endoscopy can be performed in the sickest of patients, if necessary 'on table', when other injuries or instability of the patient preclude radiological assessment.

✔ In a retrospective review of 55 trauma patients, Horwitz et al. demonstrated 100% sensitivity and 92.4% specificity for upper gastrointestinal endoscopy in confirming oesophageal perforation and although injuries were infrequent (prevalence 3.6%), no injuries were missed and the examination was safe.[10] In a similar study of 31 patients (24 of whom were intubated at the time of the examination), video endoscopy had a sensitivity of 100% and a specificity of 96% with no associated morbidity.[11] Video endoscopy has also been used to examine the oesophagogastric anastomosis post-oesophagectomy without additional morbidity.[10–12]

Computed tomography (CT)

CT is increasingly useful in patients stable enough to undergo scanning. It is especially helpful in cases of multi-trauma and in critically ill patients with an atypical presentation, but the radiology department remains a dangerous place for an unstable patient. In combination with complex interventional radiology, CT has also revolutionised the management of intrathoracic collections. It plays a significant role post-therapy, be that assessing the patient postoperatively or assessing the adequacy of non-operative management.

✔ In an intubated patient, the sensitivity of CT for spontaneous perforation is increased by placing a nasogastric tube just past the cricopharyngeus to run in a small amount of contrast media[13] (**Fig. 19.5**).

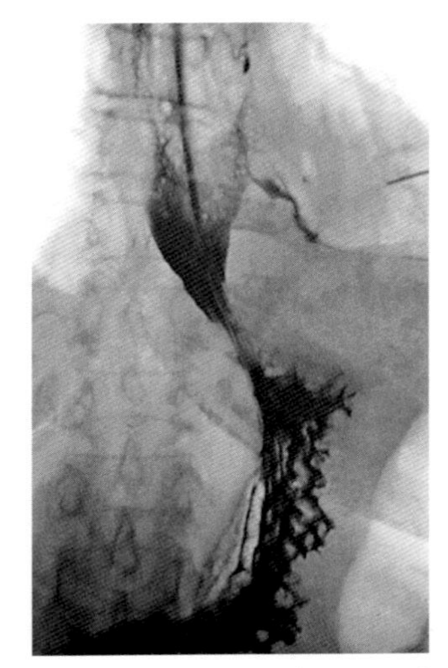

Figure 19.2 • Contrast swallow demonstrating free extravasation of contrast media after oesophageal perforation during balloon dilatation of achalasia.

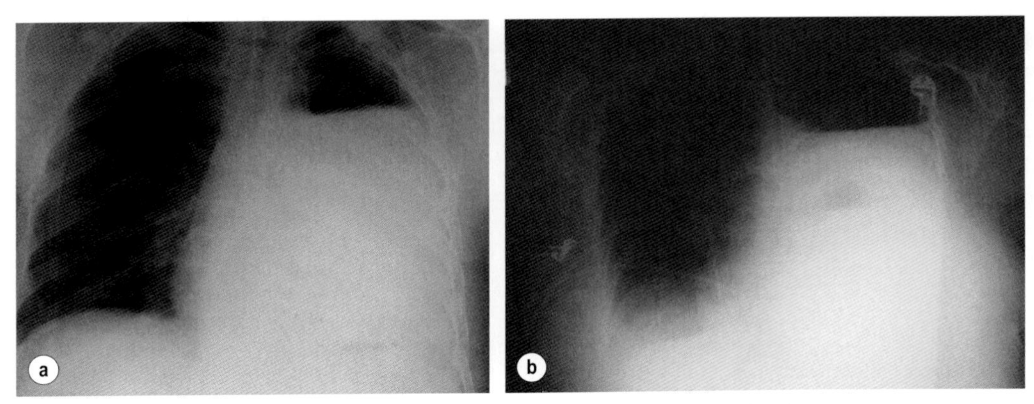

Figure 19.1 • (a,b) Typical chest radiograph findings of intrapleural oesophageal perforation.

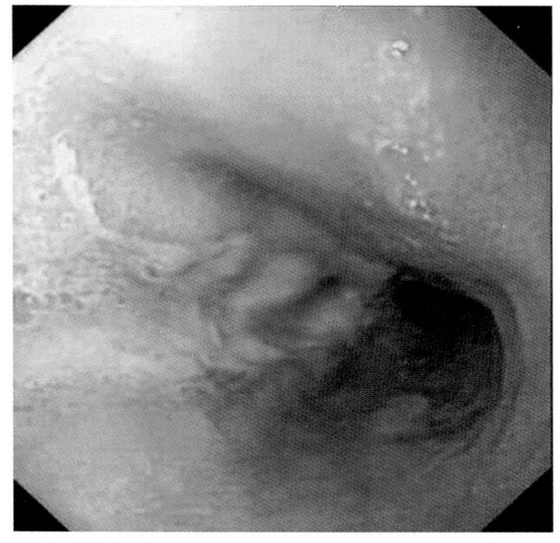

Figure 19.3 • Endoscopic appearances of full-thickness spontaneous oesophageal perforation.

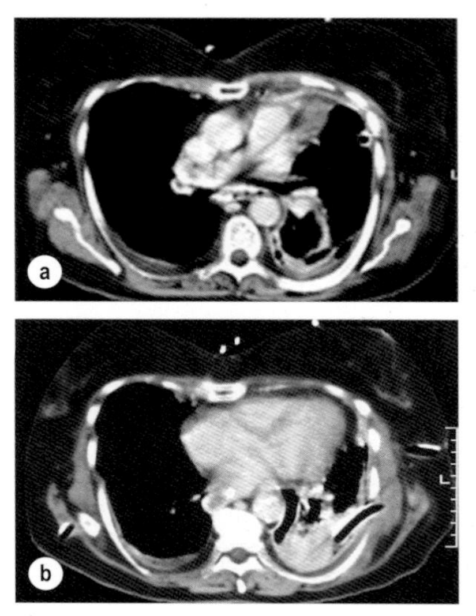

Figure 19.5 • CT appearances of spontaneous oesophageal perforation. **(a)** Left pleural hydropneumothorax. **(b)** Left basal intercostal chest drain in the same patient as in (a).

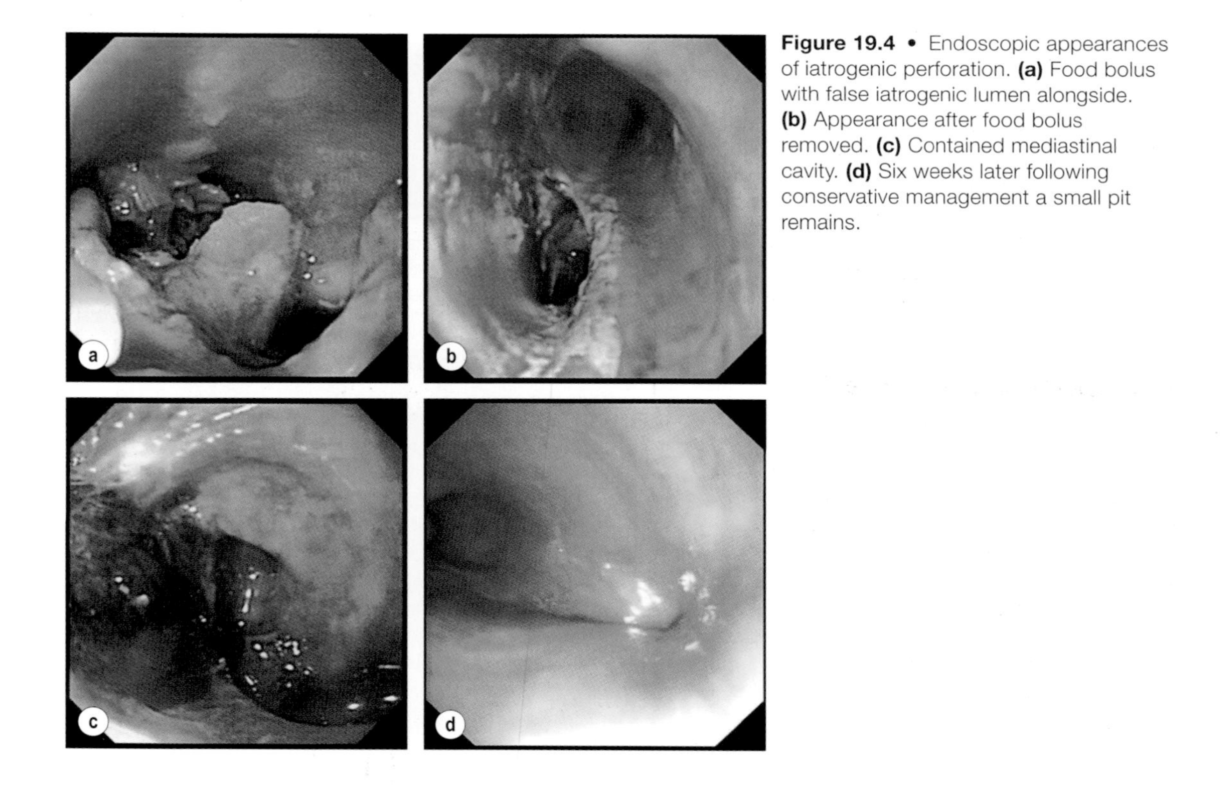

Figure 19.4 • Endoscopic appearances of iatrogenic perforation. **(a)** Food bolus with false iatrogenic lumen alongside. **(b)** Appearance after food bolus removed. **(c)** Contained mediastinal cavity. **(d)** Six weeks later following conservative management a small pit remains.

Other investigations

Thoracocentesis of frank gastric contents is diagnostic – a pH of less than 6.0, a high amylase or microscopic squamous cells in the fluid can also confirm oesophageal perforation in difficult cases. Swallowed or injected oral/nasogastric dyes, such as methylene blue, may be diagnostically useful if a communicating drain is in situ; however, dye staining can be troublesome in the operative field if surgery is subsequently required.

Management

The rarity and severe consequences of inappropriate treatment have limited the ability to evaluate management options. As a result, published observational case series often span many years, many centres, many surgeons and many techniques. Survival is dependent on controlling mediastinal and pleural contamination so surgery remains mandatory when gross contamination is present and is the mainstay for spontaneous perforation. However, non-operative treatment has become standard for iatrogenic trauma where contamination is more limited and delay in diagnosis is uncommon. Patients require a multidisciplinary approach with input from intensive care, radiology, physiotherapy and rehabilitation services. Hospitals lacking these specialist facilities or the versatile surgical cover necessary to deal with the oesophagus by abdominal or left or right thoracic operative approaches should transfer the patients at the earliest opportunity after stabilisation.

All patients with an oesophageal perforation are critically ill. The immediate priorities are the establishment of a secure and adequate airway, stabilisation of cardiovascular status and relief of pain, often using opiate-based analgesia. Regular reassessment is obligatory as an initially stable patient can rapidly decompensate. An early anaesthetic review is recommended. Box 19.3 documents the initial resuscitation.

Box 19.3 • Initial resuscitation in spontaneous oesophageal perforation

- Control of airway and administration of supplementary oxygen
- Early anaesthetic and critical care involvement and support
- Large-bore intravenous access and intravenous fluid resuscitation
- Central venous access and arterial line monitoring with or without inotropic support
- Urethral catheterisation and close monitoring of fluid balance
- Broad-spectrum antibiotic and antifungal agents
- Intravenous proton-pump inhibitors
- Strictly nil by mouth
- Large-bore intercostal chest drainage – possibly bilaterally
- Nasogastric tube (only to be placed under endoscopic vision or radiological guidance)
- Enteral access – nasojejunal tube/formal feeding jejunostomy
- Multidisciplinary approach with low threshold for aggressive/operative intervention

Non-operative management

Non-operative management, endoscopic and minimally invasive operative management have all been shown to be safe and feasible in carefully selected patients who have either been diagnosed with minimal contamination and no mediastinitis or with a contained perforation. It may also be considered in those with a delayed diagnosis who have demonstrated tolerance.[9]

Non-operative treatment comprises observation in intensive care or ward-based high-dependency units with patients kept nil by mouth and fed enterally, if necessary via a feeding jejunostomy. A nasogastric tube should be placed under endoscopic and/or radiological assistance past the perforation to decompress the stomach and to limit refluxate. Contrast radiology, endoscopy and CT are used to monitor the status of the perforation and collections should be drained. The timing of investigations is best guided by the clinical condition of the patient but weekly serial contrast or CT studies are not unreasonable. All patients should be given broad-spectrum intravenous antibiotics, antifungal and antisecretory agents. Non-operative treatment is not 'conservative'; patients require intensive observation and a low threshold for intervention, with 20% of patients requiring aggressive surgical salvage.

Iatrogenic cervical perforations are usually contained and thus managed non-operatively with percutaneous drainage of collections where necessary. Any resulting oesophagocutaneous fistulas heal rapidly in the absence of distal obstruction. Occasionally, operative prevertebral lavage, primary closure and drainage using a left lateral incision anterior to the sternocleidomastoid are required, and are well tolerated by even critically ill patients.

Criteria have been developed to aid the selection of suitable patients for non-operative management. These are detailed in Box 19.4. Case series applying these criteria demonstrate a mortality rate between zero and 16%, but numbers are small and results are skewed by both selection and publication bias.

Box 19.4 • Criteria for non-operative management of oesophageal perforation

- Perforation contained within the mediastinum
- Free drainage of contrast back into oesophagus
- No symptoms or signs of mediastinitis
- No evidence of solid food contamination of pleural or mediastinal cavities

Other factors to consider

- Perforation is controlled
- No underlying oesophageal disease
- No septic shock
- Availability for intensive observation and access to multidisciplinary care
- Low threshold for aggressive intervention
- Long delay in diagnosis such that the patient has already demonstrated tolerance
- Enteral feeding

Adjuncts to non-operative management

An endoluminal approach can be used to support patients undergoing non-operative management and can replicate some of the principles of open surgery with less associated trauma. This is pertinent in patients where the benefits of surgical exploration are outweighed by the risk and the ultimate outcome (advanced cancer) or in patients in whom the defect is small, clean and easily dealt with at the time of injury. All endoscopic approaches are technically difficult and should not be attempted by inexperienced operators unable to deal with the consequences of their actions.

Closure: clips and sealants

Endoclips are well established in closing small, clean defects after endoscopic mucosal resection or submucosal dissection for early cancer.[14,15] In the absence of significant contamination, small iatrogenic perforations may be closed immediately using endoclips in addition to supportive non-operative treatment. However, endoclipping 'en face' in the oesophagus is extremely challenging and should only be attempted by highly skilled endoscopists. It is also debatable whether this significantly alters the clinical course over a simple non-operative approach.[2] There is at least one case report of clipping a spontaneous oesophageal perforation but this cannot be recommended in the face of gross contamination.[16]

Diversion: stents

Self-expanding stents have been used to seal oesophageal perforations, chronic fistulas and even postoperative anastomotic leaks.[17–19] Stents were not designed for use in a normal oesophagus and migration rates approach 30%, and concerns have been raised in terms of extending the defect through pressure necrosis and through the trauma of their subsequent removal.[14,20] Publication bias means that failure and the consequences of failure remain unknown. There is considerable variation in the timing of stent placement and number of stents used. It is evident that the majority of cases also involve aggressive non-operative management.[21–24] It is therefore difficult to attribute successful outcomes to the stent placement alone. For example, one 'successful' report documents a patient who had five stents placed over an 8-month period before eventually proceeding to oesophagectomy at a tertiary referral centre.[21] The one prospective stenting study lists 10 patients with a Boerhaave perforation.[25] Stent migration was high (11 out of 33) and there was a 50% complication rate (bleeding/stent fracture/impacted stent) if stents were not removed before 6 weeks.

At present there is insufficient evidence to support the use of oesophageal stents in oesophageal perforations. The authors suggest that their use is highly selective and should always be viewed as a temporary solution. However, in patients whose physical condition precludes more aggressive treatments and those in whom resection is not deemed suitable, stents do offer a serious alternative. If utilised then the stent should be removed within 3 months to avoid long-term complications since the biggest concern is septic erosion into surrounding structures. This horrendous situation does not appear to be represented in the literature (**Fig. 19.6**).[25]

Drainage: repeated endoscopy

Endoscopic lavage and drainage of contained mediastinal perforations or even endoscopic placement of a vacuum sponge drainage system has been used for liquid contamination. This is certainly a novel approach but labour intensive and not suitable for gross contamination. Success may again simply reflect patients who would have done well with more simple non-operative treatment.[26,27]

✔ The authors suggest that the temporary use of covered, self-expanding metal or plastic stents as a primary treatment to seal a spontaneous perforation is limited but that they may have a place to control a postoperative leak and iatrogenic perforation.[28] Endoscopic clipping, transoesophageal debridement and mediastinal irrigation should all be viewed as experimental.

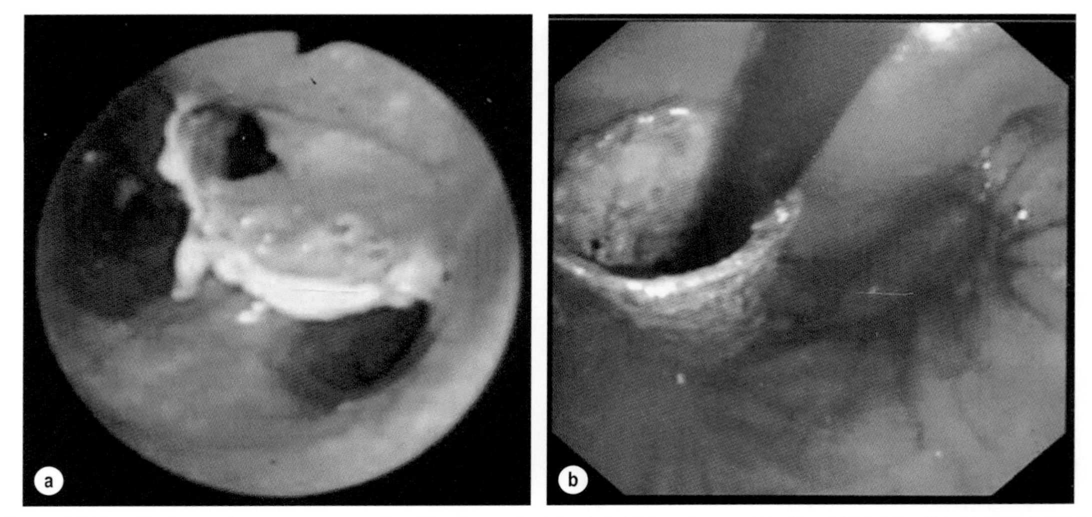

Figure 19.6 • Endoscopic appearance of septically eroded stent. **(a)** Bronchoscopic view of carina with proximal stent erosion. **(b)** J-view of distal stent clearly lying in proximal stomach allowing free reflux into airways.

Operative management

Open surgery

Surgery is advocated if the patient has overt signs of sepsis, shock, gross contamination, an obstructing pathology, a retained foreign body, a major caustic injury or has failed non-operative management. Virtually all gunshot wounds require surgery. The primary objective of surgical intervention is to restore oesophageal integrity and prevent further soiling. Thorough debridement, drainage, lavage and irrigation are more important for survival than the type of repair.[9] A feeding jejunostomy should also be fashioned as a routine to facilitate enteral feeding, usually following thoracotomy once the patient can be turned into a supine position. Management of the patients by a multidisciplinary team is again emphasised. Underlying pathology should be dealt with. Spontaneous perforation of the oesophagus carries a considerable mortality risk and a long in-hospital recovery period should the patient survive.

A posterolateral thoracotomy is used to approach the oesophagus, most commonly on the left in the seventh or eighth intercostal space. Solid debris is removed and the pleural cavity thoroughly cleaned. The mediastinal pleura is widely incised to expose the injury, and necrotic, devitalised tissue debrided. A longitudinal myotomy is made (as the mucosal injury is usually longer than the muscular one) and the oesophagus repaired.[29]

✔ Success with one surgical technique over another probably reflects the expertise and experience of the individual centre rather than a true outcome difference.

Primary repair with or without reinforcement

A simple, single- or two-layered, primary repair can be fashioned using 2/0 or 3/0 interrupted absorbable sutures with or without a small-diameter bougie (40–46 F) in situ (**Fig. 19.7**). However, primary repair is associated with a significant leak rate (20–50%) and should be reserved for those operated on rapidly with demonstrably healthy tissue and limited soiling.[30] There is circumstantial evidence that reinforcing the suture line with an onlay patch of nearby tissues (such as omentum, pleura, lung, pedicled intercostal muscle grafts, gastric fundus, pericardium or diaphragm) may reduce the leak rate.[31] Regardless, the authors would suggest that all primary repairs will leak and appropriate drains should be placed around the repair (**Fig. 19.8**).

T-tube repair

The concept of repair over a T-tube is to form a controlled oesophagocutaneous fistula.[32] A large-diameter (6–10 mm) T-tube is placed through the tear with the limbs lying beyond the boundaries of the perforation and the oesophageal wall is closed loosely around the tube with fine interrupted, absorbable sutures (**Fig. 19.9**). The authors suggest anchoring the tube to the diaphragm, as originally described, as aortic erosion due to sepsis and pressure necrosis is possible.[33] The tube is externalised and secured, a further drain is placed down to the repair, and apical and basal intercostal chest drains are sited. Healing is monitored by contrast radiology and CT scans. The T-tube is left until a defined tract is established, with the majority removed around 6 weeks.

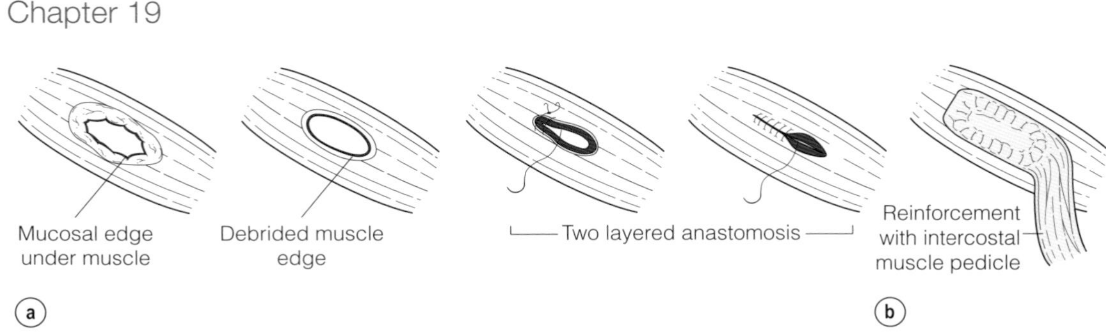

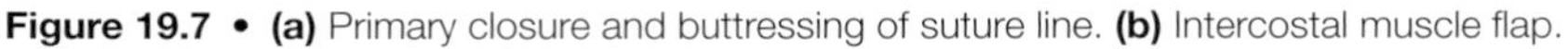

Figure 19.7 • (a) Primary closure and buttressing of suture line. **(b)** Intercostal muscle flap.

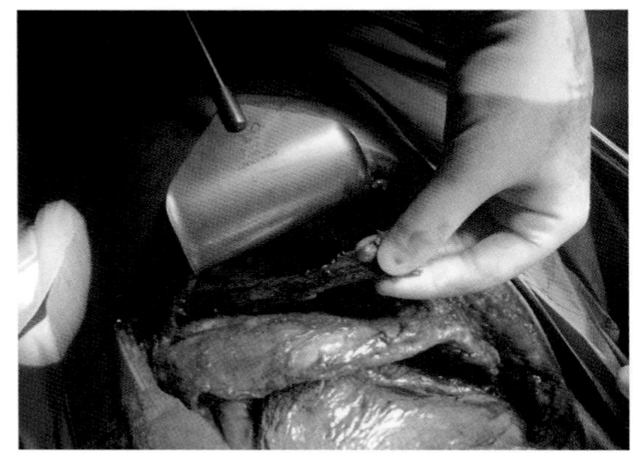

Figure 19.8 • Intraoperative photograph of raised intercostal muscle flap.

> ✔ In view of the high leak rate for primary repairs, the T-tube technique can be recommended for all patients.[6,33]

Resection

Oesophageal resection in the presence of a perforation is a major undertaking with an extremely high mortality. It is to be reserved for damage to a diseased oesophagus or in cases of extensive oesophageal trauma. This has even been performed in this setting as a minimally invasive approach.[38] If contamination is minimal then immediate reconstruction would be appropriate but a delayed approach may also be taken with limited differences in outcome.[39] The use of non-definitive exclusion and diversion techniques is mostly historical but remains in the armamentarium of an oesophageal surgeon and may occasionally be useful, such as in extensive caustic injuries.

Other approaches

Minimally invasive surgery: laparoscopic/thoracoscopic

Distal, clean and immediately recognised iatrogenic perforations may be suitable to approach laparoscopically (transperitoneally) to attempt repair and drainage by surgeons used to working at the hiatus. This requires advanced laparoscopic skills in specialist centres with appropriate facilities.[34] Equally, selected cases can be managed thoracoscopically.[35,36]

Surgical repair over a stent

In view of the high leak rate of primary repair, some authors advocate a surgical repair over a stent (sutured transluminal or externally to prevent migration). This theoretically expedites a return to enteral nutrition.[37] However, the problems of stent placement remain in terms of the risks of a foreign body in the site of sepsis.

Management of penetrating injuries

Cervical

Contained cervical perforations may be managed non-operatively irrespective of any delay, but repair should be undertaken when uncontained or in those requiring exploration for another reason, which is likely in any injury where the path traverses platysma or which passes through the mediastinum.

Thoracic

Virtually all transthoracic gunshot wounds will require surgical exploration, and life-threatening cardiovascular, pulmonary and tracheobronchial injuries take precedence. Specialist advice and input should be sought but the majority of the oesophageal injuries will be able to be dealt with using the techniques described previously. The overall mortality of penetrating thoracic oesophageal injuries is hard to ascertain but lies between 15% and 27% (lower for cervical trauma at 1–16%).[40] The morbidity arises mostly from associated spinal and airway trauma for cervical injuries and from cardiorespiratory damage in thoracic trauma.

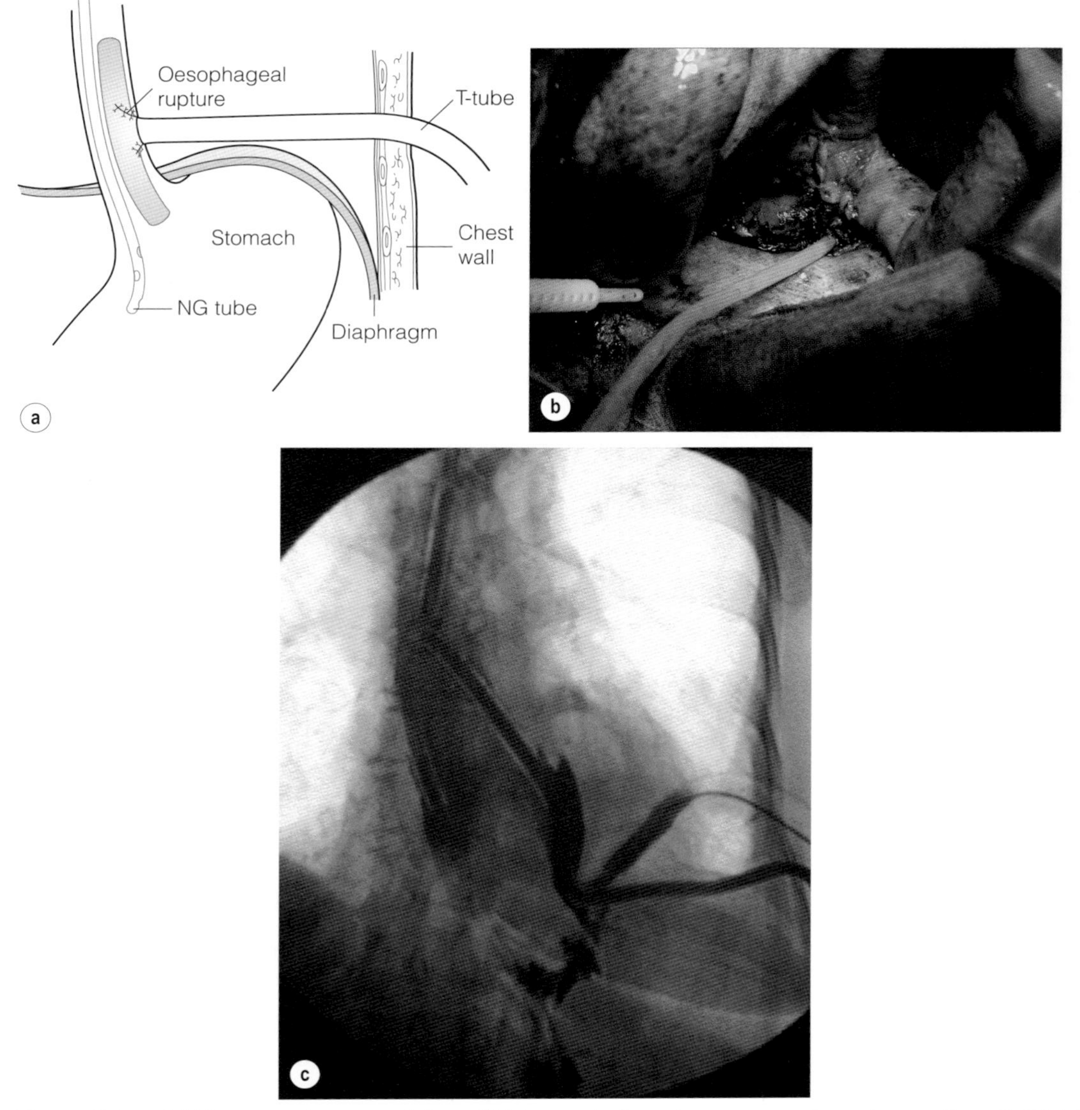

Figure 19.9 • (a) Diagrammatic representation of T-tube repair of spontaneous oesophageal perforation with T-tube in situ. **(b)** Operative photograph. **(c)** Contrast radiological image of the same patient as in (b); note additional intercostal chest drain with small contrast leak directly into this drain.

Management of underlying pathology

Patients who sustain a perforation of a malignant stricture constitute a difficult group to manage. Those who have known inoperable disease due to metastatic spread or who are unfit for surgery should be managed non-operatively, and in this situation the use of a sealing palliative stent is appropriate. In patients with less clearly defined operability most authors recommend resection with a view to control of contamination and potential cure, but this strategy carries a considerable mortality rate (11–75%).[39,41]

✔ In the presence of oesophageal cancer, the priority is to determine if the lesion was operable before the perforation, as an emergency subtotal oesophagectomy may be performed, although evidence suggests that perforation renders this a palliative resection and associated surgical mortality is high.[41,42] Every effort should be made to prevent perforation during staging endoscopic procedures.

Iatrogenic perforation of achalasia is uncommon (1–5%) and usually managed non-operatively or endoscopically as they are usually small, clean, immediately recognised and well contained. Other pathologies such as peptic stricture, infections or treatments can also predispose to perforation, e.g. radio/chemotherapy. Specific operative intervention may be required and, despite reduced contamination, the associated surgical mortality is increased. The indications for operative management are the corollary of those documented in Box 19.4.

Paraoesophageal surgery and procedural injuries

Direct oesophageal trauma is most commonly sustained during antireflux surgery, both open and laparoscopic, but the risk is low, of the order of 0–1.2%.[43] The risk increases with an intrathoracic approach, a previous hiatal operation and suturing of the wrap to the oesophagus. The majority of injuries are recognised and repaired immediately with buttressing using the fundoplication wrap. Drainage is advised and it may also be appropriate to form a feeding jejunostomy or to place a nasojejunal tube until the repair is deemed safe by contrast radiology. The mortality of unrecognised and uncontained perforations approaches 20%.

Trauma can also be sustained directly during thoracic and spinal surgery (<0.5% of procedures) or due to endotracheal intubation, nasogastric insertion and surgical tracheostomy. In ventilated patients, the clinical features of an injury may be concealed. Indirect trauma can occur through pressure necrosis or devascularisation, although the rich vascular supply of the thoracic oesophagus makes this extremely uncommmon.

Management algorithm

Diagnostic delay beyond 24 hours is classically associated with a poor outcome, but even when managed promptly and aggressively, perforation of the oesophagus, especially Boerhaave-type disruption, carries a significant mortality rate and reports to the contrary reflect selection bias. A management algorithm based on the therapeutic strategies outlined by the literature is demonstrated in **Fig. 19.10**. This is for guidance only and cases should be dealt with individually. Personal experience and expertise may well determine the best management.

Non-perforated spontaneous injuries of the oesophagus

Full-thickness oesophageal perforation contained by the mediastinal pleura is termed 'intramural rupture'.[44] This can occur spontaneously or secondary to instrumentation, food impaction or coagulopathies. Non-operative treatments with or without endoscopic adjuncts are usually successful as the perforation is contained, but a minority may require surgical intervention.[44]

'Black oesophagus syndrome' or acute oesophageal necrosis is extremely rare. This is circumferential mucosal and submucosal necrosis that ends sharply at the oesophagogastric junction in the absence of a caustic injury, most commonly presenting with upper gastrointestinal bleeding.[45] The most likely cause is vascular insufficiency from venous thrombosis as part of a 'two-hit' traumatic phenomenon associated with systemic hypotension from another cause. It has also been associated with thrombotic disorders. Diagnosis is endoscopic and treatment expectant with a low threshold for surgical resection as the condition can rapidly progress to perforation. Mortality is high, often secondary to the underlying cause.

Caustic injuries

Serious ingestion of a caustic substance is uncommon but devastating. Ingestion by children is more common and almost exclusively accidental whereas, in contrast, ingestion by adults is more often deliberate. Most caustic substances can be grouped into acids or alkalis. Dangerous acids are readily available as toilet cleaners (hydrochloric acid), battery fluid (sulphuric acid) and in metal working (phosphoric and hydrofluoric acids). In addition to local effects, ingestion of hydrofluoric acid leads to effects on metabolic calcium levels through systemic absorption, which can cause refractory cardiac dysrhythmias; specialist poisons advice is recommended and emergency personnel should take precautions, as even dermal exposure is hazardous. Strong alkalis are also readily available as cleaners and bleaches, although most household agents are only mild caustic agents.

There are two important misconceptions about caustic injuries:

Misconception 1: tissue penetration by acids is minimised by coagulative necrosis whereas alkalis

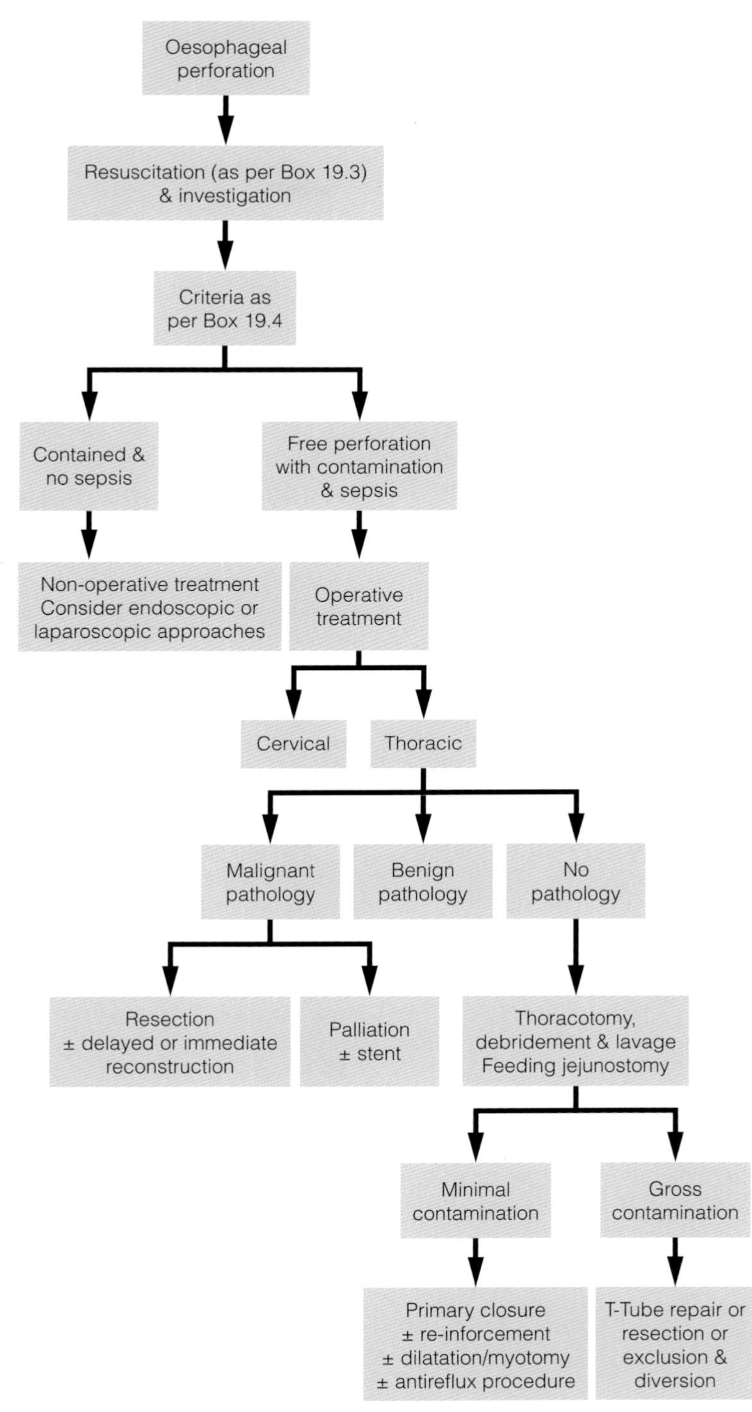

Figure 19.10 • Management algorithm for oesophageal perforation.

more rapidly penetrate transmurally through liquefactive necrosis. Although pathologically correct, this is clinically irrelevant as the ingestion of any strong caustic agent in sufficient quantity will inflict a potentially fatal oesophageal injury. Furthermore, there is evidence to suggest that strong acid ingestion is associated with greater systemic effects, a higher perforation rate and a higher mortality than alkali ingestion.[46]

Misconception 2: acid ingestion causes gastric damage whereas alkali ingestion causes oesophageal injury. Although commonly cited, there is no evidence to support this.[47,48]

The severity of any caustic injury is related to the corrosive properties, concentration, amount, viscosity and duration of contact between the particular caustic agent and the oesophageal mucosa. Intentional caustic ingestions are associated with larger ingested quantities of agent and so tend to lead to more severe injuries. In contrast, fortunately, the amount ingested accidentally by children is usually small.

Clinical presentation

Presentation can be varied and confusing. In accidental ingestion, symptoms and signs may not have developed due to rapid presentation since clinical features are dependent on the substance and the time since ingestion. Equally, the absence of oral burns or pharyngo-oesophageal symptoms does not exclude more distal injury as the caustic agent may have passed rapidly through the mouth and pharynx. Furthermore, in deliberate ingestion the clinical features may be 'underplayed' by the patients. The clinical features of a caustic injury of the oesophagus are documented in Box 19.5. Most patients survive to reach the hospital unless aspiration has occurred. Glossopharyngeal burns cause oedema that may threaten the airway and prevent clearance of secretions with drooling and hypersalivation, and injury to the epiglottis and larynx leads to stridor and a hoarse voice. Dyspnoea is uncommon unless aspiration has occurred. On inspection, oropharyngeal burns can range from mild oedema and superficial erosions to extensive mucosal sloughing and necrosis. Acid burns form a black eschar whereas alkali burns look grey and dull. Oesophageal injury is suggested by dysphagia and odynophagia, and gastric injury by epigastric pain, nausea, anorexia, retching, vomiting and haematemesis. Patients may present shocked or in respiratory distress.

Box 19.5 • Acute symptoms and signs of caustic injury of the oesophagus

- Refusal to eat or drink in children
- Facial oedema/burns
- Oropharyngeal pain
- Hypersalivation/drooling
- Stridor/hoarse voice
- Dyspnoea
- Chest pain
- Nausea and vomiting
- Epigastric pain/tenderness
- Haematemesis

Investigation and management

The immediate priorities are the establishment of a secure airway, the stabilisation of cardiovascular status and the relief of pain. Severe laryngopharyngeal burns or respiratory compromise may require early tracheal intubation and general anaesthesia. Concurrent facial or eye burns should be irrigated and ophthalmology and plastic surgery specialist involvement should be sought. Oral intake is prohibited. Gastric lavage, induced emesis, nasogastric aspiration and the use of neutralising chemicals are contraindicated. Where possible the ingested agent and amount swallowed should be identified and regional poison centres can provide information regarding the properties of specific agents. Endoscopic staging of the burn determines the optimum management, likelihood of subsequent stricture formation and is the only accurate predictor of systemic complications and death[46] (**Fig. 19.11**).

✔ All patients require admission and flexible video endoscopy of the upper gastrointestinal tract by a skilled practitioner as soon as the patient is stable, preferably within 24 hours of ingestion, to assess the stage of the oesophageal injury. A nasoenteral tube may be placed for early nutritional support – which can also act as a partial stent to prevent strictures.[47–49]

The severity of the injury is graded using a system similar to that for skin burns (Table 19.2) but differentiation between grades may be difficult, especially between second- and third-degree burns, with implications for management; consequently, some patients will benefit from repeated evaluation (Table 19.3).[50] There has been interest in the use of oesophageal endosonography to assess depth of necrosis and damage to the muscle layers, but this currently offers no advantage over conventional

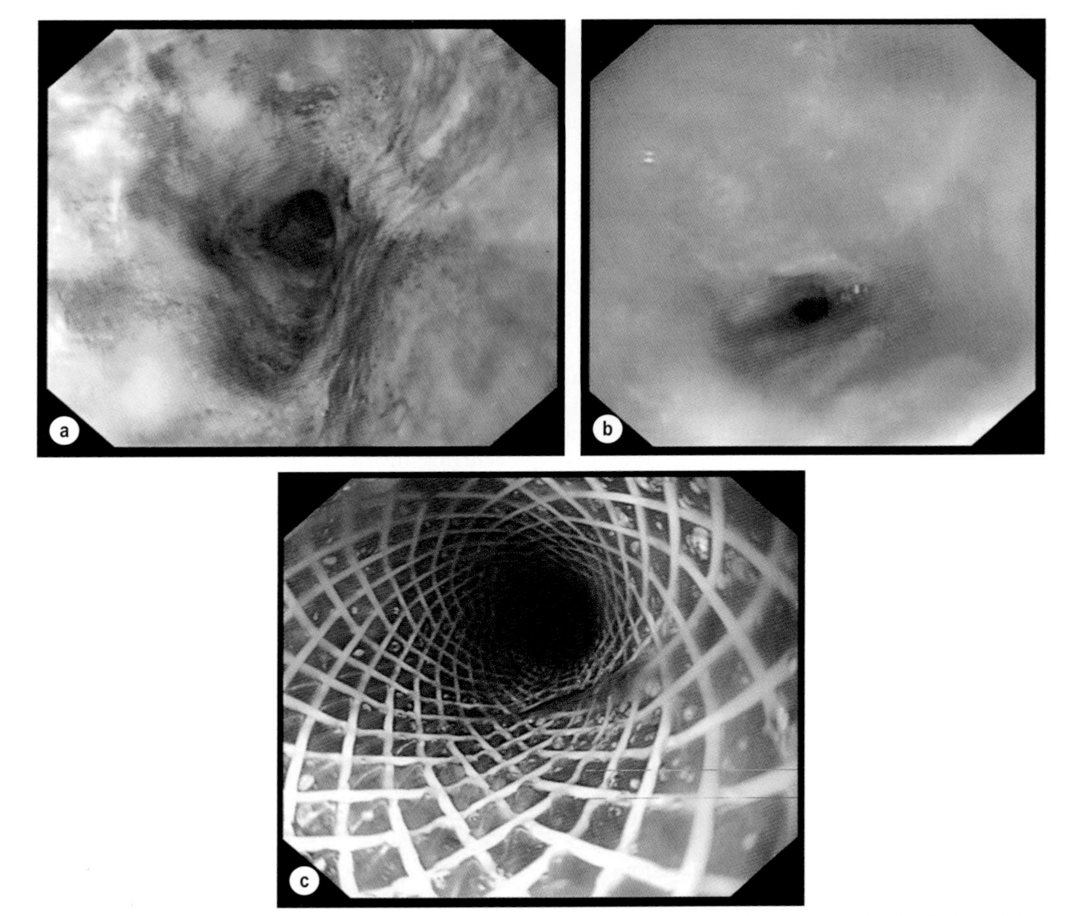

Figure 19.11 • Endoscopic appearances of caustic injury to the oesophagus. **(a)** Acute grade 3a alkali injury. **(b)** Appearance after 8 weeks with pinhole stricture. **(c)** A year later and refractory stricture treated by placement of stent.

Table 19.2 • Depth of oesophageal burn

Depth of burn	Degree of burn	Endoscopic findings
Superficial	1	Mucosal oedema and hyperaemia
Transmucosal with or without involvement of the muscularis	2a	Superficial ulcers, bleeding, exudates
	2b	Deep ulcers – focal or circumferential
Full thickness with or without adjacent organ involvement	3a	Full-thickness focal necrosis
	3b	Extensive necrosis

endoscopic assessment.[51] Equally, a modern CT grading system could be useful but is unlikely to replace an endoscopic assessment, which remains the gold standard.[52]

Most caustic injuries are managed non-operatively. The use of steroids and antibiotics during the acute phase remains controversial, with conflicting evidence regarding their benefits.

✔✔ Steroids form part of the treatment protocol of many units and research continues into their use for the prevention of strictures despite a prospective randomised, controlled trial that clearly demonstrated no benefit from steroids, with the development of oesophageal strictures related only to the severity of the corrosive injury.[53]

Patients with severe burns who are most at risk of stricture formation also represent the highest

Table 19.3 • Endoscopic staging of oesophageal caustic injury

Finding	First degree	Second degree	Third degree
Bleeding	Hyperaemia only	Mild/moderate bleeding	Moderate/severe bleeding
Oedema	Mild	Moderate	Severe
Mucosal loss	None	Mucosal ulceration or blistering	Deep ulcers
Exudate	None	Present with or without pseudomembrane	Present with or without pseudomembrane
Appearance if endoscopy delayed	None	Granulation tissue	Eschar

perforation risk and steroids may mask clinical symptoms. As such, the authors believe there is no place for steroids in the initial management of a caustic injury.

✓ Similarly, antibiotics should be reserved for those with proven infection, perforation or aspiration, and in these cases the authors suggest the additional use of antifungal agents.[54]

There are a few interesting animal-based research projects looking at other stricture-preventing medical treatments such as ibuprofen after oesophageal caustic injuries, but these have not yet been tried in a human population.[55]

Asymptomatic patients with unintentional ingestion but no oropharyngeal burns and normal or minor oesophageal findings may be discharged once they are able to take oral fluids. Intravenous fluids, analgesia, nutritional support and antisecretory agents should be given to all other patients. Patients with grade 1 and 2a burns should be admitted and observed for 5–7 days, with diet reintroduced gradually over 24–48 hours, and endoscopy or contrast radiology studies should be arranged for 6–8 weeks after discharge to assess for strictures. Suicidal/intentional injury patients require psychiatric assessment prior to discharge. It is reasonable to observe patients with grade 2b and 3 burns, continuing nasojejunal feeding and if there is no evidence of progression to perforation then clear fluids can be introduced from 48 hours, but be aware that the perforation risk is present for at least 7 days. Those who present with a perforation or deteriorate will require an emergency oesophagogastrectomy as the stomach is almost always injured. The authors do not believe that laparoscopy has a role in assessing gastric viability. Immediate reconstruction with a substernal colonic interposition graft can be performed if there is minimal local contamination but more commonly oesophagostomy and delayed reconstruction 6–8 weeks later is preferred. It is reasonable to consider resection in patients with extensive circumferential mucosal injuries in view of the problem of refractory strictures and the long-term cancer risk. The mortality for these caustic injuries is 13–40%, with the majority of deaths occurring in the adult suicidal group.[48] Mortality mainly stems from respiratory complications and delay in the aggressive surgical treatment of transmural necrosis. There is no place for 'conservative' treatment of a severe caustic oesophageal injury.

Long-term complications and outcomes

Strictures develop in 5–50% of patients, 95% of which are distal and can be graded according to the Marchand classification (Table 19.4).[56]

✓✓ Most strictures can be managed by serial Savary–Gilliard bougie dilatation.[57]

The procedure-related perforation incidence is less than 1%, but for safety the authors advise allowing approximately 6 weeks after injury before attempting dilatation. Antisecretory medication or even surgery may be required if reflux occurs after dilatation. Young patients with long, grade 3 or 4 strictures are likely to require a lifetime of repeated dilatations with a cumulative risk of iatrogenic perforation and ultimately of cancer, and in these patients other options should be considered. Surgical options are to bypass or resect the obstructive segment or to perform a stricturoplasty. Bypass avoids dissection through mediastinal fibrosis, and a retrosternal or subcutaneous route for the neo-oesophagus may avoid a thoracotomy. However, retaining the damaged oesophagus retains the long-term cancer risk and can lead to problems related to secretions and bacterial overgrowth. Thoracotomy, resection and colonic reconstruction (due to concurrent gastric damage) is therefore preferable. An alternative is an oesophageal stricturoplasty using a vascularised graft of colon, but again this retains the cancer risk. There is increasing interest in the use of removable or absorbable

Table 19.4 • The Marchand classification of oesophageal strictures

Circumferential	Length	Consistency	Grade
Incomplete	Short	Fibrotic	1
String-like circumferential	Short	Elastic	2
Complete	≤1 cm	Fibrotic	3
Complete	>1 cm	Superficial fibrosis, easily dilated, non-progressive	4a
Complete	>1 cm	Deep fibrosis, tubular, progressive, not easily dilated	4b

stents for refractory strictures but evidence is limited by numbers. However, these remain an alluring prospect and there is currently a National Institute for Health Research study investigating their use in benign oesophageal strictures.[58] There is also some evidence for the use of endoscopic triamcinolone acetonide injection into the strictured segment to augment dilatation.[59]

Cancer risk

Squamous malignant transformation of a caustically damaged oesophagus occurs in around 16%, a risk 1000 times that of the general population but with a long latent period for malignant change of between 15 and 40 years. Surveillance may be impractical with such a long latent period and the risk is not proportional to the severity of the injury. Early elective resection before transformation eliminates the risk, with low associated mortality in younger patients. In older patients, simply an awareness of the risk by clinicians and patients should lead to earlier diagnosis and an increase in the number of curative resections where deemed appropriate.

Management algorithm

An algorithm for the management of caustic injuries of the oesophagus is detailed in **Fig. 19.12**.

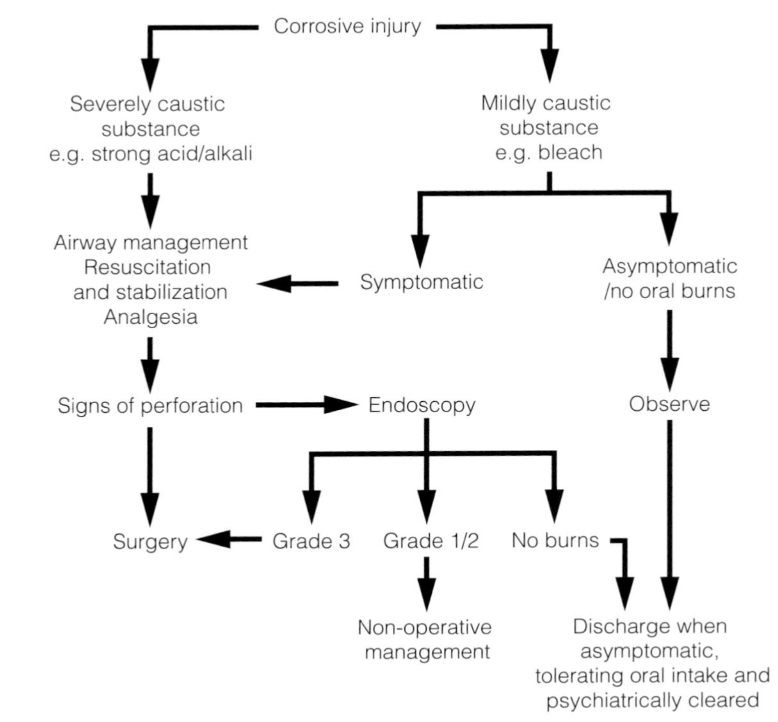

Figure 19.12 • Management algorithm for caustic oesophageal injuries.

Ingestion of foreign bodies

The oesophagus is the most common site for impaction of ingested foreign bodies within the gastrointestinal tract, accounting for 75% of cases.[60] By far the majority occur in children under the age of 10 years, with coins, toys, crayons and batteries being the commonest objects swallowed.[61] In adults, food boluses (predominantly meat) or impaction of food-related bone fragments are more common. This is especially the case in edentulous patients due to decreased palatal sensation. Cases also occur in people with mental or psychiatric difficulties, or related to drug and alcohol abuse, and in those seeking secondary gain such as prisoners, and most upper gastrointestinal units are aware of a number of recurrent offenders.

Most foreign bodies impact in the cervical oesophagus, but impaction can occur at any of the physiological narrowings: cricopharyngeus, the aortic arch, the left main bronchus and the gastro-oesophageal junction. Benign pathology accounts for some cases (e.g. Schatzki rings, peptic strictures and eosinophilic oesophagitis); in contrast, malignant strictures are uncommonly associated with impaction due to the long development phase, but there are significant food bolus impaction rates associated with palliative treatments of malignant oesophageal lesions such as self-expanding metal stents.

Clinical presentation

In over 90% there is a clear history of ingestion associated with acute dysphagia at the level of the impaction and thus a rapid diagnosis.[62] However, in young children and uncooperative adults the diagnosis may not be so clear-cut. Suspicious symptoms in children are refusal of feeds, gagging and choking, but some cases may remain concealed for months or even years and chronic aspiration or reflux may represent long-standing impaction. A high index of suspicion is also required for psychiatric patients with features suggestive of foreign body ingestion. Respiratory symptoms occur in 5–15%, especially in children and in cervical impaction, leading to coughing, wheezing, stridor and dyspnoea. In adults, acute impaction in the cervical oesophagus can cause tracheal obstruction leading to the so-called 'café coronary' or 'steakhouse syndrome'. Typically, sharp object ingestion (e.g. fish bones) can cause a persistent foreign body sensation despite easy passage through the oesophagus without impaction. Physical signs are usually limited unless impaction causes obstruction leading to drooling or perforation leading to neck swelling, erythema, tenderness, subcutaneous emphysema or systemic effects. Long-standing impaction may lead to recurrent aspiration, empyema of the lung, perioesophagitis, oesophageal stenosis or fistulation into the airways or major vessels.

Diagnosis

Plain radiographs may localise both radio-opaque and non-radio-opaque objects and are useful if perforation is suspected (**Fig. 19.13**). Both anteroposterior and lateral projections should be obtained as objects may not be visible if overlying the vertebrae,

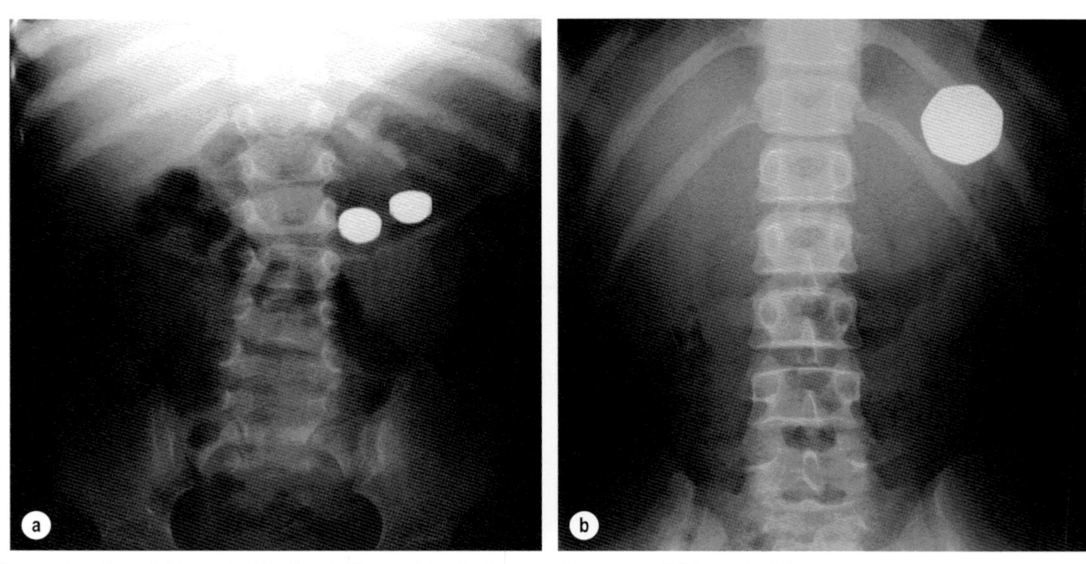

Figure 19.13 • (a) Ingested button batteries lying in the gastric antrum. **(b)** Ingested 50-pence coin.

and this also helps to distinguish whether objects are in the digestive or tracheobronchial tract. In young children and infants, extensive plain radiography may be required to confirm or refute the diagnosis of a swallowed radio-opaque foreign body. Even in the absence of symptoms or physical signs a potential history of ingestion should prompt the use of radiography, as in one study 17% of asymptomatic children with a history of coin ingestion had an impacted oesophageal coin.[63] Water-soluble contrast studies or CT scans may occasionally be required in cases of non-radio-opaque objects such as wood, aluminium, glass and plastics, but the use of hypertonic contrast media and barium should be avoided.

✔ However, flexible video endoscopy is the investigation of choice. It has been used safely for over 30 years, is associated with a diagnostic sensitivity of 86% and specificity of 63%, and allows for immediate therapeutic intervention in 95%.[64]

Management

✔ In a Western population, the majority of ingested foreign bodies will pass through the gastrointestinal tract uneventfully, with 10–20% requiring endoscopic removal due to impaction and 1% requiring surgical removal.[64,65]

The indications for urgent intervention are:

1. Airway compromise.
2. Absolute dysphagia with aspiration risk.
3. Oesophageal impaction of sharp object or button battery.
4. Oesophageal impaction of greater than 24 hours duration.

The passage of a foreign body through the oesophagus does not always indicate success as objects over 5–6 cm long or >2 cm in diameter are unlikely to pass through the pylorus or around the duodenal curves and, once impacted, endoscopic removal may be difficult. As such, expeditious retrieval while in the oesophagus is advised. Similarly, although the majority of ingested sharp objects entering the stomach will traverse the gastrointestinal tract without incident, the perforation risk (up to 35%) suggests that retrieval, if safe, should be attempted.

In all other situations, individual management strategies depend on the symptoms, objects and expertise of the receiving speciality, which includes paediatricians, surgeons and psychiatrists.

A number of techniques to dislodge food boluses without recourse to endoscopy have been reported.

✔✔ Observation of up to 24 hours is reasonable in asymptomatic patients with oesophageal coins or similar round, smooth objects as many of these will pass spontaneously.[66]

Proteolytic agents (e.g. papain) that dissolve the food bolus may cause oesophageal trauma and are dangerous if aspirated and they are not recommended. Effervescent agents, such as carbonated drinks and intravenous glucagon, which causes smooth muscle relaxation, were thought to help disimpact the food bolus but there is no good evidence to support their use.[67] Failure to progress through the gastrointestinal tract or symptomatic deterioration should prompt surgical review. Therapeutic video endoscopy is as successful in object removal as rigid endoscopy but with a significantly lower complication rate (5% vs. 10%) and avoids general anaesthesia in the majority of cases. However, in a minority, the type of object, number of objects or the inability of the patient to cooperate (i.e. young children) may dictate that general anaesthesia is required and rigid endoscopy is still useful for impaction in the pharynx as the view and access are superior, but the authors feel that it should be abandoned for distal obstructions. Patience is important in endoscopic removal but is rewarded with a high success rate (around 95%).[64] Failure is most likely to occur with long (>10 cm) or complex objects such as dental prostheses.

Smooth objects may be disproportionately difficult to retrieve; a variety of graspers, snares, magnets and baskets may be required and it is useful to practise with the proposed grasper on a duplicate foreign body prior to the actual procedure. Coins should be orientated sideways to aid passage through the cricopharyngeus and sharp or pointed objects may require an overtube or endoscopic hood for safe removal or manipulation to allow 'blunt end first' removal.

Food impactions tend to occur in the distal oesophagus and are usually accompanied by underlying pathology. Eosinophilic oesophagitis is of recent interest in this regard as a predisposing factor to acute dysphagia and food impaction. This is especially relevant as the oesophageal mucosa is thin, friable and easily traumatised by instrumentation – as such, dilatation should be avoided. Otherwise, flexible video endoscopy allows relief of the impaction and diagnosis of any underlying pathology with concurrent mucosal biopsying is necessary in all cases. Removal of the food bolus may again be achieved using a variety of techniques and tools. Larger boluses may require piecemeal removal, using an overtube if repeated intubation is required. Once the endoscope has been passed distal to the bolus then the bolus may be gently pushed into the stomach, but this technique should never be performed 'blindly'. Definitive treatment such as dilatation of a peptic stricture may be performed after successful retrieval.

'Disc' or 'button' batteries are easily ingested by curious children. Electrical discharge or release of the alkaline contents, once impacted, can lead to local damage, necrosis and perforation. As such, urgent extraction is required if lodged within the oesophagus, and plain radiographs are helpful for localisation. However, if the battery has passed on to the stomach and duodenum then 80–90% will pass without complication. As such, observation with serial radiography is used to monitor progression, reserving endoscopic or surgical intervention if the battery fails to progress out of the stomach within 48 hours, if the patient develops symptoms of intestinal injury or if the battery fragments and there is evidence of mercury toxicity.

Surgery may be necessary when endoscopy fails for large objects, for objects embedded in the oesophageal wall or when there has been an associated or iatrogenic perforation. The surgical approach depends not only on the site and severity of the injury, but also associated inflammation and any underlying oesophageal pathology. Deliberate narcotic packet ingestion is a particularly taxing scenario. The authors suggest that endoscopic removal should not be attempted as successful retrieval is outweighed by the risk of rupture.[68] Most packets will pass safely through the bowel but urgent surgery is indicated in cases where there is failure to progress, obstruction or rupture, in conjunction with medical support for absorption of relevant contents.

Summary

Oesophageal emergencies represent a widely heterogeneous group of conditions from a wide variety of insults leading to a wide spectrum of injuries. The potential for disaster is omnipresent given the fragility of the oesophageal wall, the lack of serosa, the proximity of vital organs, the inaccessibility, and the lack of symptoms and signs; these factors in combination mean that even minor injuries can be ultimately fatal. Because of the rarity of these difficult cases, most surgeons will deal with only a handful in their career; consequently, such cases are best managed by specialist units with ancillary staff who are trained, equipped and experienced to prevent potentially disastrous consequences of misdiagnosis and inappropriate management. However, the best way to improve outcomes is through prevention where possible, for example through safe and thorough training in therapeutic endoscopy, better labelling of caustic substances and development of smaller button batteries.

Key points

Oesophageal perforation

- Diagnostic error and diagnostic delay are high in spontaneous perforations.
- 75–90% of iatrogenic perforations occur distally and underlying pathology is common.
- Perforation of an oesophageal cancer renders these lesions incurable.
- Flexible video endoscopic and CT scanning are the diagnostic investigations of choice.
- Non-operative management is suitable for clean or contained perforations.
- Surgery remains the mainstay of treatment for gross contamination.

Oesophageal trauma

- Penetrating trauma is easily missed with serious injuries to surrounding viscera.
- Flexible video endoscopy and CT scanning are the investigations of choice.

Caustic injuries

- Investigation is mandatory in suspected caustic ingestion.
- Flexible video endoscopy is essential to assess the oesophagus within 24 hours of injury.
- There is no proven initial role for procrastination, steroids or antibiotics.
- Most strictures can be managed by serial Savary–Gilliard bougie dilatation.
- Reconstructive surgery should be considered in young patients with refractory strictures, also bearing in mind the long-term cancer risk.

Ingestion of foreign bodies

- Flexible video endoscopy is both the investigation and treatment option of choice.
- The majority of ingested foreign bodies will pass uneventfully.
- Observation of up to 24 hours is reasonable in asymptomatic patients with round, smooth objects.

References

1. Borotto E, Gaudric M, Danel B, et al. Risk factors of oesophageal perforation during pneumatic dilatation for achalasia. Gut 1996;39(1):9–12.
2. Fernandez FF, Richter A, Freudenberg S, et al. Treatment of endoscopic esophageal perforation. Surg Endosc 1999;13(10):962–6.
3. Hayes N, Waterworth PD, Griffin SM. Avulsion of short gastric arteries caused by vomiting. Gut 1994;35(8):1137–8.
4. Lucendo AJ, Friginal-Ruiz AB, Rodríguez B. Boerhaave's syndrome as the primary manifestation of adult eosinophilic esophagitis. Two case reports and a review of the literature. Dis Esophagus 2011;24(2):E11–5.
5. Mackler S. Spontaneous rupture of the oesophagus; an experimental and clinical study. Surg Gynecol Obst 1952;95:345–56.
6. Griffin SM, Lamb PJ, Shenfine J, et al. Spontaneous rupture of the oesophagus. Br J Surg 2008;95(9):1115–20.
7. Shenfine J, Dresner SM, Vishwanath Y, et al. Management of spontaneous rupture of the oesophagus. Br J Surg 2000;87(3):362–73.
8. Levine PH, Kelley Jr ML. Spontaneous perforation of esophagus simulating acute pancreatitis. JAMA 1965;191(4):342–5.
9. Altorjay A, Kiss J, Voros A, et al. The role of esophagectomy in the management of esophageal perforations. Ann Thorac Surg 1998;65(5):1433–6.
10. Horwitz B, Krevsky B, Buckman Jr RF, et al. Endoscopic evaluation of penetrating esophageal injuries. Am J Gastroenterol 1993;88(8):1249–53.
11. Srinivasan R, Haywood T, Horwitz B, et al. Role of flexible endoscopy in the evaluation of possible esophageal trauma after penetrating injuries. Am J Gastroenterol 2000;95(7):1725–9.
12. Griffin SM, Lamb PJ, Dresner SM, et al. Diagnosis and management of a mediastinal leak following radical oesophagectomy. Br J Surg 2001;88(10): 1346–51.
13. White CS, Templeton PA, Attar S. Esophageal perforation: CT findings. Am J Roentgenol 1993;160(4):767–70.
14. Qadeer MA, Dumot JA, Vargo JJ, et al. Endoscopic clips for closing esophageal perforations: case report and pooled analysis. Gastrointest Endosc 2007;66(3):605–11.
15. Fritscher-Ravens A, Hampe J, Grange P, et al. Clip closure versus endoscopic suturing versus thoracoscopic repair of an iatrogenic esophageal perforation: a randomized, comparative, long-term survival study in a porcine model (with videos). Gastrointest Endosc 2010;72(5):1020–6.
16. Rokszin R, Simonka Z, Paszt A, et al. Successful endoscopic clipping in the early treatment of spontaneous esophageal perforation. Surg Laparosc Endosc Percutan Tech 2011;21(6):e311–2.
17. Kiev J, Amendola M, Bouhaidar D, et al. A management algorithm for esophageal perforation. Am J Surg 2007;194(1):103–6.
18. Adam A, Watkinson AF, Dussek J. Boerhaave syndrome: to treat or not to treat by means of insertion of a metallic stent. J Vasc Interv Radiol 1995;6(5):741–6.
19. Doniec JM, Schniewind B, Kahlke V, et al. Therapy of anastomotic leaks by means of covered self-expanding metallic stents after esophagogastrectomy. Endoscopy 2003;35(8):652–8.
20. Radecke K, Gerken G, Treichel U. Impact of a self-expanding, plastic esophageal stent on various esophageal stenoses, fistulas, and leakages: a single-center experience in 39 patients. Gastrointest Endosc 2005;61(7):812–8.
21. Odell JA, DeVault KR. Extended stent usage for persistent esophageal leak. Ann Thorac Surg 2010;90: 1707–8.
22. Eubanks PJ, Hu E, Nguyen D, et al. Case of Boerhaave's syndrome treated with a self-expanding metallic stent. Gastrointest Endosc 1999;49:780–3.
23. Davies AP, Vaughan R. Expanding mesh stent in the emergency treatment of Boerhaave's syndrome. Ann Thorac Surg 1999;67:1482–3.
24. Yuasa N, Hattori T, Kobayhashi Y, et al. Treatment of spontaneous esophageal rupture with a covered self-expanding metal stent. Gastrointest Endosc 1999;49:777–80.
25. Van Heel NC, Haringsma J, Spaander MC, et al. Short-term esophageal stenting in the management of benign perforations. Am J Gastroenterol 2010;105:1515–20.
26. Loske G, Schorsch T, Müller C. Intraluminal and intracavitary vacuum therapy for esophageal leakage: a new endoscopic minimally invasive approach. Endoscopy 2011;43(6):540–4.
27. Ahrens M, Schulte T, Egberts J, et al. Drainage of esophageal leakage using endoscopic vacuum therapy: a prospective pilot study. Endoscopy 2010;42(9):693–8.
28. Petruzziello L, Tringali A, Riccioni ME, et al. Successful early treatment of Boerhaave's syndrome by endoscopic placement of a temporary self-expandable plastic stent without fluoroscopy. Gastrointest Endosc 2003;58(4):608–12.
29. Walker WS, Cameron EW, Walbaum PR. Diagnosis and management of spontaneous transmural rupture of the oesophagus (Boerhaave's syndrome). Br J Surg 1985;72(3):204–7.
30. Lawrence DR, Ohri SK, Moxon RE, et al. Primary esophageal repair for Boerhaave's syndrome. Ann Thorac Surg 1999;67(3):818–20.

31. Wright CD, Mathisen DJ, Wain JC, et al. Reinforced primary repair of thoracic esophageal perforation. Ann Thorac Surg 1995;60(2):245–9.
32. Mansour KA, Wenger RK. T-tube management of late esophageal perforations. Surg Gynecol Obstet 1992;175(6):571–2.
33. Naylor AR, Walker WS, Dark J, et al. T tube intubation in the management of seriously ill patients with oesophagopleural fistulae. Br J Surg 1990;77(1):40–2.
34. Bell RC. Laparoscopic closure of esophageal perforation following pneumatic dilatation for achalasia. Report of two cases. Surg Endosc 1997;11(5):476–8.
35. Cho JS, Kim YD, Kim JW, et al. Thoracoscopic primary esophageal repair in patients with Boerhaave's syndrome. Ann Thorac Surg 2011;91(5):1552–5.
36. Haveman JW, Nieuwenhuijs VB, Kobold JP, et al. Adequate debridement and drainage of the mediastinum using open thoracotomy or video-assisted thoracoscopic surgery for Boerhaave's syndrome. Surg Endosc 2011;25(8):2492–7.
37. Babor R, Talbot M, Tyndal A. Treatment of upper gastrointestinal leaks with a removable, covered, self-expanding metallic stent. Surg Laparosc Endosc Percutan Tech 2009;19(1):e1–4.
38. Grewal N, El-Badawi K, Nguyen NT. Minimally invasive Ivor Lewis esophagectomy for the management of iatrogenic esophageal perforation in a patient with esophageal cancer. Surg Technol Int 2009;18:82–5.
39. Orringer MB, Stirling MC. Esophagectomy for esophageal disruption. Ann Thorac Surg 1990;49(1):35–43.
40. Pass LJ, LeNarz LA, Schreiber JT, et al. Management of esophageal gunshot wounds. Ann Thorac Surg 1987;44(3):253–6.
41. Adam DJ, Thompson AM, Walker WS, et al. Oesophagogastrectomy for iatrogenic perforation of oesophageal and cardia carcinoma. Br J Surg 1996;83(10):1429–32.
42. Dresner SM, Lamb PJ, Viswanath YKS, et al. Oesophagectomy following iatrogenic perforation of operable oesophageal carcinoma. Br J Surg 2000;87(S1):29.
43. Pessaux P, Arnaud JP, Ghavami B, et al. Morbidity of laparoscopic fundoplication for gastroesophageal reflux: a retrospective study about 1470 patients. Hepatogastroenterology 2002;49(44):447–50.
44. Steadman C, Kerlin P, Crimmins F, et al. Spontaneous intramural rupture of the oesophagus. Gut 1990;31(8):845–9.
45. Moreto M, Ojembarrena E, Zaballa M, et al. Idiopathic acute esophageal necrosis: not necessarily a terminal event. Endoscopy 1993;25(8):534–8.
46. Poley JW, Steyerberg EW, Kuipers EJ, et al. Ingestion of acid and alkaline agents: outcome and prognostic value of early upper endoscopy. Gastrointest Endosc 2004;60(3):372–7.
47. Zargar SA, Kochhar R, Nagi B, et al. Ingestion of corrosive acids. Spectrum of injury to upper gastrointestinal tract and natural history. Gastroenterology 1989;97(3):702–7.
48. Zargar SA, Kochhar R, Nagi B, et al. Ingestion of strong corrosive alkalis: spectrum of injury to upper gastrointestinal tract and natural history. Am J Gastroenterol 1992;87(3):337–41.
49. Wijburg FA, Heymans HS, Urbanus NA. Caustic esophageal lesions in childhood: prevention of stricture formation. J Pediatr Surg 1989;24(2):171–3.
50. Zargar SA, Kochhar R, Mehta S, et al. The role of fiberoptic endoscopy in the management of corrosive ingestion and modified endoscopic classification of burns. Gastrointest Endosc 1991;37(2):165–9.
51. Kamijo Y, Kondo I, Kokuto M, et al. Miniprobe ultrasonography for determining prognosis in corrosive esophagitis. Am J Gastroenterol 2004;99(5):851–4.
52. Ryu HH, Jeung KW, Lee BK, et al. Caustic injury: can CT grading system enable prediction of esophageal stricture? Clin Toxicol (Phila) 2010;48(2):137–42.
53. Anderson KD, Rouse TM, Randolph JG. A controlled trial of corticosteroids in children with corrosive injury of the esophagus. N Engl J Med 1990;323(10):637–40.
    A prospective randomised, controlled trial in 60 children with caustic injuries with a follow-up of 18 years comparing a steroid and antibiotic regimen with best supportive care. No benefit was demonstrated in the steroid and antibiotic group; the development of oesophageal strictures related only to the severity of the corrosive injury.
54. Bauer TM, Dupont V, Zimmerli W. Invasive candidiasis complicating spontaneous esophageal perforation (Boerhaave syndrome). Am J Gastroenterol 1996;91(6):1248–50.
55. Herek O, Karabul M, Yenisey C, et al. Protective effects of ibuprofen against caustic esophageal burn injury in rats. Pediatr Surg Int 2010;26(7):721–7.
56. Marchand P. Caustic strictures of the oesophagus. Thorax 1955;10(2):171–81.
57. Cox JG, Winter RK, Maslin SC, et al. Balloon or bougie for dilatation of benign esophageal stricture? Dig Dis Sci 1994;39(4):776–81.
    A randomised study in 93 adult patients demonstrating a better and longer-lasting symptomatic result for lower cost with Savary–Gilliard bougie dilatation than balloon dilatation.
58. Thomas T, Abrams KR, Subramanian V, et al. Esophageal stents for benign refractory strictures: a meta-analysis. Endoscopy 2011;43(5):386–93.
59. Kochhar R, Ray JD, Sriram PV, et al. Intralesional steroids augment the effects of endoscopic dilation in corrosive esophageal strictures. Gastrointest Endosc 1999;49(4, Pt 1):509–13.
60. Webb WA. Management of foreign bodies of the upper gastrointestinal tract. Gastroenterology 1988;94(1):204–16.

61. Nadir A, Sahin E, Nadir I, et al. Esophageal foreign bodies: 177 cases. Dis Esophagus 2011;24(1):6–9.

62. Ciriza C, Garcia L, Suarez P, et al. What predictive parameters best indicate the need for emergent gastrointestinal endoscopy after foreign body ingestion? J Clin Gastroenterol 2000;31(1):23–8.

63. Hodge 3rd D, Tecklenburg F, Fleisher G. Coin ingestion: does every child need a radiograph? Ann Emerg Med 1985;14(5):443–6.

64. Li ZS, Sun ZX, Zou DW, et al. Endoscopic management of foreign bodies in the upper-GI tract: experience with 1088 cases in China. Gastrointest Endosc 2006;64(4):485–92.

65. Eisen GM, Baron TH, Dominitz JA, et al. Guideline for the management of ingested foreign bodies. Gastrointest Endosc 2002;55(7):802–6.

66. Waltzman ML, Baskin M, Wypij D, et al. A randomized clinical trial of the management of esophageal coins in children. Pediatrics 2005;116(3):614–9.

A prospective randomised controlled trial of 60 children with an asymptomatic oesophageal coin, comparing immediate endoscopic removal with observation, including radiography and endoscopic removal where deemed necessary. This demonstrated no benefit from immediate endoscopic removal and 25–30% of coins passed spontaneously without complications. They conclude that treatment could reasonably include a short period of observation, particularly in older children with distally sited coins.

67. Tibbling L, Bjorkhoel A, Jansson E, et al. Effect of spasmolytic drugs on esophageal foreign bodies. Dysphagia 1995;10(2):126–7.

A multicentre placebo-controlled trial, showing no benefit of glucagon and diazepam over a placebo treatment in the treatment of food bolus impaction.

68. Lancashire MJ, Legg PK, Lowe M, et al. Surgical aspects of international drug smuggling. Br Med J (Clin Res Ed) 1988;296(6628):1035–7.

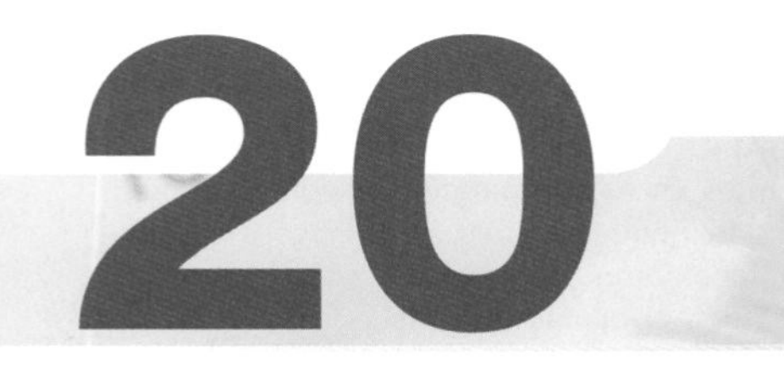

20 Bariatric surgery

Richard Welbourn

Introduction

Since its inception half a century ago, bariatric surgery (from the Greek word 'baros' for weight or pressure and '-iatric' for the medicine or surgery thereof) has grown from the preserve of a few enthusiasts to the most rapidly increasing area of surgery in developed countries. It is established that bariatric surgery is the only treatment that can result in long-lasting weight loss and improvement in obesity-related comorbidity.

Only a few operations have stood the test of time. The original jejuno-ileal bypass was abandoned due to the blind loop syndrome and resulting liver and bone metabolism problems. The vertical banded gastroplasty (VBG) has been superseded by gastric banding due to the advantage of being able to adjust the size of the gastric stoma. The gastric bypass has evolved from a continuously stapled horizontal gastroplasty and loop gastroenterostomy into a smaller pouch with a Roux-en-Y reconstruction.[1,2] The Magenstrasse and Mill procedure has evolved into the sleeve gastrectomy, an operation that is rapidly being taken up worldwide due to its perceived ease and lesser risk compared to gastric bypass.[3] Other procedures specifically for type 2 diabetes, such as duodeno-jejunal bypass and a temporary implanted endoscopic sheath that prevents absorption in the duodenum and proximal jejunum ('Endobarrier'), are being evaluated. The revolution of laparoscopic surgery has allowed most bariatric surgery to be performed laparoscopically with low mortality and morbidity. As a result, bariatric surgery is now established as a cost-effective intervention that should be increasingly provided.

Obesity as a public health problem

Obesity is a chronic, relapsing, debilitating, lifelong disease, recognised by the World Health Organisation as a global pandemic.[4] The influential Foresight report estimated that by 2010 28% of women and 33% of men in the UK would be obese, rising to 50% of women and 60% of men and, even more worrying, 25% of children as well by 2050.[5] The definitions of obesity are shown in Table 20.1. The term 'obesogenic environment' was used to describe the 'results of people responding normally to the obesogenic environments they find themselves in', given the current trends of reduced physical activity and easily available, highly advertised, relatively cheap, energy-dense foods.[6] An example of an obesogenic food environment is the observation that the price per calorie of healthy foods (whole grains, lean meats, low fat dairy, fruit and vegetables) increased to eight times the equivalent price of unhealthy foods (sweets, calorific drinks and fatty foods) between 2004 and 2008 in Seattle, USA.[7] Even payment methods have been implicated in unhealthy food choices: in a study in Buffalo, USA, buying of unhealthy compared to healthy foods significantly increased when the payment method was by card compared to cash ($P<0.01$).[8]

Table 20.1 • Definition of obesity according to body mass index

BMI (kg/m²)	WHO classification	Common clinical description
18.5–24.9	Normal range	Desirable
25–29.9	Pre-obese	Overweight
30–34.9	Obese class I	Obese
35–39.9	Obese class II	Clinically severe and complex obesity
40–49.9	Obese class III	
50 and over		Super-obesity

Adapted from Dixon JB, Zimmet P, Alberti KG et al. Bariatric surgery: an IDF statement for obese Type 2 diabetes. Diabet Med 2011; 28: 628-642.

✔✔ An estimated 1.46 billion adults (confidence interval (CI) 1.41–1.51 billion) globally were overweight in 2008 (body mass index (BMI) 25 kg/m² or over) and another 502 million obese (BMI >30), including 205 million men (CI 193–217) and 297 million women (CI 280–315 million), with another 170 million children overweight or obese.[9] In the UK, about 2% of the population, or 1.2 million people, have a BMI >40.[10]

The association between obesity and the metabolic syndrome of type 2 diabetes, hypertension, sleep apnoea and polycystic ovarian syndrome is well recognised.[11] These, together with other harmful obesity-related comorbid disease such as non-alcoholic steatohepatosis, asthma, back and lower limb degenerative problems, cancer and depression, present a massive financial burden on health services.

✔✔ The direct costs of treating these are estimated to be £5 billion per year in the UK National Health Service. This is set to double in real terms by 2050, with the indirect costs to society increasing to £50 billion.[5]

In addition, obese people are known to have higher unemployment and higher rates of claiming state benefit, and consume a disproportionate amount of the healthcare budget.[12,13]

The traditional advice 'eat less and exercise more' given to patients, based on understanding of the basic energy equation, does not work in the majority: a large study in the USA of 107 000 individuals using the Behavioural Risk Factor Surveillance System found that 63% of men and 78% of women were attempting to lose weight or maintain weight at any one time. However, 34% of men and 40% of women maintained the same energy intake despite reducing fats, and only 1 in 5 of those trying to control their weight were able to eat fewer calories and do 150 minutes exercise per week.[14]

In chronic obesity it is recognised that patients have usually missed the boat of prevention.[15] Most patients are able to diet to some extent but nearly always reach a plateau; thus a typical pattern in someone who has already become obese is a lifetime of repeated dieting and weight regain.

✔✔ Dieting decreases resting energy expenditure and basal metabolic rate, powerful physiological mechanisms that counter weight loss and encourage hunger.[16] In contrast, surgery enables weight loss usually to a far greater extent than can be achieved with dieting, and it allows weight loss to be maintained long term.[17]

It is thus not surprising that the worldwide rate of bariatric surgery has increased dramatically. In the USA, the most obese nation, the volume of surgery was 136 000 operations in 2004, while the American Society for Bariatric and Metabolic Surgery (ASMBS) estimated that 220 000 procedures were carried out in 2008.[18] This figure is similar to cholecystectomy, and at this rate of surgery the UK would be doing more than 50 000 operations per year.

Worldwide the commonest bariatric procedure is the Roux-en-Y gastric bypass (RYGB). Data from the UK and Ireland National Bariatric Surgery Registry (NBSR) indicated that in 6483 operations in 2009–10, 67% of the NHS patients had a gastric bypass, 21% gastric banding and 10.5% a sleeve gastrectomy.[19] In Europe the rate of gastric banding fell during the 2000s, having far exceeded gastric bypass during the 1990s.[20] By contrast, the popularity for banding increased in the USA after the FDA granted approval in 2001, and currently is estimated to exceed bypass (46% vs. 44%), with sleeve gastrectomy at 7.8%.[21]

Diabetes risk with obesity

Type 2 diabetes is the most important comorbid disease of obesity, affecting around 280 million people, a figure that is likely to rise to 438 million by 2030.[22] About 85% of type 2 diabetics are obese and the increased risk of becoming diabetic is estimated to be 93-fold for women and 42-fold for men who are severely obese.[23] Medical treatment cannot stop diabetes from progressing and thus the epidemic is one of the largest threats to global health in the 21st century.

Cancer risk with obesity

Obesity is the second most common cause of preventable cancer after smoking. In data from the Cancer Prevention Study II in the USA from 1982 to 1998, the relative risk (RR) of death from cancer increased above a BMI of 30 for both men and women.[24] In 900000 people the risk of most, if not all, cancers was increased in non-smokers.[25] For women with BMI >40, there was an RR of 6.25 for uterine cancer, and the overall RR was 2.51 for other cancers, in particular kidney, cervix and pancreas. For men with BMI >35, there was an RR of 4.52 for liver cancer, and for BMI >30 the RR was 1.68 for all other cancers. Thus the impact of obesity appears to be important for most, if not all, organs.

Psychosocial morbidity and prejudice

Up to 60% of bariatric patients have psychiatric disorders and substantial psychiatric comorbidity.[26] They also have impaired self-esteem, lower quality of life, and more depression and anxiety than the general population. About one-third are victims of sexual child abuse. Anti-obesity stereotypes are common in society and also in healthcare professionals: the obese are regarded as 'lazy, unmotivated and non-compliant', they 'lack self-discipline', and they face discrimination and prejudice.[26] Obesity is regarded as being 'self-inflicted' and is associated with 'moral failure and guilt', underlining the need for sensitivity and non-judgmental approaches to management.

Baseline obesity-related disease

✔✔ Data from 2559 patients in the US NIH-funded Longitudinal Assessment of Bariatric Surgery (LABS) study showed that obesity-related comorbid disease increases dramatically and highly significantly with rising BMI.[27] The *P* value for hypertension was 0.0018 and for diabetes, congestive heart failure, asthma, sleep apnoea, functional impairment, pulmonary hypertension, deep vein thrombosis (DVT)/pulmonary embolism (PE) risk and venous ulceration was $P<0.001$ after adjustment for age, sex, race and ethnicity.

Data from the NBSR

Sixteen per cent of patients with a BMI <40 had four or more comorbidities, and this rose to 37% for BMI 40–49.9, 47% for BMI 50–59.9 and 54% for BMI >60 ($P<0.01$). At baseline, 27.5% of patients had type 2 diabetes, 35.2% had hypertension, 18.2% had dyslipidaemia, 16.5% had obstructive sleep apnoea and 69% had impaired functional status on the basis of an inability to climb three flights of stairs without resting. Further, 53.9% of all patients reported some form of limiting arthritic symptoms. The high degree of disability in this population means that the dictum 'take more exercise' is not likely to be effective in weight reduction in the typical bariatric patient.

In common with the international literature, a very high proportion (80.1%) of patients undergoing bariatric surgery were female. It is not known why so few men have surgery, but men were older, heavier and had more comorbidity. For example, 43% of the men were diabetic, 50% had hypertension, 28% had dyslipidaemia and 37% had sleep apnoea ($P<0.001$). The average BMI was 50.6 compared to 47.7 in females. The differences are not simply explained by the older age of males, since on age group comparison males age 40–49 had a median of three comorbidities compared to a median of two in females of the same age group ($P<0.001$).[19]

Multidisciplinary work-up

✔✔ There is strong agreement that patients should be assessed carefully by a multidisciplinary team process that includes education sessions about the different operations and aftercare (Grade A recommendation).[28,29]

The team should include bariatric physicians, dieticians, nurse specialists, psychologists, anaesthetists and surgeons, and support groups.[29–31] Current National Institute for Clinical Excellence (NICE) guidelines, which were based on National Institutes of Health guidelines (1991), are shown in Box 20.1. It is not known what proportion of patients who

Box 20.1 • Criteria for bariatric surgery* (NICE Clinical Guideline 43, 2006)[29]

- Bariatric surgery is recommended as a treatment option for adults with obesity if all of the following criteria are fulfilled:
  - BMI of 40 kg/m² or greater, or between 35 and 40 kg/m² and weight-loss-responsive disease;
  - all appropriate measures have failed to achieve or maintain adequate, clinically beneficial weight loss for at least 6 months;
  - received or will receive intensive management in a specialist obesity service;
  - fit for anaesthesia and surgery;
  - commits to long-term follow-up.
- Bariatric surgery is also recommended as a first-line option for adults with a BMI >50 kg/m².

* SIGN (Scottish) guidelines 2010 indicate threshold for surgery is BMI >35 and one or more weight-loss-responsive comorbidities.[23]

fulfil the weight threshold for surgery would ever be suitable as patients must show that they are engaged and committed to the process and this is difficult to measure. Some believe that demonstration of weight loss before surgery is necessary to gauge this, but the evidence base for this is poor or lacking.[28] Rare endocrine causes should be excluded. Current drug or alcohol misuse and uncontrolled psychiatric disease are regarded as contraindications, as are a 'lack of comprehension of risks and lifestyle changes required', which might exclude patients with learning difficulties.[20,28] Patients should not be operated on when pregnant.[28] Crohn's disease is a relative contraindication and portal hypertension is an absolute contraindication.[20]

Optimisation of patients

Multidisciplinary teams should ensure that medical comorbidities can be identified and treated, so that high-risk patients with multiple medical comorbidities can be made as fit as possible before surgery.[28,30] This includes indentifying and treating obstructive sleep apnoea before surgery, and careful perioperative control of diabetes.[23] It is recommended that patients stop smoking at least 8 weeks before surgery.[28] Medications for epilepsy should be considered carefully as the absorption may be insufficient after gastric bypass or duodenal switch.

Obesity Surgery–Mortality Risk score (OS-MRS)

✔ This is now established as a validated tool for gastric bypass.[32] One point is scored for each of: male sex, age ≥45, BMI ≥50, presence of hypertension, known risk of DVT/PE. The possible scores range from 0 to 5. Class A (0–1 points) is low risk, class B (2–3 points) is medium risk and class C (4–5 points) is high risk. There was a 12-fold increased risk of mortality for class C patients compared to class A in the paper, which validated the score.

Thus a male patient with high BMI and hypertension, both of which are associated with central obesity, is likely to be more difficult to operate on due to the extra torque on laparoscopic instruments. Usual practice, in addition to medical work-up, is to put patients on a 'liver shrinkage diet' for at least 2 weeks before surgery, as this has been shown to reduce liver size, and probably reduces torque in central obesity (Grade B recommendation).[28,33] Weight reduction before surgery may also downgrade the risk group.

Comparisons of postoperative complications and mortality between gastric banding and bypass (or sleeve) should always take the OS-MRS into account to avoid the problem of bias, i.e. comparing apples and oranges. In the NBSR, far more bypass patients were class C than banding patients.

Current bariatric operations and surgical techniques

From a surgeon's perspective the ideal bariatric operation would provide 100% excess weight loss (EWL), complete reversal of all comorbidities, normalise functional capacity and produce no nutritional sequelae. It would also be cost-effective, provide normal quality of life and leave no loose skin. It should also need minimum resource for follow-up.

Unfortunately none provides this. A rapidly expanding literature in the last decade reflects quite variable current practice and the choice of procedure between available operations appears to be driven by patient preference, surgeon bias and local expertise.

Gastric bypass

There are several laparoscopic techniques described and there is as yet no standardisation. However, the weight loss results appear very much the same. Most agree that a short vertical lesser curvature-based gastric pouch of no more than 5–6 cm, that is separated from fundus, should be constructed, as this has been shown by MacLean and colleagues to produce weight loss over 15 years.[2] Starting just below the oblique fat pad on the lesser curve and usually taking the second branch of the left gastric artery, the pouch is made with linear staplers directed transversely over 2–3 cm then vertically up to just to the left of the angle of His, staying to the right of the posterior gastric artery if identified. Routing of the Roux limb can be retro- or antecolic and particular attention must be paid to the correct identification of the bowel limb to prevent 'Roux-en-O'[34,35] (**Fig. 20.1**).

In open surgery exact calibration of the diameter of the anastomosis of the Roux limb to the gastric pouch was thought to be critical to the rate of emptying and thus weight loss after the operation. However, as for banded gastric bypass (Fobi/Capella), there were no good data to support this.[36,37] In fact, an early study by Naslund in Sweden of 29 patients found that between-patient variation in the size of the gastric outlet did not correlate with weight loss 1 year after bypass.[38] In the UK NBSR, the techniques of pouch-enterostomy are reported as 39%

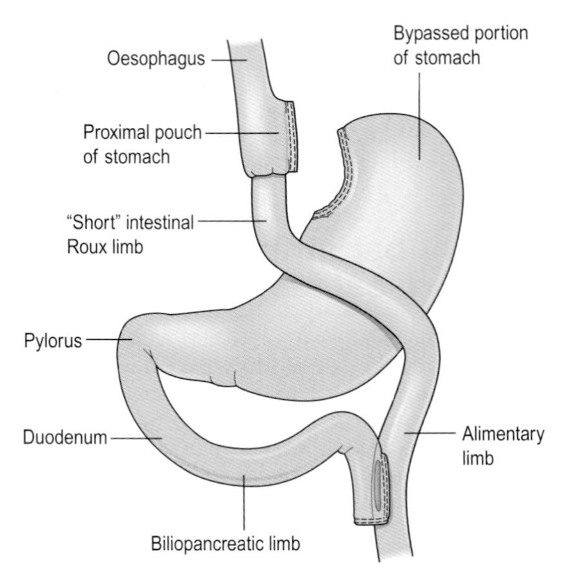

Figure 20.1 • Gastric bypass showing short vertical lesser curve-based gastric pouch with Roux-en-Y jejuno-jejunostomy.

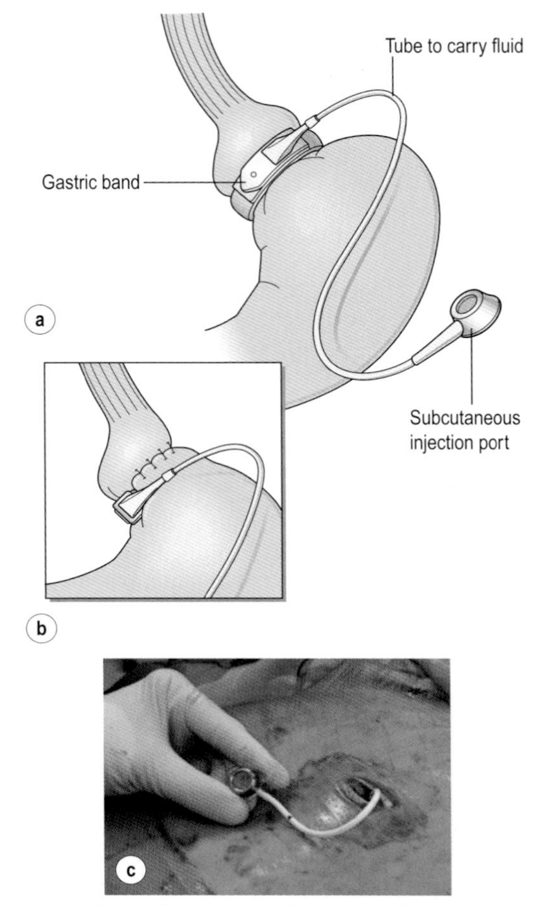

Figure 20.2 • Gastric band showing small 'virtual' pouch of stomach below gastro-oesophageal junction **(a)**, gastro-gastric tunnellating sutures **(b)** and the port used for adjustment **(c)**.

linear stapler with suture closure of the defect (after Lonroth), 23% circular stapler (after Wittgrove) and 38% hand sewn(after Higa).[19,34,35,39]

The lengths of the biliary and Roux limbs are not standardised and are impossible to measure accurately but in the US literature the biliary limb length is not usually mentioned since the assumption is that it is 'kept short' in order to reduce malabsorption of vitamins and minerals. The commonest description of the Roux limb is around 100–150 cm, after Brolin et al. in New Jersey and MacLean and colleagues in Montreal.[2,40] Limited evidence suggests that a longer Roux limb of 150 cm gives more weight loss for BMI >50, but this is not maintained in the long term. In standard bypass protein/calorie malabsorption is not the mechanism of weight loss. Since the common channel length is the determinant of available gut for absorption, and this is never measured in standard bypass, it is unlikely that longer lengths will ever be studied because of the worse nutritional consequences that would ensue.[41]

Gastric banding

The early perigastric approach for tunnelling the band posteriorly has now been abandoned as it is associated with high rates of band erosion into the stomach. The pars flaccida technique (through the window of the lesser omentum) is now preferred, keeping above the lesser omental bursa posteriorly. A band placed around the gastro-oesophageal junction would produce weight loss by dysphagia, and correct placement is just below, producing a small 'virtual pouch' of gastric mucosa above the band[20] (**Fig. 20.2**).

✔ Most choose to suture the band into place anteriorly with gastro-gastric tunnelling sutures in the belief that it reduces the risk of band slippage. In the NBSR, 99% of bands were placed by the pars flaccida technique (through the window in the lesser omentum) and 95% of bands were sutured anteriorly.[19]

The access port is usually sutured to the rectus sheath in the upper abdomen for ease of access by a non-coring, Huber needle for band adjustments. Placement of the band is just the start of the process of weight loss. Adjustments of the band are made by injecting saline progressively in order to reach the so-called 'sweet spot' of optimal restriction. A patient should probably be offered monthly clinic visits, at least for the first year. One study found that patients who attended seven or more clinics achieved 50% EWL in the first year compared to only 42% EWL in those who attended six times or fewer ($P<0.01$).[42] The ability to provide good follow-up should be part and parcel of the process, but is often lacking.[20]

Sleeve gastrectomy

Technically simpler than gastric bypass, the operation evolved from the Magenstrasse and Mill operation described by Johnston in Leeds, where the divided fundus (the 'mill') was left in continuity with the lesser curve-based tube (the 'main street').[3] In the sleeve the lesser curve-based tube is constructed over a size 32 or 34Fr bougie. The dissection uses linear stapling devices and starts 3–6 cm proximal to the pylorus upwards to just lateral to the angle of His.[43] Some descriptions of the sleeve now remove more of the antrum, leaving a true sleeve upwards from the pylorus (**Fig. 20.3**).

Sleeve gastrectomy is seen as a less risky alternative to gastric bypass, and a number of trials have now been reported (see below). The ASMBS issued an update statement on sleeve gastrectomy in October 2011, summarising the current data.[44] Himpens et al. from Belgium have the largest published series, with 5-year follow-up in which they found that 30 sleeve patients had 77.5% EWL at 3 years and 53.3% EWL at 6 years.[45] However, the starting BMI was only 39.9 and an additional 11 patients had a further bariatric procedure during follow-up, including 're-sleeve' because of weight regain. Although there is much enthusiasm for sleeve gastrectomy, the lack of long-term studies and demonstrable superiority compared to both gastric bypass and banding, together with the concern about weight regain due to expansion of the sleeve, mean this operation is unlikely to replace either in the foreseeable future. The longest follow-up so far reported is 8–9 years, when 13 patients with an initial BMI of 45.8 had 68% EWL.[46]

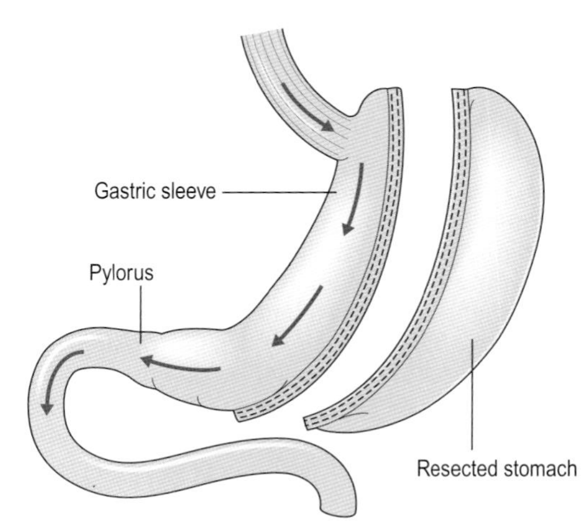

Figure 20.3 • Sleeve gastrectomy.

Biliopancreatic diversion/duodenal switch

Although the biliopancreatic diversion (BPD) described by Scopinaro in Naples produces greater weight loss than gastric bypass or banding, it requires very careful nutritional follow-up due to malabsorption, which is the mechanism of action of the operation.[31] BPD appears to be done rarely; however, its duodenal switch (DS) variant, combined with sleeve gastrectomy, is performed in a few centres.[47] DS is increasingly seen as a rescue operation for weight regain after sleeve gastrectomy.[45] All patients after DS need a high-protein diet and regular vitamin and mineral supplements with monitoring for life.

The DS variant of the BPD involves a sleeve gastrectomy followed by division of the duodenum just distal to the pylorus. The ileum is divided with a linear stapler and a duodeno-ileostomy and ileo-ileostomy are made such that the common channel for food absorption measures 75–125 cm and the alimentary channel measures 100–250 cm. The long remaining biliary limb is not measured[47] (**Fig. 20.4**).

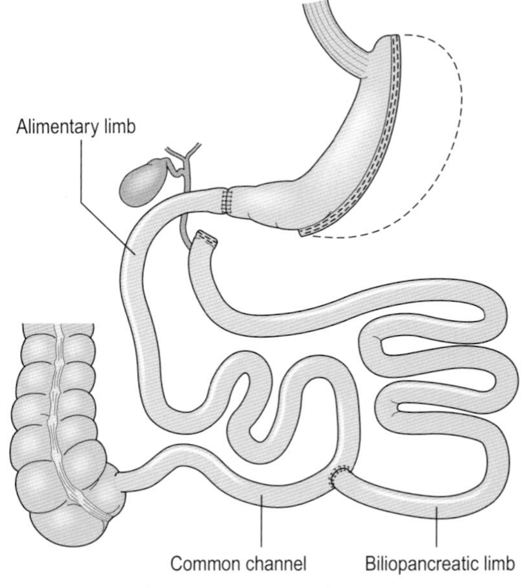

Figure 20.4 • Sleeve gastrectomy/biliopancreatic diversion with duodenal switch ('duodenal switch').

Mechanisms of bypass and banding

Both bypass and banding appear to control appetite and satiety by physiological mechanisms. In a blinded crossover trial of filling/de-filling of gastric bands, Dixon et al. demonstrated that satiety before and after eating was greater when the band was filled than when not.[48] It is proposed that stimulation of vagal afferent fibres adjacent to the band mediates the feeling of satiety, as there is no marked change, if any, in gut hormone profiles.[20]

In contrast to banding, there has been an explosion of publications demonstrating rises in gut hormone levels after gastric bypass that favour reduced appetite and early satiety. Hormones such as peptide YY (PYY), glucagon-like peptide-1 (GLP-1) and oxyntomodulin have attracted particular attention and there are currently publications exploring changes in energy expenditure and bile acids as mediators of improved insulin resistance.[49,50] In the foregut theory, diabetes has been proposed to be a disease of the duodenum and proximal jejunum, referring to the exclusion of this part of the anatomy to the passage of food in gastric bypass. In the original research, diabetic rats were made non-diabetic after duodeno-jejunal bypass, in which only the duodenum and proximal jejunum were excluded from the passage of food, leaving the stomach intact. This is the basis for the development of the duodeno-jejunal bypass in humans and the endoscopic duodenal sleeve technique (Endobarrier).[51] If current trials show success, the endoscopic sleeve could become a useful adjunct in making patients fitter for surgery.

In the distal gut theory, rapid delivery of food from the gastric pouch via the Roux limb to the terminal ileum is proposed as the mechanism by which gut hormones rise and produce early reduction in appetite and early satiety.[49] In this study, patients with good weight loss produced high levels of PYY and GLP-1 compared to patients who did not lose as much weight ($P<0.05$). In addition, in a randomised controlled trial (RCT) those receiving somatostatin after gastric bypass had attenuated gut hormone responses and experienced return of appetite compared to those receiving placebo ($P<0.05$).[49] The distal gut theory contradicts the thinking behind the banded bypass.

Weight loss outcomes

A measurement of weight loss is the most consistent variable used in reporting results of bariatric surgery, being regarded by surgeons as the paramount clinical outcome. There is, however, almost complete lack of consistency about how this is measured or presented, as illustrated in Table 20.2, in which the known RCTs of weight loss outcomes from currently performed procedures are summarised.[52] This lack of consistency leads to difficulties in combining data from studies in systematic reviews and meta-analyses, and it makes comparisons between studies and centres difficult. Most of the available evidence consists of case series (level III evidence).

✔✔ Although the long-term outcome of patients who have had gastric bands is not known, one systematic review suggests that if the band is correctly placed, the patient is well followed up and does not suffer a complication, the weight loss at 3–4 years may be similar to gastric bypass, but without the risk of the initial operation.[61] In both RCTs (see below) weight loss was better for bypass.

Enthusiasts of gastric banding maintain that since these patients lose their weight slowly over 3–4 years after surgery, differences in early EWL compared to other operations are not relevant to long-term health (although this has not been studied). The reality is that follow-up outside of funded studies is usually extremely poor, despite sometimes strenuous attempts by clinicians to make contact. In the O'Brien study, data from 3874 gastric bypass patients and 10 041 gastric band patients were analysed at 5 years, and at this time the weight status of only 4.5% of bypasses and 6.4% of bands was known. Even so, the consensus is that this is a good estimation of weight loss outcomes in practice, with some weight regain after the nadir of weight loss being usual after bypass. Most patients settle at around 55–65% EWL long term, perhaps 10% more EWL than the average band patient.

A challenge of managing gastric band patients is how to help the proportion of patients who fail to lose much weight. In the two RCTs discussed below, failure as defined by BMI >35 was found in the Italian trial in 4.2% of bypasses and 34.6% of bands ($P<0.001$). In the Californian RCT patients failing to lose the first quintile of excess weight were none for bypass and 16.7% for bands ($P<0.05$). Many patients in this position opt for revision to a gastric bypass if possible. An equally challenging group is the bypass patients who have significant weight regain at 3–4 years after the nadir of weight loss. Treatment options include adding a gastric band to the existing gastric pouch.

Band versus bypass RCTs

Two RCTs have compared gastric bypass and adjustable gastric banding. Angrisani et al. in Naples randomised 24 patients to gastric bypass and 27 patients to banding.[62] There was no mortality and

Table 20.2 • Summary of RCTs of currently performed procedures[52]

Study	Follow-up (y) (% complete)	Baseline			Intervention (sample size)	Outcome
		Mean BMI	Mean age (y)	% Female		Mean weight change
Heindorf, 1997, Denmark	0.83 (NR)	Range 40–56	Range 21–43	44	AGB (8) No surgery (8)	–26 kg +1 kg**
Langer, 2005, Australia	0.5 (NR)	48	39	90	SG (10) AGB (10)	–61.4% EWL –28.7% EWL**
Lee, 2005,* Taiwan[53]	2 (100)	44	31	69	Mini-GB (40) RYGB (40)	64.4% EWL 60.0% EWL
Himpens, 2006,* Belgium[54]	3 y (NR)	38	38	75	AGB (40) SG (40)	48% EWL 66% EWL**
O'Brien, 2006,* Australia[55]	2 (90)	33	41	76	AGB (40) No surgery (40)	87.2% EWL 21.8% EWL**
Angrisani, 2007, Italy	5 (98)	44	34	82	AGB (24) RYGB (19)	–22.1 kg –36.0 kg**
Bessler, 2007,* USA[56]	3 (NR)	59	41	65	Banded RYGB (46) Standard RYGB (44)	73.4% EWL 57.7% EWL**
Dixon, 2008,* Australia[57]	2 (92%)	37.1	46	7	AGB (30) No surgery (30)	62.5 % EWL 4.3 % EWL**
Karamanakos, 2008, Greece	1 (100)	46	34	84	SG (16) RYGB (16)	–43.6 kg –40.0 kg
Nguyen, 2009, USA	4 (69)	47	43	82	AGB (86) RYGB (111)	–45% EWL –65% EWL**
Peterli, 2009a, Switzerland	1.58 (NR)	46	41	78	SG (17) RYGB (15)	89% EWL 68% EWL
Peterli, 2009b, Switzerland	0.25 (100)	46	40	NR	SG (14) RYGB (13)	–21.6 kg –25.6 kg
Campos, 2010, USA	14d (NR)	48	44	68	RYGB (12) No surgery (10)	–9.9 kg –8.2 kg
O'Brien, 2010, Australia	2 (84)	41	17	68	AGB (25) No surgery (25)	–34.6 kg –3.0 kg**
Kehagias, 2011,* Greece[43]	3 (100)	45	35	73	RYGB (30) SG (30)	62% EWL 68% EWL
Lee, 2011,* Taiwan[58]	1 (100)	30	45	NR	Mini-GB (30) SG (30)	94% EWL 76% EWL (NS)
Søvik, 2011,* Norway/ Sweden[59]	2 (97)	55	35	68	RYGB (31) DS (29)	–50.6 kg –73.5 kg**
Woelnerhanssen, 2011,* Switzerland[60]	1 y (100)	46	38	NR	RYGB (12) SG (11)	34.5% TBWL 27.9% TBWL
Schauer, 2012,* USA	1 y (93)	36	49	66	RYGB (50) SG (49) No surgery (41)	–29.4 kg** –25.1 kg** –5.4 kg
Mingrone, 2012,* Italy	2 y (93)	45	43	53	RYGB (20) BPD (20) No surgery (20)	–33.31%** –33.82 %** –4.74 % TBWL

* Added in addition to Padwal systematic review.

** *P*<0.05.

Adv/Ev, adverse events; AGB, adjustable gastric banding; BPD, biliopancreatic diversion; DS, duodenal switch; EWL, excess weight loss; Mini-RYGB, Mini-gastric bypass; NR, not recorded; NS, not significant; RYGB, gastric bypass; SG, sleeve gastrectomy; TBWL, total body weight loss. N.B. Karamanakos and Kehagias report data from the same RCT.

one band patient was lost to follow-up. Four band patients required revision to other bariatric operations during follow-up, two for gastric pouch dilatation and two for unsatisfactory weight loss. Three bypass patients required early re-operations because of life-threatening complications (12.5%). Fifteen bypass patients (62.5%) achieved BMI <30 compared to three (11.5%) band patients ($P<0.001$). The authors concluded that gastric bypass produces better weight loss and fewer failures, acknowledging that the high complication rate was accounted for by their learning curve in the bypass operation.

Nguyen et al. in California randomised 111 patients to gastric bypass and 86 to banding.[63] There was no mortality in either group. At 4 years patients were grouped into quintiles of percentage excess weight loss (% EWL). The highest quintiles representing 60% EWL or more had 64.1% of bypass patients and 15.3% of band patients. The lowest quintiles representing <40% EWL had 5.1% of bypass patients and 50.0% of band patients ($P<0.05$). Although the authors concluded that weight loss at 4 years was superior after bypass, the follow-up rates achieved were only 83.1% for bypass and 93.3% for band, and no explanation was given for the different numbers randomised to each arm.

Given that these two procedures are the commonest in the NHS (and worldwide), the methodological weaknesses of the two RCTs limit their general applicability. A new trial comparing these head to head has recently been funded. The By-Band trial, which opened in 2012, is a multicentre RCT that aims to randomise 760 patients in the UK. The trial is designed to answer the question of whether gastric bypass is better than gastric banding in terms of health-related quality of life and at least as good as gastric banding in terms of achieving weight loss. Both aspects of this dual primary end-point need to be achieved to be certain that bypass is superior to gastric banding. They will be measured at 3 years. A cost-effectiveness analysis will also be included and it is hoped that the results will inform the debate on how bariatric services should be provided.

Band versus sleeve gastrectomy RCT

In the largest RCT, Himpens et al. in Belgium randomised 80 patients to either operation.[54] Weight loss was better for sleeve at each time point measured: 57.7% EWL vs. 41.4% EWL at 1 year and 66% EWL vs. 48% at 3 years (both $P<0.01$). Although there were several operations for complications in each group, an additional two patients in each was converted to another bariatric operation due to lack of weight loss.

Banded versus non-banded gastric bypass RCT

There has been one RCT of banded versus non-banded (standard) gastric bypass. The banded gastric bypass involves placing a silicone ring around the gastric pouch above the pouch-enterostomy anastomosis, with the intention of causing a fixed amount of restriction and thus greater weight loss. In an RCT, Bessler et al. randomised 46 patients to banded bypass and 44 to standard bypass.[56] There were no significant differences in EWL at 6, 12 and 24 months (43.1% vs. 24.7%, 64.0% vs. 57.4%, and 64.2% vs. 57.2%). However, there was a small advantage at 36 months for the banded group (73.4% vs. 57.7%, $P<0.05$), although the number available for follow-up was not specified. Other than in a few centres, this operation has not received widespread uptake and the proposed mechanism of action (hold-up of food in the pouch) is at variance with the distal gut theory.[49]

There has been one RCT of standard gastric bypass versus the so-called mini-gastric bypass. In this variant a long gastric pouch/tube (midway in length between the pouch in standard gastric bypass and that in a sleeve gastrectomy) is created and an antecolic loop gastroenterostomy is made without a Roux-en-Y. Although the weight loss outcomes are reported to be similar to standard gastric bypass, it is an uncommon operation and there has been reluctance to recognise it for credentialing purposes by the ASMBS and the American College of Surgeons (ACS).[31,53]

Sleeve versus bypass RCTs

There are at least three RCTs of sleeve gastrectomy versus gastric bypass and one of sleeve versus mini-gastric bypass. Kehagias et al. in Greece have published the longest follow-up in an RCT of bypass versus sleeve and they found no significant difference in weight loss between the two at any time point up to 3 years (3-year data: 68% EWL for sleeve and 63% EWL for bypass).[43] An earlier report of the same trial found that weight loss at 1 year was similar for the two operations and this is the general consensus for medium-term comparison of bypass with sleeve.[52]

Bypass versus duodenal switch RCT

There is one published trial, from Norway/Sweden.[59] In this study, Søvik et al. found much greater weight loss after sleeve gastrectomy with DS compared to bypass at 2 years. Cholesterol and other measures of lipid metabolism were improved more by duodenal switch but measures of vitamin

D metabolism were worse. Although quality of life was broadly similar in follow-up between the two, adverse events were more frequent after DS (62% vs. 32%, $P<0.02$). These were mainly due to the unavoidable nutritional consequences of DS and this illustrates the main challenge in follow-up after this operation.

Complications of surgery

Operative mortality

Published mortality rates after gastric banding suggest it is very safe, with about a 0.05–0.1% risk of dying. The published mortality from gastric bypass is higher at about 0.2%, with the mortality from sleeve gastrectomy between the two. The data in the table refer to large published national databases or registries reporting since 2009 (Table 20.3).[19,21,64,65]

Open bypass has higher mortality (data not shown), and the Hospital Episode Statistics (HES) data from the UK were from 2000 to 2008, when much of the surgery was not yet laparoscopic. By far the largest report of outcomes is from the Bariatric Outcomes Longitudinal Database of the ASMBS Centers of Excellence programme, in which 57918 patients had gastric bypass (54.7%), banding (39.6%) or sleeve gastrectomy (2.3%).[66] The 90-day mortality rate for those with follow-up was 0.22%, but neither mortality per procedure nor 30-day re-operation rates were presented. The ACS Bariatric Surgery Center Network reported higher morbidity, re-operation and re-intervention rates for gastric bypass than for banding, with sleeve between the two.[21] Similarly, the Michigan Bariatric Surgery Collaborative reported 30-day complication rates for bypass of 3.6% compared to 0.9% for gastric banding and 2.2% for sleeve.[67]

Gastric bypass

Early

Anastomotic leak, particularly at the pouch-enterostomy, is a feared and potentially deadly complication and may be present in up to 3%.[68] It typically occurs within 24 hours, i.e. the anastomosis is unlikely to have been water-tight initially. It is essential that a patient who has abdominal pain and a sense of 'impending doom' be considered for same-day re-laparoscopy or contrast-enhanced computed tomography (CT) scan.[68] Tachycardia is an unreliable sign, particularly when the patient is taking beta-blockers for hypertension. The pouch-enterostomy is more likely to leak than the jejuno-jejunostomy and, because of its accessibility, it is usual to do a leak test during surgery. Same-day re-operation and direct suturing or T-tube placement

Table 20.3 • Operative mortality data from UK&I National Bariatric Surgery Registry, Hospital Episode Statistics data, Longitudinal Assessment of Bariatric Surgery (USA) and American College of Surgeons Bariatric Surgical Center Network[19,21,64,65]

Primary operations		Total patients	In-hospital mortality (%)	30-day re-operation rate (%)
Gastric band	NBSR	1878	0 (0.0)	0.9
	HES	3649	3 (0.1)	N/A
	LABS	1198	0 (0.0)	0.8
	ACS	12 193	6 (0.05)	0.92
Gastric bypass	NBSR	3132*	7 (0.22)	3.4
	HES	3191*	15 (0.47)	N/A
	LABS	2975†	6 (0.20)	3.2
	ACS	14 491†	21 (0.14)	5.02
Sleeve gastrectomy	NBSR	493	0 (0)	3.1
	HES	113	1 (0.8)	N/A
	ACS	944	1 (0.11)	2.97

*Total laparoscopic/open.
†Laparoscopic only.
HES, LABS and ACS data were $P<0.05$ between groups. In the LABS study data on 117 sleeve gastrectomy patients were not analysed further. N/A, not available.

and drainage are essential due to the limited reserve in patients with severe comorbidity. Poor healing is characteristic and patients are severely catabolic, with very high energy requirements.

Bleeding from anastomoses and staple lines may present postoperatively as melaena in up to 4% and almost always settles, sometimes needing transfusion.[69] Closed loop obstruction, particularly if there is a 'Roux-en-O' or acute internal hernia, is life threatening and must be excluded or rectified quickly.

DVT/PE is still the commonest cause of mortality after bariatric surgery, probably accounting for half the deaths. It should be routine to give appropriate prophylaxis with calf compression stockings and inflatable leggings during surgery and at least one postoperative week of appropriate anticoagulant for any operation other than banding.[70] All patients should be encouraged to mobilise on the same day of surgery and enhanced recovery regimens are common. Data from the UK NBSR showed that >90% of banding patients are discharged home by 24 hours and >80% of bypass and sleeve patients are discharged home by postoperative day 3.[19]

Late

Stricture at the pouch-enterostomy occurs in up to 5%, probably depending on the technique of anastomosis and any tension.[35] It usually responds to endoscopic dilatation. Marginal ulcer is reported to occur and it may be less common if *Helicobacter pylori* infection is sought and treated preoperatively. Internal herniation with bowel ischaemia is a known serious risk as the hernia spaces made by the anatomical rearrangement enlarge as weight is lost. It is mandatory for every patient to be on lifelong vitamin and trace mineral supplementation due to the unavailability of the duodeno-proximal jejunal segment for absorption (see below).

✔ Most experts recommend prophylactic suturing of the Petersen defect (space behind the Roux limb), the mesocolic defect (in retrocolic routing) and the jejuno-jejunostomy defects with non-absorbable sutures, although there are no data to show this makes a difference.[35] An RCT based on the Swedish Registry (SOREG) is currently ongoing.

The risk of symptomatic internal hernia is at least 2% over 1–2 years after surgery.[71]

Gastric Band

Early

The re-operation rate within 30 days after banding is about 1%. It is considered mandatory to give prophylactic antibiotics. Early infection of the gastric band port wound is a potential disaster as it may indicate that the whole band is infected. After a suitable course of antibiotics a pragmatic approach (not evidence based) is to re-laparoscope and cut the band tubing as it exits the abdominal wall, completing this part of the operation before opening the infected port wound and removing the port. If the infection is localised to the port wound only, it may be possible to reconnect another port at a later date.

✔ A complication that can occur at any time after the band has been filled is acute obstruction due to a food bolus or over-filling. Every hospital should have an 'emergency de-fill box' for out-of-hours use containing a non-coring Huber needle for this purpose.[72] Patients should be educated about this possibility and know how to contact their bariatric team.

Late

Every patient must be carefully counselled about the long-term risk of re-operation. Suter et al. in Switzerland found there was a 21% cumulative re-operation rate over 7 years.[73] The real-life re-operation rate is not known since so many patients are lost to follow-up, but a realistic estimation may be 10–20% over 5–10 years. Re-operations may be minor, e.g. a needle stick injury to the tubing adjacent to the port or failure of the port membrane causing leakage and requiring local attention to replace the port or shorten the tubing. Much more serious complications are infection, requiring removal of the whole band, slippage of the position of the band around the upper part of the stomach, and erosion, where the band migrates into the lumen of the stomach.

Slippage

This typically presents at 2–3 years, and produces vomiting and loss of restriction. This is usually a non-urgent situation and treatment consists of de-filling the band, a contrast X-ray to make the diagnosis and laparoscopic repositioning of the band. Concentric pouch dilatation, sometimes with a dilated oesophagus and lack of weight loss, can be confused with slippage and may indicate lack of a satiety response from the band.

✔ Slippage can be a life-threatening emergency if there is severe abdominal pain, indicating ischaemia of the gastric pouch above the band and resulting necrosis. Treatment consists of emergency de-filling, a contrast X-ray and urgent laparoscopy. If possible, the band should be repositioned. There is no place for waiting for endoscopy to make the diagnosis.[72]

Concentric pouch dilatation, sometimes with a dilated oesophagus and lack of weight loss, can be confused with slippage and indicate lack of an appetite/satiety response from the band.

Erosion

This occurs in about 1% of patients long term and may result from, or be the cause of, port-site infection. It does not present as an emergency. Sudden loss of restriction is the norm, and a red port scar de novo is worrying for erosion. Endoscopy or contrast X-ray provides the diagnosis and band removal is usually done laparoscopically, although it can be done by endoscopy. Revision surgery, usually to convert to a gastric bypass, should be delayed for at least 6 months to allow healing.

Sleeve gastrectomy

The main early complication of sleeve is leakage along the staple line, usually at the angle of His. This is thought to be due to the relative back pressure produced by an intact pylorus against oesophageal peristalsis. With an incidence reported consistently at up to 3%, leaks can take months to heal, and many surgeons routinely use reinforcement materials or continuous suturing along the staple line to try to prevent a leak.[74] Treatment options include percutaneous drainage, endoscopic stenting, parenteral nutrition/jejunal feeding, proton-pump inhibitors and fibrin glue.

High-volume specialisation

Data from the Michigan Bariatric Surgery Collaborative assessed hospital complication rates in 15275 patients having bypass, banding and sleeve gastrectomy in 2006–2009. The overall risk for all procedures (after adjusting for comorbidity status and OS-MRS risk; see above) of serious complication was 4.0% (CI 2.8–5.3) for annual volumes of <150 cases per hospital and <100 cases per surgeon combined, compared to 1.9% (CI 1.4–2.3) for ≥300 cases per hospital and ≥250 per surgeon combined ($P<0.001$).[67] In addition to specific surgical complications, the team approach characteristic of high-volume hospitals appears to facilitate better outcomes (Grade D recommendation).[30,31] Most experts recommend round-table discussion of patients on a regular basis. Since the success of banding is completely reliant on good follow-up, the multidisciplinary team should be structured to enable this.[31] In addition, the International Diabetes Federation statement (see below) made the following comment:

✔✔ 'Bariatric surgery should be performed in high-volume centres with multidisciplinary teams.'[23]

There are a number of other case series supporting high-volume specialisation in gastric bypass surgery that also recognise the high risk of the learning curve and the need for mentoring for this operation.[75]

Comorbidity outcomes

Data from a meta-analysis of 21 studies showed improvements in diabetes, hypertension, dyslipidaemia and sleep apnoea in nearly all patients.[76] Numerous other studies show improvements in individual organ failures. For example, liver biopsies on 36 patients were assessed blindly before and 2 years after gastric banding.[77] Histology showed marked improvements in indices of grade and stage of non-alcoholic steatohepatosis ($P<0.01$). At follow-up only three patients had a fibrosis score of 2 or more compared with 18 patients at baseline ($P<001$). Another example is cardiac function; in one study 423 gastric bypass patients were compared to 733 non-operated controls with an echocardiogram at baseline and at 2 years. Left ventricular mass and right ventricular cavity area had both decreased at follow-up ($P<0.01$), and left atrial volume stayed the same in bypasses but had increased in controls ($P<0.05$), all indicating improved cardiac function.[78]

Swedish Obese Subjects study

The largest series of detailed long-term comorbidity data is the Swedish Obese Subjects (SOS) study (Table 20.4).[79] This study is also probably the best known in bariatric surgery. It was initiated in 1987, recruiting to 2001, and is a non-randomised cohort study of the effect of bariatric surgery versus

Table 20.4 • Incidence of comorbidity: 10-year data from the Swedish Obese Subjects study[79]

	Surgery (%)	Controls (%)	*P* value
Diabetes	7	24	<0.001
Recovery of diabetes	36	13	<0.001
Hypertension	41	49	= 0.13
Recovery from hypertension	19	11	= 0.02
Hyperlipidaemia	17	27	= 0.03
Recovery of hyperlipidaemia	46	24	<0.001

Reproduced from Sjöström L, Lindroos A-K, Peltonen M et al. Lifestyle, diabetes, and cardiovascular risk factors 10 years after bariatric surgery. N Engl J Med 2004; 35:2683–93. With permission from Massachusetts Medical Society.

medical therapy. At the time, before laparoscopic techniques, bariatric surgery was considered too dangerous to allow ethical randomisation between surgery and best medical therapy. Thus, 2037 patients choosing not to have surgery were matched and compared to 2010 surgical patients. Over a mean follow-up of 10.9 years (range 4.9–18.2) there was no significant weight loss in the medical group, who received all appropriate therapy for their comorbid disease. In contrast, weight loss in the surgical groups, consisting of non-adjustable gastric banding, gastric bypass and vertical banded gastroplasty, was between 13.2% and 25%. There were improvements in every variable studied, but it was noted that hypertension tended to recur, associated with advancing age of the study population.

Data from the NBSR

The proportion of patients recorded as showing no indication of comorbidities at 1 year in the NBSR is shown in Table 20.5.[19] The functional improvement was dramatic and at 2 years the rate of diabetes had fallen by 85.5%. Most of the effect of surgery in the NBSR results was from gastric bypass; in fact, for banding only dyslipidaemia and functional impairment showed significant improvement at 1 year, although all other variables showed non-significant improvement. The data are also consistent with the slower rate of weight loss universally found with gastric banding compared to RYGB.[20] Because of a lack of well-controlled randomised studies comparing the two operations, it is not clear whether the apparently slower rate of improvement in comorbidity with banding translates to different outcomes in the medium to long term.

Table 20.5 • Incidence of comorbidity: 1-year data from the UK NBSR (patients with complete follow-up, all operations)[19]

	Baseline (%)	1 year (%)	*P* value
Impaired functional status	70.7	36.2	<0.001
Diabetes	26.8	13.2	<0.001
Hypertension	31.6	20.4	<0.001
Dyslipidaemia	16.8	8.2	<0.001
Obstructive sleep apnoea	14.6	6.1	<0.001
Arthritis	53.9	41.3	<0.001
GORD	27.7	16.2	<0.001
PCOS	9.5	6.4	<0.01

GORD, gastro-oesophageal reflux disease; PCOS, polycystic ovarian syndrome.

Quality of life (QoL) after bariatric surgery

There are many studies indicating that quality of life improves after surgery compared to no surgery. Again, the largest study is the SOS, which reported that all QoL measures improved in 655 surgery patients compared to 621 controls when assessed at 2–10 years.[17] Variables included General Health Rating Index, Sickness Impact Profile, Mood Adjective Check List, and Hospital Anxiety and Depression score. Improved QoL was also found in the RCT by O'Brien et al. where band patients had improvement at 2 years in five of eight domains in the SF-36 tool – physical function, physical role, general health, vitality and emotional role.[61] Improvement in psychological functioning is not universal, however, as it also appears that there is an increased risk of suicide after surgery.[80]

Patient-reported outcomes

There is wide variation in the questionnaires used to assess health-related quality of life after bariatric surgery, with no consensus as to how the results should be reported. Poor study designs and lack of reporting integrated with clinical outcomes means there are few examples of how patient-reported outcomes have influenced practice and no data on which domains of health are important. As a result it has not been possible to produce a meta-analysis of quality-of-life studies. Thus there is a need for a core outcome set for bariatric surgery reporting that includes this variable.

Diabetes outcomes

✔✔ Bariatric surgery offers very substantial benefit for diabetes. In the RCT by Dixon et al. of gastric banding versus intensive medical therapy for recent-onset diabetes, HbA1c was lowered more with banding (7.8 ± 1.2 preop vs. 6.0 ± 0.82 postop, −1.81 ± 1.24 percentage points) than with medical therapy (7.6 ± 1.4 preop vs. 7.21 ± 1.39, −0.38 ± 1.26 percentage points, $P<0.001$). Also, there was better remission in the surgery group at 2 years (73% vs. 13%, $P<0.001$) and significantly fewer people with the metabolic syndrome (70% vs. 13%, $P<0.001$).[57]

In the systematic review of outcomes in 4070 diabetic patients by Buchwald et al., it was estimated that remission at 2 years was achieved in 57% of patients after gastric banding, 80% after gastric bypass and

95% after biliopancreatic diversion.[81] Also, HbA1c and fasting glucose levels fell significantly, indicating better diabetes control. However, the main drawback of such a meta-analysis is lack of consistent reporting of the terms used to define remission.

Given that bariatric surgery is presently only being offered to a very small proportion of those who could benefit, even in countries with highly developed healthcare, the International Diabetes Federation perceived the need in 2011 to offer international guidance.[23] The recommendations included: 'bariatric surgery is an *appropriate* treatment for type 2 diabetes and BMI ≥35 not achieving recommended treatment targets with medical therapy, especially where there is other obesity-related comorbidity' (author's italics).

Various terms for improvement of diabetes control after surgery have been used, including 'resolution' and 'cure', but 'remission' is now the preferred term. In 2009 the American Diabetes Association introduced a more strict definition of complete remission as being a return to normal measures of glucose metabolism (HbA1c <6%, fasting glucose <5.6 mmol/L) in the absence of hypoglycaemic medication over at least 1 year after bariatric surgery.[82] One study has assessed remission rates with the new definition. At 2-year follow-up in 209 diabetics, HbA1c was reduced in all surgical groups ($P<0.001$), and complete remission rates were 40.6% after gastric bypass, 7% after gastric banding and 26% after sleeve gastrectomy.[83] Although the study was not randomised, the differences between the procedures were significant ($P<0.001$).

The study by Dixon et al. in 2008 is the only randomised trial comparing diabetes outcomes between banding and intensive medical therapy. Recently, two further studies have provided randomised evidence for gastric bypass, sleeve gastrectomy and BPD as well compared to medical therapy. Both RCTs highlight the main therapeutic aim of controlling HbA1c rather than purely focusing on the ability of surgery to reduce medication usage. In the RCT by Schauer et al., HbA1c fell from 9.3 to 6.4 with gastric bypass, and 9.5 to 6.6 with sleeve gastrectomy (2.9 percentage points for both).[84] In comparison, HbA1c only fell from 8.9 to 7.5 (1.4 percentage points, both $P<0.001$) with intensive medical therapy. The primary end-point (proportion with HbA1c <6.0 at 1 year) was achieved by 42% with gastric bypass, 37% with sleeve gastrectomy and 12% with medical therapy (both $P<0.001$ compared to medical therapy).In the RCT by Mingrone et al., the starting HbA1c was 8.65±1.45, and this fell to 6.35±1.42 with gastric bypass, 4.95±0.49 with BPD and 7.69±0.57 with intensive medical therapy ($P<0.01$ between each group).[85] The primary end-point (fasting glucose <5.6 mmol/L and HbA1c <6.5% on no medication) was achieved by 75% with gastric bypass, 95% with BPD and none with medical therapy ($P<0.001$ between groups). These are the only randomised data between bypass and BPD, and suggest that the latter gives better glycaemic control. There are no randomised data studying the effect of DS on HbA1c.

The different rates of improvement/remission between operations supports the consensus that bypass (and BPD) has effects other than pure weight loss on improving glycaemic control. It is widely presumed that this is due to the postoperative rise in gut hormones such as the incretin GLP-1, which is associated with rapid improvement in diabetic control in the immediate postoperative period before significant weight loss.[86]

While all of the currently popular operations dramatically improve glycaemic control, many patients can still expect to be on diabetic medications postoperatively. Previously, surgeons tended to champion reduction in medication usage and to gauge the success of surgery in these terms. Focusing on glycaemic control (HbA1c) as well should not detract from the very substantial financial benefit of patients coming off treatment (see below). Thus, surgery is 'a component of the ongoing treatment of chronic disease management of type 2 diabetes and obesity' and patients still need long-term follow-up by interested physicians.[23]

Nutritional support in follow-up

✔ All bariatric patients should have routine metabolic and nutritional monitoring life-long (Grade A recommendation) as it is increasingly recognised that obese patients have pre-existing nutritional deficiencies that may be exacerbated by bariatric surgery, especially gastric bypass and duodenal switch.[28]

The frequency of assessment should be at least 3- to 6-monthly in the first year if there are known deficiencies, at least 6- to 12-monthly in the second year and at least annually thereafter.[28]

Recommended supplements are: multi-vitamin, calcium with vitamin D, folic acid, iron and vitamin B_{12} (Grade B recommendation). In addition, folic acid should be supplemented in all women of child-bearing age who are sexually active because of the risk of neural tube defects and the likelihood that fertility will improve after surgery (Grade A recommendation).[28]

Long-term survival benefit after surgery

Several population-based studies now indicate that bariatric surgery confers survival benefit. The SOS study was the first prospective study to show that bariatric surgery confers survival benefit; even after the 90-day mortality rate from surgery of 0.25%, 129 control patients died compared to 101 in the surgical group, hazard ratio (HR) 0.76 (95% CI 0.59–0.99), with a time to reach significance (*P*=0.04) of 13 years.[87]

Another study that also reported in 2007 was a retrospective analysis of prospectively collected data.[80] Using self-reported BMI data collected from driving licences in Utah, Adams et al. were able to match, for age, sex and BMI, 7925 patients who had undergone gastric bypass with 7925 controls. The average age was 39.5 and BMI 45.3, but it was not possible to collect data on pre- or postoperative comorbidity or BMI at follow-up. The study period was 1984–2002 and the mean follow-up was 7.1 years. Expressing mortality as deaths/10000 patient years, 37.6 patients died in the years after surgery compared to 57.1 controls (40% reduction, *P*<0.001). Disease-specific reductions in mortality were also seen for coronary artery disease (56% reduction, 2.6 vs. 5.9, *P*=0.006), diabetes (92% reduction, 0.4 vs. 3.4, *P*=0.005) and cancer (60% reduction, 5.5 vs. 13.3, *P*=0.001). The post-surgical mortality at 1 year was 0.53%, which compared to 0.52% of controls dying in the same period.

The reports described confirmed survival benefit after mainly gastric bypass surgery. O'Brien and Dixon's group in Melbourne has also reported survival benefit after gastric banding.[88] In a retrospective series of 966 operated patients followed up for 4 years, the HR for death was 0.28 (95% CI 0.10–0.85) compared to a matched cohort of 2119 community controls followed up for 12 years.

✔✔ The first systematic review and meta-analysis of long-term mortality outcomes after mainly gastric bypass and banding was published in 2011.[89] Eight studies were included, totalling 14052 surgical patients and 29970 controls, with follow-up of between 2.5 and 12 years. The odds ratio (OR) for mortality after surgery was 0.55 (CI 0.49–0.63, all eight studies), the OR for cardiovascular mortality was 0.58 (0.46–0.73, four studies) and the OR for non-cardiovascular mortality was 0.70 (0.59–0.84, four studies).

To date there are no data on survival benefit from other bariatric operations. However, a more recent study of male gastric bypass patients in Veterans Administration hospitals in the USA, who were predominantly older than in the studies above, also reported in 2011.[90] No survival benefit at 6.7 years was found in the 850 operated patients compared to 847 controls. This is the first study not to show survival benefit after bariatric surgery, possibly because of relatively high mortality in the operated patients and the relatively short follow-up.

After surgery, patients may not return to the level of risk of the general population. In Sweden 13270 bariatric surgery patients still had an HR for mortality of 1.24 (CI 1.15–1.34) when compared to 132700 individuals from the general population who did not have surgery.[91] One of the many unknowns regarding the mechanism by which surgery reduces mortality is whether any of the operations halt or reverse the characteristic microvascular changes of diabetes.

Cancer incidence after bariatric surgery

A further finding from the SOS study is the reduction in incidence of all cancers in follow-up. Using the Swedish National Cancer Registry to observe cancer incidence from 1987 to 2005, Sjöström et al. found that 117 cancers developed in 2010 operated patients compared to 169 cancers in 2037 controls (HR 0.67, *P*<0.0009).[92] Although the absolute numbers are small, Sjöström et al. found it useful to compare this effect of surgery to statin treatment, where the HR for development of fatal or non-fatal myocardial infarction was 0.80 in >90000 patients.[93]

✔✔ The Utah driving licence researchers found a similar reduction in incidence of cancer diagnoses during an average of 12.5 years follow-up in 6596 gastric bypass patients when compared to 9442 severely obese controls.[94] Using the Utah Cancer Registry, Adams et al. found the HR for cancer was 0.76 (CI 0.65–0.89, *P*=0.0006). The reduced incidence of cancer almost entirely comprised the female known obesity-related cancers; in particular, there was a 78% reduction in endometrial cancer (HR 0.22, CI 0.13–0.40, *P*<0.0001).

The risk of dying from all cancers was also decreased by 46% (HR 0.54, CI 0.37–0.78, *P*=0.001). Interestingly, the cancer mortality was also decreased in non-obesity-related cancer by 47% (HR 0.53, CI 0.31–0.91, *P*=0.02).

Cost-effectiveness of bariatric surgery

Large studies from the UK, USA and Canada have recently evaluated the economics of bariatric surgery. In 2009 the HTA programme published a systematic review in which Picot et al. analysed 5386 journal articles.[95] Of these, 26 were used in the clinical effectiveness review, including 23 RCTs. Bariatric surgery was found to be more clinically effective for weight loss than non-surgical methods, with some measures of quality of life improving but not others. In addition, cost-effectiveness was estimated using incremental cost-effectiveness ratios (ICERs) per quality-adjusted life year (Table 20.6). Particularly for longer time horizons up to 20 years, these ratios were deemed cost-effective, although not for the BMI group 30+ and <35.

Another, updated systematic review has recently reported and expressed health economic outcomes as incremental cost-utility ratios (ICURs) in 2009 US dollars.[52] ICURs ranged from $1000 to $40000 per quality-adjusted life year (QALY), and it was not possible to distinguish between different procedures. O'Brien's group has analysed the lifetime projected cost savings for recently diagnosed diabetics treated with gastric banding compared to medical therapy from their RCT, and found surgery cost less and led to more QALYs.[96] Using a different model in the USA that is based on a meta-analysis, other health economists found the cost-effectiveness over a 10-year timescale for gastric banding to be between $US11000 and 13000/QALY for patients with diabetes.[97] Gastric bypass was found to be more cost-effective at between $US7000 and 12000/QALY for diabetes, and all of these estimates were well below the threshold of cost/QALY usually used to justify expenditure.

In another study the 3651 patients in a US employer claims database of 5 million who were operated between 1999 and 2005 were matched to similarly obese non-operated controls with similar baseline comorbidity using the ICD9 code 278.01.[98] The operations were mainly gastric bypass. Total healthcare costs including hospital visits and medications were recorded during the 6 months before surgery and continuously up to 5 years. Using a model adjusted for inflation, Cremieux et al. estimated that all costs were recouped for laparoscopic bariatric surgery within 2 years and for open bariatric surgery within 4 years.

Table 20.6 • Data from UK Health Technology Assessment report 2009[93]

Baseline BMI with/ without comorbidity	Incremental cost per QALY (£)	
	2 years	20 years
BMI 40+	2000–4000	
BMI 30+ and <40 with type 2 diabetes at baseline	18930	1367
BMI 30+ and <35	60754	12763

In a study using a US insurance database of 8.5 million people, Klein et al. analysed the pre- and postoperative drug costs in diabetic patients (n=808) matched to non-operated controls (n=808).[99] They found that at 3 months after surgery insulin usage had fallen to 43% in operated patients and stayed at 84% in controls. Medication and supply costs of insulin at this time were $US33 and $US123, respectively (both P<0.001). At 6 months only 28% of operated patients still had a diagnosis of diabetes and it was found that the break-even point for the cost of surgery due to the cessation of diabetes medications alone was 26 months.

Despite the assumed benefits, the rate of bariatric surgery for the NHS in England in 2009–10 was approximately 0.30% of those who might benefit (3642 of 1.2 million). The availability of surgery appears to be no greater in other countries with a similar scale of obesity, with healthcare providers seemingly caught by the imperative to balance budgets within a 1-year timescale given that the cost of surgery may not be recouped until at least 1–2 years.[100] The case for diabetes is an illustration of this.[99] It is not known how much the willingness of healthcare systems to provide this surgery might be influenced by societal prejudice.

Wider economic benefit of bariatric surgery

The above cost-effectiveness models do not include the benefits to society as a whole, such as gainful employment after surgery. A UK Office of Health Economics (OHE) report used a novel approach in which they estimated the expected gains arising from unemployed patients going back to work.[101] The estimate was based on a study of patients who at a median 14 months follow-up after surgery increased their paid hours worked by 57% and reduced their state benefit claims by 75%.[102] The model found that if 25% of eligible patients (140000 in their estimate) received surgery the boost to the GDP would total £1.295 billion at 3 years due to increases in paid employment, with an additional £151 million being returned to the economy by reducing benefits costs. Although this was a single study, reports from at least three other European countries, including the SOS study, have also shown increases in paid work after surgery.[103–105] If the additional economic factors alone are considered, without including any cost savings from medication reduction or less hospitalisation, surgery pays for itself within 1 year.[101]

Who should have surgery?

The greater challenge is to estimate the proportion of the morbidly obese population who should be offered bariatric surgery, as there is no medical argument to limit the number treated to 1% or fewer of those who can benefit. The upper limit for how many should be treated is also unknown, but the recent Edmonton Obesity Surgery Score attempts to estimate life expectancy (akin to TMN staging) for a given level of disease.[106] After analysing data from 7967 individuals in the US NHANES studies, it was found that dying within a 20-year timescale was more likely for those scoring 2 (HR 1.57, 95% CI 1.16–2.13) and 3 (HR 2.69, 95% CI 1.98–3.67) than for those scoring 0 or 1, *irrespective* of BMI. Score 2 included established chronic disease (e.g. diabetes, hypertension, sleep apnoea, arthritis) and score 3 also included end-organ damage and significant functional limitation. Thus, if there are limited resources those likely to die earlier might be preferred for surgery, and *not* those with a high BMI but no comorbidity, in contrast to the NICE guidance.

The economic arguments for/against selection of severely obese diabetics are equally complex – although a prime target for surgery, it is not known which patient has the most to gain. Thus, a patient aged 25 with recent onset diabetes and a BMI of 50, and a newly insulin-dependent diabetic aged 50 with a BMI of 60 could both gain hugely from surgery, but from the commissioner's perspective it is not known which patient is economically the 'best bet'.

Summary

The global impact of obesity is threatening to overwhelm healthcare resources in developed countries, with the USA most affected, followed closely by Mexico and western European countries, including the UK and Ireland. Obesity can be regarded as a normal physiological response to the current environment and so the emphasis should shift from blaming the individual to the societal changes that will be needed to curb the epidemic. Reducing calorie intake is difficult, most individuals are unable to sustain weight loss through dieting and recidivism is the norm. Only surgery provides long-lasting weight loss.

Gastric bypass and banding are the commonest operations worldwide and both have been shown to reduce mortality and induce reversal of comorbidities such as diabetes. Other operations include sleeve gastrectomy, biliopancreatic diversion and its duodenal switch variant. Procedures for diabetes rather than weight loss are being promoted, such as duodeno-jejunal bypass and endoscopic duodenal sleeve. Patients must be cared for within a holistic multidisciplinary team approach since, especially for gastric banding, the operation itself is only the start of the weight loss programme. Intensive long-term follow-up should be the intention.

The evidence base for choosing a given procedure is poor and should be determined by local expertise and the ability to deliver appropriate follow-up. Available evidence suggests that specialisation improves operative outcomes, especially for bypass. Gastric banding is technically usually straightforward but the follow-up for correct band adjustment has to be intensive to get good weight loss. The long-term outcome in the community of patients with bands is not known. More long-term studies including randomised trials are needed with better follow-up to determine which procedure(s) is likely to provide the best treatment option for severe obesity on a population basis. In the UK, the By-Band randomised trial, which opened in late 2012, is intended to address the debate on gastric bypass versus gastric banding.

Key points

- Obesity is increasing and is one of the major global public health issues.
- Obesity is regarded as a normal physiological response to the current 'obesogenic' environment.
- The obese state is associated with high levels of type 2 diabetes, hypertension, sleep apnoea, cancer, functional impairment and early mortality.
- Obese individuals have poor quality of life, higher unemployment and high rates of disability benefit claims compared to non-obese individuals.

- Attempts at dieting and exercise by obese individuals rarely produce long-lasting weight loss and recidivism is very common.
- Mortality rates of bariatric surgery compare favourably to many other gastrointestinal procedures and need to be judged against the risk of not operating.
- Bariatric surgery has a cost-effectiveness of £2000–4000 per QALY for patients with BMI >40 and is thus one of the most cost-effective treatments available.
- Bariatric surgery has been shown to produce long-lasting weight loss, improvement in comorbid disease, a reduction in cancer and reduced mortality.
- Hospital and surgeon volume data suggest that better outcomes can be expected if services are centralised and there is multidisciplinary involvement.
- There are relatively few RCTs of different bariatric surgical operations and choice of procedure seems to depend largely on peer pressure, surgical and referrer choice, and local expertise.
- The loss of patients to follow-up and the few high-quality long-term follow-up studies severely hinder the quality of research into the different available procedures.
- Despite its cost-effectiveness only a small proportion of severely obese people, around 1% in the UK, receive bariatric surgery and this poses major challenges if healthcare systems are to increase its availability to those who might benefit.

References

1. Mason EE, Ito C. Gastric bypass in obesity. Surg Clin North Am 1967;47:1345–51.
2. Christou NV, Look D, MacLean LD. Weight gain after short- and long-limb gastric bypass in patients followed for longer than 10 years. Ann Surg 2006;244:734–40.
3. Johnston D, Dachtler J, Sue-Ling HM, et al. The Magenstrasse and Mill operation for morbid obesity. Obes Surg 2003;13:10–7.
4. Friedrich MJ. Epidemic of obesity expands its spread to developing countries. JAMA 2002;287:1382–6.
5. Foresight – Tackling obesity, future choices. Government Office for Science; October 2007.
   The UK government report that used sophisticated computer modelling techniques to predict the likely increase in obesity and its financial consequences.
6. Swinburn BA, Sacks G, Hall KD, et al. Obesity 1. The global obesity pandemic: shaped by global drivers and local environments. Lancet 2011;378:804–14.
7. Monsivais P, Mclain J, Drewnowski A. The rising disparity in the price of healthful foods: 2004–2008. Food Policy 2010;35:514–20.
8. Thomas M, Desai KK, Seenivasan S. How credit card payments increase unhealthy food purchases: visceral regulation of vices. J Consumer Res 2011;38:126–39.
9. Finucane MM, Stevens GA, Cowan MJ, et al. National, regional, and global trends in body-mass index since 1980: systematic analysis of health examination surveys and epidemiological studies with 960 country-years and 9·1 million participants. Lancet 2011;377:557–67.
   Data from 960 country-years and 9.1million participants were analysed to produce these estimates.
10. National Obesity Observatory. www.noo.org.uk; [accessed July 10].
    The public health observatory website that publishes rates of surgery in the different regions of the UK and also updates on the current prevalence of obesity.
11. Dixon JB, Pories WJ, O'Brien PE, et al. Surgery as an effective early intervention for diabesity: why the reluctance? Diabetes Care 2005;28:472–4.
12. Suhrcke M, McKee M, Arce RS, et al. Investment in health could be good for Europe's economies. Br Med J 2006;333:1017–9.
13. Lenzer J. Obesity related illness consumes a sixth of the US healthcare budget. Br Med J 2010;341:c6014.
14. Sedula MK, Mokdad AH, Williamson DF, et al. Prevalence of attempting weight loss and strategies for controlling weight. JAMA 1999;282:1353–8.
15. Leff DR, Heath D. Surgery for obesity in adulthood. Br Med J 2009;339:b3402.
16. Leibel RL, Rosenbaum M, Hirsch J. Changes in energy expenditure resulting from altered body weight. N Engl J Med 1995;332:621–8.
    This paper demonstrated clearly the fall in basal metabolic rate after volitional weight loss in volunteer subjects, showing that energy expenditure reduces so as to mitigate against weight loss in a period of reduced intake. It is regarded as a classic paper demonstrating the physiological difficulties in losing weight by dieting.
17. Colquitt JL, Picot J, Loveman E, et al. Surgery for obesity. Cochrane Database Syst Rev 2009;(2):CD003641.

This is the current update of the Cochrane review process enumerating extracted data from all available clinical trials by professional researchers and is a standard reference for clinical outcomes data.

18. www.win.niddk.nih.gov/publications/labs.htm; [accessed December 2011].
19. Welbourn R, Fiennes A, Kinsman R, et al. The National Bariatric Surgery Registry: First registry report to March 2010. Henley-on-Thames: Dendrite Clinical Systems; 2011.
20. O'Brien PE. Bariatric surgery: mechanisms, indications and outcomes. J Gastroenterol Hepatol 2010;25:1358–65.
21. Hutter MM, Schirmer BD, Jones DB, et al. First report from the American College of Surgeons Bariatric Surgery Center Network: laparoscopic sleeve gastrectomy has morbidity and effectiveness positioned between the band and the bypass. Ann Surg 2011;254:410–22.
22. Shaw JE, Sicree RA, Zimmet PZ. Global estimates of the prevalence of diabetes for 2010 and 2030. Diabetes Res Clin Pract 2010;87:4–14.
23. Dixon JB, Zimmet P, Alberti KG, et al. Bariatric surgery: an IDF statement for obese Type 2 diabetes. Diabet Med 2011;28:628–42.
The International Diabetes Federation is the umbrella organisation for 200 national diabetes associations in 160 countries. The working group for this statement reviewed the literature from 1991 to 2010 on diabetes and bariatric surgery before a consensus conference in Brussels in December 2010. The paper details recommendations on clinical practice and future research.
24. Adami HO, Trichopoulos D. Obesity and mortality from cancer. N Engl J Med 2003;348:1623–4.
25. Calle EE, Rodriguez C, Walker-Thurmond K, et al. Overweight, obesity, and mortality from cancer in a prospectively studied cohort of U.S. adults. N Engl J Med 2003;348:1625–38.
26. Hofman B. Stuck in the middle: the many moral challenges with bariatric surgery. Am J Bioethics 2010;10:3–11.
27. Belle SH, Chapman W, Courcoulas AP, et al. The relationship of BMI with demographic and clinical characteristics in the Longitudinal Assessment of Bariatric Surgery (LABS). Surg Obes Relat Dis 2008;4:474–80.
While the increasing level of comorbidity as the BMI rises is well established in the general population, this was the first major report showing the incidence of comorbidity for different BMI groups in patients undergoing bariatric surgery.
28. Mechanick JI, Kushner RF, Sugerman HJ, et al. AACE/TOS/ASMBS guidelines for clinical practice for the perioperative nutritional, metabolic, and nonsurgical support of the bariatric surgery patient. Endocr Pract 2008;14:S1–83.
The major evidence-based reference for bariatric surgery for clinical practice.
29. NICE. Obesity, the prevention, identification, assessment and management of overweight and obesity in adults and children, Clinical Guideline 43. National Institute for Clinical Excellence; 2006.
NICE guidance is provided in the UK for commissioning bodies but at present the NHS is not legally obliged to follow the guidance.
30. McMahon MM, Sarr MG, Clark MM, et al. Clinical management after bariatric surgery: value of a multidisciplinary approach. Mayo Clin Proc 2006;81:S34–45.
31. Kelly JJ, Shikora S, Jones DB, et al. Best practice updates for surgical care in weight loss surgery. Obesity 2009;17:863–70.
32. DeMaria EJ, Murr M, Byrne TK, et al. Validation of the obesity surgery mortality risk score in a multicenter study proves it stratifies mortality risk in patients undergoing gastric bypass for morbid obesity. Ann Surg 2007;246:578–82.
This is the paper that shows the validation of the OS-MRS. Mortality was 0.2% in class A patients compared to 2.4% in class C patients.
33. Fris RJ. Preoperative low energy diet diminishes liver size. Obes Surg 2004;14(9):1165–70.
34. Olbers T, Lonroth H, Fagevik-Olsen M, et al. Laparoscopic gastric bypass: development of technique, respiratory function, and long-term outcome. Obes Surg 2003;13:364–70.
35. Higa K, Ho T, Tercero F, et al. Laparoscopic Roux-en-Y gastric bypass: 10-year follow-up. Surg Obes Relat Dis 2011;7(4):516–25.
36. Fobi MAL, Lee H, Holness R, et al. Gastric bypass operation for obesity. World J Surg 1998;22:925–35.
37. Capella RF, Capella JF. Vertical banded gastroplasty–gastric bypass: preliminary report. Obes Surg 1991;1:389–95.
38. Naslund I. The size of the gastric outlet and the outcome of surgery for obesity. Acta Chir Scand 1986;152:205–10.
39. Wittgrove AC, Clark GW, Tremblay LY. Laparoscopic gastric bypass, Roux-en-Y: preliminary report of five cases. Obes Surg 1994;4:353–7.
40. Brolin RE, Kenler HA, Gorman JH, et al. Long-limb gastric bypass in the superobese. Ann Surg 1992;215:387–95.
41. Stefanidis D, Kuwada TS, Gersin KS. The importance of the length of the limbs for gastric bypass patients – an evidence-based review. Obes Surg 2011;21:119–24.
42. Shen R, Dugay G, Rajaram K, et al. Impact of patient follow-up on weight loss after bariatric surgery. Obes Surg 2004;14:514–9.

43. Kehagias I, Karamanakos SN, Argentou M, et al. Randomized clinical trial of laparoscopic Roux-en-Y gastric bypass versus laparoscopic sleeve gastrectomy for the management of patients with BMI <50 kg/m^2. Obes Surg 2011;21:1650–6.

44. American Society for Metabolic and Bariatric Surgery. Updated position statement on sleeve gastrectomy as a bariatric procedure. Available from http://s3.amazonaws.com/publicASMBS/GuidelinesStatements/PositionStatement/ASMBS-SLEEVE-STATEMENT-2011_10_28.pdf; 2011 [accessed December 2011].

45. Himpens J, Dobbeleir J, Peeters G. Long-term results of laparoscopic sleeve gastrectomy for obesity. Ann Surg 2010;252:319–24.

46. Sarela AI, Dexter SPL, O'Kane M, et al. Long-term follow-up after laparoscopic sleeve gastrectomy; 8–9 year results. Surg Obes Relat Dis 2012;8(6):679–84.

47. Hess DS, Hess DW, Oakley RW. The biliopancreatic diversion with the duodenal switch: results beyond 10 years. Obes Surg 2005;15:408–16.

48. Dixon AF, Dixon JB, O'Brien PE. Laparoscopic adjustable gastric banding induces prolonged satiety: a randomized blind crossover study. J Clin Endocrinol Metab 2005;90:813–9.

49. le Roux CW, Welbourn R, Werling M, et al. Gut hormones as mediators of appetite and weight loss after Roux-en-Y gastric bypass. Ann Surg 2007;246:780–5.

50. Wynne K, Park AJ, Small CJ, et al. Oxyntomodulin increases energy expenditure in addition to decreasing energy intake in overweight and obese humans: a randomised controlled trial. Int J Obes 2006;30:1729–36.

51. Rubino F, Forgione A, Cummings DE, et al. The mechanism of diabetes control after gastrointestinal bypass surgery reveals a role of the proximal small intestine in the pathophysiology of type 2 diabetes. Ann Surg 2006;244:741–9.

52. Padwal R, Klarenbach S, Wiebe N, et al. Bariatric surgery: a systematic review of the clinical and economic evidence. J Gen Intern Med 2011;26(10):1183–94.

53. Lee W-J, Yu P-J, Wang W, et al. Laparoscopic Roux-en-Y versus mini-gastric bypass for the treatment of morbid obesity. Ann Surg 2005;242:20–8.

54. Himpens J, Dapri G, Cadiere GB. A prospective randomized study between laparoscopic gastric banding and laparoscopic isolated sleeve gastrectomy. Obes Surg 2006;16:1450–6.

55. O'Brien PE, Dixon JB, Laurie C, et al. Treatment of mild to moderate obesity with laparoscopic adjustable gastric banding or an intensive medical program. A randomized trial. Ann Intern Med 2006;144:625–33.

56. Bessler M, Daud A, Kim T, et al. Prospective randomized trial of banded versus nonbanded gastric bypass for the super obese: early results. Surg Obes Relat Dis 2007;3:480–4.

57. Dixon JB, O'Brien PE, Playfair J, et al. Adjustable gastric banding and conventional therapy for type 2 diabetes. A randomized controlled trial. JAMA 2008;299:316–32.
This is the only RCT that compares banding to medical therapy for new-onset diabetics in BMI range 30–40.

58. Lee WJ, Chong K, Ser KH, et al. Gastric bypass vs sleeve gastrectomy for type 2 diabetes mellitus: a randomized controlled trial. Arch Surg 2011;146:143–8.

59. Søvik TT, Aasheim ET, Taha O, et al. Weight loss, cardiovascular risk factors, and quality of life after gastric bypass and duodenal switch. A randomized trial. Ann Intern Med 2011;155:281–91.

60. Woelnerhanssen B, Peterli R, Steinert RE, et al. Effects of postbariatric surgery weight loss on adipokines and metabolic parameters: comparison of laparoscopic Roux-en-Y gastric bypass and laparoscopic sleeve gastrectomy – a prospective randomized trial. Surg Obes Relat Dis 2011;7:561–8.

61. O'Brien PE, McPhail T, Chaston TB, et al. Systematic review of medium-term weight loss after bariatric operations. Obes Surg 2006;16:1032–40.
This systematic review compared weight loss outcomes for bypass, banding, banded bypass, and BPD with or without DS from 43 papers up to 10 years after surgery.

62. Angrisani L, Lorenzo M, Borrelli V. Laparoscopic adjustable gastric banding versus Roux-en-Y gastric bypass: 5-year results of a prospective randomized trial. Surg Obes Relat Dis 2007;3:127–32.

63. Nguyen NT, Slone JA, Nguyen X-MT, et al. A prospective randomized trial of laparoscopic gastric bypass versus laparoscopic adjustable gastric banding for the treatment of morbid obesity: outcomes, quality of life, and costs. Ann Surg 2009;250:631–41.

64. Burns EM, Naseem H, Bottle A, et al. Introduction of laparoscopic bariatric surgery in England: observational population cohort study. Br Med J 2010, Aug 26;341:c4296.

65. Flum D. Perioperative safety in the Longitudinal Assessment of Bariatric Surgery. The Longitudinal Assessment of Bariatric Surgery (LABS) Consortium. N Engl J Med 2009;361:445–54.

66. DeMaria EJ, Pate V, Warthen M, et al. Baseline data from American Society for Metabolic and Bariatric Surgery-designated bariatric surgery centers of excellence using the Bariatric Outcomes Longitudinal Database. Surg Obes Relat Dis 2010;6:347–55.

67. Birkmeyer NJ, Dimick JB, Share D, et al. Hospital complication rates with bariatric surgery in Michigan. JAMA 2010;304:435–42.

68. Lee S. Effect of location and speed of diagnosis on anastomotic leak outcomes in 3828 gastric bypass cases. J Gastrointest Surg 2007;11:708–13.

69. Nguyen NT, Longoria M, Chalifoux S, et al. Gastrointestinal hemorrhage after laparoscopic gastric bypass. Obes Surg 2004;14:1308–12.

70. Podnos YD, Jimenez JC, Wilson SE, et al. Complications after laparoscopic gastric bypass: a review of 3464 cases. Arch Surg 2003;138:957–61.

71. Ahmed AR, Rickards G, Husain S, et al. Trends in internal hernia incidence after laparoscopic Roux-en-Y gastric bypass. Obes Surg 2007;17:1563–6.

72. ASMBS position statement on emergency care of patients with complications related to bariatric surgery. Surg Obes Relat Dis 2010;6:115–7.

73. Suter M, Calmes JM, Paros A, et al. A 10-year experience with laparoscopic gastric banding for morbid obesity: high long-term complication and failure rates. Obes Surg 2006;16:829–35.

74. Casella G, Soricelli E, Rizzello M. Nonsurgical treatment of staple line leaks after laparoscopic sleeve gastrectomy. Obes Surg 2009;19:821–6.

75. Flum DR, Salem L, Elrod JA, et al. Early mortality among Medicare beneficiaries undergoing bariatric surgical procedures. JAMA 2005;294:1903–8.

76. Maggard MA, Shugarman LR, Suttorp M. Meta-analysis: surgical treatment of obesity. Ann Intern Med 2005;142:547–59.

77. Dixon JB, Bhathal PS, Hughes NR, et al. Nonalcoholic fatty liver disease: improvement in liver histological analysis with weight loss. Hepatology 2004;39:1647–54.

78. Owan T, Avelar E, Morley K, et al. Favorable changes in cardiac geometry and function following gastric bypass surgery. J Am Coll Cardiol 2011;57:732–9.

79. Sjöström L, Lindroos A-K, Peltonen M, et al. Lifestyle, diabetes, and cardiovascular risk factors 10 years after bariatric surgery. N Engl J Med 2004;35:2683–93.

80. Adams TD, Gress RE, Smith SC, et al. Long-term mortality after gastric bypass surgery. N Engl J Med 2007;357:753–61.

81. Buchwald H, Estok R, Fahrbach K, et al. Weight and type 2 diabetes after bariatric surgery: systematic review and meta-analysis. Am J Med 2009;122:248–56.e5.

82. Buse JB, Caprio S, Cefalu WT. How do we define cure of diabetes? Diabetes Care 2009;32:2133–5.

83. Pournaras DJ, Aasheim ET, Søvik TT, et al. Effect of the definition of type II diabetes remission in the evaluation of bariatric surgery for metabolic disorders. Br J Surg 2012;99:100–3.

84. Schauer PR, Kashyap SR, Wolski K, et al. Bariatric surgery versus intensive medical therapy in obese patients with diabetes. N Engl J Med 2012;366:1567–76.

85. Mingrone G, Panunzi S, De Gaetano A, et al. Bariatric surgery versus conventional medical therapy for type 2 diabetes. N Engl J Med 2012;366:1577–85.

86. Pournaras DJ, Osborne A, Hawkins SC, et al. Rapid remission of type 2 diabetes after Roux en Y gastric bypass. Ann Surg 2010;252:966–71.

87. Sjöström L, Narbro C, Sjöström CD, et al. Effects of bariatric surgery on mortality in Swedish obese subjects. N Engl J Med 2007;357:741–52.

88. Peeters A, O'Brien PE, Laurie C, et al. Substantial intentional weight loss and mortality in the severely obese. Ann Surg 2007;246:1028–33.

89. Pontiroli AE, Morabito A. Long-term prevention of mortality in morbid obesity through bariatric surgery: a systematic review and meta-analysis of trials performed with gastric banding and gastric bypass. Ann Surg 2011;253:484–7.
This is the only systematic review so far published on mortality after bariatric surgery.

90. Maciejewski ML, Livingston EH, Smith VA, et al. Survival among high-risk patients after bariatric surgery. JAMA 2011;305:2419–26.

91. Ostlund MP, Marsk R, Rasmussen F, et al. Morbidity and mortality before and after bariatric surgery for morbid obesity compared with the general population. Br J Surg 2011;98:811–6.

92. Sjöström L, Gummesson A, Sjöström CD, et al. Effects of bariatric surgery on cancer incidence in obese patients in Sweden (Swedish Obese Subjects study): a prospective, controlled intervention trial. Lancet Oncol 2009;10:653–62.

93. Preiss D, Sattar N. Lipids, lipid modifying agents and cardiovascular risk: a review of the evidence. Clin Endocrinol (Oxf) 2009;70:815–28.

94. Adams TD, Stroup AM, Gress RE, et al. Cancer incidence and mortality after gastric bypass surgery. Obesity 2009;17:796–802.
This and the SOS paper by Sjöström et al.[92] were among the first publications illustrating the powerful effect of bariatric surgery on reducing cancer incidence, which it is commented is much greater than that of statins on reducing cardiovascular events. Statins are universally accepted while bariatric surgery is not.

95. Picot J, Jones J, Colquitt JL, et al. The clinical effectiveness and cost-effectiveness of bariatric (weight loss) surgery for obesity: a systematic review and economic evaluation. Health Technol Assess 2009;13:1–214.

96. Keating CL, Dixon JB, Moodie ML, et al. Cost-effectiveness of surgically induced weight loss for the management of Type 2 diabetes: modeled lifetime analysis. Diabetes Care 2009;32:567–74.

97. Hoerger TJ, Zhang P, Segel JE, et al. Cost effectiveness of bariatric surgery for severely obese adults with diabetes. Diabetes Care 2010;33:1933–9.

98. Cremieux J, Buchwald H, Shikora SA, et al. A study on the economic impact of bariatric surgery. Am J Manag Care 2008;14(9):589–96.

99. Klein S, Ghosh A, Cremieux J, et al. Economic impact of the clinical benefits of bariatric surgery in diabetes patients with BMI ≥35 kg/m^2. Obesity 2011;19:581–7.

100. McCartney M. Slimmed down surgery. Br Med J 2010;341:c5499.

101. Office of Health Economics. Shedding the pounds, www.rcseng.ac.uk/news/docs/BariatricReport.pdf; 2010[accessed 23.11.12].

102. Hawkins SC, Osborne A, Finlay IG, et al. Paid work increases and state benefit claims decrease after bariatric surgery. Obes Surg 2007;17:434–7.

103. van Gemert WG, Adang EM, Greve JW, et al. Quality of life assessment of morbidly obese patients: effect of weight-reducing surgery. Am J Clin Nutr 1998;67:197–201.

104. Narbro K, Agren G, Jonsson E, et al. Sick leave and disability pension before and after treatment for obesity: a report from the Swedish Obese Subjects (SOS) study. Int J Obes Relat Metab Disord 1999;23:619–24.

105. Andersen JR, Aasprang A, Bergsholm P, et al. Health-related quality of life and paid work participation after duodenal switch. Obes Surg 2010;20:340–5.

106. Padwal RJ, Pajewski NM, Allison DB, et al. Using the Edmonton obesity staging system to predict mortality in a population-representative cohort of people. CMAJ 2011;83:1–8.

Index

NB: Page numbers followed by *f* indicate figures, *t* indicate tables and *b* indicate boxes.

A

B

C

D

E

F

G

H

I

J

K

L

M

N

O

P

Q

R

S

T

U

V

W

X

Z